Professional Nursing Concepts

Competencies for Quality Leadership

Welcome to *Professional Nursing Concepts: Competencies for Quality Leadership!*

Along with useful tables, charts, and figures, each chapter includes:

Chapter Objectives

Found at the beginning of each chapter, chapter objectives provide a snapshot of the key information you will encounter in each chapter. These objectives can serve as a checklist to help guide your studies.

Chapter 4

Nursing Education, Accreditation, and Regulation

CHAPTER OBJECTIVES

At the conclusion of this chapter, the learner will be able to:

- Discuss the differences between nursing education and other types of education.
- Describe the types of nursing programs and degrees.
- Identify the roles of major nursing organizations that have an impact on nursing education.
- Explain requirements and issues related to quality nursing education.
- Discuss the use of distance education in nursing programs.
- Explain the importance of lifelong learning.
- Define certification and credentialing.
- Describe the nursing education accreditation process and its importance.
- Discuss the importance of regulation and its process and critical issues.

CHAPTER OUTLINE

INTRODUCTION
NURSING EDUCATION
Nursing Education: This Is Not an English Lit Course!
A Brief History of Nursing Education
Entry into Practice: A Debate
Differentiated Nursing Practice
Types of Nursing Programs
Nursing Education Associations

123

Chapter Outline

Also found at the beginning of each chapter, chapter outlines will help keep you organized as you read. Content headers within each chapter match those in the chapter outline.

Key Terms

Listed at the beginning of and found within each chapter, these terms will help you create an expanded vocabulary in professional nursing. Visit **http://nursing.jbpub.com** to see these terms in an interactive glossary and use word puzzles to nail the definitions!

---

124 CHAPTER 4: NURSING EDUCATION, ACCREDITATION, AND REGULATION

Quality and Excellence in Nursing Education
Lifelong Learning for the Professional
Certification and Credentialing
Transforming Nursing Education
ACCREDITATION OF NURSING EDUCATION PROGRAMS
Nursing Program Accreditation: What Is It?
Nursing Program Accreditation: How Does It Work?
REGULATION
Nurse Practice Acts
State Boards of Nursing
Licensure Requirements
CONCLUSION
CHAPTER HIGHLIGHTS
LINKING TO THE INTERNET
DISCUSSION QUESTIONS
CRITICAL THINKING ACTIVITIES
CASE STUDIES
WORDS OF WISDOM
REFERENCES

KEY TERMS

- Accreditation
- Advanced practice nurse
- Apprenticeship model
- Articulation
- Associate's degree in nursing
- Baccalaureate degree in nursing
- Certification
- Continuing education
- Credentialing
- Curriculum
- Diploma school of nursing
- Distance education
- Master's degree in nursing
- Nurse externship
- Nurse Practice Act
- Nurse residency
- Practicum
- Preceptor
- Prescriptive authority
- Regulation
- Self-directed learning
- Standard
- Training

Introduction

This chapter focuses on three critical concerns in the nursing profession: (1) nursing education, (2) **accreditation** of nursing programs, and (3) regulatory issues such as licensure. These concerns are interrelated because these areas change and require input from the nursing profession. Even after graduation, nurses should be aware of educational issues, such as appropriate and reasonable accreditation of nursing programs, and ensure that regulatory issues support the criti-

---

Visit http://nursing.jbpub.com

Linking to the Internet

Follow the links provided at the end of each chapter to find a wealth of primary sources! You'll discover important associations, institutes, funds, organizations, and departments vital to professional nursing practice.

Discussion Questions

Test your knowledge and explore your understanding of key chapter content with end-of-chapter discussion questions!

Critical Thinking Activities

An integral part of the learning process, critical thinking questions and scenarios spark thought about and provide insight into nursing practice.

Case Studies with Case Study Questions

Learn how the information in this text applies to the everyday practice of the professional nurse! Found at the end of each chapter, these vignettes provide case studies from actual clinical settings. Thought-provoking questions accompany cases to facilitate higher-level thinking.

Words of Wisdom

Each chapter concludes with stories and conversations with nurses who have shared some of their experiences, insights, and advice.

Other Features Include:

Exhibit boxes are an integral part of each chapter and highlight and explain important lists, statistics, and concepts, and methods within the text.

Each chapter concludes with a series of **chapter highlights**. Like chapter objectives, chapter highlights provide an overview of the key information you should take from your reading.

for interactive exercises and additional review!

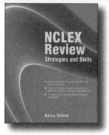
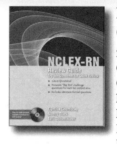
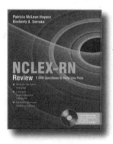
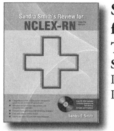
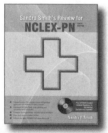
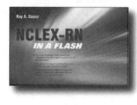

Professional Nursing Concepts

Competencies for Quality Leadership

Anita W. Finkelman, MSN, RN
Assistant Professor
University of Oklahoma College of Nursing
Oklahoma City, Oklahoma

Carole Kenner, DNS, RNC-NIC, FAAN
Dean, Professor
University of Oklahoma College of Nursing
Oklahoma City, Oklahoma

JONES AND BARTLETT PUBLISHERS

Sudbury, Massachusetts

BOSTON   TORONTO   LONDON   SINGAPORE

World Headquarters
Jones and Bartlett Publishers
40 Tall Pine Drive
Sudbury, MA 01776
978-443-5000
info@jbpub.com
www.jbpub.com

Jones and Bartlett Publishers Canada
6339 Ormindale Way
Mississauga, Ontario L5V 1J2
Canada

Jones and Bartlett Publishers International
Barb House, Barb Mews
London W6 7PA
United Kingdom

Jones and Bartlett's books and products are available through most bookstores and online booksellers. To contact Jones and Bartlett Publishers directly, call 800-832-0034, fax 978-443-8000, or visit our website www.jbpub.com.

Substantial discounts on bulk quantities of Jones and Bartlett's publications are available to corporations, professional associations, and other qualified organizations. For details and specific discount information, contact the special sales department at Jones and Bartlett via the above contact information or send an email to specialsales@jbpub.com.

The authors, editor, and publisher have made every effort to provide accurate information. However, they are not responsible for errors, omissions, or for any outcomes related to the use of the contents of this book and take no responsibility for the use of the products and procedures described. Treatments and side effects described in this book may not be applicable to all people; likewise, some people may require a dose or experience a side effect that is not described herein. Drugs and medical devices are discussed that may have limited availability controlled by the Food and Drug Administration (FDA) for use only in a research study or clinical trial. Research, clinical practice, and government regulations often change the accepted standard in this field. When consideration is being given to use of any drug in the clinical setting, the health care provider or reader is responsible for determining FDA status of the drug, reading the package insert, and reviewing prescribing information for the most up-to-date recommendations on dose, precautions, and contraindications, and determining the appropriate usage for the product. This is especially important in the case of drugs that are new or seldom used.

Production Credits
Publisher: Kevin Sullivan
Acquisitions Editor: Emily Ekle
Acquisitions Editor: Amy Sibley
Associate Editor: Patricia Donnelly
Editorial Assistant: Rachel Shuster
Associate Production Editor: Amanda Clerkin
Production Assistant: Lisa Cerrone
Senior Marketing Manager: Barb Bartoszek
V.P., Manufacturing and Inventory Control: Therese Connell
Composition: Auburn Associates, Inc.
Cover Design: Kristin E. Parker
Cover and Title Page Image: © Kurt/Dreamstime.com
Printing and Binding: Malloy, Inc.
Cover Printing: Malloy, Inc.

Library of Congress Cataloging-in-Publication Data
Finkelman, Anita Ward.
    Professional nursing concepts : competencies for quality leadership / Anita W. Finkelman and Carole Kenner.
        p. ; cm.
    Includes bibliographical references and index.
    ISBN-13: 978-0-7637-5412-9 (pbk.)
    ISBN-10: 0-7637-5412-9 (pbk.)
1. Nursing—United States. I. Kenner, Carole.   II. Title.
    [DNLM: 1.   Nursing—United States. 2.   Nurse's Role—United States.   WY 300 AA1 F499p 2009]
    RT82.F535 2009
    610.7306′9—dc22
                                                                                        2008028736
6048
Printed in the United States of America
13   12   11   10   9   8   7   6   5

Contents

Section II The Healthcare Context

Section III Core Healthcare Professional Competencies

9   Provide Patient-Centered Care   291

10   Work in Interdisciplinary Teams   333

Section IV *The Practice of Nursing Today and in the Future*

Preface

The writing of this textbook was motivated by the need to include more information in nursing education about the Institute of Medicine (IOM) reports on quality health care, with a focus on the five core competencies identified by the IOM for all healthcare professions. These concepts provide the framework for this textbook, which introduces nursing students to the nursing profession and healthcare delivery. Nursing students today are asked to cover much information in their courses and develop clinical competencies in a short period of time. It is critical that each student recognize that nursing does not happen in isolation, but rather is part of the entire healthcare experience. Nurses play critical roles in this experience through their unique professional roles and responsibilities. They are also members of the healthcare team, where they must work with others to provide and improve care.

This textbook consists of 15 chapters and is divided into four sections. Section I focuses on the profession of nursing. In these chapters, the student will learn about the dynamic history of nursing and how the profession developed; the complex essence of nursing (knowledge and caring); the controversial issue of the image of nursing; and nursing education, accreditation, and regulation.

Section II explores the healthcare context in which nursing is practiced. Health policy and political action are very important today in health care and in nursing. Students need to know about ethical and legal issues that apply to their practice now and will apply in their future as registered nurses. Students typically think of care for the acutely ill, but the health context is broader than this and includes health promotion, disease prevention, and illness across the continuum of care. Though nursing is practiced in many different settings and healthcare organizations, the final chapter in this section focuses on acute care organizations to provide the student with an in-depth exploration of one type of healthcare organization.

Section III moves the discussion to the core healthcare competencies. Each chapter focuses on one of the five core competencies: provide patient-centered care; work in interdisciplinary teams; employ evidence-based practice; apply quality improvement; and utilize informatics. Though this section covers these competencies in depth, the competencies are relevant to all the content in this textbook.

Section IV brings us to the end of this textbook, though not to the end of learning. The two chapters in this section focus on the practice of nursing today and in the future, exploring in particular the critical issues of the nursing shortage and the transformation of nursing practice.

Each chapter includes objectives, an outline of the chapter to help organize your reading, Key Terms that are found in the chapter and are defined in the Glossary, content with headers that apply to the chapter outline, and References. The end-of-chapter content includes Internet links, Discussion Questions, Critical Thinking Activities, and a Case Study with questions. In each chapter, you will also find Words of Wisdom—stories and conversations with nurses who practice, teach, manage, lead, and do much more to improve health care and ensure that patients get what they need. Above all, this textbook is patient centered. Nurses care for and about patients.

Acknowledgments

We would like to thank our families: Fred, Shoshannah, and Deborah Finkelman, and Lester Kenner. Thanks to Elizabeth Karle for assistance with research, to Kevin Sullivan for his guidance in the development of this book, and to the Jones and Bartlett editorial staff for their expertise. We also want to recognize all the students we have worked with who have taught us much about what students need to know to practice competently.

Special acknowledgment and thanks to Judy Hembd for her work on the companion Web site for this textbook.

Section

I

The Profession of Nursing

Section I of this textbook introduces the beginning nursing student to the profession of nursing. The content in this textbook is built on the Institute of Medicine core competencies for healthcare professions. Chapter 1 discusses the development and history of nursing and what it means for nursing to be a profession. The chapter concludes by discussing some issues that nursing students encounter as they enter a professional education program. Chapter 2 discusses the essence of nursing; it focuses on the need for knowledge and caring and how nursing students develop throughout the nursing education program to be knowledgeable, competent, and caring. Chapter 3 addresses the critical issue of the image of nursing—an image that is not always clear and not always positive. Chapter 4 examines nursing education (which is complex), accreditation of nursing education programs, and regulation of the practice of nursing.

Chapter 1

The Development of Professional Nursing: History, the Profession, and the Nursing Education Experience

CHAPTER OBJECTIVES

At the conclusion of this chapter, the learner will be able to:

- Identify key figures and events in nursing history
- Discuss critical nursing history themes within the sociopolitical context of the time
- Define critical professional concepts
- Discuss professionalism in nursing
- Explain the relevance of standards to the nursing profession

- Discuss the development and roles of nursing associations
- Describe the roles of the nursing student and faculty
- Identify tools for success in a nursing education program

CHAPTER OUTLINE

KEY TERMS

- ❏ Accountability
- ❏ Autonomy
- ❏ Burnout
- ❏ Clinical experience
- ❏ Clinical laboratory
- ❏ Code of ethics
- ❏ Mentor
- ❏ Mentoring
- ❏ Networking
- ❏ Nursing

- ❏ Professionalism
- ❏ Reality shock
- ❏ Responsibility
- ❏ Scope of practice
- ❏ Simulation
- ❏ Social policy statement
- ❏ Standards
- ❏ Stress
- ❏ Stress management
- ❏ Time management

Introduction

This textbook presents an introduction to the nursing profession and critical aspects of nursing care and the delivery of health care. To begin the journey to graduation and licensure, it is important to understand several aspects of the nursing profession. What is professional **nursing**? How did it develop? How can one prepare to be successful as a student, to graduate, and to obtain licensure? This chapter addresses these questions.

From Past to Present: Nursing History

Why is it important for a student eager to provide patient care to learn about nursing history? This is a legitimate question. Nursing's history provides a framework for understanding how nursing is practiced today and the societal trends that shape the profession. The characteristics of nursing as a profession and what nurses do today have roots in the past, not only the past history of nursing but also of health care and society in general. Today, health care is highly complex; diagnosis methods and treatment have been developed to offer many opportunities for prevention, treatment, and cures that did not exist even a few years ago. Understanding this growth process is part of this discussion; it helps us to appreciate where nursing is today and may provide stimulus for changes in the future. It is important to remember that "nursing is conceptualized as a practice discipline with a mandate from society to enhance the health and well-being of humanity" (Shaw, 1993, p. 1654). But the past portrayal of nurses as handmaidens and assistants to physicians has its roots in the profession's religious beginnings. So where does the story of nursing begin?

From Paternalism to Professionalism: Movement from Trained Assistants with Religious Ties to Highly Educated Individuals

The discipline of nursing slowly evolved from the traditional role of women, apprenticeship, humanitarian aims, religious ideals, intuition, common sense, trial and error, theories, and research, as well as the multiple influences of medicine, technology, politics, war, economics, and feminism (Brooks & Kleine-Kracht, 1983; Gorenberg, 1983; Jacobs & Huether, 1978; Keller, 1979; Kidd & Morrison, 1988; Lynaugh & Fagin, 1988; Perry, 1985). It is impossible to provide a detailed history of nursing's evolution in one chapter, so only critical historical events will be discussed.

Writing about nursing history itself has an interesting history (Connolly, 2004). Historians who wrote about nursing prior to the 1950s tended to be nurses, and they wrote for nurses. Though nursing, throughout its history, has been intertwined with social issues of the day, the early publications about nursing history did not link nursing to "the broader social, economic, and cultural context in which events unfolded" (Connolly, 2004, p. 10). There was greater emphasis on the "profession's purity, discipline, and faith" (Connolly, 2004, p. 10). Part of the reason for this narrowed view of the history of nursing is that the discipline of history had limited, if any, contact with the nursing profession. This began to change in the 1950s and 1960s, when the scholarship of nursing history began to grow, but very slowly. In the 1970s, one landmark publication, *Hospitals, Paternalism and the Role of the Nurse* (Ashley, 1976), addressed social issues as an important aspect of nursing history. The key issue addressed was feminism in the society at large and its impact on nursing. As social history became more important, there was increased exploration of nursing, its history, and influences on that history. In addition, nursing has been tied more to political history today. For example, it is very difficult to understand current healthcare delivery concerns without including nursing (such as the impact of the nursing shortage). This all has an impact on health policy, including legislation at the state and national levels. Chapter 5 focuses on health policy and nursing.

Schools of nursing often highlight their own history for students, faculty, and visitors to the school. This might be done through exhibits about the school's history and, in some cases, a mini-museum. This provides an opportunity to identify how the school's history has developed and how its graduates have had an impact on the community and the profession. The purpose of this chapter is to explore some of the broad issues of nursing history, but this should not replace the history of each school of nursing as the profession has developed.

NURSE LEADERS: HISTORY IN THE MAKING

Learning something about the people is one place to begin. Exhibit 1–1 provides vignettes that

---

EXHIBIT 1–1 A GLIMPSE INTO THE CONTRIBUTIONS OF NURSES

This list does not represent all the important nursing leaders but does provide examples of the broad range of contributions and highlights specific achievements.

Dorothea Dix (1840–1841)

I traveled the state of Massachusetts to call attention to the present state of insane persons confined within this Commonwealth, in cages, stalls, pens! Chained, naked, beaten with rods, and lashed into obedience. Just by bettering the conditions for these persons, I showed that mental illnesses aren't all incurable.

Linda Richards (1869)

I was the first of five students to enroll in the New England Hospital for Women and Children and the first to graduate. Upon graduation, I was fortunate to obtain employment at the Bellevue Hospital in New York City. Here I created the first written reporting system, charting and maintaining individual patient records.

Clara Barton (1881)

The need in America for an institution that is not selfish must originate in the recognition of some evil that is adding to the sum of human suffering, or diminishing the sum of happiness. Today my efforts to organize such an institution have been successful: the National Society of the Red Cross.

Isabel Hampton Robb (1896)

As the first president for the American Nurses Association, I became active in organizing the nursing profession at the national level. In 1896, I organized the Nurses' Associated Alumnae of the United States and Canada, which became the American Nurses Association. I also founded the American Society of Superintendents of Training Schools for Nurses, which became the National League of Nursing Education. Through these professional organizations, I was able to initiate many improvements in nursing education.

Sophia Palmer (1900)

I launched the *American Journal of Nursing* and served as editor in chief of the journal for 20 years. I believe my forceful editorials helped guide nursing thought and shape nursing practice and events.

Lavinia L. Dock (1907)

I became a staunch advocate of legislation to control nursing practice. Realizing the problems that students faced in studying drugs and solutions, I wrote one of the first nursing textbooks, *Materia Medica for Nurses*. I served as foreign editor of the *American Journal of Nursing* and coauthored *History of Nursing*.

Martha Minerva Franklin (1908)

I actively campaigned for racial equality in nursing and guided 52 nurses to form the National Association of Colored Graduate Nurses.

Mary Mahoney (1909)

In 1908, the National Association of Colored Graduate Nurses was formed. As the first professional Black nurse, I gave the welcome address at the organization's first conference.

Mary Adelaide Nutting (1910)

I have advocated university education for nurses and developed the first programs of this type. Upon accepting the chairmanship at the Department of Nursing Education at Teachers College, Columbia University, I became the first nurse ever to be appointed to a university professorship.

Lillian Wald (1918)

My goal was to ensure that women and children, immigrants and the poor, and members of all ethnic and religious groups would realize America's promise of "life, liberty and the pursuit of happiness." The Henry Street Settlement and the Visiting Nurse Service in New York City championed public health nursing, housing reform, suffrage, world peace, and the rights of women, children, immigrants, and working people.

Mary Breckenridge (1920)
Through my own personal tragedies, I realized that medical care for mothers and babies in rural America was needed. I started the Frontier Nursing Service in Kentucky.

Elizabeth Russell Belford, Mary Tolle Wright, Edith Moore Copeland, Dorothy Garrigus Adams, Ethel Palmer Clarke, Elizabeth McWilliams Miller, and Marie Hippensteel Lingeman (1922)
We are the founders of the Sigma Theta Tau International Honor Society of Nursing. Each of us provided insights that advanced scholarship, leadership, research, and practice.

Susie Walking Bear Yellowtail (1930–1960)
I traveled for 30 years throughout North America, walking to reservations to improve health care and the Indian Health Services. I established the Native American Nurses Association and received the President's Award for Outstanding Nursing Healthcare.

Virginia Avenel Henderson (1939)
I am referred to as the first lady of nursing. I think of myself as an author, an avid researcher, and a visionary. One of my greatest contributions to the nursing profession was revising Harmer's *Textbook of the Principles and Practice of Nursing,* which has been widely adopted by schools of nursing.

Lucile Petry Leone (1943)
As the founder of the U.S. Cadet Nurse Corps, I believe we succeeded because we had a saleable package from the beginning. The women immediately liked the idea of being able to combine war service with professional education for the future.

Esther Lucille Brown (1946)
I issued a report titled *Nursing for the Future.* This report severely criticized the overall quality of nursing education. Thus, with the Brown Report, nursing education finally began the long-discussed move to accreditation.

Lydia Hall (1963–1969)
I established and directed the Loeb Center for Nursing and Rehabilitation at Montefiore Hospital in the Bronx, New York. Through my research in nursing and long-term care, I developed a theory (core, care, and cure) that the direct professional nurse-to-patient relationship is itself therapeutic and that nursing care is the chief therapy for the chronically ill patient.

Martha Rogers (1963–1965)
I served as editor of the *Journal of Nursing Science,* focusing my attention on improving and expanding nursing education, developing the scientific basis of nursing practice through professional education, and differentiating between professional and technical careers in nursing. My book, *An Introduction to the Theoretical Basis of Nursing* (1970), marked the beginning of nursing's search for a theoretical base.

Loretta Ford (1965)
I codeveloped the first nurse practitioner program in 1965 by integrating the traditional roles of the nurse with advanced medical training and the community outreach mission of a public health official.

Madeleine Leininger (1974)
I began, and continue to guide, nursing in the recognition that the culture care needs of people in the world will be met by nurses prepared in transcultural nursing.

continues

EXHIBIT 1–1 (continued)

Florence Wald (1975)

I have devoted my life to the compassionate care for the dying. I founded Hospice Incorporated in Connecticut, which is the model for hospice care in the United States and abroad.

Joann Ashley (1976)

I wrote *Hospitals, Paternalism, and the Role of the Nurse* during the height of the women's movement. My book created controversy with its pointed condemnation of sexism toward, and exploitation of, nurses by hospital administrators and physicians.

Luther Christman (1980)

As founder and dean of the Rush University College of Nursing, I have been linked to the "Rush Model," a unified approach to nursing education and practice that continues to set new standards of excellence. As dean of Vanderbilt University's School of Nursing, I was the first to employ African-American women as faculty at Vanderbilt and became one of the founders of the National Male Nurses Association, now known as the American Assembly for Men in Nursing.

Hildegard E. Peplau (1997)

I became known as the "Nurse of the Century." I was the only nurse to serve the American Nurses Association as executive director and later as president, and I served two terms on the Board of the International Council of Nurses. My working psychiatric-mental health nursing emphasized the nurse–patient relationship.

Linda Aiken (2007)

My policy research agenda was motivated by a commitment to improving healthcare outcomes by building an evidence base for health services management and providing direction for national policy makers, resulting in greater recognition of the role that nursing care has on patient outcomes.

---

describe the contributions of some nursing leaders. People, however, do not operate in a vacuum, and neither did the nurses highlighted in this exhibit. They were influenced by their communities, the society, and the history of their time.

FLORENCE NIGHTINGALE

Let's begin with the "mother" of modern nursing throughout the world, Florence Nightingale. Most nursing students at some point say the Nightingale Pledge, which is a method for connecting the past with the present. The Nightingale Pledge is found in Box 1–1. It was composed to provide nurses with an oath similar to the physician's Hippocratic Oath. The oath was not written by Nightingale but was supposed to represent her view of nursing.

Who was this person about whom so much has been written? She has become almost the perfect vision of a nurse, but was she? Nightingale did much for nursing, but many who came after her provided even greater direction for the profession. A focus on Nightingale helps to better understand the major changes that occurred. In 1859, Florence Nightingale wrote, "No man, not even a doctor, ever gives any other definition of what a nurse should be than this—'devoted and obedient.' This definition would do just as well for a porter. It might even do for a horse. It would not do for a policeman" (Nightingale, 1860/1992). This quote clearly demonstrates that she was outspoken and held strong beliefs, though she lived during a time when this type of quote from a woman was extraordinary.

BOX 1–1 THE ORIGINAL NIGHTINGALE PLEDGE

I solemnly pledge myself before God and in the presence of this assembly, to pass my life in purity and to practice my profession faithfully. I will abstain from whatever is deleterious and mischievous, and will not take or knowingly administer any harmful drug. I will do all in my power to maintain and elevate the standard of my profession, and will hold in confidence all personal matters committed to my keeping and all family affairs coming to my knowledge in the practice of my calling. With loyalty will I endeavor to aid the physician, in his work, and devote myself to the welfare of those committed to my care.

Source: Composed by Lystra Gretter in 1893 for the class graduating from Harper Hospital, Detroit, Michigan.

Florence Nightingale was British and lived and worked in the Victorian Period during the Industrial Revolution. This is significant because during this time, the role of women, especially women of the upper classes, was clearly defined and controlled. These women did not work outside the home and maintained a monitored social existence. Their purpose was to be a wife and mother, two roles that Nightingale never assumed. Education of women was also limited. Nightingale did have some classical education supported by her father, but there was never any expectation that she would "use" the education (Slater, 1994). Nightingale grew up knowing that this was to be her life. Women of her class ran the home and supervised the servants. Though this was not her goal, the household management skills that she learned from her mother were put to good use when she entered the hospital environment. Because of her social standing, she was in the company of educated and influential men, and she learned the "art of influencing powerful men" (Slater, 1994, p. 143). This skill was used a great deal by Nightingale as she fought for reforms.

Nightingale held different views; she had "a strong conviction that women have the mental abilities to achieve whatever they wish to achieve: compose music, solve scientific problems, create social projects of great importance" (Chinn, 2001, p. 441). She felt that women should question their assigned roles, and she wanted to serve people. When she reached her twenties, she felt an increasing desire to help others and decided that she wanted to become a nurse. Nurses at this time came from the lower classes and, of course, any training for this type of role was out of the question. Her parents refused to support her goal, and because women were not free to make this type of decision by themselves, she was blocked. Nightingale became angry and then depressed. As the depression worsened, her parents finally relented and allowed her to attend nurse's training in Germany. This was kept a secret, and people were told that she was away at a spa for 3 months' rest (Slater, 1994). She was schooled in math and science, which would lead her to use statistics to demonstrate the nurse's impact on health outcomes. Had it not been for her social standing and her ability to obtain education, coupled with her friendship with Dr. Elizabeth Blackwell, nurses might well have remained uneducated assistants to doctors.

An important fact about Nightingale is that she was very religious—to the point that she felt that God had called on her to help others (Woodham-Smith, 1951). She also felt that the body and mind were separate entities, and both needed to be considered—the basis of nursing's holistic view of health. Her convictions played a major role in her views of nurses and nursing. She viewed patients as persons who were unable to help themselves or who were dying. She is quoted as saying, "What nursing has to do . . . is to put the patient in the best condition for nature to act upon him" (Seymer, 1954, p. 13). She also recognized that a patient's health depends on environmental impacts such as light, noise, smells or effluvia, and heat—something that we are just examining today in nursing and health care. In her work during the Crimean War, she applied her beliefs about the body and mind by arranging activities for the soldiers, providing them with classes and books, and she supported their connection with home—an early version of what is now often called holistic care. Later, this type of focus on the total patient would become an integral part of psychiatric-mental health nursing. Her other interest with sanitary reform grew from her experience in the Crimean War, and she worked with influential men to make changes. Nightingale, however, did not agree with the new, growing theories of contagion, but she did support the value of education in improving social problems and believed that education included moral, physical, and practical aspects (Widerquist, 1997).

Nightingale wrote four small books—or treatises, as they were called—thus starting the idea that nurses need to publish about their work. The titles of the "books" were *Notes on Matters Affecting the Health, Efficiency, and Hospital Administration of the British Army* (1858), *Subsidiary Notes as to the Introduction of Female Nursing into Military Hospitals* (1858), *Notes on Hospitals* (1859), and *Notes on Nursing* (1860). The first three focused on hospitals that she visited, including military hospitals (Slater, 1994). She kept a lot of data; her interest in healthcare data analysis helped to lay the groundwork for epidemiology, highlighting the importance of data in nursing, particularly in

a public health context. An interesting fact is that *Notes on Nursing* was not written for nurses, but rather for women who cared for ill family members. As late as 1860, she did not completely give up on the need for care provided by women as a form of service to family and friends. This book was popular when it was published because most nursing care at the time was provided by family members.

Nightingale's religious and upper-class background had a major impact on her important efforts to improve both nursing education and nursing in the hospital setting. Nurses were of the lower class, usually unschooled and often alcoholics, prostitutes, and those down on their luck. Nightingale changed all that; she believed that patients needed educated nurses to care for them, and she founded the first organized school of nursing. Nightingale's school, which opened in London in 1860, accepted women of a higher class, not alcoholics and former prostitutes as had been the case. The students were not viewed as servants, and their loyalty was to the school, not to the hospital. This point is somewhat confusing and must be viewed from the perspective that important changes were made; however, these were not monumental changes but a beginning. Even in Nightingale's school, students were very much a part of the hospital; they staffed the hospital, representing free labor, and they worked long hours. This model developed into the diploma school model—considered an apprenticeship model—though today, diploma schools have less direct relationships with the hospitals, and in some cases, they offer associate's degrees. Nightingale's students did receive training, which had not been provided in an organized manner prior to her changes. Nightingale's religious views also had an impact on her rigid educational system, and she expected students to have high moral values. Training was still based on an apprenticeship model and continued to be for some time in Britain, Europe, and, later, the United States. The structure of hospital nursing was also very rigid, with a matron in charge. This rigidity existed for decades and, in some cases, may still be present in hospital nursing organizations. Nurses in Britain, beginning to recognize the need to band together, formed the British Nurses Association. This organization took on the issue of regulating nursing practice. Nightingale did not approve of efforts by the British Nurses Association toward state registration of nurses (Freeman, 2007) mostly because she did not trust the leaders' goals regarding registration. There were no known **standards** for nursing, so how was one to be registered? Many questions were raised regarding the definition of nursing, who should be registered, and who controlled nursing. Some critics feel that Nightingale did make changes but that the way she made the changes had negative effects, including delaying the development of the profession, particularly regarding nurses' subordinate position to physicians, failing to encourage nursing education to be offered at a university level, and delaying licensure (Freeman, 2007).

Despite this criticism, Nightingale still holds an important place in nursing history. O'Rourke (2003) stated,

> *We've come a long way in 143 years. Nightingale's groundbreaking work,* Notes on Nursing: What It is and What It Is Not, *laid down the principles of nursing. Remarkably, the textbook is a classic and still in print today, more than a century later. And although Nightingale is credited with establishing the fundamentals of patient management, care, and cleanliness that have been taught in nursing schools ever since, her true legacy was far greater. She elevated nursing to a higher degree of respectability and **professionalism** than ever before with the emphasis placed on education and*

> *not just availability of a woman for work. If only she could see nurses now. In the 20th century, nursing reinforced its valued place among the professions. No longer quiet, subservient help mates, nurses of every race, class background, and gender have stepped up to leadership roles in the profession and in the healthcare industry. She would see nurses using advanced information technology to provide care, document that care, research better treatment methods, and transfer knowledge to colleagues at every level of experience, in every specialty and in every care setting imaginable. (p. 97)*

Nightingale valued data and outcomes, two key elements of today's focus on evidence-based practice.

THE HISTORY SURROUNDING THE DEVELOPMENT OF NURSING AS A PROFESSION

When nursing history is described, distinct historical periods typically are discussed: Early History (AD 1–500), Rise of Christianity and the Middle Ages (500–1500), Renaissance (mid-1300s–1600s), and the Industrial Revolution (mid-1700s–mid-1800s). In addition, the historical perspective must include the different regions and environments in which the historical events took place. Early history focuses on Africa, the Mediterranean, Asia, and the Middle East. The focus then turns to Europe, with the rise of Christianity and subsequent major changes that span several centuries. Nursing history expands as colonists arrive in America and a new environment helps to further the development of the nursing profession. Throughout all these periods and locations, wars have had an impact on nursing. As a consequence of the varied places and times in which nursing has existed, the profession has been influenced by major historical events, different cultures and languages, varying views on what constitutes disease and illness, roles of women, political issues, and location and environment. Nursing has probably existed for as long as humans have been ill; someone took care of the sick. This does not mean that there was a formal nursing position; rather, in most early cases, the nurse was a woman who cared for ill family members. The discussion begins with this group and then expands.

Early History   Early history of nursing focuses on the Ancient Egyptians and Hebrews, Greeks, and Romans. During this time, communities often had women who assisted with childbearing as a form of nursing care, and some physicians had assistants. The Egyptians had physicians, and sick persons looking for magical answers would go to them or to priests or sorcerers. Hebrew (Jewish) physicians kept records and developed a hygiene code that examined issues such as personal and community hygiene, contagion, disinfection, and preparation of food and water (Masters, 2005). This occurred at a time when hygiene was very poor, a condition that continued for several centuries. Disease and disability were viewed as curses and related to sins, which meant that afflicted persons had to change or follow the religious statutes (Bullough & Bullough, 1978). Greek mythology recognized health issues and physicians in its gods. Hippocrates, a Greek physician, is known as the father of medicine. He contributed to health care by writing a medical textbook that was used for centuries, and he developed an approach to disease that would later be referred to as epidemiology. He also developed the Hippocratic Oath (Bullough & Bullough, 1978), which is still said by new physicians today and which influenced the writing of the Nightingale Pledge. The Greeks viewed health as a balance between body and mind, which was different from earlier views related to curses and sins. Throughout this entire

period, the wounded and ill in the armies required care. Generally, in this period—which represents thousands of years and involved several major cultures that rose and fell—nursing occurred, but not nursing as it is thought of today. People took care of those who were sick and during childbirth, representing an early nursing role.

Rise of Christianity and the Middle Ages
The rise of Christianity led to more structured nursing care, but still it was far from professional nursing. Women continued to carry most of the care for the poor and the sick. The church set up a system for care that included the role of the deaconess, who provided care in homes. Women who served in these roles had to follow strict rules set by the church. This role eventually evolved into that of nuns, who began to live and work in convents. The convent was considered a safe place for women. The sick came to the convents for nursing care and also received spiritual care (Wall, 2003). The establishment of convents, which then became centers for nursing care, formed the seed for what, hundreds of years later, would become the Catholic system of hospitals that still exists today. Were men involved in nursing at this time? There were men in the Crusades who cared for the sick and injured. These men wore large red crosses on their uniforms to distinguish them from the fighting soldiers. Altruism and connecting care to religion were major themes during this period. Even Nightingale continued with these themes in her view of nursing. Disease was common and spread quickly, and medical care had little to offer in the way of prevention or cure. Institutions that were called hospitals were not like modern hospitals; they primarily served travelers and sometimes the sick (Kalisch & Kalisch, 1986).

The Protestant Reformation had a major impact on some of the care given to the sick and injured. The Catholic Church's loss of power in some areas resulted in the closing of hospitals, and some convents closed or moved. The hospitals that remained were no longer staffed by nuns but by women from the lower classes who often had major problems, such as alcoholism, or who were former prostitutes. This is what Florence Nightingale found when she entered nursing.

Renaissance and the Enlightenment   The Renaissance had a major impact on health and the view of illness. This period was one of significant advancement in science, though by today's standards, it might be viewed as limited. However, it is significant that these early discoveries led to advancements that were never thought of previously. This is the period, spanning many years, of Columbus and the American and French Revolutions. Education became important. Leonardo da Vinci's drawings of the human anatomy, which were done to help him understand the human body for his sculptures, provided details that had not been categorized before (Donahue, 1985). The 18th century was a period of many discoveries and changes (Dietz & Lehozky, 1963; Masters, 2005; Rosen, 1958):

- Jenner's smallpox vaccination method was developed during a time of high death rates from smallpox.
- Psychiatry became a specialty area.
- The pulse watch and the stethoscope were developed, changing how physical assessment was conducted.
- Pasteur discovered the process of pasteurization, which had an impact on food and milk contamination.
- Lister used some of Pasteur's research and developed approaches to antiseptic surgery. He is known as the father of surgery.
- Koch studied anthrax and cholera, both major diseases of the time, demonstrating

that they were transmitted by water, food, and clothing. He is known as the father of microbiology.
- Klebs proved the existence of the germ theory.

All these discoveries and changes had an impact on nursing in the long-term perspective and changed the sociopolitical climate of health care. Nightingale did not agree with the new theory of contagion, but over time, the nursing profession accepted these new theories, which are still critical components of patient care today. She stressed however, that the mind-body connection—*putting patients in the best light for healing*—ultimately made the difference. Discovering methods for preventing disease and using this information in disease prevention is an important part of nursing today. Community health is certainly concerned with many of the same issues that led to critical new discoveries so many years ago, such as contamination of food and water and preventing disease worldwide.

Industrial Revolution   The Industrial Revolution brought changes in the workplace, but many were not positive from a health perspective. Workplaces were hazardous and breeding grounds for spreading disease. People worked long hours and often under harsh conditions. This was a period of great exploitation of children, particularly those of the lower classes who were forced to work at very young ages (Masters, 2005). There were no child labor laws, so preteen children often worked in factories alongside adults. Some children were forced to quit school to earn wages to help support their families. Cities were crowded and very dirty, with epidemics about which little could be done. There were few public health laws to alleviate the causes. Nightingale and enlightened citizens tried to reform some of these conditions. She stated in *Notes on Nursing* (1860/1992) that "there are five essential points in securing the health of houses: Pure air, pure water, efficient drainage, cleanliness, and light." Nightingale strongly supported more efforts to promote health and felt that this was more cost-effective than treating illness—important healthcare principles today—but she did not support progressive thought at the time regarding contagion and germs. These ideas are good examples regarding how the environment and culture in which a person lives and works drives his or her views on issues and problems. If one did not know anything about the history of the time, one might wonder why Nightingale held these ideas to be important.

Colonization of America and the Growth of Nursing in the United States The initial experiences of nursing in the United States were not much different from those described for Britain and Europe. Nurses were of the lower class and had limited or no training; hospitals were not used by the upper classes, but rather the lower classes and the poor. Hospitals were dirty and lacked formal care services.

Nursing in the United States did move forward. Exhibit 1–1 describes the many contributions of nurses, demonstrating the activity and change that occurred over time. Significant steps were taken to improve nursing education and the profession of nursing. The first nursing schools—or, as they were called, training schools—were modeled after Nightingale's school. Some of the earlier schools were in Boston, New York, and Connecticut. The same approach was taken in these schools as in Britain: moral character and subservience, with efforts to move away from using lower class women with dubious histories, as was done in the early days of nursing even in the United States (Masters, 2005). Limitations regarding what women could do on their own

still constituted a major problem. Women could not vote and had limited rights. This situation did begin to change in the early 1900s when women obtained the right to vote, but only with great effort. In 1911, the American Nurses Association (ANA) began, which had been called the Nurses' Associated Alumnae (1896). This effort was led by Isabel Robb and Lavinia Dock. At the same time, the first nursing journal, the *American Journal of Nursing (AJN)*, was created through the ANA. The *AJN* was published until early 2006, when the ANA replaced it with *American Nurse Today* as its official journal. The *AJN,* the oldest U.S. nursing journal, still exists today but is not part of the ANA. Its content has always focused on the issues facing nurses and their patients.

It is notable that although some nurse leaders such as Dock were ardent suffragists, Nightingale was not interested in these ideas even though women in Britain did not have the right to vote. Nightingale felt that the focus should be on "allowing" (a permissive statement indicative of women's status) women to own property and then linking voting rights to this ownership right (Masters, 2005). What is clear is that there was communication across the ocean between nurses, and they did not always agree on the approach to take on the road to professionalism; in fact, they did not always agree within the United States. Nurse leaders and practicing nurses helped nursing to grow into a profession during times of war (the American Revolution, the Civil War, the Spanish-American War, World War I, World War II, the Korean War, the Vietnam War, and modern wars today). The Web site *Experiencing War: Women at War*, which appears in the Linking to the Internet section of this chapter, provides information about nurses who served in these wars. The Depression also had an impact, "resulting in widespread unemployment of private duty nurses and the closing of nursing schools, while simultaneously creating the increasing need for charity health services for the population" (Masters, 2005, p. 28). This meant that there were fewer student nurses to staff the hospitals, and as a consequence, nurses were hired, though at very low pay, to replace them. Up until this time, hospitals depended on student nurses to staff the hospitals, and graduate nurses served as private duty nurses in homes. Using students to staff hospitals continued until the university-based nursing effort grew; however, during the Depression, there was a greater need to replace students when schools closed. On one level, this could be seen as an improvement in care, but the low pay was difficult to overcome, resulting in a long history of low pay scales for nurses.

In 1922, the Goldmark Report, *Nursing and Nursing Education in the United States*, had a major impact on nursing education when the report recommended that university schools of nursing should be established. In 1948, a second report, the Brown Report, was critical of the quality of nursing education. This led to the implementation of an accreditation program for nursing schools, which was to be conducted by the National League for Nursing (NLN). Accreditation is a process of reviewing what a school is doing and its curriculum based on established standards. Movement toward the university setting and away from hospital-based schools of nursing, and establishment of standards with an accreditation process were major changes for the nursing profession. The ANA and the NLN continue to establish standards for practice and education and to support implementation of those standards.

In the 1940s and 1950s, other changes occurred in the healthcare system that had a direct impact on nursing. Certainly, scientific discoveries were changing care, but there were also important health policy changes. The Hill

Burton Act (1946) established federal funds to build more hospitals, and at one point in the 1980s, there were too many hospital beds. This led to hospitals laying off nurses because their salaries represented the largest operating expense. There is some belief that this decision is still impacting the current shortage; when more nurses were needed, some of the nurses who had been laid off had moved into new jobs or careers, or left the workforce. This was a period of rapid change in reimbursement for health care through the growth of health insurance and the establishment of Medicare and Medicaid. Chapter 8 discusses some of these issues in more detail.

Little has been said in this description of nursing history about the role of men and minorities in nursing; there was little in the early history, and this plagues nursing even today, though certainly there has been improvement. Segregation and discrimination existed in nursing just as it did in society at large. The National Association of Colored Graduate Nurses was closed in 1951 when the ANA began to accept African-American nurses. However, today there is still concern about the limited number of minorities in health care. The Sullivan Commission's report on health professions diversity, *Missing Persons: Minorities in the Health Professions* (Sullivan & the Sullivan Commission, 2004), is an important current document with recommendation to improve diversity in health professions and was commented on by the American Association of Colleges of Nursing (AACN, 2004).

- Health profession schools should hire diversity program managers and develop strategic plans that outline specific goals, standards, policies, and **accountability** mechanisms to ensure institutional diversity and cultural competence.
- Colleges and universities should provide an array of support services to minority

students, including **mentoring**, resources for developing test-taking skills, and application counseling.

- Schools granting baccalaureate nursing degrees should provide and support "bridging programs" that enable graduates of 2-year colleges to succeed in the transition to 4-year institutions. Graduates of associate's degree (AD) nursing programs should be encouraged and supported to enroll in baccalaureate nursing programs.

- AACN and other health profession organizations should work with schools to promote enhanced admissions policies, cultural competence training, and minority student recruitment.

- To remove financial barriers to nursing education, public and private funding organizations should provide scholarships, loan forgiveness programs, and tuition reimbursement to students and institutions.

- Congress should substantially increase funding for diversity programs within the National Health Service Corps and Titles VII and VIII of the Public Health Service Act.

Whether these recommendations and efforts to improve the number of minorities in all health professions, not just nursing, have made a difference is not yet known; it will take time to determine improvement.

The number of men in nursing has increased over the years but still lags. After the major wars—such as World Wars I and II, the Korean War, and the Vietnam War—medics came home and entered nursing programs. Men served as nurses in the early history period, such as in the Crusades, and monks provided care in convents. However, after this period, men were not accepted as nurses because nursing was viewed as a woman's role. The poet Walt Whit-man was a nurse in the Civil War. So, there were men in nursing, though few, and some were well known—though maybe not for their nursing (Kalisch & Kalisch, 1986). Early in the history of nursing schools in the United States, men were not accepted, and this may have been influenced by the sex-segregated housing for nursing students and the model of apprenticeship that focused on women (Bullough, 2006). In part this was due to nursing's religious roots, which promoted "sisters" as nurses. This made it difficult for men to come into the system and the culture—it was a women's profession. In 1940 the ANA did recognize men by having a session on men in nursing at its convention. With the return of medics from the wars and the movement of schools of nursing into more academic settings, more men began to apply. Men in nursing have to contend with male-dominated medicine, and this has had an influence on the practice. Male nurses were also able to get commissions in the military (Bullough, 2006). The changes did have an impact, but the increase in salaries and improvement in work conditions had the strongest impact on increasing men in nursing. In 2001, Boughn conducted a study to explore why women and men choose nursing. The results of this study indicated that female and male participants did not differ in their desire to care for others. Both groups had a strong interest in power and empowerment, but female students were more interested in using their power to empower others, whereas male students were more interested in empowering the profession. The most significant difference was found in the expectations of salary and working conditions, with men expecting more. This last finding is disturbing. Why would not both males and females expect higher salaries and better working conditions? Is this still part of the view of nursing and nurses from nursing's past? Luther Christman, a well-known nursing leader who served a nurse for many years, retired at age 87 but is still an active voice for the profession and for men in nursing. According to Sullivan (2002), Christman stated that "men in medicine were reluctant to give up power to women and, by the same token, women in nursing have fought to retain their power. Medicine, however, was forced to admit women after affirmative action legislation was enacted." "Sadly," Christman reported, "nursing, with a majority of women, was not required to adhere to affirmative action policies" (Sullivan, 2002, pp. 10, 12). Today, more men and minorities enter bachelor's degree programs than any other level of nursing education, as supported by national workforce data from the NLN and the AACN on an annual basis (B. Cleary, personal communication, 2007; Cleary, 2007; Sochalski, 2002). There is an organization for men in nursing, the American Assembly for Men in Nursing (http://www.aamn.org), and men are also members of other nursing organizations.

Themes: Looking into the Nursing Profession's History

Nursing's past represents a movement from a role based on family and religious ties and the need to provide comfort and care ("because that is a woman's lot in life") to an educated person representing the "glue" that holds the healthcare system together. From medieval times through Nightingale's time, nursing represented a role that women played in families to provide care. This care extended to anyone in need, but after Nightingale presented what a woman could do with some degree of education, physicians— or in many countries the term is, "doctors"— recognized that women needed to have some degree of training. Education was introduced,

but mainly to serve the need of hospitals to have a labor force. Thus, the apprenticeship model of nursing was born. Why would nursing perceive a need for greater education? Primarily because of advances in science, increased knowledge of germs and diseases, and increased training of doctors, nurses needed to understand basic anatomy, physiology, pathophysiology, and epidemiology to provide better care. To carry out a doctor's orders efficiently, nurses must have some degree of understanding of cause and effect of environmental exposures, and disease causation. Thus, the move from hospital nursing to university training occurred.

Critics of Nightingale suggest that although the "lady with the lamp" image of a nurse with a light moving about the wounded in the Crimea is laudable, it presented the nurse as a caring, take-charge person who would go to great lengths and even sacrifice her own safety and health to provide care (Shames, 1993). The message sent to the public was that nurses were not powerful. They were caring but they would not fight to change the conditions of hospitals and patient care. They instead acted, as many do today, as victims. Hospitals owned nurses and considered them cheap labor. Today, the same view is held by many. The view of health— doctors are defined by their **scope of practice** in treating diseases, whereas nurses are seen as health promoters—adds to the lesser status of nursing (Shames). The view that nurses are angels of mercy rather than well-educated professionals reinforces the idea that nurses care but really do not have to think; this view is perpetuated by advertisements that depict nurses as angels or caring ethereal humans (Gordon, 2005). Most patients, especially at 3 A.M. when few other professionals are available, hope that the nurse is more than just caring, but a critical thinker who knows when to call the rest of the team.

Professionalism: Critical Professional Concepts

Nursing is a practice profession and an applied science. To appreciate the relevance of this statement requires an understanding of professionalism and how it applies to nursing. Nursing is more than just a job; it is a professional career requiring commitment. Table 1–1 describes some differences in attitudes related to an occupation/job and a career/profession.

But what does this really mean, and why does it matter? As described previously in this chapter, getting to where nursing is today was not easy, nor did it happen overnight. Many nurses contributed to the development of nursing as a profession; it mattered to them that nurses be recognized as professionals.

Nursing as a Profession

The current definition of nursing, as defined by the ANA (2004), is "the protection, promotion, and optimization of health and abilities, preven-tion of illness and injury, alleviation of suffering through the diagnosis and treatment of human response, and advocacy in the care of individuals, families, communities, and populations" (p. 7). Box 1–2 provides several definitions of nursing that demonstrate a historical perspective.

Chapter 2 contains a more in-depth discussion of the nature of nursing, but a definition is needed in this discussion to gain a further understanding about nursing as a profession. Is nursing a profession? What is a profession? Why is it important that nursing be recognized as a profession? Some nurses may not think that nursing is a profession, but this is not the position taken by recognized nursing organizations, nursing education, and boards of nursing that are involved in licensure of nurses. Each state has its own definition of nursing that is found in the state's nurse practice act, but the ANA definition noted here encompasses the common characteristics of nursing practice.

In general, a profession—whether nursing or another profession, such as medicine, teaching, or law—has certain characteristics (Bixler &

Table 1–1 COMPARISON OF ATTITUDES: OCCUPATION VERSUS CAREER

	Occupation	Career
Longevity	Temporary, a means to an end	Lifelong vocation
Educational preparation	Minimal training required, usually associate's degree	University professional degree program based on foundation of core liberal arts
Continuing education	Only what is required for the job or to get a raise/promotion	Lifelong learning, continual effort to gain new knowledge, skills, and abilities
Level of commitment	Short-term, as long as job meets personal needs	Long-term commitment to organization and profession
Expectations	Reasonable work for reasonable pay; responsibility ends with shift	Will assume additional responsibilities and volunteer for organizational activities and community-based events

Source: From *Nursing School Success: Tools for Constructing Your Future*, by D. Wilfong, C. Szolis, and C. Haus, 2007, Sudbury, MA: Jones and Bartlett Publishers.

BOX 1–2 DEFINITIONS OF NURSING: A HISTORICAL PERSPECTIVE

The following list provides a timeline of some of the definitions of nursing over time. Key terms are bolded.

Florence Nightingale
Having "charge of the **personal health** of somebody . . . and what nursing has to do . . is to put the patient in the **best possible condition** for **nature to act upon him.**" (Nightingale, 1859, p. 79)

Virginia Henderson
"The unique function of the nurse is to assist the individual, sick or well, in the performance of those activities **contributing to health or its recovery (or to peaceful death)** and that he would perform unaided if he had the necessary strength, will or knowledge. And to do this in such a way as to **help him gain independence** as rapidly as possible." (Henderson, 1966, p. 21)

Martha Rogers
"The **process** by which this body of knowledge, **nursing science**, is used for the purpose of assisting human beings to **achieve maximum health within the potential of each person.**" (Rogers, 1988, p. 100)

American Nurses Association
Nursing is the **protection, promotion, and optimization of health and abilities, prevention of illness and injury, alleviation of suffering** through the **diagnosis and treatment of human response,** and **advocacy** in the care of individuals, families, communities, and populations. (ANA, 2004, p. 4)

International Council of Nursing
Nursing encompasses **autonomous and collaborative care** of individuals of all ages, families, groups and communities, sick or well and in all settings. Nursing includes the **promotion of health**, **prevention** of illness and the **care of ill, disabled and dying people. Advocacy,** promotion of a **safe environment**, **research,** participation in shaping **health policy** and in patient and health systems management, and education are also key nursing roles. (http://www.icn.org)

Sources: From *Notes on Nursing: What It Is and What It Is Not* (Commemorative Edition), by F. Nightingale, 1859, Philadelphia: Lippincott; *The Nature of Nursing: A Definition and Its Implications for Practice, Research, and Education,* by V. Henderson, 1966, New York: Macmillan; "Nursing Science and Art: A Prospective," by M. Rogers, 1988, *Nursing Science Quarterly*, 1, p. 99; *Nursing Scope and Standards of Practice*, by American Nurses Association, 2004, Silver Spring, MD: Author; International Council of Nursing, retrieved May 4, 2007, from http://www.icn.org

Bixler, 1959; Huber, 2000; Lindberg, Hunter, & Kruszewkski, 1998; Quinn & Smith, 1987; Schein & Kommers, 1972):

- A systematic body of knowledge that provides the framework for the profession's practice
- Standardized, formal higher education
- Commitment to providing a service that benefits individuals and the community
- Maintenance of a unique role that recognizes **autonomy**, **responsibility**, and accountability
- Control of practice responsibility of the profession through standards and a **code of ethics**
- Commitment to members of the profession through professional organizations and activities

Does nursing meet these professional characteristics?

Nursing has a standardized content, although schools of nursing may configure the content in different ways; there is consistency in content areas such as adult health, maternal–child health, behavioral or mental health, pharmacology, assessment, and so on. The National Council Licensure Examination (NCLEX) covers standardized content areas. This content is based on *systematic, recognized knowledge*—or "information that is synthesized so that relationships are identified and formalized" (ANA, 2004, p. 48)—that is required for practice and expected to be offered in higher education programs. Chapter 4 discusses nursing education in more detail. The focus of nursing is practice—care provided to assist individuals, families, communities, and populations.

Nursing as a profession has a social contract with society, as described in *Nursing's* **Social Policy Statement** (ANA, 2003): "The authority for the practice of professional nursing is based on a social contract that acknowledges professional rights and responsibilities as well as mechanisms for accountability" (p. 2). Nurses make contributions to society (the community in which nurses practice), and because of this, nurses have a relationship to the society and its culture and institutions. Nurses do not operate in a vacuum, without concern for what the individuals in a community and the community need. Understanding needs and providing care to meet those needs are directly connected to the social context of nursing. There are critical value assumptions related to the contract between nursing and society that provide an explanation of the importance of this contractual relationship (ANA, 2004, p. 3):

- Humans manifest an essential unity of mind, body, and spirit.
- Human experience is contextually and culturally defined.
- Health and illness are human experiences. The presence of illness does not preclude

health, nor does optimal health preclude illness.
- The relationship between nurse and patient occurs within the context of the values and beliefs of the patient and the nurse.
- The interaction between nurse and patient occurs within the context of the values and beliefs of the patient and the nurse.
- Public policy and the healthcare delivery system influence the health and well-being of society and professional nursing.

Autonomy, responsibility, and accountability are intertwined with the practice of nursing and are critical components of a profession. Autonomy is the "freedom to act on what you know" (Kramer & Schmalenberg, 2002, p. 36). It is the right to make a decision and take control. Nurses have a distinct body of knowledge and develop competencies in nursing care that should be based on this nursing knowledge. When this is accomplished, nurses can then practice nursing. "Responsibility refers to being entrusted with a particular function" (Ritter-Teitel, 2002, p. 34). "Accountability means being responsible and accountable to self and others for behaviors and outcomes included in one's professional role. A professional nurse is accountable for embracing professional values, maintaining professional values, maintaining competence, and maintenance and improvement of professional practice environments" (Kupperschmidt, 2004, p. 114). A nurse is also accountable for the outcomes of the nursing care that he or she provides; what nurses do must mean something (Finkelman, 2006). The nurse is answerable for the actions that he or she takes. How are accountability and responsibility different? A nurse often delegates a task to another staff member, telling him or her what to do and when. The staff member assigned the task is responsible for performing the task and for the performance. The nurse who delegated the task to the staff person is accountable for the decision to delegate the task. Delegation is discussed in more detail in Chapter 10.

Sources of Professional Direction

Professions develop documents or statements about what the members feel is important in order to guide their practice, to establish control over practice, and to influence the quality of that practice. What are some of the important sources of professional direction for nurses?

1. *Nursing's Social Policy Statement* (ANA, 2003) is an important document that has been mentioned several times in this chapter. It describes the profession of nursing and its professional framework and obligations to society. The statement has been revised three times, in 1980, 1995, and 2003 (the current edition). This document informs consumers, government officials, other healthcare professionals, and other important stakeholders about nursing and its definition, knowledge base, scope of practice, and regulation.

2. *Nursing: Scope and Standards of Practice* (ANA, 2004) is another important document that has been developed by the ANA and its members. Nursing standards, which are "authoritative statements defined and promoted by the profession by which the quality of practice, service, or education can be evaluated" (ANA, 2004, p. 49), are critical to guiding safe, quality patient care. Standards describe minimal expectations. "We must always remember that as a profession the members are granted the privilege of self-regulation because they purport to use standards to monitor and evaluate the actions of its members to ensure a positive impact on the public it

serves" (O'Rourke, 2003, p. 97). "Standards guide practice, and the profession has generic standards that apply to all nurses, as well as specialty standards. They are developed by professional organizations, legal sources such as state nurse practice acts and federal and state laws, regulatory agencies such as accreditation bodies and federal and state agencies, and healthcare facilities, and are supported by scientific literature" (Finkelman, 2006, p. 263).

The standards include a scope of practice statement that describes the "who, what, where, when, why, and how" of nursing practice. The definition of nursing is the critical foundation. As noted in Box 1–2, the definition of nursing has evolved and will most likely continue to evolve over time as needs change and healthcare delivery and practice evolve. Nursing knowledge and the integration of science and art, which is discussed in more detail in Chapter 2, is part of the scope of practice, along with the definition of the "what and why" of nursing. Nursing care is provided in a variety of settings by the professional registered nurse (RN), who may have an advanced degree and specialty training and expertise. There is additional information about the standards, as well as the nurse's roles and functions throughout this text. Part of being a professional is having a commitment to the profession: a commitment to lifelong learning, adhering to standards, maintaining membership in professional organizations, publishing, and ensuring that nursing care is of the highest quality possible.

To go full circle and return to the social contract, nursing care must be provided and should include consideration of health, social, economic, legislative, and ethical factors. Content related to these issues is discussed in other chapters in this text. Nursing is not just about making someone better; it is about health education, assisting patients and families in making health decisions, providing direct care and supervising others who provide care, assessing care and applying the best evidence in making care decisions, communicating and working with the treatment team, developing a plan of care with a team that includes the patient and family, evaluating patient outcomes, advocating for patients, and much more.

Chapter 12 discusses safe, quality care in more detail, but as the student becomes more oriented to nursing education and nursing as a profession, it is important to recognize that establishing standards is part of being in a profession. The generic standards and their measurement criteria, which apply to all nurses, are divided into two types of standards: standards of practice and standards of professional performance. The major content areas of the standards follow (ANA, 2004, p. 3).

Standards of Practice (competent level of practice based on the nursing process)

1. Assessment
2. Diagnosis
3. Outcomes Identification
4. Planning
5. Implementation (coordination of care, health teaching and health promotion, consultation, and prescriptive authority)
6. Evaluation

Standards of Professional Practice (competent level of behavior in the professional role)

7. Quality of Practice
8. Education
9. Professional Practice Evaluation
10. Collegiality
11. Collaboration
12. Ethics
13. Research
14. Resource Utilization
15. Leadership

   Nursing specialty groups, and in some cases, in partnership with the ANA, have developed specialty standards, such as those for cardiovascular nursing, neonatal nursing, and nursing informatics. However, all nurses must meet the generic standards regardless of their specialty.

3. The *Code of Ethics for Nurses with Interpretive Statements* (ANA, 2001) assists the profession in controlling its practice. This code is a "list of provisions that makes explicit the primary goals, values, and obligations of the profession" (ANA, 2004, p. 47). Implementation of this code is an important part of nursing's contract with society. As nurses practice, they need to reflect these values. Chapter 6 focuses on ethical and legal issues related to nursing practice and describes the code in more detail.

4. State boards of nursing also play an important role in providing sources of professional direction. Each state board operates under a state practice act, which allows the state government to meet its responsibility to protect the public—in this case, the health of the public—through nursing licensure requirements. Regulation is discussed in more detail in Chapter 4. Each nurse must practice, or meet the description of, nursing as identified in the state in which he or she practices. Some exceptions are discussed in Chapter 4.

Nursing Associations

Nurses have a history of involvement in organizations that foster the goals of the profession. The presence of professional associations and organizations is one of the characteristics of a profession.

A professional organization is a group that has specific goals, objectives, and functions that relate to the mission of a specific profession. Typically, membership is open to members of that profession and requires payment of dues. Some organizations have more specific membership requirements or may be by invitation only. Nursing has many organizations at the local, state, national, and international levels, and some organizations function on all these levels.

PROFESSIONAL ASSOCIATION ACTIVITIES

Professional organizations often publish journals and other information related to the profession and offer continuing education opportunities through meetings, conferences, and other formats. As discussed previously, many of the organizations, particularly ANA, have been involved in developing professional standards.

Professional education is a key function of many organizations. Some organizations, through lobbying and advocacy, are very active in policy decisions at the government levels and in taking political action to ensure that the profession's goals are addressed. Some of the organizations are involved in advocacy in the work environment, with the aim of making the work environment better for nurses.

MAJOR NURSING ASSOCIATIONS

The following description highlights some of the major nursing organizations (keep in mind that many professional organizations exist). Organizations that focus on nursing specialties have expanded. Other organizations related to nursing education are described in Chapter 4. Exhibit 1–2 provides a list of some of these organizations and their Web sites.

EXHIBIT 1–2 SPECIALTY NURSING ORGANIZATIONS

Academy of Medical-Surgical Nurses, http://www.medsurgnurse.org/
Academy of Neonatal Nursing, http://www.academyonline.org/
American Academy of Ambulatory Care Nursing, http://www.aaacn.org/
American Academy of Nurse Practitioners, http://www.aanp.org/
American Academy of Nursing, http://www.aannet.org/
American Assembly for Men in Nursing, http://aamn.org/
American Association for the History of Nursing, http://www.aahn.org/
American Association of Colleges of Nursing, http://www.aacn.nche.edu/
American Association of Critical-Care Nurses, http://www.aacn.org/
American Association of Diabetes Educators, http://www.diabeteseducator.org/
American Association of Legal Nurse Consultants, http://www.aalnc.org/
American Association of Managed Care Nurses, http://www.aamcn.org/
American Association of Neuroscience Nurses, http://www.aann.org/
American Association of Nurse Anesthetists, http://www.aana.com/
American Association of Nurse Attorneys, http://www.taana.org/
American Association of Occupational Health Nurses, http://www.aaohn.org/
American Association of Spinal Cord Injury Nurses, http://www.aascin.org/
American College of Nurse-Midwives, http://www.acnm.org/
American College of Nurse Practitioners, http://www.acnpweb.org/
American Holistic Nurses' Association, http://www.ahna.org/
American Nephrology Nurses' Association, http://www.annanurse.org/

continues

EXHIBIT 1–2 (continued)

American Nurses Association, http://www.nursingworld.org/

American Nurses Foundation, http://www.nursingworld.org/anf/

American Nursing Informatics Association, http://www.ania.org/

American Organization of Nurse Executives, http://www.aone.org/

American Psychiatric Nurses Association, http://www.apna.org/

American Public Health Association – Public Health Nursing, http://www.apha.org/

American Radiological Nurses Association, http://www.arna.net/

American Society of PeriAnesthesia Nurses, http://www.aspan.org/

American Society of Plastic Surgical Nurses, http://www.aspsn.org/

Association of Camp Nurses, http://www.campnurse.org/

Association of Nurses in AIDS Care, http://www.anacnet.org/

Association of PeriOperative Registered Nurses, http://www.aorn.org/

Association of Pediatric Oncology Nurses, http://www.apon.org/

Association of Rehabilitation Nurses, http://www.rehabnurse.org/

Association of Women's Health, Obstetric and Neonatal Nurses, http://www.awhonn.org/

Commission on Graduates of Foreign Nursing Schools, http://www.cgfns.org/

Council of International Neonatal Nurses, http://www.coinnurses.org/

Developmental Disabilities Nurses Association, http://www.ddna.org/

Emergency Nurses Association, http://www.ena.org/

Home Healthcare Nurses Association, http://www.hhna.org/

Hospice and Palliative Nurses Association, http://www.hpna.org/

Infusion Nurses Society, http://www.ins1.org/

International Association of Forensic Nurses, http://www.iafn.org/

International Council of Nurses, http://www.icn.ch/

International Society for Psychiatric-Mental Health Nurses, http://www.ispn-psych.org/

International Transplant Nurses Society, http://itns.org/

National Alaska Native American Indian Nurses Association, http://www.nanainanurses.org/

National Association of Clinical Nurse Specialists, http://www.nacns.org/

National Association of Geriatric Nursing Assistants, http://www.nahcacares.org/

National Association of Hispanic Nurses, http://thehispanicnurses.org/

National Association of Neonatal Nurses, http://www.nann.org/

National Association of Orthopaedic Nurses, http://www.orthonurse.org/

National Association of Pediatric Nurse Practitioners, http://www.napnap.org/

National Association of School Nurses, http://www.nasn.org/

National Black Nurses Association, http://www.nbna.org/

National Council of State Boards of Nursing, https://www.ncsbn.org/

National Gerontological Nursing Association, http://www.ngna.org/

National League for Nursing, http://www.nln.org/

National Nursing Staff Development Organization, http://www.nnsdo.org/

National Student Nurses Association, http://www.nsna.org/

Oncology Nursing Society, http://www.ons.org/

Pediatric Endocrinology Nursing Society, http://www.pens.org/

Society of Gastroenterology Nurses and Associates, http://www.sgna.org/

Society of Pediatric Nurses, http://www.pedsnurses.org/

Society of Trauma Nurses, http://www.traumanurses.org/
Society of Urologic Nurses and Associates, http://www.suna.org/
Society for Vascular Nursing, http://www.svnnet.org/
State Nurses Associations
http://www.nursingworld.org/functionalmenucategories/aboutana/whoweare/cma.aspx
Transcultural Nursing Society, http://www.tcns.org/
Wound, Ostomy and Continence Nurses Society, http://www.wocn.org

American Nurses Association The ANA is the organization that represents all RNs in the United States, but not all RNs belong to ANA. How does it represent nurses who are not members? It does so because it is viewed by many in government and business as the voice of nursing. It represents 2.7 million RNs through its 54 constituent state and territorial associations, but the actual membership is only 150,000 (ANA, 2007). This shift in membership must be considered in light of generational issues. New nurses typically do not join organizations, and there is continual unrest regarding the perception by some nurses of ANA's lack of response to vital nursing issues. In addition to being a professional organization, the ANA is also a labor union, which is not true for most nursing professional organizations. Participation in the labor union is optional for members, and each state organization's stance on unions has an impact. ANA's major publication is *American Nurse Today*. Other goals and activities of the organization are (ANA, 2007):

- Ensuring availability of an adequate supply of highly skilled and well-trained nurses
- Advancing the profession through its standards of nursing practice, promoting the economic welfare of the profession in the workplace, and projecting a positive and realistic view of nursing
- Lobbying Congress and regulatory agencies on healthcare issues that impact nurses and consumers' health care

- Participating in health policy-making through its political and legislative program
- Participating in the expansion of the scientific and research base for nursing practice

The ANA has three affiliated organizations: the American Nurses Foundation (ANF), the American Academy of Nursing (AAN), and the American Nurses Credentialing Center (ANCC).

American Nurses Foundation The ANF is the national philanthropic organization that promotes the nursing profession. Since 1955, the ANF has awarded more than $3.5 million for more than 950 research grants (ANF, 2007).

American Academy of Nursing The AAN was established in 1973, and it serves the public and the nursing profession through its activities to advance health policy and practice (AAN, 2007). The Academy is considered the think tank for nursing. Membership is by invitation to become an Academy Fellow. Fellows may then list "FAAN" in their credentials. There are approximately 1,500 fellows. This is a very prestigious organization, and fellows have demonstrated their leadership. Examples of some of AAN's current projects are coordination of the John A Hartford Foundation's Building Academic Geriatric Nursing Capacity; Raise the Voice Campaign for Transforming America's Healthcare System; Commission on Workforce; Workforce Commission Committee on the

Preparation of the Nursing Workforce; and the Health Disparities Task Force.

American Nurses Credentialing Center   The ANCC was established by the ANA in 1973 to develop and implement a program that would provide tangible recognition of professional achievement (ANCC, 2007). Through this program, many nurses meet certification requirements and pass certification exams in specific nursing practice areas, such as pediatric nurse practitioner, adult psychiatric and mental health clinical specialist, nursing administration-advanced, gerontological nurse, informatics nurse, and many more. After receiving certification, nurses must continue to adhere to specific requirements, such as completion of continuing education. ANCC includes five major activities (ANCC, 2007):

1. Certifying healthcare providers
2. Accrediting educational providers, approvers, and programs
3. Recognizing excellence in nursing and healthcare services (Magnet Recognition Program)
4. Educating the public and collaborating with organizations to advance the understanding of credentialing services.
5. Supporting credentialing through research, education, and consultative services

National League for Nursing   The NLN is the nursing organization that focuses on excellence in nursing education. Its membership is primarily composed of schools of nursing and nurse educators. The NLN began in 1893 as the American Society of Superintendents of Training Schools. Its major publication is *Nursing Outlook*. It holds a number of educational meetings annually and provides continuing education and certification for nurse educators. The organization

has six major goals (NLN, 2007):

1. Nursing Education: Set standards for excellence and innovation.
2. Faculty Development: Promote nurse educator professional growth and improvement.
3. Research in Nursing Education: Promote evidence-based teaching practices.
4. Data Collection: Provide and interpret nursing workforce and nurse educator workforce data.
5. Assessment and Evaluation: Develop and provide comprehensive evaluation and assessment of educational outcomes and practice competencies.
6. Public Policy: Advocate for public policy related to education.

American Association of Colleges of Nursing   The AACN is the national organization for educational programs at the baccalaureate level and higher. The organization is particularly concerned with development of standards and resources and promotes innovation, research, and practice to advance nursing education (AACN, 2007). The organization represents over 600 schools of nursing at the baccalaureate and higher levels. The dean or director of a school of nursing serves as a representative to the AACN. The organization holds annual meetings for nurse educators that focus on different levels of nursing education. The AACN has most recently been involved in creating and promoting new roles and educational programs, which will be discussed in other chapters. These roles are the Clinical Nurse Leader and the Doctor of Nursing Practice. The major AACN publication is the *Journal of Professional Nursing*. The organization's three major goals are to (AACN, 2007):

1. Provide strategic leadership that advances professional nursing education, research, and practice

2. Advance academic leadership to meet the challenges of changing healthcare and higher education systems
3. Institute innovative strategies to recruit a highly qualified and diverse nursing workforce, including faculty, sufficient to meet societal needs

National Organization for Associate Degree Nursing The National Organization for Associate Degree Nursing (N-OADN) represents AD nursing itself, AD nursing programs, and individual member nurse educators. The organization focuses on enhancing the quality of AD nursing education, strengthening the professional role of the AD nurse, and protecting the future of AD nursing in the midst of healthcare changes. Its major goals are to (N-OADN, 2007):

1. Educate students and promote AD nursing programs at community colleges nationwide
2. Provide a forum for discussion of issues impacting AD education and practice
3. Develop partnerships and increase communication with other professional organizations
4. Increase public understanding of the role of the AD nurse
5. Participate at national and state levels in the formation of healthcare policy
6. Facilitate legislative action supportive of the goals of N-OADN

Sigma Theta Tau International Sigma Theta Tau International (STTI) is a not-for-profit international organization based in the United States. The nursing honor society, STTI was created in 1922 by a small group of nursing students at what is now the Indiana University School of Nursing. Its mission is to provide leadership and scholarship in practice, education, and research to improve health of all people (STTI, 2007). Membership in this organization is by invitation to baccalaureate and graduate nursing students who demonstrate excellence in scholarship and to nurse leaders who demonstrate exceptional achievements in nursing. STTI has 405,000 members, 130,000 of whom are active members, and 92 countries are represented in its membership. Chapters are formed by schools of nursing through which the work of the organization takes place. There are 451 chapters, which include schools in Australia, Botswana, Brazil, Canada, Ghana, Hong Kong, Japan, Mexico, Pakistan, Singapore, South Africa, South Korea, Swaziland, Sweden, Taiwan, Tanzania, and the United States. This is an important organization, and students should learn more about their school's chapter (if the school has one) and aspire to an invitation for induction into STTI. Inductees meet specific academic and leadership standards. The major STTI publications are the *Journal of Nursing Scholarship, Reflections on Nurs-ing Leadership*, and the newest publication, *Worldviews on Evidence-Based Nurs-ing*. The organization manages the major online library for nursing resources, the Virginia Henderson International Nursing Library, through its Web site.

International Council of Nurses The International Council of Nurses (ICN), founded in 1899, is a federation of 128 national nurses associations representing millions of nurses worldwide (ICN, 2007). This organization is the international voice of nursing and focuses on activities to better ensure quality care for all and sound health policies globally. Its three major goals are:

1. To bring nursing together worldwide
2. To advance nurses and nursing worldwide
3. To influence health policy.

ICN focuses primarily on professional nursing practice (specific health issues, International Classification of Nursing Practice), nursing regulation (regulation and credentialing, ethics, standards, continuing education), and socioeconomic welfare for nurses (occupational health and safety, salaries, migration, and other issues). The ICN headquarters is in Geneva, Switzerland. Nurses from many countries work within the organization.

National Student Nurses Association   The National Student Nurses Association (NSNA), the organization for student nurses, has a membership of 45,000 students enrolled in diploma, associate's degree, baccalaureate, and generic graduate nursing programs (NSNA, 2007). It is a national organization with chapters within schools of nursing. Its major publication is *Imprint*. It is helpful for students to get involved in the NSNA program in their schools. Joining the NSNA is a great way to get involved and to begin to develop professional skills needed for the future (such as learning more about being a leader and a follower, critical roles for practicing nurses). The NSNA Web site (http://www.nsna.org) provides an overview of the organization and its activities. Attending a national convention is a great way to find out about nursing in other areas of the country and to network with other nursing students. Annual conventions attract over 3,000 nursing students and are held at different sites each year. Through NSNA, students can also get involved in the NSNA Leadership U (http://www.nsnaleadershipu.org). Through this program, students have the opportunity to be recognized for the leadership and management skills that they develop in NSNA and to earn academic credit for this experience.

Why Belong to a Nursing Association?

Belonging to a nursing association requires money for membership and commitment to the association. Commitment involves being active, which means that it takes time. Membership and, it is hoped, active involvement can help nurses develop leadership skills, improve **networking**, and find **mentors**. Additionally, membership gives nurses a voice in professional issues and, in some cases, health policy issues, and it provides opportunities for professional socialization and development. Nurses who attend meetings, hold offices, and serve on committees or as delegates to large meetings benefit more from membership than those who do not participate. Submitting abstracts for a presentation or poster at a meeting is excellent experience for nurses and also provides additional opportunities for networking with other nurses who might also provide resources and mentoring for professional development.

Joining a professional organization and becoming active in the work of such an organization is a professional obligation. Nurses represent the single largest voting block in any state. By using this political power through nursing and other professional organizations, healthcare reform could be accomplished. Yet as nurses, we have failed to pull together. Membership in a professional organization is one way to accomplish "one strong voice."

Students can begin to meet this professional obligation by joining local student organizations and developing skills that can then be used after graduation, when they join professional organizations. What are the skills that might be learned? Students can learn about serving as a committee member and even chairing a committee. Organization communication methods can be observed, and the student can participate in the processes.

Nursing organizations give members the opportunity to participate in making decisions about nursing and health care in general. As new nurses enter the profession today, they find a healthcare system that is struggling to improve its quality and safety and keep up with medical changes; one of the key issues impacting this struggle is the nursing shortage. This is a topic that will come up again in this book. To demonstrate the critical concern about this issue, the following is an example of how professional organizations can come together and advocate for patient care.

The Americans for Nursing Shortage Relief (ANSR) Alliance represents a diverse cross-section of healthcare and professional organizations. The ANSR includes 45 nursing organizations that collectively represent nearly all the nation's 2.9 million nurses, healthcare providers, and supporters of nursing issues who have united to address the national nursing shortage. The ANSR published a consensus document with recommendations to the U.S. Congress (2007) and stated that "the U.S. continues to be challenged by a chronic nursing shortage of RNs that was first noted in 1998 and is currently showing no signs of abating." It will have a negative impact on healthcare delivery in the foreseeable future. Nursing is one of the largest healthcare professions, with an estimated 2.9 million licensed RNs in the United States (Steiger, Bausch, Johnson, & Peterson, 2006). Nurses work in a variety of settings, including public health, long-term care, and hospitals. Advanced practice nurses (nurse practitioners, nurse midwives, clinical nurse specialists, and certified registered nurse anesthetists) practice in numerous settings, including primary care, hospitals, and surgical care facilities. Approximately three out of five jobs are in hospitals (Bureau of Labor Statistics, 2007). A federal report published in 2004 estimates that by 2020, the national nurse shortage will increase to more than 1 million full-time nurse positions. According to these projections, which are based on the current rate of nurses entering the profession, only 64% of projected demand will be met (Health Resources and Services Administration, 2004). According to Auerbach, Buerhaus, and Staiger:

> *A recent study that uses different assumptions published in Health Affairs has adjusted the demand projection to 340,000 nurses by 2020. In either scenario, the short-age presents an extremely serious challenge to healthcare access and quality patient care. Even considering only the smaller projection of vacancies, this shortage still results in a frightening gap in nursing service, essentially three times the 2001 nursing shortage.* (2007, p. 185)

The recommendations in the document were evidence based and cost-effective, and pertain to four areas:

- Building capacity of nursing education programs and enhancing nursing research
- Strengthening the capacity of the nation's nursing public health infrastructure
- Helping to retain nurses, with an emphasis on the older nurse
- Expanding recruitment of new nurses, with an emphasis on diversity

In conclusion, nursing is a profession, meeting all the requirements for a profession. It did not start out being viewed as such, as the review of nursing history describes earlier in this chapter, but it has grown to be recognized as a profession with a "body of knowledge reflective of is dual components of science and art" (American Nurses Association, 2004, p. 10). O'Rourke explains that the profession of nursing "subscribes to the notion that the service orientation and ethics of its members is the basis for justifying the privilege of self-regulation," and "that the profession is responsible for developing a body of knowledge and techniques that can be applied in practice along with providing the necessary training to master such knowledge and skill" (2003, pp. 97–98). Chapter 2 explores the art and science of the profession of nursing.

Your Pursuit of a Profession: Making the Most of Your Educational Experience to Reach Graduation and Licensure

Beginning a nursing program is a serious decision. It means that the student has chosen to become a professional RN. This text introduces the nursing student to the profession and provides an orientation regarding a variety of important material that will be covered in more depth in future courses. One topic that needs to be addressed in the initial stages of a student's nursing education is how to make the most of the experience in order to reach the goal of graduation and licensure to practice as a professional RN. The following content discusses the roles of the student and faculty, tools for success, different teaching and learning approaches used in nursing education, and caring for self. This is all critical content—maybe not something a student will be tested on, but content that will provide some guidance for how to navigate through the nursing education process effectively. This will be different from other educational experiences that a student has had.

Roles of the Student and the Faculty

Nonnursing educational experiences are quite different from nursing educational experiences. Nursing education has two major components: didactic or content-focused experiences, and clinical experiences. The latter is divided into laboratory and **simulation** experiences, and experiences with patients in clinical settings. More will be discussed about this experience

later in this section. The student has a very active role in the learning process and needs to take responsibility for learning; this cannot be passive learning. Students who ask questions, read and critique, apply information even if it is risky, and are interested in working with others—not just patients and their families, but also fellow students and faculty—will be more successful. Students who wait to be told what to do and when to do it will not be as successful.

Nursing faculty facilitate student learning. This is done by developing course content and by using teaching and learning strategies to assist the student in learning the required content. Faculty develop learning situations in the **clinical laboratory** and in clinical settings by guiding students to practice and become competent in areas of care delivery. The best learning takes place when faculty and students work together and communicate about needs and expectations. Faculty members not only plan for a whole group of students but also assess learning needs of individual students and work with them to meet the course and program objectives. Becoming an RN is more than just graduating from a nursing program. New graduates must pass the NCLEX, which is not offered by the school of nursing but rather through the National Council of State Boards of Nursing. Regulation and licensure are discussed in more detail in Chapter 4. Throughout the nursing program, students may be offered opportunities to complete practice exams and receive feedback. In addition, course exam questions are typically written in the formats found in the NCLEX, such as application of knowledge questions rather than questions relating to memorized content. This is often difficult for new nursing students because they are accustomed to taking exams that focus less on application and that do not build on knowledge gained from course to course. For example, students take anatomy and physiology and are then expected to apply this information later for exams on clinical content. The student learns about blood flow through the heart, and then in adult health content, he or she is expected to understand this content and apply it to providing care to a patient with a myocardial infarction (a heart attack). Months or even a year may elapse between when the student completes the anatomy and physiology course, and when he or she takes an adult health course or cares for a patient with a myocardial infarction. Key to success with faculty is communication—ask questions, ask for explanation if confused, meet course requirements when due, and use the faculty as a resource to enhance learning.

Tools for Success

What tools does a student need for success in a nursing program? Organization and **time management** are very important. Whereas in the past, the student may have gone to class for a few hours a day, in nursing, some courses will meet once or several times a week for several hours. Some courses may be taught online, requiring some attendance in a classroom setting, or maybe none. In addition, the clinical component of the program has a major impact on a student's schedule. Students also need to prepare for clinical and work this into their schedules to meet their course requirements. Study skills and test

taking skills are critical. This educational experience will not be without some **stress**, so students who develop **stress management** skills to help them cope will find that the experience can be handled better. Box 1–3 provides some links to Web sites with tools for student success.

TIME MANAGEMENT

Time management is not difficult to define, but it is difficult to achieve. Learning how to manage time and requirements is also very important to effective nursing practice. Time management skills in school are not different from what is required for clinical practicum and after graduation in practice. Review Figure 1–1, which describes how to get started with time management.

There never is enough time, it seems, and no one can make more time, so it is best to figure out how to make the most of available time. Everyone has felt unproductive or guilty of squandering time. What is productivity? In simple terms, it is the ratio of inputs to outputs. What does the person put into a task or activity (resources such as time, energy, money, giving up doing something else, and so forth) that then leads to outcomes or results? For example, one student studies 12 hours for an exam and gives up going to a film with friends, and another student studies 5 hours and goes to the same film. These two students put different levels of resources into exam preparation, and they get

---

BOX 1–3 LINKS FOR STUDENT SUCCESS

- Overcoming Procrastination
  http://ub-counseling.buffalo.edu/stressprocrast.shtml
- Test Taking Strategies
  http://www.d.umn.edu/kmc/student/loon/acad/strat/test_take.html
- Test Taking Checklist
  http://www.d.umn.edu/kmc/student/loon/acad/strat/testcheck.html

Figure 1–1 Getting started with time management.

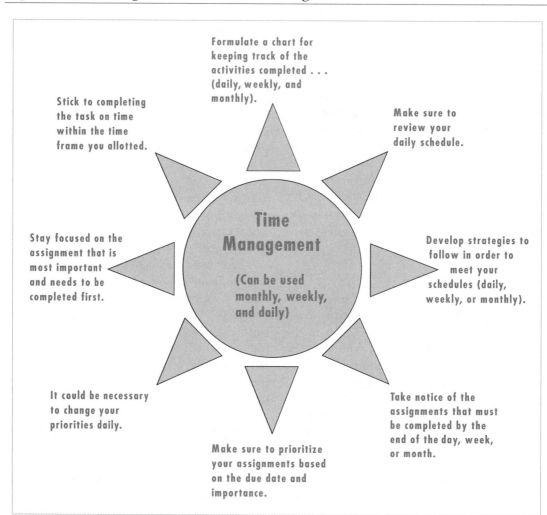

Source: From *Nursing School Success: Tools for Constructing Your Future*, by D. Wilfong, C. Szolis, and C. Haus, 2007, Sudbury, MA: Jones and Bartlett Publishers.

different results—the first student makes an A on the exam and the second a B. The second student then has to decide if it was worth it. Should more time be spent on studying for exams and the personal schedule arranged to allow for some fun, but after exams? Or is the B acceptable? This is a more global perspective of time man-

agement, but time management also gets to the details of how one uses time, to efficiency and effectiveness. How does a student understand more about his or her use of time?

Time analysis is used to assess how one uses time. The student might keep a log for a week and record all activities, including time spent on each activity and interruptions. If a student commits to doing this, he or she needs to be honest so that the data truly reflect activities. After the data are collected, the student needs to analyze them with these questions:

- What were your activities, and how long did each take?
- Do you see a difference on certain days as to activities and time?
- What did you complete, and what did you not complete? Can you identify reasons?
- Did you set any priorities, and did you adhere to them?
- What type of interruptions did you have? How many were really important and why?
- Did you procrastinate? Are there certain activities that you put off more than others? Why?
- Did you jump from one task to another?
- Look at your telephone calls, e-mails, and so on. What impact did these have on your time?
- Did you spend time getting ready to do a task, to communicate with others, and so on? Was some of this required, or could it have been done more effectively?
- Did you take breaks? (Breaks are important.) How many breaks did you take, how long were they, and what did you do?
- Did you consult your calendar?

Nurses need to be able to plan their day's work and still be flexible because changes will occur. They set priorities and follow through, evaluate how they use their time, and cut down on wasted time so that care can be delivered effectively and in a timely manner. They use communication effectively and prepare for procedures and other care delivery activities in an organized manner so that they are not running back and forth to get supplies and so on. They handle interruptions by determining what is important and what can wait. All this relates to the student's need to assess time management and learn time management skills.

Technology has made life easier and more organized in some respects, with computers, cell phones with multiple capabilities, personal digital assistants (PDAs), e-mails, text messaging, and more. However, these new resources can also interfere with time management; a person stops what he or she is doing to answer an e-mail or a text message that just arrived, or he or she may spend so much time synching all this technology that the work does not get done. Managing time today means managing personal technology, too.

There are some common problems that people have with time management. Consider these examples and how they might apply.

- No planning—not using a calendar effectively.
- Not setting goals and priorities.
- Allowing too many interruptions.
- Getting started without getting ready.
- Inability to say "no," often leading to overcommitment. (This is often the most common problem.)
- Inability to concentrate.
- Insufficient rest, sleep, exercise, and unhealthy diet making one tired.
- High stress level.
- Too much socializing when work needs to be done—not knowing how to find the right balance.
- Ineffective use of communication tools—e-mail, computer and Internet, cell phone, and so on.
- Too much crisis management—waiting too long, then it is a crisis to get the work done.
- Inability to break down large projects into small steps.

- Wasting time—little tasks, procrastination.

Other more serious problems can have a major impact on time management. These occur when the student does not feel competent or does not know what is expected. Students often experience these problems, although they may not know it or want to admit it. Both of these feelings can lead to problems with time management as students struggle to feel better and/or try to figure out what they are supposed to do. What should students do if they know they have one or both of these feelings? They need to talk to their faculty openly about their concerns. They need to also know that they are not expected to be perfect; the educational process is focused on helping them to gradually build their competence. In some cases, perfectionism actually becomes a barrier to completing a task; the student may fear that the task will not be completed perfectly, so he or she avoids the task. Benner (2001) described the experience of moving from novice to expert in nursing, a practice profession. Beginners or novices have no experience as nurses and thus must gain clinical knowledge and expertise (competence) over time. A beginning student may enter a nursing program with some nursing care experience, such as nursing aide experience. That student may then be at a different novice level but still a novice. A graduate will not be an expert; this comes with time and experience. This can be difficult for students who may have felt that they were competent in understanding the content after a course such as American History or Introduction to Sociology. Nursing competency, however, is built over time. Each course and its content are relevant to subsequent courses. There is no neat packaging that allows one to say, "I have mastered all there is to know about nursing."

Another component to time management is goal setting and priorities. This helps to organize a person's time and focus activities. Students need to consider what is needed now and what is needed later. This is not always easy to follow; sometimes a student might prefer to work on a task that is not due for a while, avoiding work that needs to be done sooner. Sometimes writing down goals and priorities and putting them where they can be seen helps to center time management. Delegation plays a major role in health care and is related to time management. One of the key issues when prioritizing is who should be doing the task. Perhaps someone else is a better choice to complete the task; in this case, the task may be delegated.

Tasks and activities can be dissected. Consider the needs of the task, when it is due, how long it will take, how critical it is or what impact it will have, and what the consequences are if it is postponed or not completed. Large projects are best broken into smaller parts or steps. For example, a major paper should be broken into steps, such as identifying the topic or problem, working with a team (if a team assignment), researching for the paper, writing the paper (which should begin with an outline), reviewing and editing, and polishing the final draft. Building in deadlines for the steps will better ensure that the final due date is met. Many large papers or projects in nursing courses cannot be completed overnight. They may require active learning, such as interviews, assessments, and other types of activities. A presentation may need to be developed after the paper is written or a poster designed. Often this type of work is done with a team of students, which is important because nurses work on teams. This takes more time because team members have to learn to work together, develop a team work plan, and meet if necessary. Some team assignments are now done virtually through online activities in which students never physically meet at the same time. Getting prepared for clinical is also a larger task that will be described later in this chapter. All this takes organization.

Some strategies for improving time management that students can consider include the following:

- Use a calendar or electronic method for a calendar; update it as needed.
- Decrease socializing at certain times to improve production.
- Limit use of cell phone, text messaging, and e-mails during specific times.
- Identify typical interruptions and control them.
- Anticipate—flexibility is necessary because something can happen that will disturb the plan.
- Determine the best time to read, study, prepare for an exam, write papers, and so on. Some people do better in early morning, others late at night. Know what works best.
- Work in blocks of time, minimizing interruptions.
- Develop methods for note taking and organizing learning materials to decrease the need to hunt for these materials.
- Conquer procrastination. Try dividing tasks into smaller parts to get a project done.
- Come prepared to class, clinical laboratory, and clinical settings. Preparation means that less time will be spent figuring out what needs to be done.
- Do the right thing right, working effectively and efficiently.
- Develop a daily time management plan (see Figure 1–2).
- Remember that time management is not a static process but a dynamic process; time management needs will change.

Figure 1–2 Daily time management worksheet.

Primary Task		Projected Start Time	Projected Finish Time	Actual Time Taken to Complete Task

Secondary Task				

Source: From *Nursing School Success: Tools for Constructing Your Future*, by D. Wilfong, C. Szolis, and C. Haus, 2007, Sudbury, MA: Jones and Bartlett Publishers.

Figure 1–2 describes a daily time management worksheet.

STUDY SKILLS

Study skills are developed over time; however, this does not mean that they cannot always be improved. This is the time to review study skills and determine what can be done to improve them.

What is included in study skills? Typical components are reading, using class time effectively, preparing written assignments and team projects, and preparing for discussions, quizzes, and exams. In nursing, clinical preparation, discussed later in this chapter, is also a key area.

Preparation: Students need to prepare for class, whether a face-to-face class, seminar, or online course. The first issue is what to prepare. The guide for this involves the focus for the experience and its objectives. The type of format also influences preparation—for example, preparing for a class session with 60 students as compared with a seminar of 10 students. The latter is the experience in which the student will undoubtedly be expected to respond to questions and discuss issues. The larger class may vary; it could be a straight lecture, with little participation expected, or it could include participation. The student needs to be clear on the expectations. The course syllabus and related documents should explain this. If they do not, the student is responsible for asking about expectations or for clarification of confusing expectations. The student then needs to complete work that is expected prior to the class or experience.

Reading: There is much reading to do in a nursing program, from textbooks and published articles to Internet resources and handout materials that faculty may provide. It is very easy to get overwhelmed. Explore the textbook(s) for the course from front to back. Sometimes students do not realize that a textbook has a valuable glossary or appendix that could help them. Review the table of contents to become familiar with the content. Some faculty may assign specific pages rather than entire chapters, so making note of the details of a reading assignment is critical. Look at a chapter to get familiar with its structure. Typically, there are objectives and key terms; content divided into sections; additional elements, such as exhibits, figures, and boxed information; and then the summary, learning activities, and references. Increasing numbers of textbooks have a Web site with additional information. Some books are now published as e-books, which are highly interactive and can be downloaded to computers and PDAs. This trend is likely to grow.

Yes, this is all overwhelming, and where does one begin? Reading focuses on four goals. (1) Learning information for recall, which is memorizing. This is important for some content, but if it is the only focus of reading, the student will not be able to apply the information and build on learning. (2) Comprehension of general principles, facts, and examples. (3) Critical evaluation of the content. Ask questions and challenge the content. Does it make sense? (4) Application of content, which is critical in nursing, a practice-oriented profession. A student may be taking a course in maternal-child content and be expected to apply that content in clinical in a pediatric unit.

How can a student develop more effective reading skills? As noted in the previous section on time management, time is precious. The student should not waste time reading ineffectively but rather should accomplish specific goals in a timely manner. What is the best way to tackle that chapter that looks so long and complex?

- Take a quick look at the chapter—objectives, terms, and major headers—and compare with course content expectations. Pay particular attention to the chapter outline, if there is one, and the summary, conclusions, and/or key points at the end of the chapter.

- Read through the chapter, not for details but to get a general idea of the content.
- Go back and use a marker to highlight key concepts, terms, and ideas. If this is done first, some students overmark. Using different colors for different levels of content may be useful for some. You will need to go back and study the content; just highlighting is not studying.
- Note exhibits, figures, and boxes. (This is when it is important to check the reading assignment. Does it specify pages, or content to read or ignore?)
- Some students make notes in the margins.

Figures 1–3 and 1–4 provide two different formats for organizing notes if they are taken. The first format can be used to take notes in class, too.

Using Class Time Effectively: Attending any class can be a positive or negative learning experience. Preparation is important. In addition, how the student approaches the class is important. If the student has trouble concentrating, sitting in the back of the room may not be the best approach. Sitting with friends can be helpful, but if it means that the student cannot concentrate, alternatives need to be considered. It is difficult to disconnect from other issues and problems, but class time is not the place to focus on them. One of the most common issues in class involves students who use class time to prepare for another class—working on assignments, studying for an exam, and so on. In the end, the learning experience on both ends is less effective. Students waste their time if they come to class without completing the reading, analyzing the content, or preparing assignments. A second element of preparation for class and other learning experiences involves bringing needed resources, such as the textbook, a notebook, assignments, and so on. In some schools, laptops may be used,

---

Figure 1–3 Taking two-column notes.

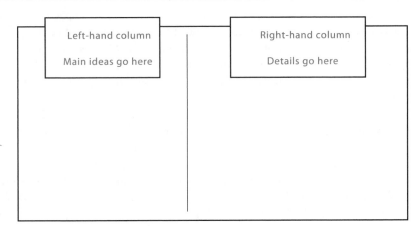

Source: From *Nursing School Success: Tools for Constructing Your Future*, by D. Wilfong, C. Szolis, and C. Haus, 2007, Sudbury, MA: Jones and Bartlett Publishers.

Figure 1–4 Unit organizer.

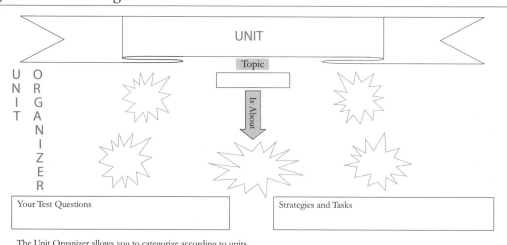

The Unit Organizer allows you to categorize according to units.
Steps to create a Unit Organizer:
1. Break down each topic in that unit.
2. Describe the content material related to each topic.
3. Formulate test questions for each topic.
4. List the strategies and tasks needed to successfully learn the material.

Source: From *Nursing School Success: Tools for Constructing Your Future*, by D. Wilfong, C. Szolis, and C. Haus, 2007, Sudbury, MA: Jones and Bartlett Publishers.

so planning for access if the battery runs out is important. Learning will be compromised if a student uses electronic equipment such as a laptop, PDA, or cell phone for purposes that do not involve course content.

If a course has face-to-face sessions, taking notes is important. Figure 1–4 provides one method for organizing notes. It is critical to find a way that works for the individual student. Some students may be more visual learners, and thus they may draw figures and charts to help them remember something. Going back and reviewing notes soon after a class session will help students to remember items that may need to be added and to recall information long term. As notes are taken in class, include comments from faculty that begin with "This is important," "You might want to remember this," and so on. Questions that faculty might ask should

be noted. It is easy to get addicted to PowerPoint slide presentations and think that if one has these in a handout, learning has taken place. This presentation content is only part of the content that nursing students are expected to learn. Students need to pay attention to content found in reading assignments, research, written assignments, and clinical experiences.

Using the Internet: The Internet has become a critical tool in the world today. Chapter 13 includes more information about technology. As students increasingly use the Internet to get information, it is important that they visit reputable Web sites. Government sites are always appropriate sources, and professional organization sites also have valuable and appropriate information. See who sponsors the site. Bias is a concern; for example, a pharmaceutical company site will praise its own products. When was the site last updated? Sites that are not updated regularly have a greater chance of including outdated information. In addition, the Internet is now used frequently for literature searches, usually through university libraries that offer online access to publications. Students need to learn about the resources available to them through their school libraries.

Preparing Written Assignments, Team Projects, and for Discussions: The critical first step for any assignment is to understand the assignment—what is expected. The student then completes the assignment based on those expectations. If the assignment describes specific areas to cover in a paper, this should be an important part of the outline for the paper—and these areas may even be used as key headers in the paper. If students have questions about the assignment, they should ask ahead of time. For some assignments, students can select the topic. If possible, selecting a topic similar to one used for a different assignment might save some time, but this does not mean that the student may repeat the assignment. Plagiarism, and submitting the same paper or assignment for more than one course, is not acceptable. The student needs to be aware of the school's honor code. Correct grammar, spelling, writing style, and citation format are critical for every written assignment. Nurses need to know how to communicate both orally and in written form.

Students will have assignments that require that they work with a team or group of students. Some students do not like doing this, but it provides a great opportunity to learn about working on teams, which is important in nursing. Teamwork requires clear communication among members and an understanding of the expectations for the work that the team needs to do. Effective teams spend time organizing their work and determining how they will communicate with one another. Conflicts may occur, and

these need to be dealt with early. Chapter 10 provides information about teams that applies to all teams, including student teams. If the team must document its work and evaluate peer members, this must be done honestly, with appropriate feedback and comments about the work. This is not easy to do. The team must decide how to do the assignment, which might involve analysis of a case, a paper, a poster, a presentation, an educational program, or another type of activity. Having a clear plan of what needs to be done, by whom, and when will help guide the work and decrease conflict. Everyone is busy, and preventing conflict and miscommunication will decrease the amount of time needed to do the work. If there are serious problems with communication or equality in workload that the team cannot resolve, faculty should be consulted for guidance.

Preparing for and Taking Quizzes and Exams: Quizzes and exams are inevitable. Students who routinely prepare for them will have less pressure at quiz or exam time. This takes discipline. Building review into study time, even if for a short period, does make a difference. As is true for any aspects of a learning experience, knowing what is expected comes first. What content will be covered in a specific quiz or exam? What types of questions are expected, and how many? The most common types of questions in nursing are multiple choice, true-false, essay, and some fill-in-the-blank and multiple-section questions, though the latter two are less common. The first quiz or exam is always the hardest, as students get to know the faculty and the style of questions. Some faculty may provide a review guide, which should be used. One aspect of nursing exams that seems to be a problem for new students is the number of application questions. Preparing for a nursing exam by just memorizing facts will not have a positive result. The student does need to know factual information, but he or she also must know how to use that information in examples. Before a major exam, getting enough rest is important. Fatigue interferes with functioning—reading, thinking, managing time during the exam, and so on. Eating also is important. Students usually know how they respond if they eat too little or too much before an exam.

A second common exam-taking problem is the inability to read the question and the possible choices. Students skip over words and think something is there that is not. They may not be able to define all the words in the question and do not identify the key words. Reading the question and the choices carefully will make a difference; students should identify the key words and define them. A student who does not know the answer to a question should narrow the choices by eliminating answers that he or she does understand or thinks might be wrong. Then, the student should look for qualifiers such as "always," "all," "never," "every," and "none" because these indicate that the answer is not correct. Figure 1–5 describes a system for preparing for multiple-choice exams.

Essay questions require different preparation and skills. Students need to have a greater in-depth understanding of the content to respond to an essay question. Some questions may ask for opinions. In all cases, it is important to be clear and concise, provide rationales, include content relevant to the question and to the material being covered in the course, and to present the response in an organized manner. Reading the question is also important; it is easy to not answer a question by providing irrelevant information. Sometimes the directions may give guidelines as to length, but in many cases, this must be judged according to what is required to answer the question. The amount of space provided on the exam may be a good indication. Grammar, spelling, and writing style are important. Jotting down a quick outline will help in focusing the writing and managing time. It is important for a student to review his or her essay response to make sure the question (or questions) has been answered. As is true for all types of exams, the student must pace the work based on the allotted time. Spending a lot of time on questions that may be difficult is unwise. The student can return to difficult questions and should keep this tactic in mind when managing time during the exam.

Study skills also include organizing. Retaining information from one course to another is important. Nursing education does not come in packages that one closes up before moving on to the next package. Learning flows from one course to another, and students need to build on their knowledge and competencies. Improvement and growth are the goals.

NETWORKING AND MENTORING

Professional nurses use networking and mentoring to develop themselves and to help peers. Students need to understand what these are and begin to work toward using networking and mentoring.

Networking is a strategy that involves using any contact that might be helpful. Using the networking strategy is a skill that takes time to develop. Going to any professional meeting offers opportunities to network. Students can begin to network in student organization activities, whether local, statewide, or national. Networking allows a person to meet and communicate with a wide variety of people, exchange ideas, explore new approaches, and obtain information that might be useful. Some of the networking skills that are important are meeting new people, approaching an admired person, learning how to start a conversation and keep it going, remembering names, asking for contact information, and sharing, because networking works both ways. Networking can take place

Figure 1–5 Multiple-choice tests.

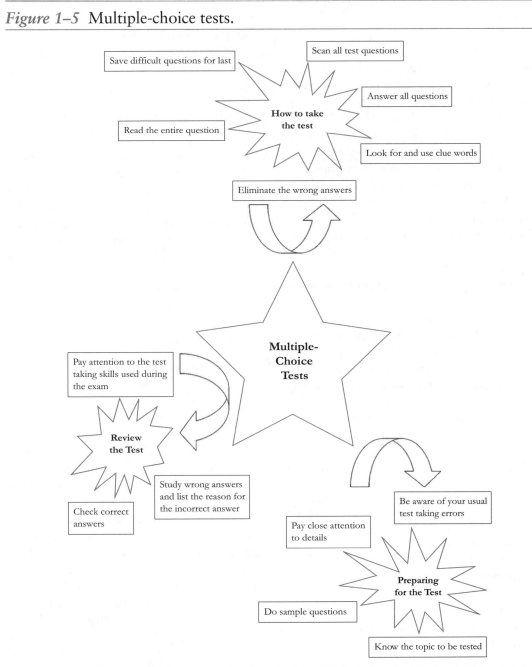

Source: From *Nursing School Success: Tools for Constructing Your Future*, by D. Wilfong, C. Szolis, and C. Haus, 2007, Sudbury, MA: Jones and Bartlett Publishers.

anywhere: in school, in a work setting, at a professional meeting or during organizational activities, and in social situations.

Mentoring is a career development tool. A mentor–mentee relationship cannot be assigned or forced. A mentor is a role model and a career advisor. The mentee has to feel comfortable with the mentor and usually chooses him or her. The mentor, of course, must agree. A mentorship can be short term or long term. It does take some time to develop the mentor–mentee relationship. Today, the relationship could actually occur virtually. Why should a student just entering a nursing education program think about a mentor? One does not know when a possible mentor might be met. Students can keep their eye out for possible mentors. The mentor may be a nurse who works in an area where the student has clinical. New graduates can benefit from a mentorship relationship to help guide them in early career decisions; a mentor can give them constructive feedback about their strengths and limitations, and suggest improvement strategies. The mentor does not make decisions for the mentee, but rather serves as a sounding board to discuss options and allow the mentee to benefit from the mentor's expertise. The mentor acts as a guide and a teacher.

What are the characteristics of an effective mentor?

- Expert in an area related to the mentee's needs and interests
- Honest and trustworthy
- Professional
- Supportive
- An effective communicator
- A teacher and motivator
- Respected and influential
- Accessible

The mentor should not have a formal relationship, such as a supervisory or managerial relationship, with the mentee. This could cause stress and not allow the mentor and mentee to communicate openly without concern about possible repercussions. There may come a time when a past supervisor becomes a mentor to a former employee.

Nursing Education: Different Teaching and Learning Approaches

As a new student begins a nursing program, it usually quickly becomes clear that it is different from past learning experiences. Competencies need to be developed to provide safe, quality care to patients, communities, and populations. Nursing education not only uses traditional didactic learning experiences, which may be offered through face-to-face classes or seminars or online, but also depends greatly on practice in the clinical laboratory using simulation and in clinical settings with patients. What does this mean to the student?

CLINICAL LABORATORY AND SIMULATION LEARNING

Schools of nursing use a variety of methods for teaching clinical competencies. A competency is an expected behavior that a student must demonstrate. Two methods that have become more common in nursing education are the clinical laboratory (lab) and simulation learning, which is often combined with the lab experience. The clinical lab is a classroom in a lab that is configured to look like a hospital. The lab may be a hospital room, a room with multiple beds, or a specialty room such as a procedure room or operating room. Some schools have areas that look like a patient's home so that students can practice care that would be provided on a home visit. The lab has the same equipment and supplies that are used in a healthcare setting. Students are assigned specific time in the lab as part of a course. There might be some didactic (content) delivered prior to the lab experience. Students are expected to come to the lab prepared (for example, having completed a reading assignment, viewed a video, or completed online learning activities). Preparation makes the lab time more effective, and students will be able to practice applying what they have learned. Students need to be motivated and self-directed learners; this is true for any learning experience in the nursing program. Schools have different guidelines about dress and behavior in the lab. In some schools, the lab is treated as if it were clinical, with dress and behavior expectations, such as wearing the school uniform or a lab coat, and meeting all other uniform requirements related to appearance and professional behavior in the clinical setting. What does the student learn in the lab? Most procedures and related competencies can be taught in a lab, such as health assessment, wound care, catheterization, medication administration, enema, general hygiene, and much more. Complex care can also be practiced in the lab setting using teams of students. Some schools are developing interdisciplinary simulation experiences that involve medical, pharmacy, and respiratory therapy students. These can be very important experiences and improve interdisciplinary teamwork.

Simulation plays a critical role in competency development. Practice is important, but guided practice is even more important, and ideally, this should be risk free. Practicing on a real patient carries risk. It is not realistic to expect that a student will be able to provide care without some degree of harm potential the first time care is given. For this reason, practicing in a setting without a real patient allows students to gain competence and self-confidence. Simulation is an attempt "to replicate some or nearly all of the essential aspects of a clinical situation so that the situation may be more readily understood and managed when it occurs for real in clinical" (Morton, 1995, p. 76). There are levels of simu-

lations, from low fidelity to high fidelity. The difference is in how close the simulated scenario comes to reality (Jeffries & Rogers, 2007). Simulation is used with nursing students at all levels. Beginning students learn basic competencies in low-fidelity scenarios in which they practice skills and provide care in "a safe environment that allows them to make mistakes, learn from those mistakes, and develop confidence in their ability to approach patients and practice in the clinical setting" (Hovancsek, 2007, p. 4). How is this done? Exhibit 1–3 describes the types of simulators and simulations that a school might use.

Simulation allows faculty to design learning experiences that meet a variety of learning styles—visual, auditory, tactile, or kinesthetic—and give students time to incorporate their learning. Time is devoted to discussing the care provided without concern for the care that needs to be provided, as would occur in a clinical setting. Students can work alone, with faculty, and with other students. Faculty can better control the types of experiences that students may need, whereas in the clinical setting, it is not always easy to find a patient who needs a specific procedure or has certain complex care needs at one time. Simulation is active learning, which helps the student improve critical thinking (Billings & Halstead, 2005). Critical thinking and clinical reasoning and judgment are discussed in more detail in Chapter 9.

CLINICAL EXPERIENCES

Clinical experiences, or practicum, are part of every nursing program. This experience occurs when students with faculty supervision provide care to patients. This care may be provided to individual patients or to their families or significant others (e.g., providing care to a patient after surgery and teaching the family how to provide care after discharge), to communities (e.g.,

EXHIBIT 1–3 TYPES OF SIMULATORS AND SIMULATIONS

Type	Definition	Example
Task Trainer	Part of a mannequin designed for a specific psychomotor skill	Ear model, central/PICC line dressing model, Leopold palpitation model
Mannequin	Passive full body mannequin with exchangeable parts (e.g., wounds)	Resusci® Anne, age-specific mannequins (baby, geriatric)
Basic Simulator	Full body simulator with installed human qualities (breath sounds, childbirth)	VitalSim™ child and infant, Nursing Anne, Noelle™ birthing simulator
Patient Simulator	Full body simulator that can be programmed to respond to affective and pyschomotor changes	SimMan®, Human Patient Simulator™
Computer Assisted Instruction (CAI)	Passive and interactive programmable software	Fetal monitoring, ABG interpretation
Virtual Reality	Complete simulated environment that includes audio, visual, tactile, hardware, electronics, and software	Virtual hospital/nursing home, IV simulator, robotics, data gloves
Standardized Patient (SP)	Individual who is trained to portray a patient or teach students using the SP as a teaching tool	Scenarios related to invasive and noninvasive physical examination, interview, patient education, and discharge planning
Web-based Simulation	Multimedia and interactive information accessed from around the world	Access via hyperlinks to virtual clinical environments in action (e.g., time lapse demonstration of the development of pressure sore)
Blended Simulation	Use of multiple types of simulation to provide a comprehensive learning experience	SP: interview, simulator: physical examination and intervention; SP: education and discharge planning

Source: "Setting Up a Simulation Laboratory, by D. Spunt, 2007, *Simulation in Nursing Education*, ed. P. Jeffries (p. 113). New York: National League for Nursing. Reprinted with permission.

working with a school nurse in a community), or to groups of the population (e.g., developing a self-management education program for a group of patients with diabetes). Some nursing programs begin this experience early in the program and others later, but all must have it. Typically, these practica are conducted in blocks of time— for example, students are in clinical two days a week for 6 hours each day. Faculty may be present the entire time or may be available at the site or by telephone. The amount of supervision depends on the level and competency of the student, the type of setting, and the objectives of the experience. The clinical setting may also dictate the student-faculty ratio and supervision. The settings are highly variable—a hospital, clinic, physician's office, school, community health service, patient home, rehabilitation center, long-term care facility, senior center, child daycare center, or mental health center, among others. In some practica, a student may work with a group of students, and in others, the student may be alone; for example, the student may be assigned to work with a school nurse.

Going to clinical requires preparation. In many experiences, the student must go to clinical before the clinical day begins (sometimes the day before) to obtain information about patient(s) and to plan the care for the assigned time. This is done so that the student is ready to provide care; he or she should understand the patient's (or patients') history and problems, laboratory work, medications, procedures, and critical care issues, and plan for care effectively. Often this is a written plan that is evaluated by the faculty. It might take the form of a nursing care plan or a concept map. These methods are discussed in Chapter 9. Students who arrive at clinical unprepared will be unable to meet the requirements for that day.

Another important aspect of clinical experiences relates to professional responsibilities and appearance. When a nursing student is providing care, the student is representing the profession. The student needs to meet the school's uniform requirement for the assigned experience, be clean, and meet safety requirements (such as appearance of hair) to decrease infection risk. Students who come to clinical not meeting these requirements may be required to go home. Making up clinical experiences is very difficult, and in some cases impossible, because it requires reserving a clinical site again and securing faculty time, student time, and so on. Minimizing absences is critical; however, if the student is sick, he or she should not care for patients. Schools have specific requirements related to illness and clinical experiences that should be fol-

lowed. The student should show up for every clinical experience dressed appropriately, prepared, and with any required equipment, such as a stethoscope. In addition, the student needs to be on time; set the alarm with plenty of preparation time, and plan for those delays in traffic. All this relates to the practicing nurse—employers expect nurses to come to work dressed as required, prepared, and on time.

Caring for Self

Caring for others is clearly the focus of nursing. The process of caring for others can be a drain on the nurse. Students quickly discover that they are very tired after a long day in clinical. Some of this is due to the number of hours and the pace, but stress also has an impact. When students graduate and practice, they find that the stress does not disappear, and in some cases, it may increase, particularly during early years of practice. Nurses often feel that they must be perfect. They may feel guilty when they cannot do everything they think they should be doing, both at work with patients and in their personal lives. There is still much to learn about nursing, working with others, pacing oneself, and figuring out the best way to mesh a career with a personal life—finding a balance and accepting that nursing is not a career of perfection. Be aware of **burnout**, which is a "syndrome manifested by emotional exhaustion, depersonalization, and reduced personal accomplishments; it commonly occurs in professions like nursing" (Garrett & McDaniel 2001, p. 92). A work-life balance is "a state where the needs and requirements of work are weighed together to create an equitable share of time that allows for work to be completed and a professional's private life to get attention" (Heckerson & Laser, 2006, p. 27).

Learning how one routinely responds to stress and developing coping skills to manage stress can make a major impact and, it is hoped, prevent burnout later. Symptoms such as headaches, abdominal complaints, anxiety, irritability, anger, isolation, and depression can indicate a high level of stress. How does stress affect the body? A review of anatomy and physiology provides some answers. When a person experiences stress, the hormones adrenaline and cortisol trigger the body to react and alert the nervous, endocrine, cardiovascular, and immune systems. This is actually helpful because it helps a person to cope with the stress, but the problem occurs when these stress responses happen frequently and over a period of months or years. Stress can be felt from a real or imagined threat, and the person feels powerless. Exposure to constant or frequent stress can lead to chronic stress, which can have an overall impact on a person's health.

The best time to begin stress management is now. Strategies for coping with stress can be found in a great variety of resources. Box 1–4 identifies some Web sites that provide general information about stress.

Using the following guide can help prevent and reduce stress.

- Set some goals to achieve a work–life balance.
- Use effective time management techniques and set priorities.
- Prepare ahead of time for assignments, quizzes, and exams.

Box 1–4 Links to Help Cope with Stress

- Understanding and Dealing with Stress
  http://www.mtstcil.org/skills/stress-intro.html
- Stress Busters
  http://stressrelease.com/www/strssbus.html
- Preventing Burnout
  http://www.coping.org/growth/burnout.htm

- Ask questions when confused and ask for help—do not view this as a sign of weakness, but rather strength.
- Take a break—a few minutes can do wonders.
- Get an appropriate amount of exercise and sleep, and eat a healthy diet. (Watch excessive use of caffeine.)
- Practice self-assertion.
- When you worry, focus on what is happening rather than what might happen.
- When you approach a problem, view it as an opportunity.
- Use humor. "We all need to laugh together at our imperfections, and finding humor in our common experiences ties us closer together. Laughter lends us mutual support and encouragement as we perform difficult jobs" (Porter-O'Grady, 1999, p. 4).
- Set aside some quiet time to just think—a short period can be productive.
- Care for self.

When students approach their first nursing job after graduation, many experience **reality shock**. This is a shock-like reaction that occurs when an individual who has been educated in a nursing education system with one view of nursing encounters a different view of nursing witnessed in the practice setting (Kramer, 1985). Students do not have to experience reality shock. One preventive measure is to develop greater stress management during the nursing education experience. This will not make the difference between a student's **clinical experience** and the real world of work disappear, but it will help the new graduate cope with this change in roles and views of what is happening in the healthcare delivery system. More and more institutions are creating externship and residency programs to guide new graduates through the first year of transition to graduate nursing status. Chapters 14 and 15 discuss these programs in more detail. Nursing, unlike medicine, pushes its "young" out of the nest without the safety net of a residency period (Goode, 2007). This year-long mentoring program is one attempt to increase retention of new nurses and assist them in gaining confidence in their skills (Goode, 2007).

Conclusion

This chapter has highlighted the history of nursing, societal trends, and other influences that shape nursing as a profession. It has presented an overview of the remainder of this book. Professional nursing includes many key aspects that will be discussed in more detail: art and science of nursing; the image of nursing; education; critical issues related to health care, such as those involving consumers; the continuum of care; the healthcare delivery system; policy, and legal and ethical concerns; the five core competencies; and current issues regarding the practice of nursing.

CHAPTER HIGHLIGHTS

1. Nursing history provides a framework for understanding how nursing is practiced today.
2. The history of nursing is complex and has been influenced by social, economic, and political factors.
3. Florence Nightingale played a major role in changing the view of nursing and education to improve care delivery.
4. A profession must meet the following characteristics:
    a. An identified systematic body of knowledge that provides the framework for the profession's practice.
    b. Standardized formal higher education.
    c. A commitment to providing a service that benefits individuals and the community.
    d. Maintenance of a unique role that recognizes autonomy, responsibility, and accountability.
    e. Control of practice responsibility of the profession through its standards and code of ethics.
    f. Commitment to members of the profession through professional organizations and activities.
5. The sources of professional direction were outlined, such as ANA documents that describe the scope of practice, accountability, and ethical code.
6. The rationale for belonging to professional organizations and their role in shaping nursing as a profession were outlined.
7. The educational experience—which included discussion of the different types of educational programs, licensure requirements, and tools for success—was described.

Linking to the Internet

- American Association for the History of Nursing
  http://www.aahn.org
- Directory of Links
  http://dmoz.org/Health/Nursing/History/
- Bates Center for the Study of Nursing History, University of Pennsylvania
  http://www.nursing.upenn.edu/history/
- Experiencing War: Women at War (Includes nurses)
  http://www.loc.gov/vets/stories/ex-war-womenatwar.html

DISCUSSION QUESTIONS

1. How might knowing more about nursing history impact your personal view of nursing?
2. How did the image of nursing in Nightingale's time impact nursing from the 1860s through the 1940s?
3. How would you compare and contrast accountability, autonomy, and responsibility?
4. Based on content in this chapter, how would you define *professionalism* in your own words?
5. Why are standards important to the nursing profession and to healthcare delivery?
6. Review the ANA standards of practice and professional performance. Are you surprised by any of the standards? If so, why?
7. How would you explain to someone who is not in health care the reason that nursing emphasizes its social policy statement?
8. What role should professional organizations play in getting nursing greater status within health care?
9. Why is stress management important to nurses?

CRITICAL THINKING ACTIVITIES

1. Describe how the Nightingale Pledge has relevance today and how it might be altered to be more relevant. Work with a team of students to accomplish this activity and arrive at a consensus statement.
2. Interview two nurses and ask them if they think nursing is a profession, and the rationale for their viewpoint. How does what they say compare with what you have learned about professionalism in this chapter?
3. Write your own definition of nursing. Work on this definition throughout this course as you learn more about nursing. Save the final draft, and at the end of each semester or quarter, go back to your definition and make any changes you feel are necessary. Keep a draft of each definition so that you can see your changes. When you graduate, review all your definitions; see how you have developed your view of professional nursing. Ideally, you would then review your definition again 1 year postgraduation.
4. Develop a study plan for yourself that incorporates information about tools for success. Include an assessment of how you use your time.
5. Attend a National Student Nurses Association meeting at your school. What did you learn about the organization? What did you observe in the meeting about leadership and nursing? Do you have any criticisms of the organization, and how might it be improved?
6. Review the Words of Wisdom from a new graduate found in this chapter. What thoughts do you have about her comments? How might you use her advice?

CASE STUDY

Bowers, Lauring, and Jacobson (2001) conducted a study to better understand how nurses manage their time in long-term care settings. Data indicated that the nurses attempted to create new time when time was short. As students, you will be confronted with issues of time when you begin your clinical experience, and then throughout your career as a nurse. Consider the following information from this study as listed in Table 1–2 below.

Case Questions

1. Consider your own schedule for a week. How would these strategies apply to your own personal methods for handling your time? What impact do they have on your time management, both positive and negative?
2. Keep this list, and when you begin your clinical experience, consider whether you are using these strategies to "create more time." Can time really be created?

Sources:
Bowers, B., Lauring, C., & Jacobson, N. (2001). How nurses manage time and work in long-term care. Journal of Advanced Nursing, 33(4), 484–491.

Table 1–2

Strategy	Description
Longevity	Increasing the pace of work has consequences, such as less time to really talk to patients. This also results in an increased focus on technical or visible and urgent tasks and less focus on surveillance and follow-up. For nurses, this means increased frustration and lower morale.
Working Faster	Combining or bundling tasks is done to complete work more quickly and to reduce interruptions. This can lead to errors when tasks are bundled together that may not fit well, and the nurse cannot focus.
Changing Sequence of Tasks	The order of some tasks may be changed in an attempt to create more time. One will fall behind by doing something just in case there is an interruption later.
Communicating Inaccessibility	Minimizing some activities or eliminating them altogether to get more time typically relates to communication with patients and families. The message is, "I don't have time for this." Avoid those activities that nurses have control over and are viewed as ineffective communication.
Converting Wasted Time	Find ways to use wasted time or down time; this can be helpful if done right—for example, doing a quick assessment of a patient while waiting for him or her to take oral medications.
Negotiating "Actual Time"	Nurses tried to maximize their "actual work time" by coming in early, skipping lunch and breaks, and so on.

Source: How nurses manage time and work in long-term care, by Bowers, B., Lauring, C., & Jacobson, N., (2001), *Journal of Advanced Nursing, 33*(4), 484–491.

WORDS OF WISDOM

Jamie White, MSN, RN
Staff Nurse, Neonatal Intensive Care Unit,
The University of Oklahoma Medical
Center, Oklahoma City, Oklahoma

What would have made the transition to your first nursing job easier?

Transition to my job was very easy. What made it this way was working in the unit for a year and a half as a nurse partner and clerk. If you already know the basics of the unit, then transition is much easier.

What things were included in your education that were most helpful? Least helpful?

The most helpful educational tool was the group work. Nursing is all about being a member of a team and relying on others to help you perform your job more efficiently. The other helpful experience was how nursing school changes your mindset of school and work. Nursing is ever-changing and so is nursing school. I remember being stressed out my first semester due to the ever-changing environment and no clear line. Now, I understand why it's that way because nursing is that way. I cannot tell you the least helpful, only because everything I thought at the time had no purpose I found the purpose when I entered the field.

What advice would you give entering students?

My advice would be to come into nursing if you truly want to touch people's lives. Nursing is full of frustrations and politics, but if you are in it for the love of people, then you will do fine. The best feeling I get is to hand a family their sick infant for the first time and to see the hope, fear, and love that is expressed.

References

American Academy of Nursing. (2007). Retrieved April 17, 2007, from http://www.aannet.org

American Association of Colleges of Nursing. (2004, September 20). *AACN endorses the Sullivan Commission Report on increasing diversity in the health professions* (Press Release). Washington, DC: Author.

American Association of Colleges of Nursing. (2007). Retrieved May 15, 2007, from http://www.aacn.nche.edu

American Nurses Association. (2001). *Code of ethics for nuses with interpretive statements*. Silver Spring, MD: Nursesbooks.org.

American Nurses Association. (2003). *Nursing's social policy statement*. Silver Spring, MD: Author.

American Nurses Association. (2004). *Nursing: Scope and standards of practice*. Silver Spring, MD: Author.

American Nurses Association. (2007). Retrieved May 15, 2007, from http://www.nursingworld.org

American Nurses Credentialing Center. (2007). Retrieved April 17, 2007, from http://www.nursecredentialing.org

American Nurses Foundation. (2007). Retrieved May 15, 2007, from http://www.nursingworld.org/anf/

Americans for Nursing Shortage Relief. (2007). *Alliance Assuring Quality Healthcare for the United States: Building and Sustaining an Infrastructure of Qualified Nurses for the Nation Consensus Document*. New York: National League for Nursing.

Ashley, J. (1976). *Hospitals, paternalism, and the role of the nurse*. New York: Teachers College Press.

Auerbach, D. I., Buerhaus, P. I., & Staiger, D. O. (2007). Better late than never: Workforce supply implications of later entry into nursing. *Health Affairs, 26,* 178–185.

Benner, P. (2001). *From novice to expert* (Commemorative Edition). Upper Saddle River, NJ: Prentice Hall Health.

Billings, D., & Halstead, J. (2005). *Teaching in nursing: A guide for faculty* (2nd ed.). Philadelphia: W.B. Saunders.

Bixler, G., & Bixler, R. (1959). The professional status of nursing. *American Journal of Nursing, 59,* 1142–1147.

Boughn, S. (2001). Why women and men choose nursing. *Nursing and Healthcare Perspectives, 22,* 14–19.

Bowers, B., Lauring, C., & Jacobson, N. (2001). How nurses manage time and work in long-term care. *Journal of Advanced Nursing, 33,* 484–491.

Brooks J. A., & Kleine-Kracht, A. E. (1983). Evolution of a definition of nursing. *Advances in Nursing Science, 5*(4), 51–63.

Bullough, V. (2006). Nursing at the crossroads: Men in nursing. In P. Cowen & S. Moorhead (Eds.), *Current issues in nursing* (7th ed., pp. 559–568). St. Louis, MO: Mosby.

Bullough, V., & Bullough, B. (1978). *The care of the sick: The emergence of modern nursing*. New York: Prodist.

Bureau of Labor Statistics, U.S. Department of Labor. (2007). Registered nurses. In *Occupational outlook handbook, 2006-2007 edition*. Retrieved January 15, 2007, from http://www.bls.gov/oco/ocos083.htm

Chinn, P. (2001). Feminism and nursing. In J. Dochterman & H. Grace (Eds.). *Current issues in nursing* (6th ed., pp. 441–447). St. Louis, MO: Mosby.

Cleary, B. (2007, July). Report given at the American Academy of Nursing Workforce Commission Committee on Preparation of the Nursing Workforce, Chicago, IL.

Connolly, C. (2004). Beyond social history: New approaches to understanding the state and the state in nursing history. *Nursing History Review, 12*, 5–24.

Dietz, D., & Lehozky, A. (1963). *History and modern nursing*. Philadelphia: F. A. Davis.

Donahue, M. (1985). *Nursing: The finest art*. St. Louis, MO: Mosby.

Finkelman, A. (2006). *Leadership and management in nursing*. Upper Saddle River, NJ: Pearson Education.

Freeman, L. (2007). Commentary. *Nursing History Review, 15*, 167–168.

Garrett, D., & McDaniel, A. (2001). A new look at nurse burnout. *Journal of Nursing Administration, 31*, 91–96.

Goode, C. (2007, July). Report given at the American Academy of Nursing Workforce Commission Committee on Preparation of the Nursing Workforce, Chicago, IL.

Gordon, S. (2005). *Nursing against the odds*. Ithaca, NY: Cornell University Press.

Gorenberg B. (1983). The research tradition of nursing: An emerging issue. *Nursing Research, 32*, 347–349.

Health Resources and Services Administration. (2004) *What is behind HRSA's projected supply, demand, and shortage of registered nurses?* Retrieved February 26, 2007, from http://bhpr.hrsa.gov/healthworkforce/reports/behindrnprojections/4.htm

Heckerson, E., & Laser, C. (2006). Just breathe! The critical importance of maintaining a work-life balance. *Nurse Leader, 4*(12), 26–28.

Hovancsek, M. (2007). Using simulation in nursing education. In P. Jeffries (Ed.), *Simulation in nursing education* (pp. 1–9). New York: National League for Nursing.

Huber, D. (Ed.). (2000). *Leadership and nursing care management*. Philadelphia: W. B. Saunders.

International Council of Nurses. (2007). Retrieved May 15, 2007, from http://www.icn.ch/

Jacobs, M. K., & Huether, S. E. (1978). Nursing science: The theory practice linkage. *Advances in Nursing Science, 1*, 63–78.

Jeffries, P., & Rogers, K. (2007). Evaluating simulations. In P. Jeffries (Ed.), *Simulation in nursing education* (pp. 87–103). New York: National League for Nursing.

Kalisch, P., & Kalisch, B. (1986). *The advance of American nursing* (2nd ed.). Boston: Little, Brown.

Kaufman, M. (Ed.). (1988). *Dictionary of American nursing biography*. Westport, CT: Greenwood Press.

Keller, M. C. (1979). The effect of sexual stereotyping on the development of nursing theory. *American Journal of Nursing, 79*, 1584–1586.

Kidd, P., & Morrison, E. (1988). The progression of knowledge in nursing: A search for meaning. *Image, 20*, 222–224.

Kramer, M. (1985). Why does reality shock continue. In J. McCloskey & H. Grace (Eds.), *Current issues in nursing* (pp. 891–903). Boston: Blackwell Scientific.

Kramer, M., & Schmalenberg, C. (2002). Staff nurses identify essentials of magnetism. In M. McClure & A. Hinshaw (Eds.), *Magnet hospitals revisited* (pp. 25–59). Washington, DC: American Nurses Association.

Kupperschmidt, B. (2004). Making a case for shared accountability. *Journal of Nursing Administration, 34*, 114–116.

Lindberg, B., Hunter, M., & Kruszewski, K. (1998). *Introduction to nursing* (3rd ed.). Philadelphia: Lippincott.

Lynaugh J. E., & Fagin, C. M. (1988). Nursing comes of age. *Image, 20*, 184–190.

Masters, K. (2005). *Role development in professional nursing practice*. Sudbury, MA: Jones and Bartlett.

Morton, P. (1995). Creating a laboratory that simulates the critical care environment. *Critical Care Nursing, 16*(6), 76–81.

National Association for Associate Degree Nursing. (2007). Retrieved May 15, 2007, from http://www.noadn.org/all.php?l=certification&x=0

National League for Nursing. (2007). Retrieved May 15, 2007, from http://www.nln.org

National Student Nurses Association. (2007). Retrieved April 17, 2007, from http://www.nsna.org

Nightingale, F. (1992). *Notes on nursing: What it is, and what it is not* (Commemorative Edition). Philadelphia: Lippincott Williams & Wilkins. (Original work published 1860).

Nightingale, F. (1858). *Notes on matters affecting the health, efficiency, and hospital administration of the British army*. Harrison and Sons.

Nightingale, F. (1858). *Subsidiary notes as to the introduction of female nursing into military hospitals*. London: Longman, Green, Longman, Roberts, and Green.

Nightingale, F. (1859). *Notes on hospitals*. Harrison and Sons.

O'Rourke, M. (2003). Rebuilding a professional practice model. The return of role-based practice accountability. *Nursing Administrative Quarterly, 27*, 95–105.

Perry J. (1985). Has the discipline of nursing developed to the stage where nurses do "think nursing"? *Journal of Advanced Nursing, 10*, 31–37.

Porter-O'Grady, T. (1999). Laughter lightens our load. *Nursing Management, 39*(9), 4.

Quinn, C., & Smith, M. (1987). *The professional commitment: Issues and ethics in nursing.* Philadelphia: W. B. Saunders.

Ritter-Teitel, J. (2002). The impact of restructuring on professional nursing practice. *Journal of Nursing Administration, 32*, 31–41.

Rosen, G. (1958). *A history of public health.* New York: M.D. Publications.

Schein, E., & Kommers, D. (1972). *Professional education.* New York: McGraw-Hill.

Seymer, L. (Ed.). (1954). *Selected writings on Florence Nightingale.* New York: Macmillan.

Shames, K. H. (1993). *The nightingale conspiracy: Nursing comes to power in the 21st century.* Montclair, NJ: Enlightenment Press.

Shaw, M. (1993). The discipline of nursing: Historical roots, current perspectives, future directions. *Journal of Advanced Nursing, 18*, 1651–1656.

Sigma Theta Tau International. (2007). Retrieved May 15, 2007, from http://www.nursingsociety.org

Slater, V. (1994). The educational and philosophical influences on Florence Nightingale, an enlightened conductor. *Nursing History Review, 2*, 137–151.

Sochalski, J. (2002). Nursing shortage redux: Turning the corner on an enduring problem. *Health Affairs, 21*, 157–164.

Steiger, D. M., Bausch, S., Johnson, B., & Peterson, A. (2006). *The registered nurse population: Findings from the March 2004 National Sample Survey of Registered Nurses.* Health Resources and Services Administration, U.S. Department of Health and Human Services. Retrieved April 17, 2007, from http://bhpr.hrsa.gov/healthworkforce/rnsurvey04/

Sullivan, E. (2002). In a woman's world. *Reflections on Nursing Leadership, 28*(3), 10–17.

Sullivan, L., & the Sullivan Commission. (2004). *Missing persons: Minorities in the health professions.* Battle Creek, MI: W. K. Kellogg Foundation.

Wall, B. (2003). Science and ritual: The hospital as medical and sacred space, 1865–1920. *Nursing History Review, 11*, 51–68.

Widerquist, J. (1997). Sanitary reform and nursing. *Nursing History Review, 5*, 149–159.

Woodham-Smith, C. (1951). *Florence Nightingale: 1820-1910.* New York: McGraw-Hill.

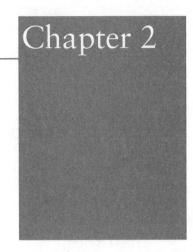

Chapter 2

The Essence of Nursing: Knowledge and Caring

CHAPTER OUTLINE

KEY TERMS

- Advocate
- Caring
- Change agent
- Collaboration
- Competency
- Counselor
- Critical thinking
- Educator
- Entrepreneur
- Identity
- Intuition
- Intrapreneur
- Knowledge
- Knowledge worker

- Knowledge management
- Leadership
- Manager
- National Institute of Nursing Research
- Provider of care
- Reality shock
- Reflective thinking
- Research
- Researcher
- Role
- Role transition
- Scholarship
- Status
- Theory

Introduction

In 2007, Dr. Pamela Cipriano, editor-in-chief of *American Nurse Today*, wrote an editorial in honor of Nurses Week entitled, "Celebrating the Art and Science of Nursing." This is the topic of this chapter, though the title is "The Essence of Nursing: Knowledge and Caring." **Knowledge** represents the science of nursing, and **caring** represents the art of nursing. Along with this editorial and the theme of Nurses Week 2007, described in Box 2–1 (both of which are directly related to this chapter), is the 2006 publication by Nelson and Gordon, *The Complexities of Care: Nursing Reconsidered*. Nelson and Gordon stated, "Because we take caring seriously we (the authors) are con-

Box 2–1 National Nurses Week 2007 Theme Is Nursing: A Profession and a Passion

Often described as an art and a science, nursing is a profession that embraces dedicated people with varied interests, strengths and passions because of the many opportunities the profession offers. As nurses, we work in emergency rooms, school based clinics, and homeless shelters, to name a few. We have many roles—from staff nurse to educator to nurse practitioner and nurse researcher—and serve all of them with passion for the profession and with a strong commitment to patient safety.

Source: "The American Nurses Association Underscores Importance of Nursing Profession During National Nurses Week," by the American Nurses Association, February, 22, 2007. (Press Release)

cerned that discussions of nursing care tend to sentimentalize and decomplexify the skill and knowledge involved in nurses' interpersonal or relational work with patients" (p. 3). An example of a statement about Nurses Week appears in Box 2–1.

The authors make a strong case about the concern that nurses themselves devalue the care they provide, particularly regarding the knowledge component of nursing care and technical competencies needed to meet patient care needs and focus on the caring. This chapter explores the knowledge and caring of nursing practice. Both must be present, and both are important for safe, quality nursing care. Content includes the effort to define nursing, knowledge and caring, **competency, scholarship** in nursing, the major nursing **roles**, and **leadership**.

Nursing: How Do We Define It?

Definitions of nursing were briefly discussed in Chapter 1, but defining nursing is relevant to this chapter and requires further exploration. Can nursing be defined, and if so, why is it important to define it? Before this discussion begins, the student should review his or her personal definition of nursing that was written as part of Critical Thinking Activities in Chapter 1. Students may find it strange to spend time on

the question of a definition of nursing, but the truth is, there is no universally accepted definition. The easy first approach to developing a definition is to describe what nurses do; however, this approach leaves out important aspects and essentially reduces nursing to tasks. More consideration needs to be given to (1) what drives nurses to do what they do, (2) why they do what they do (rationales, evidence-based practice [EBP]), and (3) what is achieved by what they do (outcomes; Diers, 2001). Diers noted that even Florence Nightingale's and Virginia Henderson's definitions, as described in Chapter 1, are not definitions of what nursing is, but more what nurses do. Henderson's definition is more of a personal concept than a true definition. Henderson even said that what she wrote was not the complete definition of nursing (Henderson, 1991). Diers also commented that there really are no full definitions for most disciplines. So why is nursing so concerned with a definition? Having a definition serves several purposes that really drive what that definition will look like (Diers). These purposes are:

- Providing an operational definition to guide **research**
- Acknowledging that changing laws requires a definition that will be politically

accepted—for example, in relationship to a nurse practice act

- Convincing legislators about the value of nursing—for example, to gain funds for nursing education
- Explaining what nursing is to consumers/patients (though no definition is totally helpful because patients/consumers will respond to a description of the work, not a definition)
- Explaining to others in general what one does as a nurse (then the best choice is a personal description of what nursing is)

One could also say that a definition is helpful in determining what to include in a nursing curriculum, but nursing has been taught for years without a universally accepted definition. The American Nurses Association (ANA, 2004) defines nursing as "the protection, promotion, and optimization of health and abilities, prevention of illness and injury, alleviation of suffering through the diagnosis and treatment of human response, and advocacy in the care of individuals, families, communities, and populations" (p. 7). What do some of the critical terms in this definition mean?

- *Promotion of health*: Development of attitudes and behaviors that help a person maintain or improve well-being, for example, learning about nutrition and changing diet. (Protection and optimization relate to this.)
- *Health*: "An experience that is often expressed in terms of wellness and illness, and may occur in the presence or absence of injury" (ANA, 2004, p. 48).
- *Prevention of illness and injury*: Interventions taken to keep illness or injury from occurring, for example, immunization for tetanus or teaching parents how to use a car seat.

- *Illness*: "The subjective experience of discomfort" (ANA, 2004, p. 48).
- *Injury*: Harm to the body, for example, a broken arm due to a fall from a bicycle.
- *Diagnosis*: "A clinical judgment about the patient's response to actual or potential health conditions or needs" (ANA, 2004, p. 47).
- *Human response*: "Nursing diagnoses are often called *human responses* because we, as nurses, focus on how people respond to changes in health or life circumstances—for example, how they are responding to illness or becoming a parent" (Alfaro-LeFevre, 2006, p. 106).
- *Treatment*: To give care through interventions—for example, administering medication, teaching a patient how to give himself or herself insulin, wound care, preparing a patient for surgery, ensuring that the patient is not at risk for an infection, and so on.
- *Advocacy*: The act of pleading for or supporting a course of action on behalf of individuals, families, communities, and populations—for example, a nurse who works with the city council to improve health access for a community.

Six essential features of professional nursing have been identified from definitions of nursing (ANA, 2003, p. 5):

- Provision of a **caring relationship** that **facilitates** health and healing
- Attention to the **range of human experiences and responses** to health and illness within the physical and social environments
- **Integration of objective data with knowledge** gained from an appreciation of the patient's or group's **subjective experience**

- Application of scientific knowledge to the processes of diagnosis and treatment through the **use of judgment and critical thinking**
- **Advancement of professional nursing knowledge** through **scholarly inquiry**
- **Influence on social and public policy** to promote social justice

In this list, terms that indicate the importance of knowledge and caring to nursing are in bold. Knowledge and caring are the critical dyad in any description or definition of nursing, and they both relate to nursing scholarship and leadership.

The North American Nursing Diagnosis Association (2003); describing nursing interventions, the Nursing Interventions Classification (McCloskey & Bulechek, 2002), and the Nursing Outcomes Classification all reflect attempts to define the work of nursing (Moorehead, Johnson, & Maas, 2007). These initiatives are led by the Iowa Intervention Project and are discussed in more detail in Chapter 9. Maas (2006) discussed the importance of these initiatives, which she described as the building blocks of nursing practice theory, and noted that "rather than debating the issues of definition, nursing will be better served by focusing those energies on its science and the translation of the science of nursing practice" (p. 8). The conclusion is that (1) no universally accepted definition of nursing exists, though several definitions have been developed by nursing leaders and nursing organizations; (2) individual nurses may develop their own personal description of nursing to use in practice; and (3) a more effective focus is the pursuit of nursing knowledge to build nursing scholarship. The first step is to gain a better understanding of knowledge and caring in relationship to nursing practice.

Knowledge and Caring: A Total Concept

Understanding how knowledge and caring form the critical dyad for nursing is essential to providing effective, safe, quality care. Knowledge is specific information about something, and caring is behavior that demonstrates compassion and respect for another. But these are very simple definitions. The depth of nursing practice goes beyond basic knowledge and the ability to care. Nursing encompasses a distinct body of knowledge coupled with the art of caring. As stated in Butcher, "A unique body of knowledge is a foundation for attaining the respect, recognition, and power granted by society to a fully developed profession and scientific discipline" (2006, p. 116). Critical thinking is used by nurses as they apply knowledge, evidence, and caring to the nursing process and become competent. Critical thinking is discussed more in Chapter 9. Experts like Dr. Patricia Benner who led the Carnegie Foundation Study (Benner, 2007) suggest that we often use the term *critical thinking*, but there is high variability and little consensus on what constitutes critical thinking. Clinical reasoning and judgment are very important and include critical thinking. Few of our educational activities really promote this type of reasoning.

Knowledge

Knowledge can be defined and described in a number of ways. There are five ways of knowing (Carper, 1978; Cipriano, 2007) that are useful in understanding how one "knows" something. A nurse might use all or some of these ways of "knowing" when providing care.

1. *Empirical knowing* focuses on facts and is related to quantitative explanations—predicting and explaining.

2. *Ethical knowing* focuses on a person's moral values—what should be done.
3. *Personal knowing* focuses on understanding and actualizing a relationship between a nurse and a patient, including knowledge of self (nurse).
4. *Aesthetic knowing* focuses on the nurse's perception of the patient and the patient's needs, emphasizing the uniqueness of each relationship and interaction.
5. *Synthesizing,* or pulling together the knowledge gained from the four types of knowing, allows the nurse to understand the patient better and to provide higher quality care.

The ANA (2003) identified the key issues related to the knowledge base for nursing practice, both theoretical and evidence-based knowledge. This is the basic knowledge that every nurse should have to practice. Nurses use this knowledge base in collaboration with patients to assess, plan, implement, and evaluate care.

- Promotion of health and safety
- Care and self-care processes
- Physical, emotional, and spiritual comfort, discomfort, and pain
- Adaptation to physiologic and pathophysiologic processes
- Emotions related to experiences of birth, growth and development, health, illness, disease, and death
- Meanings ascribed to health and illness
- Decision making and the ability to make choices
- Relationships, role performance, and change processes within relationships
- Social policies and their effects on the health of individuals, families, and communities
- Healthcare systems and their relationships with access to, and quality of, health care
- The environment and the prevention of disease

KNOWLEDGE MANAGEMENT

Knowledge work plays a critical role in healthcare delivery today, and nurses are **knowledge workers**. Forty percent or more of workers in knowledge-intense businesses, such as a healthcare organization, are knowledge workers (Sorrells-Jones, 1999). **Knowledge management** includes both *routine work* (such as taking vital signs, administering medications, and walking a patient) and *nonroutine work*, which (1) involves exceptions, (2) requires judgment and use of knowledge, and (3) may be confusing or not fully understood. In a knowledge-based environment, a person's title is not as important as the person's expertise, and use of knowledge and learning take center stage. Knowledge workers actively use

- Collaboration
- Teamwork
- Coordination
- Analysis
- Critical thinking
- Evaluation
- Willingness to be flexible

Knowledge workers recognize that change is inevitable and that the best approach is to be ready for change and look at it as an opportunity for learning and improvement. Nurses use knowledge daily in their work—both routine and nonroutine—and must have the characteristics of the knowledge worker. They work in an environment that expects healthcare providers to use the best evidence in providing care. "Transitioning to an evidence-based practice requires a different perspective from the traditional role of nurse as 'doer' of treatments and procedures based on institutional policy or personal preference. Rather, the nurse practices as a 'knowledge worker' from an updated and ever-changing knowledge base" (Mooney, 2001, p. 17). The knowledge worker focuses on acquiring, analyzing, synthesizing, and applying evidence to guide practice decisions (Dickenson-Hazard,

2002). The knowledge worker uses synthesis, competencies, multiple "intelligences," mobile skill set, outcome practice, and teamwork, as opposed to the old skills of functional analysis, manual dexterity, fixed skill set, process value, process practice, and unilateral performance (Porter-O'Grady & Malloch, 2007). This nurse is a clinical scholar. This nurse is valued by the employer and patients for what he or she knows and how this knowledge is used to meet patient care outcomes—not just for technical expertise or caring, though these are also important (Kerfoot, 2002). This change in a nurse's work also is reflected in the Carnegie Foundation Report, as reported by Patricia Benner (2007). Benner suggested that instead of focusing on content, nurse educators need to focus on teaching the skills of how to access information, use and manipulate data (such as those data available from patient information systems), and document in the electronic interdisciplinary format.

CRITICAL THINKING, REFLECTIVE THINKING, AND INTUITION: IMPACT ON KNOWLEDGE DEVELOPMENT AND APPLICATION

Critical thinking, **reflective thinking**, and **intuition** are different approaches to thinking and can be used together. Nurses use all of them to explore, understand, develop new knowledge, and apply knowledge. What do they mean, and how are they used in nursing?

Critical Thinking Critical thinking is clearly a focus of nursing. Even the ANA standards state that the nursing process is a critical thinking tool, though not the only one used in nursing (ANA, 2004). This skill uses "purposeful, informed, outcome-focused (results-oriented) thinking that requires careful identification of key problems, issues, and risks involved" (Alfaro-LeFevre, 2006, p. 30). Alfaro-LeFevre identified four key critical thinking components of critical thinking.

1. Critical thinking characteristics (attitudes/behaviors)
2. Theoretical and experiential knowledge (intellectual skills/competencies)
3. Interpersonal skills/competencies
4. Technical skills/competencies

In reviewing each of these components, one can easily see the presence of knowledge, caring (interpersonal relationships, attitudes), and technical expertise.

A person uses four key intellectual traits in critical thinking (Paul, 1995). Each of the traits can be learned and developed.

1. Intellectual humility: Willingness to admit what one does not know. (This is difficult to do, but it can save lives. A nurse who cannot admit that he or she does not know something and yet proceeds is taking a great risk. It is important for students to be able to use intellectual humility as they learn about nursing.)
2. Intellectual integrity: Continual evaluation of one's own thinking and willingness to admit when thinking is not adequate. (This type of honesty with self and others can make a critical difference in care.)
3. Intellectual courage: Ability to face and fairly address ideas, beliefs, and viewpoints for which one may have negative feelings. (Students enter into a new world of health care and do experience confusing thoughts about ideas, beliefs, and viewpoints, and sometimes their personal views may need to be put aside in the interest of the patient and safe, quality care.)
4. Intellectual empathy: Conscious effort to understand others by putting one's own feelings aside and imagining oneself in another person's place.

Critical thinking skills that are important to develop are affective learning; applied moral reasoning and values (relates to ethics); comprehension; application, analysis, and synthesis; interpretation; knowledge, experience, judgment, and evaluation; learning from mistakes when they happen; and self-awareness (Finkelman, 2001). This type of thinking helps to reduce dichotomous thinking and groupthink. Dichotomous thinking leads one to look at an issue, situation, or problem as "one way or the other," such as good or bad, black or white. This limits choices. Groupthink occurs when all group or team members think alike. One might say that this is great, because they are all working together. However, groupthink limits choices, open discussion of possibilities, and the ability to consider alternatives. Problem solving is not critical thinking, but effective problem solvers use critical thinking. A combination of the two results in the following process (Finkelman, 2001, p. 196):

1. Seek the best information and data possible to allow you to fully understand the issue, situation, or problem. Questioning is critical. Examples of some questions that might be asked are: What is the significance of _____? What is your first impression? What is the relationship between _____ and _____? What impact might _____ have on _____? What can you infer from the information/data?
2. Identify and describe any problems that require analysis and synthesis of information—thoroughly understand the information/data.
3. Develop alternative solutions—more than two is better because this forces you to analyze multiple solutions even when you discard one of them. Be innovative and move away from only proposing typical or routine solutions.

4. Evaluate the alternative solutions and consider the consequences for each one. Can the solutions really be used? Do you have the resources you need? How much time will it take? How well will the solution be accepted? Identify pros and cons.
5. Make a decision, choosing the best solution, though there is risk in any decision making.
6. Implement the solution but continue to question.
7. Follow up and evaluate; plan for evaluation from the very beginning.

Self-assessment of critical thinking skills is an important part of using critical thinking. How does one use critical thinking, and is it done effectively?

Reflective Thinking   Throughout one's nursing education experience and practice, reflective thinking needs to become a part of daily learning and practice. Conway (1998) noted that nurses who used reflective thinking implemented care based on the individualized care needs of the patient, whereas nurses who used reflective thinking less tended to provide illness-oriented care. Reflection is seen as a part of the art of nursing, which requires "creativity and conscious self-evaluation over a period of time" (Decker, 2007, p. 76). Reflection helps nurses cope with unique situations. This type of thinking uses Carper's (1978) ways of knowing discussed earlier in this chapter. Using these four ways of knowing, the following questions might be asked (Johns, 2004, p. 18):

- *Empirical*: "What knowledge informed or might have informed you?"
- *Aesthetic*: "What particular issues seem significant to pay attention to?"
- *Personal*: "What factors influenced the way you felt, thought, or responded?"

- *Ethical*: "To what extent did you act for the best and in tune with your values?"; which leads to
- *Reflection*: "How might you respond more effectively given this situation *again?*"

The skills needed for reflective thinking are the same skills required for critical thinking: the ability to monitor, analyze, predict, and evaluate (Pesut & Herman, 1999), and to take risks, be open, and have imagination (Westberg & Jason, 2001). Guided reflection with faculty who assist students in using reflective thinking during simulated learning experiences can enhance student learning and help students learn reflective learning skills. It is recommended (Decker, 2007; Johns, 2004) that this process be done with faculty to avoid negative thoughts that a student may experience. The student should view the learning experience as an opportunity to improve and to see the experience from different perspectives. Some strategies that might be used to develop reflective thinking are keeping a journal, engaging in one-to-one dialogue with a faculty facilitator, engaging in e-mail dialogues, and participating in structured group forums. Group forums help students learn more about constructive feedback and can also be done online with discussion forums. Reflective thinking strategies are not used for grading or evaluation, but rather to help the student "think about" the experience in an open manner.

Intuition   Intuition is part of thinking. Including intuition in critical thinking helps to expand the person's ability "to know" (Hansten & Washburn, 2000). The most common definition of intuition is having a "gut feeling" about something. Nurses have this feeling as they provide care—"I just have this feeling that Mr. Wallace is heading for problems." It is hard to explain what this is, but it happens. A definition

that might be applied is "insightful sense of knowing without conscious use of reason" (Rubenfeld & Scheffer, 2006, p. 20). Rubenfeld and Scheffer described a variety of thoughts that a person may apply to intuition (Rubenfeld & Scheffer, 2006, p. 24):

- I felt it in my bones.
- I couldn't put my finger on why, but I thought; instinctively I knew.
- My hunch was that; I had a premonition/inspiration/impression.
- My natural tendency was to _____.
- Subconsciously I knew that _____.
- Without thought I figured out _____.
- Automatically I thought that _____.
- While I couldn't say why, I thought immediately _____.
- My sixth sense said I should consider _____.

Is intuition science? No, it is not, but sometimes intuition can stimulate research and lead to greater knowledge and questions to explore. Intuition is related to experience. A student would not likely experience intuition about a patient care situation, but over time, as nursing expertise is gained, intuition may be experienced. Benner's (2001) work *From Novice to Expert* suggests that intuition is really the putting together of the whole picture based on scientific knowledge and clinical expertise, not just a hunch.

Caring

There is no universally accepted definition for caring in nursing, but it can be described from four perspectives (Mustard, 2002). The first is the *sense of caring*, which is probably the most common perspective for students to appreciate. This perspective emphasizes compassion, or being concerned about another person. This type of caring may or may not require knowledge and expertise, but in nursing, effective caring requires knowledge and expertise. The second perspective is *doing for other people what they cannot do for themselves.* Nurses do this all the time, and it requires knowledge and expertise to be effective. The third perspective is to *care for the medical problem,* and this too requires knowledge of the problem, interventions, and so on, as well as expertise to provide the care. Providing wound care or administering medications is an example of this type of caring. The last perspective is "*competence in carrying out all the required procedures, personal and technical, with true concern for providing the proper care at the proper time in the proper way*" (*italics added;* Mustard, p. 37). A nurse can be caring and yet not use all four perspectives of caring (Pellegrino, 1985). Caring practices have been identified by the American Association of Critical-Care Nurses in the organization's Synergy Model for Patient Care (2005, p. 1) as "nursing activities that create a compassionate, supportive, and therapeutic environment for patients and staff, with the aim of promoting comfort and healing and preventing unnecessary suffering." This model is discussed more in Chapter 15.

Nursing theories often have a focus on caring. Theories are discussed later in this chapter. One in particular is known for its focus on caring—Watson's Theory on Caring. Watson (1979) defined nursing "as the science of caring, in which caring is described as transpersonal attempts to protect, enhance, and preserve life by helping find meaning in illness and suffering, and subsequently gaining control, self-knowledge, and healing" (Scotto, 2003, p. 289).

Patients today need "caring." They feel isolated and often confused with the complex medical system. Many have chronic illness such as diabetes, arthritis, and cardiac problems that require long-term treatment, and these patients need to learn how to manage their illnesses and be supported in the self-management process.

(See Chapter 9 for more information on self-management and chronic illness as it relates to patient-centered care.) Even many cancer patients who have longer survival rates today are now described as having a chronic illness. How do patients view caring? Patients may not see the knowledge and skills that nurses need, but they can appreciate when a nurse is there with them. The nurse–patient relationship can make a difference when the nurse uses caring consciously (Schwein, 2004). Characteristics of this relationship are as follows:

- Being physically present with the patient
- Having a dialogue with the patient
- Showing a willingness to share and hear—to use active listening
- Avoiding assumptions
- Maintaining confidentiality
- Showing intuition and flexibility
- Believing in hope

Caring is "offering of self. This means offering the intellectual, psychological, spiritual, and physical aspects one possesses as a human being to attain a goal. In nursing, this goal is to facilitate and enhance patients' ability to do and decide for themselves (i.e., to promote their self-agency)" (Husted & Husted, 2001). According to Scotto, "Nurses must prepare themselves in each of the four aspects to be competent to care" (2003, p. 290). The following describes the four aspects identified by Scotto (pp. 290–291).

1. The *intellectual aspect* of nurses consists of an acquired, specialized body of knowledge, analytical thought, and clinical judgment, which are used to meet human health needs.
2. The *psychological aspect* of nurses includes the feelings, emotions, and memories that are part of the human experience.
3. The *spiritual aspect* of nurses, as for all human beings, seeks to answer the questions, "Why? What is the meaning of this?"

4. The *physical aspect* of nurses is the most obvious. Nurses go to the patients' homes, the bedside, and a variety of clinical settings where they offer strength, abilities, and skills to attain a goal. For this task, nurses first must care for themselves, and then they must be accomplished and skillful in nursing interventions.

For students to be able to care for others, they need to care for themselves. This is also important for practicing nurses. Chapter 1 includes some content about caring for self and stress management. It takes energy to care for another person, and this is draining. Developing positive, healthy behaviors and attitudes now can protect a nurse later when more energy is required in the practice of nursing.

As students begin their nursing education program (and indeed throughout the program), the issue of the difference between medicine and nursing often arises. Caring is something that nurses do, or so nurses say. Many physicians would say that they also care for patients and have a caring attitude. Is nursing the only healthcare professional who can say that caring is part of the profession? No, not really. However, what has happened with nursing (which may not have been so helpful) is that when caring is discussed in relation to nursing, it is described only in emotional terms (Moland, 2006). This ignores that caring often involves competent assessment of the patient to determine what needs to be done, and the ability to provide care; all of this requires knowledge. The typical description of medicine is "curing," and for nursing, it is "caring." This type of extreme dichotomy is not helpful for either profession individually and also has an impact on the interrelationship between the two professions, adding conflict and difficulty in communication to the interdisciplinary team.

The use of technology in health care has increased steadily in the last 50 years, particu-larly since the end of the 20th century. Nurses work with technology daily, and more and more care involves some type of technology. This has had a positive impact on care; however, some wonder about the negative impact of technology on caring. Does technology put a barrier between the patient and the nurse that interferes with the nurse–patient relationship? Because of this concern, "nurses are placing more emphasis on the 'high touch' aspect of a 'high tech' environment, recognizing that clients (patients) require human interactions, such as warmth, care, acknowledgement of self-worth, and collaborative decision-making" (Kozier, Erb, & Blais, 1997, p. 10). There must be an effort to combine technology and caring because both are critical to positive patient outcomes. This is referred to as "technological competency as caring" in nursing (Locsin, 2005). Nurses who use technology but ignore the patient as a person are just technologists; they are not nurses who use knowledge, caring, critical thinking, technological skills, and recognition of the patient as a person as integral parts of the caring process (Locsin, 1995).

Competency

Competency is the behavior that a student is expected to demonstrate. The National Council of State Boards of Nursing (NCSBN) defines competency as encompassing knowledge and skills, with an emphasis on interpersonal, decision-making, and psychomotor skills (1996). The ultimate goal of competence is to promote patient safety. Today the phrase "continued competency" is used to denote the need for a nurse to engage in lifelong learning and commit to demonstrating a certain level of competency throughout one's career (NCSBN, 1996). Competency levels change over time as students gain more experience. Development of competencies continues throughout a nurse's career. Nurses in practice have to meet certain competencies to continue practice. This is typically done through meeting staff development requirements. Students, however, must meet competencies to progress through the nursing program and graduate. Competencies include elements of knowledge, caring, and technical skills. Porter-O'Grady (2001) discussed the changes that nursing is confronting and will confront in the 21st century and concluded that nursing will increasingly focus on:

- Facilitating access
- Interpreting information
- Advising and guiding consumers in sorting through increasingly complex therapeutic choices
- Educating the consumer (patient) in the use and application of new therapies
- Partnering with the consumer and the consumer's significant support persons in making choices that fit lifestyle, and discussing therapeutic options and the activities related to genomic options and choices

These activities need to be included in nursing student competencies to prepare nurses for current and future practice.

The Institute of Medicine (IOM) identified five core competencies for the health professions (2003a). After a number of IOM reports identified serious problems with health care, including errors and poor-quality care, an initiative was developed to identify core competencies for all healthcare professions, including nursing, and build a bridge across the quality chasm to improve care. It is hoped that these competencies will have an impact on education for, and practice in, health professions. All the core competencies are covered in more depth in Section III of this textbook. The core competencies are:

1. Provide patient-centered care—Identify, respect, and care about patients' differences, values, preferences, and expressed needs; relieve pain and suffering; coordinate continuous care; listen to, clearly inform, communicate with, and educate patients; share decision making and management; and continuously advocate disease prevention, wellness, and promotion of healthy lifestyles, including a focus on population health. *The description of this core competency relates to content found in definitions of nursing, nursing standards, nursing social policy statement, and nursing theories. (See Chapter 9.)*

2. Work in interdisciplinary teams—Cooperate, collaborate, communicate, and integrate care in teams to ensure that care is continuous and reliable. *There is much knowledge available about teams and how they impact care. Leadership is a critical component of working on teams—as team leader and as followers or members. Many of the major nursing roles that are discussed in this chapter require working with teams. (See Chapter 10.)*

3. Employ evidence-based practice—Integrate best research with clinical expertise and patient values for optimum care, and participate in learning and research activities to the extent feasible. *EBP has been mentioned in this chapter about knowledge and caring as it relates to research. (See Chapter 11.)*

4. Apply quality improvement—Identify errors and hazards in care; understand and implement basic safety design principles, such as standardization and simplification; continually understand and measure quality of care in terms of structure, process, and outcomes in relation to patient and community needs; and design and test interventions to change processes and systems of care, with the objective of improving quality. *Understanding how care is provided and problems in providing care often lead to the need for additional knowledge development through research. (See Chapter 12.)*

5. Utilize informatics—Communicate, manage knowledge, mitigate error, and support

decision making using information technology. *This chapter focuses on knowledge and caring, both of which require use of informatics to meet patient needs. (See Chapter 13.)*

Scholarship in Nursing

There is a great need to search for better solutions and knowledge and to disseminate knowledge. This discussion about scholarship in nursing explores the meaning of scholarship, the meaning and impact of **theory** and research, use of professional literature, and new scholarship modalities.

What Does Scholarship Mean?

The American Association of Colleges of Nursing (AACN) defines scholarship in nursing "as those activities that systematically advance the teaching, research, and practice of nursing through rigorous inquiry that: (1) is significant to the profession, (2) is creative, (3) can be documented, (4) can be replicated or elaborated, and (5) can be peer-reviewed through various methods" (1999, p. 1). The common response to the question of which activities might be considered scholarship is research. Boyer (1990), however, questioned this view of scholarship, suggesting that other activities are scholarly. These include

1. *Discovery*, in which new and unique knowledge is generated (research, theory development, philosophical inquiry)
2. *Teaching*, in which the teacher creatively builds bridges between his or her own understanding and the students' learning
3. *Application*, in which the emphasis is on the use of new knowledge in solving society's problems (practice)
4. *Integration*, in which new relationships among disciplines are discovered (publishing, presentations, grant awards, licenses, patents or products for sale; must involve

two or more disciplines, thus advancing knowledge over a broader range)

These four aspects of scholarship are critical components of academic nursing and support the values of a profession committed to both social relevance and scientific advancement.

Some nurses think that the AACN definition of scholarship limits scholarship to educational institutions only. Mason (2006) commented that this is a problem for nursing; science needs to be accessible to practitioners. She defined scholarship as "an in-depth, careful process of exploring current theory and research with the purpose of either furthering the science or translating its findings into practice or policy" (Mason, 2006, p. 11). The better approach, then, is to consider scholarship in both the education and practice arenas and still emphasize that nursing is a practice profession that must be patient centered. Nursing theory and research have been mentioned in this chapter and by Mason as part of knowledge and caring, and scholarship of nursing. Understanding what they are and how they have an impact on practice is important if all nurses are to be scholars and leaders.

Nursing has a long history of scholarship, though some periods more than others seem to have been more active in terms of major contributions to nursing scholarship. Exhibit 2–1 describes some of the milestones that are important in understanding nursing scholarship.

Nursing Theory

A simple description of a theory is "words or phrases (concepts) joined together in sentences, with an overall theme, to explain, describe, or predict something" (Sullivan, 2006, p. 160). Theories help nurses understand and find meaning in nursing. Nursing has a number of theories that have been developed since Nightingale's contributions to nursing, particularly during the 1960s–1980s, and there is variation in

EXHIBIT 2–1 A BRIEF HISTORY OF SELECT NURSING SCHOLARSHIP MILESTONES

1850	Nightingale conducted first nursing search by collecting healthcare data during the Crimean War.
1851	Florence Nightingale, age 32, went to the Institution of Deaconesses at Kaiserswerth to train in nursing. At that time the model was to study spirituality and healing, a result of Dr. Elizabeth Blackwell's influence.
1854–56	Nightingale applied knowledge of statistics and care training. She took charge of lay nurses and the Anglican sisters; nurses had to wear uniforms: loose gray dresses, a jacket, cap, and sash. This dress was practical because halls and rooms were drafty and cool.
1854–55	Nightingale created the first standards for care.
1860	The first training school was founded in London.
1860	*Notes on Nursing* by Nightingale was published.
1860	Prior to the 1860s and the Civil War, religious orders (primarily of the Catholic Church) cared for the sick. These early times were characterized by several significant historical events: • A lack of organized nursing and care led to the development of Bellevue Hospital, which was founded in 1658 in New York. • In 1731 the Philadelphia Almshouse was started by the Sisters of Charity, spearheaded by Elizabeth Ann Bayley Seton, a physician's daughter who married, was widowed, and then entered religious life and provided nursing care. • Charity Hospital in New Orleans, Louisiana, was founded in 1736 and funded by private endowment.
1860–65	The Civil War broke out. Dorothea Dix, Superintendent of Female Nurses for the Union Army, needed help with the wounded. She set the first qualifications for nurses.
1860s	Dr. Elizabeth Blackwell, first female U.S. physician, started the Women's Central Association for Relief in New York City, which later became the Sanitary Commission. Also: • The New England Hospital for Women and Children in Boston, Massachusetts, opened in 1860. During its early years there was no structured care. • Woman's Hospital of Philadelphia opened in 1861, also with no structured care. • In 1863, the state of Massachusetts began the first board of nursing, the first attempt at regulation of the practice of nursing.
1870s	The first nursing school graduate was Linda Richards in 1873 from the New England Hospital for Women and Children in Boston, Massachusetts. Other items of note: • Although a plea for attention to the hospital environment had been made by Nightingale, it wasn't until the 1870s that lights were introduced. • Written patient cases were instituted during this time, replacing the verbal reports previously used. • Hospitals began to examine the causes of mortality among their patient population. • Mary Mahoney, the first black nurse, graduated in 1879.
1873	Three nursing schools were founded: • The Bellevue Training School in New York City, New York. • The Connecticut Training School in New Haven, Connecticut. • The Boston Training School in Boston, Massachusetts.
1882	Clara Barton, a schoolteacher, founded the American Red Cross.
1885	The first nursing text was published: *A Textbook of Nursing for the Use of Training Schools, Families and Private Students.*

1884	Alice Fisher, a Nightingale-trained nurse, came to the United States.
1884	Isabel Hampton Robb wrote *Nursing: Its Principles and Practice for Hospital and Private Use.*
1890s	The Visiting Nurses Group started in England.
1893	The American Society of Superintendents of Training Schools was formed. Other events of note include:

- The Henry Street Settlement, a community center in New York City, was founded by Lillian Wald. This was the beginning of community-based care.
- The Nightingale Pledge was written by Mrs. Lystra E. Gretter as a modification of the doctor's Hippocratic Oath. The pledge was written for the Committee for the Farrand Training School for Nurses, Detroit, Michigan.

1897	The University of Texas at Galveston moved undergraduate nursing education into the university setting.
1900	The first graduate nursing degree was offered by Columbia Teachers College. In addition:

- As nursing moved from a practice-based discipline to a university program, subjects such as ethics were introduced for the first time. Isabel Hampton Robb, considered the architect of American nursing, wrote *Nursing Ethics*, the first ethics text for nurses.
- Both textbooks and journals for nurses became available. Among the first of the journals was the *American Journal of Nursing*.

1901	Mary Adelaide Nutting started a 3–6-month preparatory course for nurses; by 1911, 86 schools had some form of formalized and structured nurse training.
1907	Mary Adelaide Nutting became the first nursing professor and began the first state nursing association in Maryland. At this time nursing was moving toward a more formal educational system, similar to that of the discipline of medicine. A professional organization at a state level gave recognition to nursing as a distinct discipline.
1907	Now a distinct discipline, nursing needed standards to guide practice and education. Isabel Hampton Robb wrote *Educational Standards for Nurses.*
1908	Other professional organizations grew, beginning with the National Association of Colored Graduate Nurses.
1909	The first bachelor's degree program in nursing was started at the University of Minnesota.
1900s–1940s	As nursing became more ensconced in university settings, nursing research was another area viewed as necessary for a well-educated nurse to study. The first research focused on nursing education.
1911	The concept of specialties within nursing began with Bellevue Hospital's midwifery program.
1912	The American Society of Superintendents of Training Schools became the National League for Nursing Education (NLNE). Also:

- The National Organization for Public Health Nursing was founded.
- The *Public Health Nursing* journal was started.

1917	The National League for Nursing Education identified its first *Standard Curriculum for Schools of Nursing*, a remedy for the lack of standards in nursing education.
1920	The first master's program in nursing began at Yale School of Nursing.
1922	Sigma Theta Tau International (STTI), the nursing honor society, was formed.
1923	The Goldmark Report called for nursing education to be separate from (and precede) employment; it also advocated nursing licensure and proper training for faculty at nursing institutions.
1925	Mary Breckenridge founded the Frontier Nursing Service in Kentucky. Her intent was to provide rural healthcare; this organization was the first to employ nurses who could also provide midwifery services.

continues

Exhibit 2–1 (continued)

1925	As the status of women increased, nurses were among the first women to lead the women's rights movements in the United States.
1930	A total of 41 (out of 48) states have regulatory state boards of nursing.
1900–30s	A shortage of funds put nursing education under the control of doctors and hospitals. This situation resulted from:
	• Leaders believing that the only way to change was to organize.
	• The need to provide protection for the public from poorly educated nurses.
	• A lack of sanitation.
	• Schools providing cheap services for hospitals.
1931	The Association of Collegiate Schools of Nursing is formed, eventually the Department of Baccalaureate and Higher Degrees of the NLN.
1934	New York University and the Teachers College start PhD and EdD in programs in nursing.
1940	Nursing Council on National Defense, formed after World War I (1917–1918), underwent changes during 1940.
1942	American Association of Industrial Nurses (AAIN) was founded.
1948	The Brown Report recommended that nursing education programs be housed in universities; this report also formed the basis for evaluating nursing programs.
1950	Graduate nursing education started with the clinical nurse specialist.
1954	The University of Pittsburgh started a PhD program in nursing (academic doctorate).
1956	Columbia University granted its first master's degree in nursing.
1950s–1960s	Early nursing theory was developed.
1950	The American Nurses Association (ANA) published the first edition of the *Code for Nurses*.
1952	The NLNE changed its name to the National League for Nursing (NLN).
1952	Initial publication of *Nursing Research* under the direction of the ANA.
1952	Mildred Montag started the first associate's degree nursing programs. These were designed as pilots to create a technical nurse below the level of the professional nurse, but with training beyond that of a practice nurse.
1955	American Nurses Foundation was formed to obtain funds for nursing research.
1960	The doctorate in nursing science (DNS) degree was started at Boston University (professional doctorate).
1960s	Federal monies were made available for doctoral study for nurse educators.
1963	The initial publication of the *International Journal of Nursing Studies* was available.
1964	The first nurse practitioner program was instituted by Loretta Ford at the University of Colorado.
1965	The first nursing research conference was held.
1965	The ANA made the statement that a baccalaureate degree should represent the entry level for nursing practice.
1967	The STTI launched the initial publication of *Image*.
1969	The American Association of Colleges of Nursing formed with 123 members to serve as representation for bachelor's degree and higher education nursing programs.
1970s–90s	This marked the period of development that saw the birth of most nursing theories; some of these theories were tested and expanded upon.
1973	The first nursing diagnosis conference was held.
1973	The American Academy of Nursing was formed under the aegis of ANA to recognize nursing leaders.
1973	The ANA published the first edition of *Standards of Nursing Practice*.
1978–79	Several new nursing research journals had their initial publication.

1985	The National Center for Nursing Research was established at the National Institutes of Health, later to become the National Institute of Nursing Research.
1990s	Evidence-based practice began to become a major focus.
1993	The ANA published its position statement on nursing education.
1993	The Commission on Collegiate Nursing Education was formed to accredit nursing programs, with an emphasis on bachelor's and master's degree programs.
1993	The Cochrane Collaborative was formed for systematic reviews and was named after British epidemiologist Archie Cochrane.
1996	The Joanna Briggs Institute for Evidence-Based Practice was founded in Adelaide, Australia.
1997	The National League for Nursing Accrediting Commission became a separate corporation from the NLN.
1995	The ANA published the first edition of *Nursing's Social Policy Statement*.
1999	The American Association of Colleges of Nursing (AACN) published its position statement on nursing research.
2004	The NLN established Centers for Excellence in Nursing Education to recognize exemplar schools of nursing.
2004	The AACN endorsed the development and called for pilot schools to create the Clinical Nurse Leader (CNL).
2004	The Columbia University School of Nursing offered the first doctor of nursing practice (DNP) degree.
2007	The NLN established the Academy of Nursing Education to recognize nursing education leaders.

the theories. This surge in development of nursing theories was related to the need to "justify nursing as an academic discipline"—the need to develop and describe nursing knowledge (Maas, 2006, p. 7). Some of the major theories are described in Exhibit 2–2 from the perspective of how each description, beginning with Nightingale, responds to the concepts of

- The person
- The environment
- Health
- Nursing

Over the last decade, there has been less emphasis placed on nursing theory in nursing education (Butcher, 2006; DeKeyser & Medoff-Cooper, 2002). This change has been controversial. Theories may be used to form frameworks for research studies and to test their applicability. In addition, practice is not often guided by one of the nursing theories (Butcher, 2006). In

hospitals and other healthcare organizations, the nursing department may identify a specific theory on which the staff base their mission. In these organizations, it is usually easy to see how the designated theory is present in the official documents about the department, but it is not always so easy to see how the theory impacts the day-to-day practice of nurses in the organization. It is important to remember that theories do not tell nurses what they must do or how they must do something; rather, they are guides—abstract guides. Figure 2–1 (p. 73) describes the relationship between theory, research, and practice.

Most of the nursing theories were developed in the 1970s–1990s, so what might some of the issues of future theories be? In 1992, the following were predicted as possible areas to be included in nursing theories (Meleis, 1992):

1. The human science underlying the discipline that "is predicated on understanding

EXHIBIT 2–2 OVERVIEW OF MAJOR NURSING THEORIES & MODELS

Theories and Models	Person	Environment	Health	Nursing
Systematic Approach to Health Care Florence Nightingale	Recipient of nursing care	External (temperature, bedding, ventilation) and internal (food, water, and medications)	Health is "not only to be well, but to be able to use well every power we have to use" (Nightingale, 1969, p. 24).	Alter or manage the environment to implement the natural laws of health
Theory of Caring in Nursing Jean Watson	A "unity of mind body spirit/nature" (Watson, 1996, p. 147) (human)	A "field of connectedness" at all levels (p. 147)	Harmony, wholeness, and comfort	Reciprocal transpersonal relationship in caring moments guided by curative factors
The Science of Unitary Human Beings Martha E. Rogers	An irreducible, irreversible, pandimensional, negentropic energy field identified by pattern; a unitary human being develops through three principles: helicy, resonancy, and integrality (Rogers, 1992) (human being)	An irreducible, pandimensional, negentropic energy field, identified by pattern and manifesting characteristics different from those of the parts and encompassing all that is other than any given human field (Rogers, 1992)	Health and illness area a part of a continuum (Rogers, 1970)	Seeks to promote symphonic interaction between human and environmental fields, to strengthen the integrity of the human field, and to direct and redirect patterning of the human and environmental fields for realization of maximum health potential (Rogers, 1970)
Self-Care Deficit Nursing Theory Dorothea E. Orem	A person under the care of a nurse; a total being with universal, developmental needs, and capable of self-care (patient)	Physical, chemical, biologic, and social contexts with which human beings exist, environmental components include environmental factors, environmental conditions, and developmental environment (Orem, 1985)	"A state characterized by soundness or wholeness of developed human structures and of bodily and mental functioning" (Orem, 1995, p. 101)	Therapeutic self-care designed to supplement self-care requisites. Nursing actions fall into one of three categories: wholly compensatory, partly compensatory, or supportive educative system (Orem, 1985)
The Roy Adaptation Model Callista Roy	"A whole with parts that function as a unity" (Roy & Andrews, 1999, p. 31) (human system)	Internal and external stimuli; "the world within and around humans as adaptive systems" (p. 51)	"A state and process of being and becoming an integrated and whole human being" (p. 54)	Manipulation of stimuli to foster successful adaptation
The Neuman Systems Model Betty Neuman	A composite of physiological, psychological, sociocultural, developmental, and spiritual variables in interaction	All internal and external factors of influences surrounding the client system	A continuum of wellness to illness	Prevention as intervention; concerned with all potential stressors

Theories and Models	Person	Environment	Health	Nursing
	with the internal and external environment; represented by central structure, lines of defense, and lines of resistance			
Systems Framework and Theory of Goal Attainment Imogene M. King	A personal system that interacts with interpersonal and social systems (human being)	A context "within which human beings grow, develop, and perform daily activities" (King, 1981, p. 18). "The internal environment of human beings transforms energy to enable them to adjust to continuous external environmental changes" (p. 5).	"Dynamic life experiences of a human being, which implies continuous adjustment to stressors in the internal and external environment through optimum use of one's resources to achieve maximum potential for daily living" (p. 5)	A process of human interaction; the goal of nursing is to help patients achieve their goals.
Behavioral Systems Model Dorothy Johnson	A biophysical being who is a behavioral system with seven subsystems of behavior (human being)	Includes internal and external environment	Efficient and effective functioning of system; behavioral system balance and stability	An external regulatory force that acts to preserve the organization and integrity of the patient's behavior at an optimal level under those conditions in which the behavior constitutes a threat to physical or social health or in which illness is found (Johnson, 1980, p. 214)
Theory of Human Becoming Rosemarie Parse	An open being, more than and different than the sum of parts in mutual simultaneous interchange with the environment who chooses from options and bears responsibility for choices (Parse, 1987, p. 160)	In mutual process with the person	Continuously changing process of becoming	Use of true presence to facilitate the becoming of the participant
Transcultural Nursing Model Madeleine Leininger	Human beings, family, group, community, or institution	"Totality of an event, situation, or experience that gives meaning to human expressions, interpretations, and social interactions in physical, ecological, sociopolitical, and/or	"A state of well-being that is culturally defined, valued, and practiced" (Leininger, 1991, p. 46)	Activities directed toward assisting, supporting, or enabling with needs in ways that are congruent with the cultural values, beliefs, and lifeways of the *continues*

EXHIBIT 2–2 (continued)

Theories and Models	Person	Environment	Health	Nursing
		cultural settings" (Leininger, 1991, p. 46)		recipient of care (Leininger, 1995)
Interpersonal Relations Model Hildegard Peplau	"Encompasses the patient (one who has problems for which expert nursing services are needed or sought) and the nurse (a professional with particular expertise)" (Peplau, 1952, p. 14).	Includes culture as important to the development of personality	"Implies forward movement of personality and other ongoing human processes in the direction of creative, constructive, productive, personal, and community living" (Peplau, 1952, p. 12).	The therapeutic, interpersonal process between the nurse and the patient

Sources: Johnson, D. (1980). The behavioral systems model for nursing. In J. Riehl & C. Roy (Eds.), Conceptual models for nursing practice (2nd ed., pp. 207–216). New York: Appleton-Century-Crofts; King, I.M. (1981). A theory of nursing: Systems, concepts, process. New York: Wiley; Leininger, M. M. (1991). Culture care diversity and universality: a theory of nursing. New York: National League for Nursing; Leininger, M. M. (1995). Transcultural nursing perspectives: Basic concepts, principles, and culture care incidents. In M.M. Leininger (Ed.), Transcultural nursing: concepts, theories, research, and practices (2nd ed., pp. 57–92). New York: McGraw-Hill; Nightingale, F. (1969). Notes on nursing: What it is and what it is not. New York: Dover; Orem, D. (1985). Nursing: Concepts of practice (3rd ed.). St. Louis, MO: Mosby; Orem, D. (1995). Nursing: Concepts of practice (5th ed.). St. Louis, MO: Mosby; Parse, R.R. (1987). Nursing science: Major paradigms, theories, and critiques. Philadelphia: Saunders; Peplau, H. (1952). Interpersonal relations in nursing. New York: G. P. Putnam's Sons; Rogers, M. E. (1970). An introduction to the theoretical basis of nursing. Philadelphia: F.A. Davis; Rogers, M. E. (1992). Nursing science and the sapce age. Nursing Science Quarterly, 5, 27–34; Roy, C., & Andrews, H. A. (1999). The Roy Adaptation Model. New York: Appleton-Lange; Watson, J. (1996). Watson's philosophy and theory of human caring in nursing. In J. P. Riehl-Sisca (Ed.), Conceptual models for nursing practice (pp. 219–235). Norwalk, CT: Appleton & Lange, as cited in K. Masters (2005), Role development in professional nursing practice. Sudbury, MA: Jones and Bartlett.

the meanings of daily lived experiences as they are perceived by the members or the participants of the science" (p. 112).

2. The increased emphasis on the practice-orientation, or actual, rather than "ought-to-be," practice.

3. The mission of nursing to develop theories to empower nurses, the discipline, and clients (patients).

4. "Acceptance of the fact that women may have different strategies and approaches to knowledge development than men" (p. 113).

5. Nursing's attempt to "understand consumers' experiences for the purpose of empowering them to receive optimum care and to maintain optimum health" (p. 114).

6. "The effort to broaden nursing's perspective, which includes efforts to understand the practice of nursing in third world countries" (p. 114).

These potential characteristics of nursing are somewhat different from past theories. Consumerism is highlighted through better understanding consumers and empowering them. Empowering nurses is also emphasized. The suggestion that women nurses and men nurses might approach care issues differently is very new and has not really been addressed. The sixth characteristic listed above is highly relevant today, with the increase in globalization. Developed and developing countries can share information via the Internet in a matter of seconds.

Figure 2–1 The relationships of theory, research, and practice.

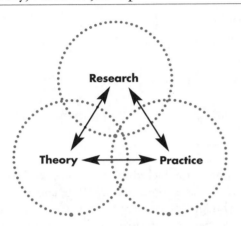

Source: From *Evidence-Based Practice for Nurses: Appraisal and Applications of Research*, by N.A. Schmidt and J.M. Brown, 2009, Sudbury, MA: Jones and Bartlett Publishers.

There are fewer boundaries than ever before; better communication and information exchange is possible. A need certainly exists because the nursing issues and care problems are worldwide. A global effort to solve these problems on a worldwide scale is absolutely necessary. Take for example, issues such as infectious diseases, which can quickly spread from one part of the world to another in which the disease is relatively unknown due to the ease of travel. In conclusion, it is not really clear what role nursing theories might play and how theories might change.

Nursing Research

Nursing research is "a methodological examination that uses regimented techniques to resolve questions or decipher dilemmas" (Boswell & Cannon, 2007, p. 346). The major purpose of doing research is to expand nursing knowledge to improve patient care and outcomes. It helps to explain and predict care that nurses provide. There are two major types of research: basic and applied. Basic research is done to gain knowledge for

knowledge's sake; however, basic research results may then be used in applied or clinical research.

> *For too long, nursing has sustained the myth of the theory practice gap and promulgated science as distinct from the discipline's art or practice. The **researcher** has been portrayed as the producer who hands down scientific knowledge to the clinician: as the applier of knowledge, sometimes supplier of ideas or researchable problems, and maybe even tester of knowledge, but rarely the producer. This traditional model of nursing knowledge production not only misrepresents and constrains the knowledge potential in nursing, but it marginalizes the practitioner and distances patients from knowledge development. (Reed, 2006, p. 36)*

This type of approach separates the practitioner from the research process too much. Nursing needs to know more about "whether and how nurses produce knowledge in their practice" (Reed, p. 36). Nursing, and all health care, needs to be patient-centered (Institute of Medicine, 2003a), and research should not be an exception. This does not mean that there is no need for research in administration/management and in education, because there are critical needs in these areas, but it does mean that nursing needs to gain more knowledge about the nursing process with patients as the center. Because of these issues, EBP has become more central in practice.

The research process is similar to the nursing process in that there is a need to identify a problem using data, determine goals, describe what will be done, and then assess results. Exhibit 2–3 identifies the steps in the research process and is discussed in more detail in Chapter 11.

Researchers take time to develop research proposals that describe in detail what they plan to do in a study. These proposals are also used to request funding in the form of grants. This is a complicated and time-consuming process. If funding is received, the study is conducted, but

---

Exhibit 2–3 Steps in the Research Process

1. State the research problem or question.
2. Describe the purpose of the study.
3. Review the literature.
4. Apply a theoretical framework. (Some studies do not include this step.)
5. Formulate hypotheses and variables.
6. Describe the research design: data collection methods.
7. Select the setting and the sample and ensure that ethical requirements are met.
8. Collect the data.
9. Analyze the data.
10. Report on the findings or results.

---

it must follow the proposal or plan. Funding typically is given for a time period, such as a year or several years. Results are then disseminated through published articles, poster presentations, and podium presentations. Today, there is increasing emphasis on the difference that research makes on practice.

The National Institute of Nursing Research

Beginning with the initial work of Nightingale when she collected data during the Crimean War to improve care, nursing slowly moved toward research. In 1946, the Division of Nursing was created on the federal level, and with this funding, nursing research was formalized (Boswell & Cannon, 2007). Almost 10 years later, in 1955, the Nursing Research Study Section was established by the National Institutes of Health (NIH), but the critical major change was the creation of the National Center of Nursing Research at the NIH in 1985. This center became the **National Institute of Nursing Research** (NINR) in 1993. Box 2–2 describes the NINR mission, its major strategies, and its major research areas.

The focus of nursing research has shifted from development of the profession to an emphasis on clinical research to improve nursing practice. In the last 10 years, there has been increased emphasis on including EBP. The budget for NINR was $16 million in 1986, and in 2005, the budget increased to $127,134,000. Seventy-three percent of this budget goes to extramural funding, which is research support for studies that are done outside the NIH (Butcher, 2006)—for example, at a college of nursing, hospital, or community healthcare site. The federal government, through Congress, funds NINR in the NIH budget. The NINR budget is very large, but it still is not sufficient to fund all the needed research.

Evidence-Based Practice

As discussed, research results that can make a difference in health care in general, and in nursing in particular, need to be implemented in practice. It takes too long for this to happen. EBP is the major initiative to increase the use of best practice or evidence in making clinical decisions. EBP requires that nurses "integrate best research with clinical expertise and patient values for optimum care" (IOM, 2003a, p. 4). It is important to note that this definition of EBP includes more that just research results. Best practice clinical decisions also require healthcare provider expertise and patient assessment, and also must include the patient's perspective (patient preferences and values). A critical question is, How much EBP is actually being used? Pravikoff et al. (2005) conducted a study to

---

BOX 2–2 THE NATIONAL INSTITUTE OF NURSING RESEARCH: MISSION, STRATEGIES, RESEARCH AREAS

The National Institute of Nursing Research

The mission of the National Institute of Nursing Research (NINR) is to promote and improve the health of individuals, families, communities, and populations. NINR supports and conducts clinical and basic research and research training on health and illness across the life span. The research focus encompasses health promotion and disease prevention, quality of life, health disparities, and end-of-life. NINR seeks to extend nursing science by integrating the biological and behavioral sciences, employing new technologies to research questions, improving research methods, and developing the scientists of the future.

Strategies for Building the Science
- Integrating biological and behavioral science for better health
- Adopting, adapting, and generating new technologies for better health care
- Improving methods for future scientific discoveries
- Developing scientists for today and tomorrow

NINR's Research Program is guided by four strategies intended to advance science:

- Integrating biology and behavior
- Designing and using new technology
- Developing new tools
- Preparing the next generation of nurse scientists

Areas of Research Emphasis
- Promoting health and preventing disease
- Improving quality of life
- Eliminating health disparities
- Setting directions for end-of-life research

Source: Department of Health and Human Services (DHHS), National Institutes of Health (NIH), National Institute of Nursing Rsearch (NINR). Retrieved May 31, 2007, from http://www.ninr.nih.gov/

---

assess the readiness of U.S. nurses for EBP, and the results indicated that nurses are not using research evidence in their practice. This was a disappointing finding, but not surprising. Research done for research's sake, without ever making it into practice, might as well not be done. There are growing efforts to change this by increasing EBP content, not just research content, in all levels of nursing education, undergraduate through graduate. Efforts are also being made to improve staff development on EBP so that nurses in practice can gain essential competencies to increase EBP in clinical settings. Chapter 11 discusses EBP in more detail; employing EBP is one of the five core health care professions competencies. In this chap-

ter, it is important to recognize that research cannot be discussed without considering EBP; research and EBP should be interconnected. As discussed, science must be accessible (Mason, 2006). EBP provides methods for making science more accessible to the practitioner who does not have a lot of time to pore through research study reports to determine what works and what does not, and to compare one study with another in detail.

It is easy to confuse research utilization and EBP. Research utilization usually involves using knowledge gained from one study, with limited regard to provider expertise, patient assessment, and patient preferences and values. EBP is a much more organized approach to getting research into practice, as will be discussed in Chapter 11.

Sigma Theta Tau International (STTI) offers a nursing continuing education course that focuses on EBP: Clinical Scholars at the Bedside. The relationship between the content of this chapter and the content of Clinical Scholars at the Bedside is evident in the module titles described in Box 2–3.

Professional Literature

Professional literature is an important part of nursing scholarship, but it is important to remember that "because of the changing health care environment and the proliferation of knowledge in health care and nursing, much of the knowledge acquired in your nursing education program may be out of date 5 years after you graduate" (Zerwekh & Claborn, 2006, p. 197). This literature is found in textbooks and in professional journals. The literature provides a repository of nursing knowledge that is accessible to nursing students and nurses. It is important that nurses keep up with the literature in

their specialty areas, given the increased emphasis on EBP.

Textbooks typically are a few years behind current information because of the length of the publication schedule. Although this is improving, it still takes significantly longer to publish a textbook than a journal. It is also more expensive to publish a book, so new editions do not come out annually. The content found in textbooks provides the background information and detail on particular topics. A textbook is peer reviewed when content is shared with experts on the topic for feedback to the author(s). Today, many textbook publishers offer companion Web sites to provide additional material and, in some cases, more updated content or references. E-books are on the horizon, and this might reduce the delay in getting textbooks published and provide a method for updating content quickly.

Content in journals is typically more current and usually focuses on a very specific topic in less depth as compared with a textbook. Journals with higher quality articles are peer reviewed. This means that submitted manuscripts are reviewed by several nurses who have expertise in the man-

---

BOX 2–3 EXAMPLE OF A CONTINUING EUCATION PROGRAM PROMOTING CLINICAL SCHOLARS AT THE BEDSIDE

Sigma Theta Tau International offers a continuing education course for nurses, Clinical Scholars at the Bedside, which focuses on evidence-based practice. Content includes the following modules:

- Clinical Scholars at the Bedside: An EBP Mentorship Model for How Nurses Work Today
- Origins and Aspirations: Conceiving the Clinical Scholar Model
- Observation: Conceptualizing a Researchable Clinical Issue
- Analysis: What's All the Speak About Critique?
- Synthesis and Evaluation: The Clinical Scholar Model in Practice
- Critiquing Clinical Guidelines
- Creating the Clinical Scholar Student: Collaboration Between Education and Practice
- Curiosity and Reflective Thinking: Renewal of the Spirit
- Dear Diary: Rewards and Challenges of Applying Evidence

Source: Sigma Theta Tau International. Retrieved June 1, 2007, from http://www.nursingknowledge.org/Portal/main.aspx? PageID=36&SKU=67128&WT.mc_id=&WT.desvid=954750955

uscript's topic. A consensus is then reached with the editor regarding whether to publish the manuscript. Online access to journal articles has increased accessibility to nurses. Journals are often published by nursing professional organizations.

In 2005, there were 190 nursing journals in continual print, and 15 of them focus on research (University of Adelaide Library Guides, 2005). Who writes for all these journals, and who writes nursing textbooks? Any nurse with expertise in an area can submit for publication. The profession needs more nurses publishing, particularly in journals. Exhibit 2–4 identifies examples of nursing journals.

New Modalities of Scholarship

Scholarship, as noted previously, includes publications, copyrights, licenses, patents, or products for sale. Nursing is expanding into a number of new modalities that can be considered scholarship. Many of these modalities relate to Web-based learning—including course development and learning activities, and products such as case software for simulation experiences—and involve other technology, such as personal digital assistants and podcasting. Most of these new modalities relate to teaching and learning in academic programs, though many are now expanding into staff development and continuing education. In developing these modalities, nurses are creating innovative teaching methods, developing programs and learning outcomes, improving professional development, and applying technical skills. When interdisciplinary approaches are used, integrative scholarship occurs. The STTI course on EBP described in Box 2–3 uses the Web to provide broader access to this critical content.

Multiple Nursing Roles and Leadership

Nurses use knowledge and caring as they provide care to patients; however, there are other aspects of nursing that are important. Nurses hold multiple roles, sometimes at the same time. As nurses function in these roles, they need to demonstrate leadership.

Key Nursing Roles

Before discussing nursing roles, it is important to discuss some terminology related to roles. A role can vary depending on the context, but a commonly accepted definition is "behavior oriented to the patterned expectation of others" (Merton, 1968, p. 110). Merton indicated that role and **status** are connected. Status is a position in a social structure, with rights and obligations—for example, a nurse manager. Role expectations are the norms, expected behaviors, attitudes, and cogni-

---

EXHIBIT 2–4 EXAMPLES OF NURSING JOURNALS

- *American Journal of Nursing*
- *American Nursing Today*
- *Emergency Room Nursing*
- *Home Healthcare Nurse*
- *Journal of Cardiovascular Nursing*
- *Journal of Nursing Administration*
- *Journal of Nursing Care Quality*
- *Journal of Nursing Informatics*
- *Journal of Nursing Scholarship*
- *Journal of Pediatric Nursing*
- *Journal of Perinatal and Neonatal Nursing*
- *Journal of Professional Nursing*
- *Journal of Psychiatric Nursing*
- *Nursing Management*
- *Nursing Outlook*
- *Nursing Research*
- *Nursing2008*
- *Oncology Nursing*
- *Online Journal of Nursing*
- *World Views of Evidence-Based Nursing*

tions of the person in the role (Kozier et al., 1997). As a person takes on a new role, he or she experiences **role transition**. Nursing students are in role transition as they gradually learn the nursing roles. All nursing roles are important in patient care, and typically these roles are interconnected in practice. Students learn about the roles and what is necessary to be competent to meet role expectations, and **identity** also is involved. "Identity is foundational to professional nursing practice. Identity in nursing can be defined as the development within nurses of an internal representation of people-environment interactions in the exploration of human responses to actual or potential health problems. Professional identity is foundational to the assumption of various nursing roles" (Ohlen & Segesten, 1998, as cited in Cook, Gilmer, & Bess, 2003, p. 311).

Nursing is a complex profession and involves multiple types of consumers of nursing care (e.g., individuals, families, communities, and populations), multiple types of problems (e.g., physical, emotional, sociological, economical, and educational), and multiple settings (e.g., hospitals, clinics, communities, and schools), and specialties within each of these. Some roles do not focus so much on direct patient care, such as teaching, administration, and research roles. Different levels of knowledge, caring, and education may be required for different roles. There are many nursing roles, and all of them require leadership. What are the key roles found in nursing?

PROVIDER OF CARE

The **provider of care** role is probably what students think nursing is all about, and this is the role typically seen in the hospital setting. One might call this the traditional role of the nurse (Zerwekh & Claborn, 2006). Caring is attached most to this role, but knowledge is critical to providing safe, quality care. When the nurse is described, it is often the caring that is most emphasized—less emphasis on the knowledge and expertise is required, and more emphasis on the emotional side of caring. Providing care has moved far beyond the hospital, with nurses providing care in clinics, schools, the community, homes, industry, and at many more sites.

EDUCATOR

Nurses spend a lot of time teaching—teaching patients, families, communities, and populations. What do they teach? Nurses as **educators** focus on health promotion and prevention, and helping the patient (individuals, families, communities, and populations) cope with illness and injury. Teaching needs to be planned and based on needs, and nurses must know about teaching principles and methods. Some nurses teach other nurses and healthcare providers in healthcare settings, which is called staff development or staff education. Other nurses teach in nursing schools.

COUNSELOR

Nurses may act as a **counselor**, providing advice and counseling to patients, families, communities, and populations. This is often done in conjunction with other roles.

MANAGER

Nurses act as **managers** daily in their positions even if they do not have a formal management position. Management is the process of getting something done efficiently and effectively through and with other people. Nurses might do this by ensuring that a patient's needs are addressed. For example, he or she may ensure that the patient receives needed laboratory work or a rehabilitation session. The nurse plans who will give care (and when and how), evaluates results, and so forth. Managing care involves critical thinking, planning, decision making, delegating, collaborating, coordinating, communicating, and working with interdisciplinary teams. Much of this will be discussed in later chapters. Leadership is also a critical component.

RESEARCHER

Only a small percentage of nurses are actual nurse researchers; however, nurses participate in research in other ways. The most critical is by using EBP, which is discussed in more detail in Chapter 11 as one of the five core health care professional competencies. Some nurses now hold positions in research studies that may or may not be nursing research studies. These nurses assist in data collection and even manage data collection projects.

COLLABORATOR

Every nurse is a collaborator. "Collaboration is a cooperative effort that focuses on a win-win strategy. **Collaboration** depends on each individual recognizing the perspective of others who are involved and eventually reach a consensus of common goal(s)" (Finkelman, 2006, p. 71). A nurse collaborates with other healthcare providers, members of the community, government agencies, and many more.

CHANGE AGENT (INTRAPRENEUR)

It is difficult to perform any of the nursing roles without engaging in change. This change may be found in how care is provided, where care is provided and when, to whom care is provided, and why. Change is normal today. The healthcare delivery system experiences constant change. Nurses deal with it wherever they work, but they may also initiate change for improvement. When a nurse is a **change agent** within the organization where he or she works, the nurse is an **intrapreneur**. This requires risk and the ability to see change in a positive light. An example of a nurse acting as a change agent would be a nurse who sees the value in extending visiting hours in the intensive care unit. He or she reviews the literature on this topic to support

EBP and then approaches management with the suggestion about making a change.

ENTREPRENEUR

The **entrepreneur** role is not as common as other roles, but it is increasing. The entrepreneur works to make changes in a broader sense. Some examples are nurses who are healthcare consultants and legal nurse consultants, and nurses who establish businesses related to health care, such as a staffing agency, a business to develop a healthcare product, or a healthcare media business.

PATIENT ADVOCATE

Nurses serve as the patient and family **advocate**. The nurse may advocate on behalf of an individual, a family, a community, or a population. In this role, the nurse is a change agent and a risk taker. The nurse speaks for the patient but does not take away the patient's independence. A nurse caring for a patient in the hospital might advocate with the physician to alter care in order to allow a dying patient to spend more time with family. A nurse might advocate for better health coverage by writing to the local congressman or attending a meeting about care in the community. Additional information about advocacy is included in Chapters 6 and 9.

To meet the demands of these multiple roles, nurses need to be prepared and competent. Prerequisites and the nursing curriculum, through content, simulation laboratory experiences, and clinical experiences, help students to transition to these roles. The prerequisites provide content and experiences related to biological sciences, English and writing, sociology, government, languages, psychology, and mathematics and statistics. In nursing, course content relates to the care of a variety of patients in the hospital, in homes, and in communities; planning and implementing care; communication and interpersonal relationships; culture; teaching; community health;

epidemiology; issues related to safe, quality care; research and EBP; health policy; and leadership and management.

As discussed earlier in this chapter, this content relates to the knowledge base noted by the ANA's social policy statement. When students transition to the work setting as registered nurses, they should be competent as beginning nurses; however, the transition is often difficult. **Reality shock** may occur. This is a shocklike reaction that occurs when a new nurse is confronted with the realities of the healthcare setting and nursing, which are typically very different from what the nurse has experienced in school (Kramer, 1985). Knowledge and competency are important, but new nurses also need to build self-confidence, and they need time to adjust to the differences. Some schools of nursing, in collaboration with hospitals, now offer internship or residency-type programs for new graduates to decrease the reality shock. The major nursing roles that students learn about in their nursing programs are important in practice, but it is important for students to learn more about being an employee, working with and in teams, communicating in real situations, and functioning in complex organizations.

More nurses work in hospitals, particularly new graduates, than in other healthcare settings, though this number is decreasing. Hospital care has changed over the last 10 years, with sicker patients in the hospital for shorter periods and with greater use of complex technology. The healthcare delivery system is discussed in more detail in Chapter 6. These changes have an impact on what is expected of nurses: competencies. Nurses need to have clinical knowledge and communication competencies to be able to (Grando, 2001, p. 16):

1. Monitor and care for patients
2. Counsel patients' families
3. Interface and collaborate with other healthcare providers as part of healthcare team
4. Keep up with rapid technological advances
5. Effectively use information systems to manage patient care
6. Participate in clinical research

Nursing roles are influenced by nursing standards, nurse practice acts, professional ethics, and the nursing process. This topic is discussed in Chapter 9, which focuses on the first core healthcare professional competency: providing patient-centered care. Health policy also has an impact on roles; for example, legislation and changes in state practice guidelines were required before the advanced practice nurse could have prescriptive authority (ability to prescribe medications). This type of change in role requires a major advocacy effort from nurses and nursing organizations.

The Importance of Leadership to Nursing Roles: An Introduction

Many theories about leadership can apply to nursing. One theory that has become important to nursing is transformational leadership (Burns, 1985). The IOM (2003b) suggested that transformational leadership provides a patient safety net. This type of leadership focuses on:

- Developing a vision (a view of what could be) and working toward that vision
- Viewing the total picture
- Accepting change and making the most of it
- Guiding and rewarding staff
- Encouraging staff to be self-aware and willing to take risk; empowering staff (Burns; Barker, Sullivan, & Emery, 2006)

Transformational qualities are very important to the success of the transformational leader. These qualities are honesty, energy, self-confidence, commitment, and self-direction. This type of leader, however, does not ignore typical leadership functions, such as making decisions, taking responsibility for actions, planning, and all the activities required to accomplish the job.

Managers are part of every organization; however, not all managers are leaders. The major management functions are:

- Planning
- Organizing
- Leading
- Controlling

Reviewing what the transformation leader does and the qualities of this leadership indicates that leadership is more than these four functions. Typically, management is thought of as a formal

position, such as a nurse manager who has authority because of his or her position; however, leadership does not require a formal position. Leaders can be found anywhere, and they gain authority from the ability to influence others.

Nursing leadership is an important component of the profession, and it impacts, and is impacted by, nursing knowledge and caring. The American Organization of Nurse Executives (AONE) has identified guiding principles for future patient care delivery. These principles are a good example of the extent to which knowledge and caring are interrelated in nursing, and the importance of leadership. See Exhibit 2–5, which describes these principles.

Why should a student be concerned about leadership when entering a nursing program?

EXHIBIT 2–5 AONE GUIDING PRINCIPLES FOR FUTURE PATIENT CARE DELIVERY

Guiding Principle #1: The Core of Nursing is Knowledge and Caring.
The actual work that nurses do will change, but core values will remain.

Guiding Principle #2: Care is User-Based.
Care will be directed in partnership with the patient/client or population needs and will be respectful of the diversity of health belief models of all users.

Guiding Principle #3: Knowledge is Access Based.
The knowledge base of the nurse will shift from "knowing" a specific body of knowledge to "knowing how to access" the evolving knowledge base to support the needs of those for whom care is managed.

Guiding Principle #4: Knowledge is Synthesized.
The processing of accessed knowledge will shift the work of the nurse from critical thinking to "critical synthesis." Synthesis occurs as care is coordinated across multiple levels/disciplines/settings.

Guiding Principle #5: Relationships of Care.
Our knowledge and the care provided are grounded in the relationships with our patients/clients/populations. The relationship will be multidisciplinary and include the full societal scope of generations, diversity, and interdependency.

Guiding Principle #6: The "Virtual" and the "Presence" Relationship of Care.
The relationships will be dramatically changed by the increased application of technology, causing us to further define the relationship context as being "virtual" or "physical presence" and knowing when each is required.

Guiding Principle #7: Managing the Journey.
The work of the nurse in the future will be to partner with the patient/client to manage their journey in accordance with their needs and desires and available resources.

Source: The American Organization of Nurse Executives (AONE), 2005, *Voice of Nursing Leadership,* 5(2), p. 3. Reprinted with permission.

Students need to begin developing leadership qualities and competencies during their nursing education experience. This will allow new graduates to be more effective early after graduation and may help to decrease reality shock. Students have many opportunities to observe managers and leaders in the practice setting and even in the educational program. Leaders use reflective thinking and critical thinking. Leaders understand the importance of nursing knowledge and its relationship to nursing scholarship. Leaders advocate for EBP and the need for greater knowledge development through research. Leaders care about patients, families, and significant others, and their coworkers and colleagues. Leaders are effective in their roles and use leadership qualities to improve in whatever role they may be in. There are more staff nurses than there are managers, but this does not mean that every staff nurse could not be a leader. Students will observe and interact with managers in clinical settings who are not leaders. When this happens, students need to consider why this is so and how that manager could have demonstrated leadership. This type of reflection will help students develop leadership competencies. Students can take advantage of a variety of other opportunities to develop leadership, as mentioned in Chapter 1. Students may participate in the National Student Nurses Association or other campus organizations. Leadership competencies are not unique to nursing; they are generic and can be learned and used anywhere. "In today's increasingly less hierarchical and more lateral organizational structures, leadership is not about position of authority, as much as it is a role of influence. Staff nurses can and must lead through teamwork, the development of better practices, through the development of centrality of communication networks, and in contributing to the strategic management of units and departments" (Ferguson & Brindle, 2000, p. 5).

Conclusion

This chapter has highlighted the definitions of nursing, the changing skills sets needed by nurses, transformational leadership and ties to patient safety, ways of knowing, and the need for a movement toward nurses as knowledge workers.

CHAPTER HIGHLIGHTS

1. The definition of nursing is variable.
2. The need to define nursing relates to the ability to describe what nursing is and what it does.
3. The six professional characteristics of nursing according to the ANA (2003) are:
   a. Provision of a **caring relationship** that **facilitates** health and healing
   b. Attention to the **range of human experiences and responses to** health and illness within the physical and social environments
   c. **Integration of objective data with knowledge** gained from an appreciation of the patient's or group's **subjective experience**
   d. **Application of scientific knowledge** to the processes of diagnosis and treatment through the **use of judgment and critical thinking**
   e. **Advancement of professional nursing knowledge** through **scholarly inquiry**
   f. **Influence on social and public policy** to promote social justice
4. Competency is defined by and related to the new skills that nurses need to function in today's healthcare environment.
5. The movement toward preparing nurses as knowledge workers is discussed.
6. The key roles of the nurse are care provider, educator, manager, advocate, counselor,

researcher, change agent (intrapreneur), and entrepreneur.

7. Transformational leadership is described as it relates to the new healthcare environment.

8. Differences between management and leadership are described.

Linking to the Internet

- National Institutes of Health
  http://www.nih.gov
- National Institute of Nursing Research
  http://www.ninr.nih.gov/
- American Nurses Association
  http://www.nursingworld.org
- North American Nursing Diagnosis (NANDA) International
  http://www.nanda.org/html/about.html
- Nursing Interventions Classification (NIC)
  http://www.nursing.uiowa.edu/
  excellence/nursing_knowledge/clinical_
  effectiveness/nic.htm
- Nursing-Sensitive Outcomes Classification (NOC)

  http://www.nursing.uiowa.edu/
  excellence/nursing_knowledge/clinical_
  effectiveness/nocpubs.htm
- Omaha Nursing Classification System for Community Health
  http://www.himss.org/content/files/
  ImplementationNursingTerminology
  Community.pdf
- International Classification for Nursing Practice (ICNP®)
  http://www.icn.ch/icnp.htm
- Our Concept of Critical Thinking
  http://www.criticalthinking.org/aboutCT/
  ourConceptCT.cfm
- Defining Critical Thinking
  http://www.criticalthinking.org/about
  CT/definingCT.cfm
- Sigma Theta Tau International: Nursing Knowledge International
  http://www.nursingknowledge.org/
  Portal/main.aspx?PageID=32
- Nursing Theory Information
  http://www.sandiego.edu/academics/
  nursing/theory/

DISCUSSION QUESTIONS

1. Discuss the relationship between knowledge and caring in nursing.
2. How might knowing the definition of nursing impact how you practice?
3. What is meant by knowledge worker?
4. What are the characteristics of a transformational leader?
5. What are the characteristics of a nurse manager?
6. Describe the nurse's role in today's healthcare system.
7. Why are competencies important?
8. Discuss the difference between management and leadership.
9. Why should a staff nurse demonstrate leadership?
10. Discuss the role of critical thinking in nursing education and why there is little agreement about what constitutes critical thinking.

CRITICAL THINKING ACTIVITIES

1. Based on what you have learned about critical thinking, assess your own ability to use critical thinking. Write down your strengths and limitations regarding using critical thinking. Determine several strategies that you might use to improve your critical thinking. Write down these strategies and track your improvement over the semester. Use the critical thinking Web link to guide you in this activity.

2. Review the descriptions of the nursing theories found in Exhibit 2–2. Compare and contrast the theories in relationship to views of person, environment, health, and nursing. Identify two similarities and dissimilarities in the theories. Select a theory that you feel represents your view of nursing at this time. Why did you select this theory?

3. Caring is a concept central to nursing. Review the description of the nursing theories found in Exhibit 2–2. Identify which theories emphasize caring, and describe how this is demonstrated in the theory.

4. Go to the National Institute of Nursing Research Web site (http://www.ninr.nih. gov/AboutNINR/) and click Mission & Strategic Plan. Explore Ongoing Research Interests. What are some of the interests? Do any of them intrigue you? If so, why? Now click Nursing Research—Making a Difference. What can you learn about past and current nursing research? Did you think of these areas of study as part of nursing before this course? Why or why not? What impressed you about the research? Do you think these results are practice oriented?

5. Describe someone you think demonstrates leadership qualities. Explain why you think he or she demonstrates leadership. (You do not have to choose a nurse.)

6. What does caring mean to you? How does your view of caring compare with what you have learned in this chapter?

7. Do you think nursing scholarship is important? Provide your rationale for your response.

8. Select one of the major nursing roles and describe it and why you would want to function in this role.

9. Interview a staff nurse, nurse manager, and educator and ask for their definition of nursing. Compare your answers. Why do you believe there are differences?

10. Ask a consumer to describe the role of a nurse; then compare it with your view of nursing. Is it similar or different, and why?

CASE STUDY

A Historical Event to Demonstrate Importance of the Art and Science of Nursing, Nursing Roles, and Leadership

The following case is a true story. After reading the case, respond to the questions.

In the 1960s, something significant began to happen in hospital care and, ultimately, in the nursing profession. But first, let's go back to the 1950s for some background information. There was increasing interest in coronary care during this time, particularly for acute myocardial infarctions (AMIs). It is important to remember that changes in health care are certainly influenced by changes in science and technology, but incidents and situations within the country as a whole also drive change and policy decisions. This situation was no exception. Presidents Eisenhower and Johnson both had AMIs, which received a lot of press coverage. The mortality rate from AMIs was high. There were also significant new advances in care monitoring and interventions: cardiac catherization, cardiac pacemakers, continuous monitoring of cardiac electrical activity, portable cardiac defibrillator, and external pacemakers. This really was an incredible list to come onto the scene at the same time.

Now, what was happening with nursing in the 1950s regarding the care of cardiac patients? Even with advances, nurses were providing traditional care, and the boundaries between physicians and nurses were very clear.

Physicians

Examined the patient
Took the EKG
Drew blood for lab work
Diagnosed cardiac arrhythmias
Determined interventions

Nurses

Made the patient comfortable
Took care of the patient's belongings
Answered the family's questions
Took vital signs (blood pressure, pulse, respirations)
Made observations and documented them

In the 1960s, change began to happen. Bethany Hospital in Kansas City had a physician, Dr. Hughes Day, who had an interest in cardiac care. The hospital redesigned its units, moving away from open wards to private and semiprivate rooms. This was nice for the patients, but it made it difficult for nurses to observe patients. (This is a good example of how environment and space impact care.) Day established a Code Blue to provide response to patients having critical cardiac episodes. This was a great idea but often came too late for many patients who were not observed early enough. He also instituted monitoring of patients with cardiac problems who were unstable. Another good idea, but what would happen if there was a problem? Who would intervene, and how? Day would often be called, even at home at night, but how could he get to the hospital in time in such a critical situation? Nurses had no training or experience with the monitoring equipment or in recognizing arrhythmias, or knowledge about what to do if there were problems. Day (1972) was beginning to see that his ideas needed revision.

At the same time that Day was exploring cardiac care, Dr. L. Meltzer was involved in similar activity at the Presbyterian Hospital in Philadelphia. Each did not know of the work that the other was doing. Meltzer went about the problem a little differently. He knew that a separate unit was needed for cardiac patients, but he was less sure about how to design it and how it would function. Meltzer approached the Division of Nursing, U.S. Public Health Services, for a grant to study the problem. He wanted to establish a two-bed cardiac care unit (CCU). His research question was, Will nurse monitoring and intervention reduce the high incidence of arrhythmic deaths from AMIs? At this time, and good for nursing, Faye Abdella, PhD, RN, was leading the Division of Nursing. She really liked the study proposal but felt that there was something important missing. To receive the grant, Meltzer needed to have a nurse lead the project. Meltzer proceeded to look for that nurse. He turned to the University of Pennsylvania and asked the dean of nursing for a recommendation. Rose Pinneo, MSN, RN, a nurse who had just completed her master's and had experience in cardiac care, was selected. Meltzer and Pinneo became a team. Pinneo liked research and wanted to do this kind of work By chance, she had her opportunity. What she did not know was that this study and its results would have a major impact on the nursing profession.

Dr. Zoll, who worked with Meltzer, recognized the major issue: Nurses had no training in what would be required of them in the CCU. This represented a major shift in what nurses usually did. If this was not changed, no study could be conducted based on the research question that they had proposed. Notably, Meltzer proposed a new role for nurses in the CCU:

- The nurse has specific skills in monitoring patients using the new equipment.
- RNs would provide all the care. Up until this time, the typical care organization was a team of licensed practical nurses and aides, who provided most of the direct care, led by an RN (team nursing). This had to change in the CCU.
- RNs would interpret heart rhythms using continuous-monitoring EKG data.
- RNs would initiate emergency interventions when needed.
- The RN, not the MD, is central to CCU care 24-7.

There were questions as to whether RNs could be trained for this new role, but Meltzer had no doubt that they could be.

In 1963, Rose Pinneo entered the picture. Based on Meltzer's plan and the new role, she needed to find the nurses for the units. She wanted nurses who were ready for a challenge and who were willing to learn the new knowledge and skills needed and to collect data. Collecting data would be time consuming, plus the nurses had to provide care in a very new role. The first step after finding the nurses was training. This too was unique. It was interdisciplinary, and it took place in the clinical setting, the CCU. Clinical conferences were held to discuss patients and their care once the unit opened.

The nurses found that they were providing care for highly complex problems. They were assessing and diagnosing, intervening, and having to help patients with their psychological responses to having had an AMI. Clearly, knowledge and caring were important, but added to this was curing. With the interventions that nurses initiated, they were saving lives. Standing orders telling nurses what to do in certain situations based on data they collected were developed by Meltzer and used. House staff, physicians in training,

began to turn to the nurses to learn because the CCU nurses had experience with these patients. Meltzer called his approach the scientific team approach. Ten years later, he wrote, "Until World War II even the recording of blood pressure was considered outside the nursing sphere and was the responsibility of a physician. As late as 1962, when coronary care was introduced, most hospitals did not permit their nursing staff to perform venipunctures or to start intravenous infusions. That nurses could interpret the electrocardiograms and defibrillate patients indeed represented a radical change for all concerned" (Meltzer, Pinneo, & Kitchell, 1972, p. 8).

What were the results of this study? Nurses could learn what was necessary to function in the new role. Nurses who worked in CCU gained autonomy, but now the boundaries between physicians and nurses were less clear, and this began to spill over into other areas of nursing. There is no doubt that nursing began to change. CCUs opened across the country. They also had an impact on other types of intensive care.

Case Questions

If you do not know any terms in this case, look them up in a medical dictionary.

1. Based on this case, discuss the implications of the art and science of nursing.
2. What were the differences in how Dr. Day and Dr. Meltzer handled their interests in changing cardiac care?
3. Who led this initiative? Why is this significant?
4. Compare and contrast the changes in nursing roles before the Melzer and Day studies. What was the role supported by their work?
5. What about this case is unique and unexpected?
6. What does this case tell you about the value of research?

Sources:

Day, H. (1972). History of coronary care units. *American Journal of Cardiology, 30,* 405.

Meltzer, L., Pinneo, R., & Kitchell, J. (1972). *Intensive coronary care: A manual for nurses.* Philadelphia: Charles Press.

WORDS OF WISDOM

Nancy Batchelor, MSN, RNC, CNS
Assistant Professor of Clinical Nursing,
University of Cincinnati College of Nursing
Staff Nurse, Hospice of Cincinnati, East
Inpatient Unit, Cincinnati, Ohio

Hospice nursing is different from any other type of nursing. Some feel that it is a ministry. The focus is on providing holistic care for the patient diagnosed with terminal disease and the family. Hospice and palliative care nurses care for patients who have incurable disease. The hospice nurse manages symptoms to allow the patient the highest quality of life possible while moving along life's continuum toward death. Hospice and palliative care nursing is a growing specialty, and it will continue to grow as the population ages and as individuals cope with chronic disease. Hospice and palliative care nurses deliver care based on principles identified by Florence Nightingale: caring, comfort, compassion, dignity, and quality.

As a hospice inpatient care center nurse, I care for my patients using the above principles. Besides using my technical nursing skills, I am able to spend time with them doing the "little things" that make them more comfortable—whether it is holding their hand, giving a massage, sharing a snack, reminiscing about their lives, alleviating the burden of care from the family, praying, or just providing a caring presence. Depending on the situation, I may prepare my "angels in waiting" to return home with family, to a level of long-term care, or to the hereafter. I feel totally blessed and privileged to minister: to alleviate suffering, to facilitate bereavement, and to prepare for transition from life to death.

References

Alfaro-LeFevre, R. (2006). *Applying nursing process. A tool for critical thinking.* Philadelphia: Lippincott Williams & Wilkins.

American Association Colleges of Nursing. (1999, March). *Position statement on defining scholarship for the discipline of nursing.* Washington, DC: Author.

American Association of Critical Care Nurses. (2005). *The AACN synergy model for patient care.* Aliso Viejo, CA: Author.

American Nurses Association. (2003). *Nursing's social policy statement.* Silver Spring, MD: Author.

American Nurses Association. (2004). *Nursing: Scope and standards of practice.* Silver Spring, MD: Author.

Barker, A. M., Sullivan, D. T., & Emery, M. J. (2006). *Leadership competencies for clinical managers: The renaissance of transformational leadership.* Sudbury, MA: Jones and Bartlett.

Benner, P. (2001). *From novice to expert: Excellence and power in clinical nursing practice* (Commemorative Edition). Upper Saddle River, NJ: Prentice Hall.

Benner, P. (2007, June). *Educating nurses: Teaching and learning a complex practice of care.* Based on the Carnegie Foundation Study. Presented at the fifth annual conference of State Nursing Workforce Centers, San Francisco, CA.

Boswell, C., & Cannon, S. (2007). *Introduction to nursing research: Incorporating evidence-based practice.* Sudbury, MA: Jones and Bartlett.

Boyer, E. (1990). *Scholarship reconsidered: Priorities for the professionate.* Princeton, NJ: Carnegie Foundation for the Advancement of Teaching.

Burns, J. (1985). *Leadership.* New York: Harper Collins.

Butcher, H. (2006). Integrating nursing theory, nursing research, and nursing practice. In J. P. Cowen & S. Moorehead (Eds.), *Current issues in nursing* (7th ed., pp. 112–122). St. Louis, MO: Mosby.

Carper, B. (1978). Fundamental patterns of knowing in nursing. *Advances in Nursing Science, 17*(4), 73–86.

Cipriano, P. (2007). Celebrating the art and science of nursing. *American Nurse Today, 2*(5), 8.

Conway, J. (1998). Evolution of the species "expert nurse." An examination of practical knowledge held by expert nurses. *Journal of Clinical Nursing, 7*(1), 75–82.

Cook, T., Gilmer, M., & Bess, C. (2003). Beginning students' definitions of nursing: An inductive framework of professional identity. *Journal of Nursing Education, 42*(7), 311–317.

Decker, S. (2007). Integrating guided reflection into simulated learning. In P. Jeffries (Ed.), *Simulation in nursing education* (pp. 73–85). New York: National League for Nursing.

DeKeyser, F., & Medoff-Cooper, B. (2002). A non-theorist's perspective on nursing theory: Issues in the 1990s. *Scholarly Inquiry for Nursing Practice: An International Journal, 15*, 329–341.

Dickenson-Hazard, N. (2002). Evidence-based practice: "The right approach." *Reflections in Nursing Leadership, 28*(2), 6.

Diers, D. (2001). What is nursing? In J. Dochterman & H. Grace (Eds.), *Current issues in nursing* (pp. 5–13). St. Louis, MO: Mosby.

Ferguson, S., & Brindle, M. (2000). Nursing leadership: Vision and the reality. *Nursing Spectrum, 10*(21DC), 5.

Finkelman, A. (2001, December). Problem-solving, decision-making, and critical thinking: How do they mix and why bother? *Home Care Provider,* 194–199.

Finkelman, A. (2006). *Leadership and management in nursing.* Upper Saddle River, NJ: Pearson Education.

Grando, V. (2001). Staff nurses working in hospitals. In J. P. Cowen & S. Moorehead (Eds.), *Current issues in nursing* (7th ed., pp. 14–18). St. Louis, MO: Mosby.

Hansten, R., & Washburn, M. (2000). Intuition in professional practice: Executive and staff perceptions. *Journal of Nursing Administration, 30*, 185–189.

Henderson, V. (1991). *The nature of nursing: Reflections after 25 years.* Geneva, Switzerland: International Council of Nurses.

Husted, G., & Husted, J. (2001). *Bioethical decision making in nursing and health care: A symphonological approach* (3rd ed.). New York: Springer.

Institute of Medicine. (2003a). *Health professions education: A bridge to quality.* Washington, DC: National Academies Press.

Institute of Medicine. (2003b). *Keeping patients safe: Transforming the work environment of nurses.* Washington, DC: National Academies Press.

Johns, C. (2004). *Becoming a reflective practitioner* (2nd ed.). Malden, MA: Blackwell.

Kerfoot, K. (2002). The leader as chief knowledge officer. *Nursing Economics, 20*(1), 40–41, 43.

Kozier, B., Erb, G., & Blais, K. (1997). *Professional nursing practice: Concepts and perspectives.* Menlo Park, CA: Addison Wesley Longman.

Kramer, M. (1985). Why does reality shock continue? In J. McCloskey & H. Grace (Eds.), *Current issues in nursing* (pp. 891–903). Boston: Blackwell Scientific.

Locsin, R. (1995). Machine technologies and caring in nursing. *Image: Journal of Nursing Scholarship, 27*, 201–203.

Locsin, R. (2005). *Technological competency as caring in nursing. A model for practice.* Indianapolis, IN: Sigma Theta Tau International.

Maas, M. (2006). What is nursing, and why do we ask? In P. Cowen & S. Moorhead (Eds.), *Current issues in nursing* (7th ed., pp. 5–10). St. Louis, MO: Mosby.

Mason, D. (2006). Scholarly? *AJN* is redefining a crusty old term. *American Journal of Nursing, 106*(1), 11.

McCloskey, J., & Bulechek, G. (Eds.). (2002). *Nursing interventions classification (NIC): Iowa intervention project* (3rd ed.). St. Louis, MO: Mosby.

Meleis, A. (1992). Directions for nursing theory development in the 21st century. *Nursing Science Quarterly, 5*, 112–117.

Merton, R. (1968). *Social theory and social structure.* Glencoe, IL: Free Press.

Moland, L. (2006). Moral integrity and regret in nursing. In S. Nelson & S. Gordon (Eds.), *The complexities of care: Nursing reconsidered* (pp. 50–68). Ithaca, NY: Cornell University Press.

Mooney, K. (2001). Advocating for quality cancer care: Making evidence-based practice a reality. *Oncology Nursing Forum, 28*(Suppl. 2), 17–21.

Moorehead, S., Johnson, M., & Maas, M. L. (Eds.) (2007). *Nursing outcomes classification* (4th ed.). St. Louis, MO: Mosby.

Mustard, L. (2002). Caring and competency. *JONA's Healthcare Law, Ethics, and Regulation, 4*(2), 36–43.

National Council of State Boards of Nursing. (1996). *Definition of competence and standards for competence.* Chicago: Author.

Nelson, S., & Gordon, S. (Eds.). (2006). *The complexities of care: Nursing reconsidered.* Ithaca, NY: Cornell University Press.

North American Nursing Diagnosis Association. (2003). *Nursing diagnoses: Definitions and classification 2003–2004.* Philadelphia: Author.

Ohlen, J., & Segesten, K. (1998). The professional identity of the nurse: Concept analysis and development. *Journal of Advanced Nursing, 28*, 720–727.

Paul, R. (1995). *Critical thinking: How to prepare students for a rapidly changing world.* Santa Rosa, CA: Midwest Publishing.

Pellegrino, E. (1985). The care ethic. In A. Bishop & J. Scudder (Eds.), *Caring, curing, coping: Nurse, physician, and patient relationships.* Tuscaloosa: University of Alabama Press.

Pesut, D., & Herman, J. (1999). *Clinical reasoning: The art and science of critical and creative thinking*. Albany, NY: Delmar.

Porter-O'Grady, T. (2001). Profound change: 21st century nursing. *Nursing Outlook, 49*, 182–186.

Porter-O'Grady, T., & Malloch, K. (2007). *Quantum leadership: A resource for health care innovation* (2nd ed.). Sudbury, MA: Jones and Bartlett.

Pravikoff, D., Tanner, A. B., & Pierce, S. T. (2005). Readiness of U.S. Nurses for Evidence-Based Practice. *American Journal of Nursing, 105*(9), 40–50.

Reed, P. (2006). The practitioner in nursing epistemology. *Nursing Science Quality, 19*(1), 36–38.

Rubenfeld, M., & Scheffer, B. (2006). *Critical thinking tactics for nurses*. Sudbury, MA: Jones and Bartlett.

Schwein, J. (2004). The timeless caring connection. *Nursing Administration Quarterly, 28*(4), 265–270.

Scotto, C. (2003). A new view of caring. *Journal of Nursing Education, 42*, 289–291.

Sorrels-Jones, J. (1999). The role of the chief nurse executive in the knowledge-intense organization of the future. *Nursing Administration Quarterly, 23*(3), 17–25.

Sullivan, A. (2006). Nursing theory. In J. Zerwekh & J. Claborn (Eds.), *Nursing Today* (pp. 159–178). St. Louis, MO: Elsevier.

University of Adelaide Library Guides. (2005). *Nursing journal contents*. Retrieved May 23, 2005, from http://www.library.adelaide.edu.au/guide/med/nursing/nursjnl.html

Watson, J. (1979). *Nursing: The philosophy and science of caring*. Boston: Little, Brown.

Westberg, J., & Jason, H. (2001). *Fostering reflection and providing feedback*. New York: Springer.

Zerwekh, J., & Claborn, J. (2006). *Nursing today: Transition and trends*. St. Louis, MO: W. B. Saunders.

Chapter 3

The Image of Nursing: What It Is and How It Needs to Change

CHAPTER OBJECTIVES

At the conclusion of this chapter, the learner will be able to:

- Discuss critical issues related to visibility of nursing
- Describe the current and past image of nursing and critical related issues
- Describe advertising and media and how they relate to the nursing image
- Discuss the advantages and disadvantages of the Johnson & Johnson campaign
- Explain the importance of the following nursing initiatives and their relationship to image: Nurses for a Healthier Tomorrow, Nursing's Agenda for the Future, and the Institute of Medicine's *Quality Series* reports
- Discuss strategies that impact image: generational issues, power and empowerment, and professional presentation

OUTLINE

KEY TERMS

- ❏ Advertising
- ❏ Advocacy
- ❏ Assertiveness
- ❏ Colleagueship
- ❏ Empowerment

- ❏ Image
- ❏ Influence
- ❏ Power
- ❏ Powerlessness

Introduction

Image may appear to be an unusual topic for a nursing textbook, but it is not. Image is part of a profession. It is the way a person appears to others, or, in the case of the profession, the way that profession appears to other disciplines and to the general public—consumers of health care. Image and the perception of the profession impact recruitment of students, the view of the public, funding for nursing education and research, relationships with healthcare administrators and other healthcare professionals, government agencies and legislators at all levels of government, and, ultimately, the profession's self-identity. Just like individuals may feel depressed or less effective if others view them negatively, professionals can experience similar reactions if their image is not positive. It impacts everything the profession does or wishes to do.

The content in this chapter focuses on the image of nursing from the perspectives of how the profession views its own image and how those outside the profession view nursing and nurses. Image is a part of any profession. How nurses view themselves—their professional self-image—has an impact on professional self-esteem. How one is viewed has an impact on whether others seek that person out and how they view the effectiveness of what that person might do. The content in this chapter includes discussion about the importance of visibility, the current image of nursing, various nursing initiatives that relate to image, and the importance of the media and of **advertising** nursing. Examples of strategies that may impact image are described, particularly generational issues, **power** and **empowerment**, and examples are given regarding how nurses present themselves to communicate the value of the profession. Every time a nurse says to family, friends, or in public that he or she is a nurse, he or she is representing the profession and has an impact on the image of nursing. Buresh and Gordon stated, "We cannot expect outsiders to be the guardians of our visibility and access to public media and health policy arenas. We must develop the skills of presenting ourselves in the media and to the media—We have to take the responsibility for moving from silence to voice" (Buresh & Gordon, 2000, as cited in Benner, 2005, p. 15).

Visibility: Good or Bad?

"Although nurses comprise the majority of healthcare professionals, they are largely invisible. Their competence, skill, knowledge, and judgment are—as the word 'image' suggests—only a reflection, not reality" (Sullivan, E. J., 2004, p. 45). The public views of nursing and nurses are typically based on personal experiences with nurses, which can lead to a narrow view of a nurse often based only on a brief personal experience. This experience may not provide an accurate picture of all that nurses can and do provide in the healthcare delivery process. In addition, this view is impacted by the emotional response of a person to the situation in which he or she encountered a nurse. But the truth is that most often, the nurse is invisible. Consumers may not recognize that they are interacting with

a nurse, or they may think someone is a nurse who is not. When patients go to their doctor's office, they interact with staff, and often these patients think that they are interacting with a registered nurse (RN). Most likely, they are not, and the staff person is a medical aide of some type, or maybe a licensed practical/vocational nurse. When in the hospital, patients interact with many staff, and there is little to distinguish one from another, so patients may refer to most staff as nurses.

This does not mean that the public does not value nurses—quite the contrary. When a person tells another that he or she is a nurse, the typical response is positive. However, many people do not know about the education required to become a nurse and to maintain current knowledge, or about the great variety of educational entry points into nursing that all lead to the RN qualification. Consumers generally view nurses as "good people" who care for others. The annual Gallup Poll lists nursing on the annual list of occupations rated for honesty and ethical standards by 4 out of 5 Americans. This high vote of confidence has been a consistent result in the poll over time (Saad, 2006). What is not mentioned is that knowledge and competency are required to do the job.

Each year there is an annual National Nurses Week, and within this week is a designated National Nurses Day, May 6, just as there is an annual recognition week for many workers and professionals. This period was chosen because it coincides with Florence Nightingale's birthday, May 12, which is International Nurses Day. Nursing, primarily through the American Nurses Association (ANA), identifies an annual theme and issues that are emphasized during the week. In 2007, as part of Nurses Week, the ANA and the Congressional Nursing Caucus (nurses who are in Congress) held a luncheon briefing for Congress that focused on an important nursing concern: safe patient handling. Invited guests were congressional staff who dealt with health issues. "Over the past decade, attention has been given to the health and safety concerns among healthcare workers. Despite the recognition that manual patient handling is a high-hazard task, the incidence of musculoskeletal disorders persists at high rates for nurses and other healthcare personnel" (ANA, 2007a). Nurses Week is also used as an opportunity to recognize nurses in practice and to advertise the profession of nursing, increasing its visibility and portraying a positive image. In 2007, ANA president Rebecca M. Patton, MSN, RN, CNOR, stated in her letter about this special annual event, "I hope you take time to reflect on how rewarding a nursing career can be, and to share your passion for nursing with others. This week is an opportunity to take stock, and take pride in what you accomplish as nurses, and hopefully to inspire others to choose this challenging and fulfilling profession" (ANA, 2007b). Why would a profession with an effective image make this type of statement? It should not need to do this; however, the nursing profession does need to be reminded of these issues and to step up and be more visible.

During the week, healthcare organizations typically hold special celebrations to honor nurses, give out awards for leadership and other accomplishments, and announce via the media (such as local newspapers, radio, and TV) how proud they are of their nurses. Stories and photos that are provided to the media tend to focus on caring—a nurse holding a patient's hand or talking to a patient. This is not to say that this type of image is not important in nursing, because it is; however, it portrays a limited image of nursing. There is less recognition of the other complex professional aspects of nursing. The critical question about the visibility of nursing is, Who is driving the image and its accuracy?

Why Is It Important for Nurses to Be More Visible?

Students may wonder why it is so important for nurses to be more visible. They chose nursing, so they know that it is an important profession. However, when they enter nursing, many students also have a narrow view of the profession, much closer to what is portrayed in the media—the nurse who cares for others with less understanding of the knowledge base required and competency needed to meet the complex needs of patients. There is limited recognition that nursing is a scientific field. The profession needs to be more concerned about visibility because nursing is struggling to attract qualified students and keep current nurses in practice.

The nurse's voice is typically silent, and this has demoralized nursing (Pike, 2001). This is a strong statement and may be a confusing one. What is the nurse's voice? It is the "unique perspectives and contributions that nurses bring to patient care" (Pike, 2001, p. 449). Nurses have been silent about what they do and how they do it, but this has been a choice that nurses have had—to be silent or to be more visible. External and internal factors have impacted the nurse's voice and this silence. The external factors are (Pike, 2001):

- Historical role of nurse as handmaiden (*not an independent role*)
- Hierarchical structure of healthcare organizations (*has often limited the role of nursing in decision making*)
- Perceived authority and directives of physicians (*has limited independent role of nurses*)
- Hospital policy (*has often limited nursing actions*)
- Threat of disciplinary or legal action or loss of job (*might limit a nurse when he or she needs to speak out—advocate*)

The internal factors to consider are:

- Role confusion
- Lack of professional confidence
- Timidity
- Fear
- Insecurity
- Sense of inferiority

Nurses who can deal with the internal factors can be more visible and less silent about nursing. These factors combined have damaged nurses' professional self-esteem, so nurses are less likely to present themselves in a positive light (Pike, 2001). This loss of professional pride and self-esteem can also lead to a more serious professional problem: Nurses feel like victims and then act like victims. Victims do not take control, but rather see others in control; they abdicate responsibility. They play passive-aggressive games to exert power. This can be seen in the image of nurses, which is predominantly driven by forces outside the profession. This also has an impact on the nurse's ability to collaborate with others—other nurses and other healthcare professionals. It is much easier for nurses to feel like victims, and this has also had an impact on nurses viewing physicians in a negative light, emphasizing that physicians have done this "to us." As a consequence, nurses have problems saying that they are colleagues with other healthcare professionals and acting like colleagues. "**Colleagueship** involves entering into a collaborative relationship that is characterized by mutual trust and response and an understanding of the perspective each partner contributes" (Pike, 2001, p. 449). Colleagues:

- Do not let inter- or intraprofessional competition and antagonism from the past drive the present and future
- Integrate their work to provide the best care

- Acknowledge that they share a common goal: quality patient care
- Recognize interdependence
- Share responsibility and accountability for patient care outcomes
- Recognize that collegial relationships are safe
- Handle conflict in a positive manner

What is unexpected is how nurses' silence may actually have a negative impact on patient care. "The choice a nurse makes about how he/she defines his/her professional self affects not only his/her morale but also the nature of care the patients receive" (Pike, 2001, p. 451). It influences how a nurse might speak out to get the care that a patient needs; how effective a nurse can be on the treatment team; and how nurses participate in healthcare program planning on many levels. Each nurse has the responsibility and accountability to define himself or herself as a colleague; empowerment is part of this process (empowerment is discussed in more detail later in this chapter).

Visibility also has an impact on consumers and how they view nurses. As health care changes—and it will most likely experience greater changes in the future to address healthcare reimbursement—nurses need to be actively involved in this process: in policy and funding decisions and regarding any aspect of changes that impact nursing care and broader healthcare issues. If nurses are not viewed as vital members of the healthcare team and are seen only as team members who hold a patient's hand or serve as "an angels of mercy," they will not be more visible in the critical process of change. Chapter 5 includes content about health policy and **advocacy**, which is directly impacted by the visibility of nursing. What is its image, and will that image empower the profession? Does nursing have anything to offer when healthcare issues are addressed? Yes it does, but nurses need to become more effective in communicating what nursing has to offer.

Current Image of Nursing and How It Is Impacted by Past Images

The role of nursing has experienced many changes, and many more will occur. How has nursing responded to these changes and communicated them to the public and other healthcare professionals? Suzanne Gordon, a journalist who has written a lot about the nursing profession, noted that often it is the media that is accused of representing nursing poorly, when in reality, the media is reflecting the public image of nursing (Buresh & Gordon, 2006). Nurses have not taken the lead in standing up and discussing their own image of nursing—what it is and what it is not. It is not uncommon for a nurse to refuse to talk to the press because he or she feels no need, or sometimes because of the fear of reprisal from his or her employer. When nurses do speak to the press, often when being praised for an action, they say, "Oh, I was just doing my job." This statement undervalues the reality that critical quick thinking on the part of nurses daily saves lives. What is wrong with taking that credit? Because of these types of responses in the media, nursing is not directing the image, but rather accepting what is described as nursing by those outside the profession.

Gordon and Nelson commented that nursing needs to move "away from the 'virtue script' toward a knowledge-based identity" (2005, p. 62). The "virtue script" continues to be present in current media campaigns that are supported by the profession. For example, a video produced by the National Student Nurses Association mentions knowledge but not many details, and instead it includes statements such as "[nursing is a] job where people will love you" (Gordon & Nelson, 2005). How helpful is this approach? Is this view

of being loved based on today's nursing reality? Nursing practice involves highly complex care; it can be stressful, demanding, and at times rewarding, but it is certainly not as simple as "everyone will love you." Why do nurses continue to describe themselves in this way? "One reason nurses may rely so heavily on the 'virtue script' is that many believe this is their only legitimate source of status, respect, and self-esteem" (Gordon & Nelson, 2005, p. 67). This, however, is a view that perpetuates the victim mentality.

The connection of nursing with the "angel" image is not helping the profession. There needs to be a more contemporary image of nursing to attract the next generation of nurses. People have many career options today, and most want careers that are intellectually stimulating. How do nurses describe what they do? Frequently, they tell stories of hand-holding and emotional experiences with patients, leaving out the knowledge-based care that requires high levels of competency. At the same time, nurses are confronting heavy pressure to demonstrate how nursing impacts patient outcomes. However, it is difficult to respond to this pressure if nurses themselves do not appreciate, and articulate to others, their role and the knowledge and competency required to provide effective nursing care. Nurses must remember that, in general, the public wants a competent nurse regardless of whether he or she is warm and friendly.

How Do Nurses View Themselves?

Current data indicate that the number of nurses in the United States is very high compared with other countries and growing, but still there is a shortage. The National Sample Survey of Registered Nurses is conducted every 4 years by the Health Resources and Services Administration (U.S. Department of Health and Human Services, 2006). This report presents an overview of the personal, professional, and employment characteristics of the 2.9 million RNs residing in the

United States as of March 2004. The profession is not taking full advantage of these statistics to leverage **influence**. More details about the survey are described in Exhibit 3–1.

In 2006, Cohen (2007) conducted a survey of emergency room nurses, asking questions about what the nurse participants thought mattered. A total 331 nurses responded to the following issues and questions:

1. How we present ourselves to patients and families
2. How we dress
3. How skilled we appear to be at our jobs
4. Misinformation from TV and other media
5. Whether we introduce ourselves as nurses
6. How we appear to get along with co-workers
7. Whether we belong to the Emergency Nurses Association *(This survey was given only to nurses who worked in emergency departments.)*
8. How we act around the nursing station, and so on.
9. Whether the patient and family feel that we care
10. How easily the patient and family can read our name tags

The results indicated that nurses thought Items 1–6, 8, and 9 were 75%–98% important to the image of nursing. Forty-five percent thought that Item 10 had a great effect on image, and 17% thought that Item 7 had a great effect on image. Most of the nurses in the sample were older than 30 years of age, with only 9% younger than 30, and 59.3% had more than 10 years of experience. The nurses were asked what change they thought would be the most important. Though the responses were varied for all 10 items, 8% indicated that dress was most important, and 3% responded that changing nurses' attitudes was most important. One conclusion from this result could be that the participants did not have a consensus opinion about what might improve the image of nursing.

Accessing Image and Increasing Visibility

How do the public, government agencies, and other healthcare professionals learn about nurs-

---

EXHIBIT 3–1 DATA ON THE NURSING PROFESSION: 2004

- Number of licensed registered nurses (RNs) in the United States grew by almost 8% between 2000 and 2004, to a new high of 2.9 million.
- Average age of RNs climbed to 46.8 years, the highest average age since the first comparable report was published in 1980.
- Just over 41% of RNs were 50 years of age or older (33% in 2000 and 25% in 1980).
- Only 8% of RNs were under the age of 30, compared with 25% in 1980.
- Average annual earnings for RNs were $57,785.
- Real earnings (comparable dollars over time) have grown almost 14% since 2000, the first significant increase in more than a decade.
- Employment in nursing rose to more than 83% of RNs with active licenses, the highest since 1980.
- RNs with master's or doctorate degrees rose to 376,901, an increase of 37% from 2000.

Source: Department of Health and Human Services (DHHS), Health Resources and Services Administration. The 2004 National Sample Survey of Registered Nurses. Retrieved July 9, 2007, from http://bhpr.hrsa.gov/healthworkforce/rnsurvey04/

ing? How do those who might want to enter the profession learn about nursing? Where could one get an accurate snapshot of nursing?

Advertising Nursing

Advertising is done by employers and schools of nursing for recruitment, and professional organizations advertise to make nursing more visible. Why advertise nursing? This is a reasonable question and one that the profession needs to understand. Goals for any initiative need to come from understanding the need, and goals for advertising nursing are no different. There are a number of reasons for advertising nursing. First, of course, is the need to attract more qualified people to nursing and to attract minorities and men to the profession. Second, advertising has an impact on other groups that need to know about nursing—what nurses do and the impact that nurses have on health care and outcomes. These groups include policy makers, healthcare organizations, insurers, educators, school counselors who may direct students into nursing, and the consumer. Given these two clear needs, any advertising campaign should offer messages to multiple groups. Even when a school of nursing uses advertising to recruit students, it also advertises about nursing in general to the public. This makes the advertising complex. The following exemplar illustrates one complex, multipronged campaign that has received positive and negative reviews.

Exemplar: *Johnson & Johnson Campaign: Discover Nursing*

Johnson & Johnson (J&J) funded an advertising campaign to promote nursing as a career. The initiative, called Campaign for Nursing's Future, was started several years ago. The ads are sentimental, and the theme is "the importance of a nurse's touch." "In them, we see caring young nurses helping patients ranging from a newborn to an older man. The spots are certainly well-produced. And they do include a few elements that suggest the nurses have some skill. But sadly, the ads rely mainly on the same kind of unhelpful angel and maternal imagery that infected the Campaign's original 'Dare to Care' ads. And that era's four-minute Recruitment Video, complete with the gooey theme song, is still circulating. Of course, "caring" is an important part of nursing. But everyone knows that, and we believe that only greater understanding that nurses actually save lives and improve patient outcomes will attract the resources nursing needs in the long term" (Center for Nursing Advocacy, 2006).

Despite negative critique by the Center for Nursing Advocacy and others, J&J has contributed to the positive image of nursing by its involvement in the following initiatives:

- Funding a nursing Web site in collaboration with the Center for Nursing Advocacy
- Raising funds for faculty fellowships and student scholarships
- Sponsoring a recruiting video, *Nurse Scientists: Committed to the Public Trust*. This video focuses on demonstrating how nurses can be scholars, particularly in the areas of cancer, HIV, geriatrics, and domestic violence

The J&J campaign's (Gordon & Nelson, 2005; response from Donelan, Buerhaus, Ulrich, Norman, & Dittus, 2005) theme was "caring and compassion" and included two 30-second television advertisements; five videos; eight million pieces of recruitment materials distributed to hospitals, nursing schools, and junior and senior high schools; a Web site; regional celebrations that raised scholarship and fellowship funds; training materials for students distributed on the Web site; and continuing education activities offered through *Nursing Spectrum.* Written materials were offered in English and Spanish. The cost of this campaign was $30 million.

This was an extremely complex, robust, and multifaceted advertising campaign. But was it successful? The evaluation team looked at awareness of, and solutions to, the nursing shortage, the profession's image, learning and work environments, and awareness of the J&J campaign.

It is clear that Americans are more aware of the nursing shortage and concerned about what it means to patient care, often because of a negative experience in a short-staffed hospital. Ninety percent of nurses who were aware of the J&J campaign felt that it had a positive impact on the public image of nursing, the number of students applying to nursing schools, recognition by healthcare organizations, and local and regional efforts to promote nursing. Ninety percent of students applying to nursing said that the campaign made them feel better about nursing; the campaign did not seem to push potential applicants into a decision to enter nursing, however, but rather made them more aware.

A key concern with the J&J campaign continues to be its limited focus on caring and compassion. Will this type of initiative—which may not be as reality based as it needs to be—lead to problems when those who use this limited view of nursing to make a decision to enter nursing and then find out that the view was not accurate, describing only one aspect of the profession (Gordon & Nelson, 2005)? A second J&J campaign focused more on the knowledge and technology required for nursing.

The Role of Media

Does the media really influence the image of nursing? "The news media can confer status upon issues, persons, organizations, or social movements by singling them out for attention. Audiences apparently subscribe to the circular belief that if something matters, it will be the focus of mass media attention" (Lazarsfeld & Merton, 1971, as cited in Kalisch & Kalisch, 2005, p. 12). Today, the media is a powerful force. Through a great variety of media methods, people can find information quickly; it is accessible anywhere, even on a cell phone. The media focuses not only on news but also on related information in broad areas, including health care and entertainment, and also provides information to viewers. The media is interested in more than the news and weather. But if the media is to accurately portray nursing as more than just caring, we as nurses must provide the information. We must inform the public about our actions and activities and not be shy about taking credit when we deserve it.

MEDIA: TELEVISION, RADIO, FILM, INTERNET, BOOKS, AND MAGAZINES

Healthcare issues can be found in all types of media, news, and entertainment (film and television), and in publications such as magazines and books. How much is focused on nursing, and how is nursing portrayed? How can the profession keep up with the media and know what the trends are? This is very important because the profession needs information about the current media image(s) of nursing in order to advocate for change if it is required.

The Center for Nursing Advocacy, founded in 2001, was initially created to consider the nursing shortage. This organization approaches the nursing shortage problem from the perspective of the impact of nursing's image on the ability to attract qualified students to the profession and retain them long term. The center has been active in identifying media examples in which nursing is portrayed positively and negatively and to mobilize nurses to respond. These examples are made public through the center's Web site (http://nursingadvocacy.org). The center also develops campaigns to push for changes in media (television, radio, advertising, film, magazines, and so forth). The major functions of the Web site are to (Buresh & Gordon, 2006, p. 201):

1. Track depictions of nurses in the news, entertainment, and advertising media
2. Serve as an early warning system to alert nurses to problematic media images of nurses and mobilize them to respond so that creators of such images withdraw or amend them
3. Maintain an accessible archive of materials and reports on significant studies and developments in nursing

In 2006, the center was successful in influencing the Coors Brewery to change its ads, which featured "naughty nurse" imagery (Cohen, 2007). Exhibit 3–2 describes examples of negative images in the media as identified in the cen-

EXHIBIT 3–2 GOLDEN LAMP AWARDS

Best Media

John Blanton, *The Wall Street Journal,* "There and Back Again," Apr. 24. *Journal* editor Blanton resigned from the paper and became a nurse in a post-9/11 search for meaning. His piece focuses on the crushing workload and fear of error he faced as a new burn unit nurse. It has extensive descriptions of the complexity and importance of nursing care, and it ably describes Blanton's transition from novice toward higher competence.

Rachel Gotbaum, WBUR, "Nursing a Shortage: Inside Out," Jan. 19. This extensive radio documentary on National Public Radio's Boston affiliate examines the causes and effects of the nursing shortage, as well as possible solutions. Its three 9-minute segments and supplementary WBUR Web site materials rely heavily on nursing scholars and executives.

Allison Van Dusen, *Forbes,* "TV's Medical Missteps," Sept. 20. This piece discusses the accuracy of popular health-related dramas and the common depiction of physicians doing things that nurses really do. It also makes a point rarely seen in the media: that nurse characters often endure slurs from physicians like House without response, reinforcing the image of nurses as meek servants and suggesting that the slurs are rude but basically accurate.

Suzanne Gordon, *Yankton Press and Dakotan* (SD), "TV Nurses Don't Represent Reality," May 9. The journalist's op-ed described a Hollywood vision of care in which "nurses barely exist." She observed that *Grey's* has hardly ever shown nurses "doing the work they would actually do," like monitoring the patient during surgery or afterward, or preventing life-threatening errors and complications.

Media reports on the violence and stress that nurses confront worldwide. These pieces addressed the extraordinary physical and emotional challenges that nurses face in the modern healthcare workplace.

Dan Lothian, *CNN,* "Nurses Confront Violence on the Job," July 12.

K. Nancoo-Russell, *The Freeport News* (Bahamas), "Nurses Should Not Have to Work in Fear, Official Says," May 8.

BBC News, "Stress 'Harms Nurses' Sex Lives," May 28.

Siddhartha D. Kashyap, *Times News Network* (India), "For Nurses, There's Stress Everywhere," May 26.

Articles addressing the interaction of nursing and new technology. These pieces took a thought-provoking look at how nurses influence and cope with the increasing role of advanced technology in patient care.

Susan Kreimer, *Dallas Morning News,* "Nurses Bridge Gap Between IT, Care: Brave New Paperless World Opens Opportunities for More Nurse Informaticists," Apr. 30.

Sindya N. Bhanoo, *The Baltimore Sun,* "Nurses Cast Wary Eye on High-Tech Advances: Robots, Electronic Records and Hand-Held Devices Streamline Care but Hinder Bedside Manner, Some Say," Aug. 27.

Best efforts to remedy poor media portrayals of nursing 2007
Johnson & Johnson, *Campaign for Nursing's Future,* **Andrea Higham,** Director; two television commercials, mid-late 2007. The campaign's two new television recruiting commercials made it clear that nurses save lives and improve outcomes, a marked improvement over its 2004–2006 efforts. The spots even offered some specific examples, like defibrillation and ventilation.

Worst Media Depictions of Nursing 2007
Grey's Anatomy. Executive Producers: Shonda Rhimes, Mark Gordon, Betsy Beers, Jim Parriott; ABC; each episode aired in 2007. The massively popular drama showed physicians providing all significant health care, including much that nurses really do, while nurses were peripheral subordinates. In the Jan. 25 episode, "Great Expectations," physicians were punished by having to perform seemingly grotesque, trivial nursing tasks, with no hint that the tasks might be important to patient outcomes. Episodes late in the year with OR nurse Rose did little to help; we learned that Rose attended college and that she could flirt with McDreamy, but the only expertise she displayed was in computer repair. (http://www.nursingadvocacy.org/action/letters/2005/greys_anatomy/greys.html)

Private Practice. Executive Producers: Shonda Rhimes, Mark Gordon, Marti Noxon, and Mark Tinker; ABC; "In Which We Meet Addison, a Nice Girl from Somewhere Else," Sept. 26; "In Which Sam Receives an Unexpected Visitor," Oct. 3; "In Which Addison Finds the Magic," Oct. 10; "In Which Addison Has a Very Casual Get Together," Oct. 17; "In Which Addison Finds a Showerhead," Oct. 24. This new show included wide-eyed mid-wifery student Dell Parker, perhaps the least knowledgeable major nurse character in recent primetime history. Dell was the receptionist for the seven physician characters who provided all-important health care. Early episodes also featured relentless mockery of nurse midwifery, including super OB Addison asking whether *midwifery* was even a word. (http://www.nursingadvocacy.org/media/tv/2007/private_practice.html)

Kelly Ripa, *LIVE with Regis and Kelly,* **shows broadcast Mar. 15 and Apr. 26.** Ripa initially made comments suggesting that she would act as an erotic "sponge bath nurse" to aid the recovery of cohost Regis Philbin after his open-heart surgery. The show's attempt to make amends involved lengthy glorification of Regis's physicians as brilliant life-savers, then having his nurses stand by mutely to receive generic thanks, reinforcing the sense that they were noble but low-skilled handmaidens.

Public communications following Governor Jon Corzine's near-fatal car crash that plainly told the public that physicians did everything that mattered in his recovery.

Governor Jon Corzine and the U.S. Department of Transportation. Television and radio commercials, May. These commercials encouraging seatbelt use gave credit for Corzine's recovery to "a remarkable team of doctors," "a series of miracles," and a "ventilator" in the ICU where he spent 8 days but failed to credit any of the many nurses who kept him alive. Corzine refused to respond to any one of the 150 nursing supporters who contacted him to object to these ads. (http://www.nursingadvocacy.org/news/2007/may/corzine.html)

continues

Exhibit 3–2 (continued)

House. Executive Producers: David Shore, Paul Attanasio, Katie Jacobs, and Bryan Singer; Fox, all 2007 episodes. This popular drama continued to present hospital care as an exercise in physician diagnosis, and nurses as mute, ignorant servants. "Insensitive," broadcast Feb. 13, suggested that the most prestigious nurse practitioner preparation is nondegree training to which entry can be had at the whim of physicians, rather than graduate degree programs at major universities. In "The Jerk," May 15, nurses were portrayed as physician handmaidens who performed menial assistive tasks but panicked in an emergency, relying on physicians to supply all the thinking, expertise, and courage.   (http://www.nursingadvocacy.org/action/letters/house/house.html)

Scrubs. Executive Producer: Bill Lawrence; NBC; "His Story IV," Feb. 1. Although this show has run helpful plot-lines for nurses, this episode featured chief of medicine Bob Kelso replacing nurse manager Carla Espinosa during her maternity leave. It told viewers that physicians supervise nurses and can become nurse managers at will; that nursing is for women, so men who do it should be mocked; that nurses are low-skilled handmaidens; and that physicians take the lead in patient monitoring, though nurses actually do that.
(http://www.nursingadvocacy.org/action/letters/scrubs/scrubs.html)

Atul Gawande, MD, *The New Yorker,* "The Way We Age Now: Medicine Has Increased the Ranks of the Elderly. Can It Make Old Age Any Easier?" Apr. 30. This long article about the shortage of geriatricians clearly suggested that only physicians can deliver expert care to the elderly, despite the long history of nurses taking the lead on this care. One striking passage described a 3-week training program in which physicians taught nurses to recognize basic issues in geriatrics as a sad stopgap, implying that nurses have no independent expertise or experience in geriatric care, though they in fact provide the vast majority of it. Of course, the piece consulted no nurses.
(http://www.nursingadvocacy.org/action/letters/scrubs/scrubs.html)

Will Shortz (puzzle master), *New York Times,* Feb. 26 and Mar. 16 crossword puzzles. The most prominent cross-word in the world first sought the answer "RN" with the clue "ICU helpers." Of course, that is a grotesque distortion of ICU care, in which highly skilled nurses take the lead. Rather than respond directly to the concerns of nurses, the crossword later sought "RN" with the clue "Hosp. workers." That clue, although accurate, is consistent with the earlier one and does nothing to address the disrespect it conveyed.

Gracie. Directed by Davis Guggenheim; story by Andrew Shue, Ken Himmelman, and Davis Guggenheim; screenplay by Lisa Marie Petersen and Karen Janszen; June. This earnest soccer movie used the main character's mother, a nurse, to show that past generations of ambitious women were stuck in dead-end loser jobs. But today, we learn, girls can actually achieve something worthwhile in work and in life. Yay.

Source: Courtesy of The Association of Educational Publishers, 2008. Retrieved March 10, 2008, from http://www.nursingadvocacy.org/press/releases/golden/lamp_awards.html

---

ter's Golden Lamp Awards for the worst and best views of nursing.

Use of Media by Nurses

In 1997, Sigma Theta Tau International (STTI), in collaboration with University of Rochester School of Nursing, conducted a study on nursing in the media called the Woodhull Study. The study concluded that nurses are health care's invisible partner (Sieber, Powers, Baggs, Knapp, & Sileo, 1998). In the study, a month's worth of healthcare media coverage was reviewed. The results indicated that there was a serious deficit in nurses' presence in the media. Journalists typically rely on physicians when they want statements about health care; most would not even think of asking a nurse for an interview. After this study, the ANA established a source called

"RN=Real News" to increase nurses' presence in the media (Stewart, 1999). What types of nurses might be sought by news media? Representatives of nursing professional organizations, education administrators and faculty, and nurses who deliver direct care are of particular interest to local news publications and broadcasts.

MEDIA TRAINING

The ANA, through its Web site, "RN=Real News," provides guidelines for media input (ANA, 2007c). "The media is the primary means by which consumers and policy makers obtain information about healthcare, about registered nurses, and about the nursing profession. While the situation is gradually improving, RNs continue to be under-represented in media coverage of health issues—even where nurses are the primary experts" (Stewart, 2007). STTI is another organization that offers media training. Nurses need to pay attention to positive images and note the type of image portrayed. Is it an accurate image? For example, a nurse may be portrayed as a caring individual in a television series, but there is little (if any) emphasis on the knowledge and competency, resulting in an inaccurate portrayal of nursing. Nurses also need to consider whether nursing is left out when it should be present.

Any nurse who becomes involved with the media needs to remember that he or she is an expert and thus must demonstrate professionalism and expertise. Reminding oneself that the public trusts nurses may help decrease anxiety when interacting with the media. Certainly, preparing for an interview is important, and if the topic is known, one can consider what types of questions might be asked. Most people who are interviewed by the media have an agenda—the message that they want to communicate through the media to the audience, which is usually more than just understanding an issue—and

action is usually a goal. Listening carefully to the question is very important because it often indicates what the reporter thinks about the issue. At no time should the nurse interviewee become angry or defensive, even if the reporter gives good reason for this type of response. Keeping anger and defensiveness under control is important. A thoughtful, clear answer is the best approach, one backed up by facts. If the answer to a question is not known, the nurse should say so and then follow up with required information. Many nursing organizations provide information and training for nurses who may become involved with the media and are looking for nurses who want to do this type of work for the profession. Buresh and Gordon (2006, p. 23) identified three tiers or modes of communication that are important to consider when educating the public about nursing:

1. Public communication through professional self-presentation.
2. Public communication through anecdotal descriptions of nursing.
3. Public communication through the mass media.

All three of these modes are addressed in this chapter.

Initiatives That Impact Image

Is the profession adequately influencing how nursing is viewed and maximizing its visibility? Influence is related to power—the power to cause others to agree to a certain direction. Influence is tied to image. "Your identity as a nurse goes with you wherever you are whether you are aware of it or not. How we present ourselves is an outward expression of our inner experience. Our beliefs about ourselves color all that we do and say" (Sullivan & the Sullivan Commission, 2004, p. 8). Influence is related to how a person communicates with, and gains support from, others. Influence requires relationships, because it happens between people. A person can be influential in one area but not in others. For example, a nurse with expertise in pediatric nursing may be able to influence policy makers about a new policy related to child health but have no influence when it comes to funding education for nurse anesthetist programs. Buresh and Gordon asked, "How can nurses end the silence about nursing and tell a credible compelling story about their work?" (2006, p. 21):

1. Nurses must inform the public about nursing.
2. Every nurse must make public communication and education about nursing an integral part of his or her nursing work.
3. Nurses must communicate in ways that highlight nurses' knowledge rather than their virtues.

Nursing Initiatives to Address the Visibility of the Profession

The nursing profession has developed a number of initiatives to focus on the profession and its needs—image, the nursing shortage, and the nursing faculty shortage. These issues are interconnected. When developing these initiatives, the profession is standing up for change and directing its own public image. Though there are 2.4 million jobs for RNs, making nursing the largest healthcare occupation, the shortage is a critical issue for the profession and the public (U.S. Department of Labor, 2006). The profession needs to take advantage of its strength in numbers to influence health care and its own image.

Nurses for a Healthier Tomorrow

Nurses for a Healthier Tomorrow (NHT) is a coalition of 43 nursing and healthcare organizations that work together in developing a communications campaign to attract people to the nursing profession (NHT, 2007). The goal of this campaign is to address the nursing shortage from the standpoint of the faculty shortage. If there are not enough nursing faculty members, schools of nursing cannot admit more students. NHT's initial campaign was called "Nursing. It's Real. It's Life." Its focus was on attracting people to nursing. The 2004 campaign, "Nursing education . . .pass it on" included a series of ads to attract nurses to nursing faculty positions.

Nursing's Agenda for the Future (2002)

Nursing's Agenda for the Future (ANA, 2002) is an initiative developed by the ANA in collaboration with 13 other nursing organizations. The final document describes nursing's desired future state with objectives and strategies. What is the vision of nursing? What should it look like, and where should it be by 2010? The desired future state of nursing was described as follows:

> *Nursing is the pivotal healthcare profession, highly valued for its specialized knowledge, skill and caring in improving the health status of the public and ensuring safe, effective, quality care. The profession mirrors the diverse population it serves and provides leadership to create positive changes in health policy and delivery systems. Individuals choose nursing as a career, and remain in the profession, because of the opportunities for personal and professional growth, supportive work environments and compensation commensurate with roles and responsibilities. (ANA, 2002, p. 2)*

Ten major domains are covered in the description and are based on other professional literature, particularly the Institute of Medicine's (IOM) *Crossing the Quality Chasm: A New Health System for the 21st Century* (2001). This agenda is discussed in more detail in Chapter 15.

Introductory content related to all the domains is found throughout this textbook. The 10 domains are:

1. Leadership and planning
2. Economic value
3. Delivery systems
4. Work environment
5. Legislation/regulation/policy
6. Public relations/communication
7. Professional/nursing culture
8. Education
9. Recruitment/retention
10. Diversity

RAISE THE VOICE CAMPAIGN

The American Academy of Nursing launched a campaign, Raise the Voice, to increase the visibility of nursing (2007). Academy president Linda Burns-Bolton, PhD, RN, has challenged nursing to begin to "call the circle"?in other words, to seek opportunities to participate in interdisciplinary and corporate boards by first inviting others to meet with nursing leaders. Nursing no longer needs to wait to be invited but should call the meeting. These activities will "raise the voice" of nursing and increase its visibility.

INSTITUTE OF MEDICINE QUALITY SERIES REPORTS

In 1999, the IOM began to publish a series of reports that looked at the U.S. healthcare system and the quality and safety issues related to care. Chapter 12 discusses many of the reports in detail. Relevant to the topic of this chapter is the 2004 IOM report that focuses on nursing and the nurse's work environment. The report emphasizes the major role that nurses have in health care in any setting and that nurses spend more time with patients than other healthcare professionals. No other report in this series focuses on one healthcare professional group.

Having nursing highlighted—and done so in a positive manner that includes important recommendations for making the work environment more conducive to effective nursing care—is a major step forward in clarifying the public image of nursing and emphasizing that nurses have an important impact on patient outcomes.

Strategies That Impact Image

Many strategies could be taken to improve the image of nursing. Several examples of these strategies are described in this section, including those involving generational issues, power and empowerment, **assertiveness**, advocacy, and the need for more men and minorities in nursing.

Generational Issues in Nursing: Impact on Image

Nursing today is composed of four generations: (1) Traditional, (2) Baby Boomers, (3) Generation X, and (4) Generation Y. Box 3–1 identifies the time frames for these generations.

Why are generational issues important? The generations are part of the image of nursing. When a person thinks of a nurse, what generation or age group does he or she envision? Most people probably do not realize that there is no one age group, but several. Nurses in these four generations are different from one another. What impact does this have on the image of nursing? This means that the image of nursing is one of multiple age groups with different historical backgrounds. How they each view nursing can be quite different, and their educational backgrounds vary a great deal, from nurses who entered nursing through diploma programs to nurses who entered through baccalaureate programs. Some of these nurses have seen great changes in health care, and others see the current status as the way it has always been. Technology, for example, is frequently taken for granted. Some nurses have seen

---

BOX 3–1 CURRENT GENERATIONS IN NURSING

- Traditional Generation   Born 1930–1940
- Baby Boomers   Born 1940–1960
- Generation X   Born 1960–1980
- Generation Y   Born 1980–present
  (Millennnials)

---

great changes in the roles of nurses to other nurses who take the roles for granted—for example, the advanced practice nurse. If one asked a nurse in each generation for his or her view of nursing, the answers might be quite different. If these nurses then tried to explain their views to the public, the perception of nursing would most likely consist of multiple images.

The situation of multiple generations in one profession provides opportunities to enhance the profession through the diversity of the age groups and their experiences, but it also has caused problems in the workplace. What are the characteristics of the groups? How well do they mesh with the healthcare environment? How well do they work together? The following list provides a summary of some of the characteristics of each generation (American Hospital Association, 2002; Bertholf & Loveless, 2001; Finkelman, 2006; Gerke, 2001; Santos & Cox, 2002; Ulrich, 2001; Wieck, Prydun, & Walsh, 2002).

1. *The traditional, silent, or mature generation, born 1930–1940*: This generation is important now because of its historical impact on nursing but is not currently in practice. This group of nurses was hard working, loyal, and family focused and felt that the duty to work was important. Many served in the military in World War II. This period was prior to the "women's liberation" movement. These characteristics had

an impact on how nursing services were organized and on the expectations of management of nurses. Some of this impact has been negative, such as the emphasis on bureaucratic structure, and difficult to change in some healthcare organizations.

2. *Baby Boomers, born 1940–1960*: This generation, currently the largest in the work arena, is also the group moving toward retirement. This will lead to an even greater nursing shortage problem. This is the generation that grew up in a time of major changes: "women's lib," the civil rights movement, and the Vietnam War. They had less opportunity than nurses today; typical career choices for women were teaching or nursing. This began to change during this period as the women's liberation movement grew. In this generation, fewer men went into nursing, as was true of the previous generation. This group's characteristics include independence, acceptance of authority, loyalty to employer, workaholic tendency, and less experience with technology, though many in this group have led the drive for more technology in nursing. This generation has been more materialistic and competitive and appreciates consensus leadership; it is a generation in which a person chose a career and then stuck to it, even if he or she was not very happy.

3. *Generation X (Gen-X), born 1960–1980*: The presence of Generation X, along with Generation Y, is growing in nursing. They will assume more nursing leadership roles as the Baby Boomers retire. They are more accomplished in technology and very much involved with computers and other advances in communication and information; they have experienced much change in these areas in their lifetimes to date. These

nurses want to be led, not managed, and they have not yet developed high levels of self-confidence and empowerment. What do they want in leaders? They look for leaders who are motivational, who demonstrate positive communication, who appreciate team players, and who exhibit good people skills—leaders who are approachable and supportive. Baby Boomers would not look for these characteristics in a leader. Gen-Xers typically do not join organizations (implications for nursing organizations), do not feel that they must stay in the same job for a long time (implications for employers), and feel that they want a balance between work and personal life (not as willing to "bring home work"). They are more informal, pragmatic, technoliterate, independent, creative, intimidated by authority, and loyal to those they know, and they appreciate diversity more. By contrast, Baby Boomers with whom the Gen-Xers are working often see things very differently; Baby Boomers are more loyal to their employer, stay in the job longer, are more willing to work overtime (though they are not happy about it), and have a greater long-term commitment. All this can cause problems between the two generations, with Baby Boomers often in supervisory positions and Gen-Xers in staff positions but moving into more leadership positions.

4. *Generation Y (Nexters, Millennials), born 1980–present*: This is the generation primarily entering nursing now, though second-career students and older students are also entering the profession. Millennials' characteristics are optimism, civic duty, confidence, achievement, social ability, morality, and diversity. In work situations, they demonstrate collective action, optimism, tenacity, multitasking, and a high level of technology skill, and they are also more trusting of centralized authority than Generation X. Typically, they handle change better, take risks, and want to be challenged. This generation is connected to cell phones, iPods, and personal digital assistants; they are tech savvy and multitask. Sometimes this makes it difficult for them to focus on one task.

In a profession with representatives from multiple generations, it is necessary to recognize that this diversity means great variation in positive and negative characteristics; some will pull the profession back if allowed, and some will push the profession forward. "In the workplace, differing work ethics, communication preferences, manners, and attitudes toward authority are key areas of conflict" (Siela, 2006, p. 47). This also has an impact on the profession's image; it is not a profession of one type of person or one age group. People in all the major age groups are entering nursing. As one generation moves toward retirement, the next generation will undoubtedly have an impact on the image of nursing, but this impact needs to be driven by nurses, not others. It is also critical that gender role stereotyping be avoided and neutralized to increase the strength of nurses as one group of professionals, while still recognizing that these differences exist and how they might impact the profession.

Power and Empowerment

Power and empowerment are connected to the image of nursing. How one is viewed can impact whether the person is viewed as having power—power to influence, to say what the profession is or is not, and to influence decision making. Nurses typically do not like to talk about power; they find this to be philosophically different from their view of nursing (Malone, 2001). This belief, viewing power only in the negative, acts as a barrier to success as a healthcare professional. But what are power, **powerlessness**, and empowerment? To feel like one is not listened to or viewed positively can make a person feel powerless. Many nurses feel that they cannot make an impact in clinical settings, and they are not listened to or sought out for their opinion. This powerlessness can result in nurses feeling like victims. This feeling can act against nurses when they do not take on issues such as the image of nurses and when they allow others to describe what a nurse is or to make decisions for nurses. All this only worsens their image. What nurses want and need is power—to be able to influence decisions and have an impact on issues that matter. It is clear that power can be used constructively or destructively (such as for the person's own good), but the concern here with the nursing profession is constructively using power deconstructively. Fisher compared power and influence. Power is about control to reach a goal. Influence, which is on the same continuum as power, is "a dynamic process; it seeks not to control but to set in place an interdependence that fosters cooperation" (1996, p. 114). There is more than one type of power, as described in Box 3–2, and the type has an impact on how it can be used to reach goals or outcomes.

Empowerment is an important issue with nurses today. To empower is to enable to act—a critical need in the nursing profession. Empowerment is "an interrelationship between authority, resources, timely and accurate information, and accountability. A nurse manager who is providing staff an environment in which empowerment is valued works to see that all four of these elements are present for staff in their daily work environment" (Finkelman, 1996, p. 1–1:6). Basically, empowerment is more than just saying you can participate in decision making; staff need more than words. Empowerment is needed in day-to-day practice as nurses meet the needs of patients in hospitals, in the community, and in home settings. What does empowerment really offer staff? Bennis and Goldsmith (1997) identified some of the benefits of empowerment for staff:

- Staff feel significant because they make a difference in the organization and in its success.
- The organization emphasizes that learning and competence are critical. Failure is not an issue because mistakes are seen as opportunities for improvement.
- Staff who are empowered usually feel that their work is exciting.

Box 3–2 Types of Power

- **Informational Power:** Arises from the ability to access information and share information.
- **Referent Power:** A type of informal power that exists when others recognize that a person has special qualities and is admired; others are willing to follow that person.
- **Expert Power:** A person is respected for his or her expertise—and others will follow. The person may or may not be in a management position; staff may follow another staff member because they feel that person has expertise.
- **Coercive Power:** Power is based on punishment when someone does not do what is desired; result might be loss of raise or promotion, a decision made by a supervisor who has formal power.
- **Reward Power:** When a person's power comes from his or her ability to reward others when they do as expected. In this case, the person would have to be in a position of authority—for example, a manager.
- **Persuasive Power:** This type of power occurs when a person uses persuasion to influence others.

Staff who feel empowered feel that they are respected and trusted to be active participants. Staff who feel empowered also demonstrate a positive image to other healthcare team members, patients and their families, and the public. Nurses who do not feel empowered will not be effective in demonstrating a positive image in that they will not be able to communicate that nurses are professionals with much to offer.

Control over the profession is a critical issue that is also related to the profession's image. Who should control the profession, and who does? This is related to independence and autonomy—key characteristics of any profession. Some questions typically asked about control and the profession have yet to fully be resolved (Lindberg, Hunter, & Kruszewski, 1998, p. 397):

1. What services should nurses provide? *(There have been many role changes, and many more to come. These changes are not easily resolved.)*
2. How should nurses be educated? *(The issue of the entry-level degree continues to be unresolved.)*
3. What payment should nurses receive for their services? *(There is much to be done regarding this question.)*
4. What should be the influence of organized nursing on American healthcare policy? *(Nursing is certainly more involved in healthcare policy today, but far from where it should be as the largest healthcare profession.)*

A question missing from this list is, "What should be the image of nursing?" Nursing as a profession does not appear to have a consensus about this image, given that the types of advertising and responses to these initiatives vary. In addition, the image of nursing has a direct impact on the four preceding questions. Nursing needs to control the image and visibility of the profession and, in doing so, may have more control over the solutions for the four questions.

- If nurses had a more realistic image, it would be easier to support the types of services that nurses offer to the public.
- If nurses had a more realistic image, it would be easier to support an entry-level baccalaureate degree to provide the type of education needed.
- If nurses had a more realistic image, it would be easier to support the need for reimbursement for nursing services, which are much more than hand holding.
- If nurses had a more realistic image, it would be easier to participate in the healthcare dialogue on the local, state, national, and international levels to influence policy.

Assertiveness

Assertiveness is demonstrated in how a person communicates—direct, open, and appropriate in respect of others. When a person communicates in an assertive manner, his or her verbal and non-verbal communication is congruent, making the message clearer, and often includes "I" statements. Assertive and aggressive communications are not the same. Assertive persons are better able to confront problems in a constructive manner and do not remain silent. The problems that the profession has with image have been influenced by nursing's silence—the inability to be assertive. Smith (1975) identified some critical rules related to assertive behavior that can easily be applied to the difficulties that nursing has had with changing its image and visibility.

1. Avoid overapologizing.
2. Avoid defensive, adverse reactions, such as aggression, temper tantrums, backbiting, revenge, slander, sarcasm, and threats.
3. Use body language—such as eye contact, body posture, gestures, and facial expressions—that is appropriate to and that matches the verbal message.

4. Accept manipulative criticism while maintaining responsibility for your decision.
5. Calmly repeat a negative reply without justifying it.
6. Be honest about feelings, needs, and ideas.
7. Accept and/or acknowledge your faults calmly and without apology.

Other examples of assertive behavior are (Katz, 2001, p. 267):

- Expressing feelings without being nasty or overbearing
- Acknowledging emotions but staying open to discussion
- Expressing self and giving others the chance to express themselves equally
- Using "I" statements to defuse arguments
- Asking and giving reasons

Advocacy

Advocacy is speaking for something important, and it is one of the major roles of a nurse. Typically, one thinks of advocacy for the patient and family; however, nurses also need to be advocates for themselves and for the profession. To do this successfully, nurses need to feel empowered and be assertive. All nurses represent nursing—acting as advocates—in their daily work and in their personal lives. When someone asks, "What do you do?" the nurse's response is a form of advocacy. The goal is to have a positive, informative, and accurate response.

The White Female Face of Nursing: It Needs to Change

There is no question that the majority of nurses are White females, and there is also no question that this needs to change. There has been an increase in the number of male and minority nurses, but not enough. There is a greater need to actively seek out more male and minority students (Cohen, 2007). Men and minorities in nursing need to reach out and mentor student nurses and new nurses to provide them with the support they need as they enter a profession predominantly composed of White women. There needs to be more media coverage regarding the role of men and minorities in nursing; for example, when photos are used in local media, and in media in general, they should have a more diverse representation of the profession.

Men in Nursing

Men still constitute a very small percentage of the total number of RNs living and working in the United States, although their numbers have continued to grow (U.S. Department of Health and Human Services, 2006). In 2000, 146,902 (5.4%) of RNs were men. In 2004, 5.8% (168,181 RNs) were male (see Table 3–1).

Data from 2005–2006 indicated that men represented 12.1% of new graduates (National League for Nursing, 2008). Male RNs are more likely to be younger than female RNs, with 30.1% of male RNs under the age of 40 compared with 26.1% of female RNs, and 65.7% of male RNs under the age of 50 compared with 57.4% of female RNs. Male RNs are more likely to be employed in nursing (88.4%) compared with female RNs (82.9%). Male and female RNs also differ with respect to the type of program in which they received their initial nursing education. Male and female RNs differ in the proportions graduating with either a diploma or an associate's degree, with males more often receiving an associate's degree than a diploma. And now that there are accelerated bachelor's degree programs, more men are coming into the profession after several years in computer science, law, engineering, and other programs. Approximately 13.5% of male RNs graduated from diploma programs, compared with 25.9% of female RNs, and 52.0% of male RNs graduated from associate's degree programs, compared with 41.6% of female RNs.

Table 3–1 HRSA Data: The RN Population by Gender, Racial/Ethnic Background, and Age

Gender, racial/ethnic background and age group	Total			Employment status					
				Employed in nursing			Not employed in nursing		
	Number in sample	Estimated Number	Percent	Number in sample	Estimated Number	Percent	Number in sample	Estimated Number	Percent
Total	35,635	2,909,357	100.0	30,233	2,421,351	100.0	5,402	488,006	100.0
Gender									
Male	2,166	168,181	5.8	1,937	148,642	6.1	229	19,539	4.0
Female	33,454	2,740,144	94.2	28,283	2,271,717	93.8	5,171	468,427	96.0
Not known	15	1,033	0.0	13	993	0.0	2	40	0.0
Racial/ethnic background									
White(non-hispanic)	29,561	2,380,529	81.8	24,958	1,966,330	81.2	4,603	414,199	84.9
Black/African American (non-hispanic)	1,297	122,495	4.2	1,146	106,644	4.4	151	15,850	3.1
Asian (non-hispanic)	963	84,383	2.9	863	75,943	3.1	100	8,440	1.7
Native Hawaiian/ Pacific Islander (non-hisp)	65	5,594	0.2	55	4,613	0.2	10	981	0.2
American Indian/Alaska native (non-hisp)	157	9,453	0.3	141	8,347	0.3	16	1,106	0.2
Hispanic/Latino (any race)	512	48,009	1.7	450	42,262	1.7	62	5,747	1.2
Two or more races (non-hispanic)	519	42,244	1.4	451	35,554	1.5	68	5,690	1.2
Not known	2,561	217,651	7.5	2,169	181,658	7.5	392	35,993	7.4
Age group									
Less than 25	609	61,778	2.1	588	59,592	2.5	21	2,186	0.4
25–29	2,117	171,659	5.9	1,981	159,676	6.6	136	11,983	2.5
30–34	3,053	243,182	8.4	2,794	221,052	9.1	259	22,130	4.5
35–39	3,646	289,525	10.0	3,280	256,967	10.6	366	32,557	6.7
40–44	4,996	408,248	14.0	4,481	360,249	14.9	515	47,999	9.8
45–49	6,407	508,708	17.5	5,718	449,797	18.6	689	58,910	12.1
50–54	5,816	463,565	15.9	5,160	406,748	16.8	656	56,817	11.6
55–59	4,099	338,078	11.6	3,361	271,264	11.2	738	66,814	13.7
60–64	2,477	210,196	7.2	1,667	136,191	5.6	810	74,006	15.2
65 and over	2,085	185,254	6.4	928	75,305	3.1	1,157	109,949	22.5
Not known	330	29,165	1.0	275	24,511	1.0	55	4,655	1.0
Average age		46.8			45.4			54.1	
Median age		47.0			46.0			55.0	

NOTE: Estimated numbers may not equal totals, and percents may not add to 100 because of rounding.

Source: From *The Registered Nurse Population: Findings From the March 2004 National Sample Survey of Registered Nurses,* by U.S. Department of Health and Human Resources, Health Resources and Services Administration, Bureau of Health Professions. June 2006, Washington, DC: Author.

Men in nursing have worked to develop support for men who decide to enter the profession. One type of support is the American Assembly of Men in Nursing (2007). The goals of this organization are to:

1. Encourage men of all ages to become nurses and join together with all nurses in strengthening and humanizing health care;
2. Support men who are nurses to grow professionally and demonstrate to each other and to society the increasing contributions being made by men within the nursing profession;
3. Advocate for continued research, education and dissemination of information about men's health issues, men in nursing, and nursing knowledge at the local and national levels;
4. Support members' full participation in the nursing profession and its organizations and use this Assembly for the limited objectives stated above.

The ANA, as well as many state nursing organizations, has supported the theme of men in nursing and has gone as far as creating a "Men in Nursing" calendar to depict the various types of nursing that men do, and the different types of men attracted to nursing.

MINORITIES IN NURSING

Along with a limited number of men in nursing is the problem of limited minority representation in the profession. Comparisons of the racial/ethnic composition of the RN population in 2004 with previous years should be interpreted with caution (U.S. Department of Health and Human Services, 2006). Unlike earlier versions of the National Sample Survey of Registered Nurses, which included a single question and asked the respondent to choose only one racial/ethnic background, the 2000 and 2004 surveys

collected this information in two questions. Respondents were asked to indicate whether their ethnic background was either Hispanic or Latino; they were also asked to identify all races that described themselves. The survey information was aggregated into categories similar to those reported in previous years, with one additional category to delineate Hispanic and non-Hispanic RNs who reported two or more races. In 2004, the number of nurses in the two or more races, non-Hispanic category was estimated to be 41,244, or 1.4% of the RN population. In 2004, 7.5% of RNs (217,651) did not specify their combined racial/ethnic background, and in 2000, only 1.1% of RNs did not specify their combined racial/ethnic background. The number of nurses identifying their combined racial/ethnic background as one or more non-White groups, Hispanic, or Latino numbered 311,177 (10.7%) in 2004. This change is a decrease of 22,190 RNs from 2000, but nearly triple the number of non-White, Hispanic, or Latino nurses in 1980. See Figure 3–2.

In 2000, 12.4% of all RNs (333,368) came from one or more of the identified racial and ethnic non-White, Hispanic, or Latino groups. It must be noted that this apparent decline may be a result of an increase in the proportion of RNs who did not completely specify their combined racial or ethnic background. In the past, non-White, Hispanic, or Latino RNs have grown at a greater rate than White non-Hispanic RNs for all the years from 1980 to 2000, except the period from 1984 to 1988. These growth rates were particularly pronounced between 1996 and 2000, when the number of non-White, Hispanic, or Latino RNs increased about 35.3%, whereas the number of White non-Hispanic RNs increased by 1.7%. Most of the increase in the RN population between 1996 and 2000 was a result of the growth in the non-White.

Figure 3–2 HRSA data: The RN poulation by race/ethnicity.

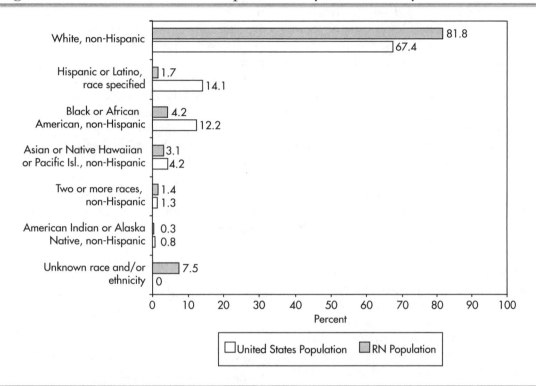

Source: From *The Registered Nurse Population: Findings From the March 2004 National Sample Survey of Registered Nurses*, by U.S. Department of Health and Human Resources, Health Resources and Services Administration, Bureau of Health Professions. June 2006, Washington, DC: Author.

Hispanic, or Latino nurse population (which increased by 87,003 RNs).

Fifty-one percent of those who specified ethnicity but not race (15,231) indicated that they are Hispanic or Latino. Of the estimated 128,645 who specified race but not ethnicity, 78.2% are White, and 21.8% (28,067) are racial minorities. Of these RNs who specified race but not ethnicity, 56.3% are Black or African American, 4.6% are American Indian or Alaska Native, 29.3% are Asian or Other Pacific Islander, and the remain-

ing RNs checked two or more races. Therefore, a total of 354,475 (12.2% of the RN population) can be considered minority by race and/ or ethnicity. However, for the purposes of clarity and consistency, in this narrative report on minority comparison with White non-Hispanic RNs, only RNs with both race and ethnicity provided are generally being compared in the text, charts, and tables.

Hispanic or Latino RNs still remain the most underrepresented group of nurses when compared with their representation in the U.S. population. After adjusting for those Hispanic or Latino RNs who provided no response to the question on race, only 2.2% of the RN population were Hispanic or Latino nurses, although Hispanics or Latinos constitute 14.1% of the general population. Of the 7.5% of respondents who did not specify one or both of race and ethnicity, 6.4% of respondents were of unknown ethnicity in 2004.

The Sullivan Commission (Sullivan & the Sullivan Commission, 2004) explored the critical issue of the need for more minorities in healthcare professions and made recommendations to work on this problem. The final report stated,

> *Diversity is a critical part of the mission of healthcare and the national challenge of preparing our nation's future workforce. America's success in improving health status and advancing the health sciences is wholly dependent on the contributions of people from a myriad of diverse backgrounds and cultures, including Latinos, Native Americans, African Americans, European Americans, and Asian Americans. The lack of diversity is a key barrier to ensuring a culturally competent healthcare system at the provider, organizational, and system levels. It diminishes our nation's capacity to eliminate racial and ethnic health disparities and compromises our national capacity to advance the health sciences. (p. 28)*

Professional Presentation: Increasing Visibility and Professional Growth

How might you represent the profession? Every nurse represents the profession every day at work. The profession is communicated through dress, appearance, name tags and credential identification, how one communicates and introduces oneself, and how one performs and provides care. Nurses also represent the profession in nonwork

settings and in their personal lives as soon as they say that they are an RN. People then look at them differently and most likely have certain expectations. Most nurses have experienced being asked many health questions by family members and consumers who want advice even though the nurse is not in a working role. Nurses have to know how to respond to these questions and be professional in their response. Nurses who complain about their work or joke about patient care issues when they think they are in a neutral situation, such as a social setting, are still representing the profession. Consumers will take note of these comments and nonverbal communication. Nurses really never stop being nurses no matter what role or occupation they are in; this is a characteristic of a profession, just like a physician or a lawyer is never "not" a physician or lawyer even if his or her main job is as an editor or legislator. What are some issues that might come up as a nurse becomes a visible representative of the profession?

What Do You Wear to Work as a Nurse?

If one took a tour of a hospital today, could RNs be easily identified? Most likely not. In fact, it can be difficult to identify the roles of any staff members in the hospital, from the doctors and nurses to the staff who clean the units. Nurses' uniforms have changed over time. The image of the nurse in a white uniform—typically a woman in a dress with a cap and white stockings and shoes—is long past. Prior to the all-white uniform, the nurse's uniform was gray or blue, similar to a nun's habit and to the uniforms worn during Florence Nightingale's time (Tobin, 2006). But in the 1980s, even the all-white uniforms (dresses) began to change. White pantsuits became more common, and soon after that, scrubs became the uniform of the day and continue to be. Why scrubs? They are cheaper, easier to clean, and more comfortable. Colors are wide open, and in some cases, lab coats are worn over the scrubs. At the same time that nurses began to wear scrubs, others who worked in health care also changed to scrubs, adding to the confusion (Tobin, 2006). Then came the prints—animals, cartoon characters, flowers, and so on. How comfortable are adult patients when a nurse comes in wearing scrubs with animals or cartoon characters and says, "I will be your nurse today"? What impression does this give? Another problematic aspect of this change in uniform is less control over dress code; consistency is now lacking in a dress and appearance code: Hair length and style, appropriate jewelry, and style of shoes are not as carefully assessed. One can see scrubs that look like they just came out of the washer, wrinkled and thrown on in haste. Hospitals are full of staff who all look alike; wearing scrubs in different colors and patterns, with or without lab coats, but mostly all in scrubs. Staff, patients, families, and visitors cannot tell one type of staff member from another. The results of a 1997 study about uniforms (Mangum, Garrison, Lind, & Hilton) indicated that the best first impression was given by a white-pants uniform with a stethoscope rather than colored scrubs or white pants with a colored top, both of which scored lowest. In the last 5–10 years, some hospitals have returned to requiring that RNs wear all white, even if all-white scrubs, and limiting white to just RNs; however, this is not common. Recently, the wearing of shoes called Crocs came up as an issue in the United Kingdom (British Broadcasting Corporation, 2007). Some hospitals are telling staff that they cannot wear these clogs because there is concern about infection control and, in some cases, static electricity buildup. Body fluids and needles might drop into the holes in the shoes, representing a safety risk. The goal is to prevent infection, maintain health and safety, and keep professional image.

REPRESENTING THE PROFESSION: PUBLIC COMMUNICATION SKILLS

Presentations   Nurses represent the profession in a variety of settings. The most common place is in professional meetings, typically nursing meetings. Nurses need to participate more in interdisciplinary meetings where they represent the profession, and they could do much to improve the image of nursing with other healthcare professionals, communicating what nurses can do. Presentations require certain skills: developing a clear message verbally and nonverbally; using effective presentation methods such as PowerPoint slides; using storytelling during presentations; demonstrating a professional physical appearance (dress, body language, and so on); and generally showing competency in delivering presentations. Nurses who want to take an active role in the profession should develop these skills. It is important that nurses acknowledge their credentials when they are listed in programs and introduced. Some nurses also speak to consumer-focused groups such as Parent Teacher Associations, disease-focused organizations (e.g., Arthritis Foundation, American Diabetes Association), religious groups, and community organizations. The same advice is important in this type of setting. Additionally, the nurse presenter must be able to speak to the consumers in language that is understood but not talk down to the audience. This takes practice. Consumers who learn from nurses about health care will have a better understanding of the complex role of nursing. Some nurses speak directly with the media (important issues related to media communication were discussed earlier in this chapter). All these efforts increase the awareness of nursing among the public and other healthcare professionals. See Exhibit 3–3 for a description of public speaking skills.

EXHIBIT 3–3 PREPARING A PRESENTATION
_____

- Prepare an outline for the presentation considering the objectives, audience, location, and time.
- Develop the content for the presentation.
- Develop audiovisuals to support the content.
- If the presentation is offered for continuing education credit, information about your résumé and content must be prepared and shared with the continuing education provider. You should be informed about this prior to the presentation.
- Consider the physical attire for the presentation (type of meeting, time of day, weather, and the image that you want to exhibit).
- Practice your presentation, keeping in mind the time factor. Your actual presentation will probably take longer than your practice presentations. It is best not to memorize a presentation or read it word for word, but rather to present it in a more natural manner. This takes practice. Consider how you will cue yourself about content during the presentation.
- If you are using slides and the slides are on a computer monitor in front of you, do not look at the large audience screen, but at the computer monitor.
- If you must change the slides yourself, practice doing this. If someone else is changing the slides, confirm with that person as to how you want this done. This is easy to do yourself if you have a computer.
- Consider if the audience will have a copy of the slides or other handouts. If there are a lot of different handouts, decide how you will identify them during the presentation; for example, color-code paper or use number labels to refer to them during the presentation. You will need to prepare the handouts and give them to the sponsoring organization. In some cases, you may bring them with you to the presentation. This needs to be clarified depending on the presentation location and audience.
- At the beginning of your presentation, thank the organization and any specific persons who influenced your presentation. In some cases, employer and/or grant funding must be acknowledged, and this is easily done on an initial slide.
- Keep aware of time. You may have someone give you a cue as time is running out.
- Will there be a question-and-answer portion to the presentation? If so, how long will it be, and who will lead it? In some situations, the person who introduced you will actually call on the audience for questions, and you will just answer the questions. If you are doing both, remember to look around the audience to include everyone. Note the required time limit and meet it. If questions are asked without a microphone, repeat the questions so that everyone can hear them.
- If the organization is recording your presentation, the organization should ask for your permission to do so.

Storytelling with a Hook   Storytelling can be an effective communication tool to clarify confusing messages (Finkelman, 2006). Why would storytelling apply to the topic of the image of nursing? When the issue of image is assessed, a critical point is what type of message is being communicated about nursing. The message is not clear and often not based on the reality of nursing practice. Storytelling is needed and is used, but the stories may not be as realistic as they should be. What types of stories are most effective? "Typically, stories that have the perspective of a single protagonist who was in a predicament that was prototypical of the organization (profession) are most successful" (Denning, 2001 as cited in Finkelman, 2006, p. 116). The story needs to be familiar, grab attention, and be brief and to the point. Storytelling can be used in public presentations by nurses to better explain what nurses do; in communication with policy makers such as legislators (Chapter 5 includes more detailed content about political advocacy); and in advertising. In the latter two, the stories must be very brief and make the message clear in a short period of time. Every nurse should be a storyteller—in his or her personal life as he or she interacts with others and explains nursing. The selection of the story makes a difference. Nurses tend to choose the stories that pull at heart strings and may not really give a view of all that is required to be a nurse: knowledge and competency. Nurses need to rethink the stories that they are using. When an intensive care nurse describes an experience of personal communication with a dying patient but leaves out all the other aspects of care that he or she provides, what message does this send?

Conclusion

What can individual nurses do to influence the image of nursing? It is often easy to assume that professional issues, such as the image of nursing, can be responded to only by the "profession" as a whole. However, many nursing issues require individual nurses to take action in response. The image of nursing is certainly impacted by broad concerns, such as content in television, film, or advertising. But much of the image of nursing comes from the day-to-day personal contact that the public has with nurses and that the nurse has with other healthcare professionals in the workplace. The following are some actions that individual nurses should consider.

- Critically assess the actions that you take that might impact the image of nursing.
- Maintain dress standards that display a professional image. Healthcare organizations need to review and revise dress codes and enforce them.

- Consider what you say when you "complain" about work in the work setting and in your personal life.
- Consider how you would respond to the question, "Why didn't you go into medicine?"
- Do you speak with enthusiasm about your work and about being a nurse?
- How do you present yourself to patients and family members? Do you give your full name? Do you say you are an RN? Do you let them know your role?
- Remember that nonverbal communication can sometimes be more important than verbal communication. What are people seeing when you talk about nursing?
- Write letters when you read about, see, or hear nurses portrayed in a negative light in the media. Include information about the positive qualities of nurses and what nurses do. Do not forget to describe the education that is required to be a nurse.
- Define unacceptable workplace behaviors and hold staff accountable (Cohen, 2007, p. 25).
- Educate, educate, educate. The public knows little about nursing except to say that nurses care for patients. The public needs to know about the high level of education and technological competency required, the different levels of nursing education, including graduate school programs, different nursing roles, and the impact that nurses have on patient outcomes.
- Post, circulate, and advertise nursing's accomplishments (Cohen, 2007, p. 26). For example, submit articles to local newspapers about what the professions is doing. Speak to civic and community groups about nursing.
- Learn communications skills so that you are empowered to respond to negative comments in a manner that stops behaviors that

negatively impact the nursing image. (Cohen, 2007, p. 26).

CHAPTER HIGHLIGHTS

1. The image of nursing is formulated in many ways by the public, the media, interdisciplinary colleagues, and nurses.
2. Nursing's image as a profession has both positive and negative aspects.
3. Nurses tend to act as victims in many situations and convey this to other constituencies.
4. The visibility of nursing's contribution to health care is often hidden.
5. The historical roots that described nurses as handmaidens still influence our visibility as a profession.
6. The lack of visibility leads to a lack of confidence among nurses regarding their contribution to the health profession.
7. The role of the media through newspapers, TV programs, and ads has a powerful influence on how nurses are viewed.
8. Generational differences among nurses that impact nursing are voice and visibility.
9. Empowerment is a critical issue for nurses and must be addressed before the image of nursing will improve.
10. Two other critical issues, assertiveness and advocacy, impact nursing's image.
11. A change in nursing is the inclusion of more men and minorities. Although still not reflective of the populations we serve, the numbers of men and minorities are increasing. The image of nursing is moving away from a predominantly White female profession.
12. Our actions, attire, and method of telling our story, and how we present ourselves to the public are important in changing the image of nursing.

Linking to the Internet

- American Nurses Association Press Releases
  http://www.nursingworld.org/FunctionalMenuCategories/MediaResources/PressReleases.aspx
- Nurses Week
  http://www.nursingworld.org/pressrel/nnw/
- Center for Nursing Advocacy (View current the Golden Lamp Awards
  http://www.nursingadvocacy.org/news/news.html
- Nursing the Ultimate Adventure pamphlet NSNA
  http://www.nsna.org/pdf/career/tools.pdf
- American Assembly of Men in Nursing
  http://aamn.org/
- For information on a career as a registered nurse and nursing education, contact the National League for Nursing
  http://www.nln.org
- For additional information on registered nurses, including credentialing, contact the American Nurses Association
  http://nursingworld.org
- For information on the NCLEX-RN exam and a list of individual state boards of nursing, contact the National Council of State Boards of Nursing
  http://www.ncsbn.org
- For information on obtaining U.S. certification and work visas for foreign-educated nurses, contact the Commission on Graduates of Foreign Nursing Schools
  http://www.cgfns.org
- For a list of accredited clinical nurse specialist programs, contact the National Association of Clinical Nurse Specialists
  http://www.nacns.org/cnsdirectory.shtml
- For information on nurse anesthetists, including a list of accredited programs,

contact the American Academy of Nurse Practitioners
http://www.aanp.org
- For information on nursing career options, financial aid, and listings of bachelor's degree, graduate, and accelerated nursing programs, contact the American Association of Colleges of Nursing
http://www.aacn.nche.edu

DISCUSSION QUESTIONS

1. Why is the image of nursing important to the profession? To health care in general?
2. What role do you think you might have as a nurse in influencing the image of nursing? (Provide specific examples.)
3. What is your opinion about nursing uniforms?
4. What stimulated your interest in nursing as a profession? Was the image of nursing in any way related to your decision, and in what way did it impact your decision?

CRITICAL THINKING ACTIVITIES

1. Complete a mini-survey of six people and ask them to describe their image of nursing and nurses. Try to pick a variety of people. Summarize your data and analyze them to determine if there are themes and unusual views. How does what you learned relate to the content in this chapter? List the similarities and differences, and then discuss with a group of your classmates.
2. In teams, develop a presentation to be delivered to a group of high school students who are interested in all types of healthcare professions. Plan a 10-minute presentation, and provide a written outline and five PowerPoint slides. Deliver this presentation in class. Consider creativity, realistic content, and how you might grab an audience whose members are not sure that nursing is the direction they will choose. Do some research on effective presentations and use the guide provided in Exhibit 3–3. Critique presentations, both content and presentation style. At the conclusion of the presentations, students should vote for the presentation that they think would be most effective in illustrating a positive, accurate image of nursing that would grab attention.
3. Conduct a survey for a week of local media (newspapers, television, radio) to identify examples of when nurses might have participated in news stories about health topics.
4. Analyze a television program that focuses on a healthcare situation/storyline. How are nurses depicted compared with other healthcare professionals? Compose a letter to the program describing your analysis, and document your arguments to support your viewpoint. This could be done with a team of students; watch the same program and then discuss opinions and observations.

5. Design a print ad that could be used by your school of nursing to recruit students. This can be done with a team of students or individually. Include content and graphics.
6. Develop a survey that would determine what hospital staff think about uniforms. If possible, conduct the survey and share information with the class. Discuss the results.

CASE STUDY

"Dr. Finkelman, this is Nurse Kenner. I am so sorry to bother you. I know it is late. I am calling because I am very concerned about Mr. T. He is 2 days post-op, and he is complaining of cramping and nausea and is bloated. When I listen for bowel sounds, I hear nothing. I know you are very busy, and it is 2 a.m., but he is so uncomfortable. Do you think maybe you could help?"

Case Questions

1. What image is portrayed by this phone conversation when the nurse calls the resident?
2. How does the language chosen impact the image that you have of this nurse?
3. Listen in your clinical settings for such conversations. What strategies might you use to change the image of this nurse?

WORDS OF WISDOM

Jamie White, RN, MSN
Staff Nurse Neonatal Intensive Care Unit
OU Medical Center
Oklahoma City, Oklahoma
Now that you have graduated, either for the first time or with an advanced degree, what do you perceive as the image of nursing by your colleagues (across disciplines) and the public?

The image of nursing across the disciplines is one of respect. Most of your colleagues value your opinion and knowledge about your patients. The image of the public is often naïve.

What do you believe practicing nurses and nurse educators should do to improve the image of nursing?

Nurse educators and practicing nurses need to join together and support each other. We also need to promote critical thinking, leadership, and encourage each other to be strong patient advocates. By doing this, patient outcome may improve, resulting in a more complete picture of nursing to our patients, which diffuses to the public. Also, spending more time with our patients in conversation leads to a more positive image portrayed to our patients.

References

American Academy of Nursing. (2007). *Raise the voice.* Retrieved August 26, 2007, from http://www.aannet.org

American Assembly of Men in Nursing. (2007). Retrieved August 5, 2007, from http://aamn.org/

American Hospital Association. (2002). *In our hands: How hospital leaders can build a thriving workplace.* Chicago: Author.

American Nurses Association. (2002). *Nursing's agenda for the future: A call to the nation.* Washington, DC: Author.

American Nurses Association. (2007a). *Celebrating 2007 Annual Nurses Week.* Washington, DC: Author.

American Nurses Association. (2007b). *President's letter.* Retrieved July 2, 2007, from http://www.nursingworld.org/pressrel/nnw/rpatton.htm

American Nurses Association. (2007c). *RN=Real News: Media relations and you.* Retrieved August 18, 2008, from http://www.nursingworld.org/mods/archive/mod230/cernver.htm

Benner, P. (2005). Commentary by Patricia Benner. *Nursing Education Perspectives, 26*(1), 14–15.

Bennis, W., & Goldsmith, J. (1997). *Learning to lead.* Reading, MA: Perseus Books.

Bertholf, L., & Loveless, S. (2001). Baby Boomers and Generation X: Strategies to bridge the gap. *Seminars for Nurse Managers, 9,* 169–172.

British Broadcasting. (BBC). *Crocs cause nurse safety concern.* Retrieved September 5, 2007, from http://news.bbc.co.uk/2/hi/health/6979400.stm

Buresh, B., & Gordon, S. (2006). *From silence to voice: What nurses know and must communicate to the public* (2nd ed.). Toronto, Ontario, Canada: Canadian Nurses Association.

Center for Nursing Advocacy. (2006, May 10). *Johnson & Johnson campaign.* Retrieved July 9, 2007, from http://www.nursingadvocacy.org

Cohen, S. (2007). The image of nursing. *American Nurse Today, 2*(5), 24–26.

Donelan, K., Buerhaus, P. I., Ulrich, B. T., Norman, L., & Dittus, R. (2005). Awareness and perceptions of the Johnson & Johnson Campaign for Nursing's Future: Views from nursing students, RNs, and CNOs. *Nursing Economics, 23,* 150–156.

Finkelman, A. (1996). *Psychiatric nursing administration manual.* Gaithersburg, MD: Aspen.

Finkelman, A. (2006). *Leadership and management in nursing.* Upper Saddle River, NJ: Pearson Education.

Fisher, M. (1996). Dynamics of implementation. In M. Fisher (Ed.), *Redesigning the nursing organization* (pp. 114–130). Albany, NY: Delmar.

Gerke, M. (2001). Understanding and leading the quad matrix: Four generations in the workplace. *Seminars for Nurse Managers, 9,* 173–181.

Gordon, S., & Nelson, S. (2005). An end to angels. *American Journal of Nursing, 105*(5), 62–69.

Institute of Medicine. (2001). *Crossing the quality chasm: A new health system for the 21st century.* Washington, DC: National Academies Press.

Institute of Medicine. (2004). *Keeping patients safe: Transforming the work environment of nurses.* Washington, DC: National Academies Press.

Kalisch, P., & Kalisch, B. (2005). Perspectives on improving nursing's public image. *Nursing Education Perspectives, 26*(1), 10–17.

Katz, J. (2001). *Keys to nursing success.* Upper Saddle River: NJ: Prentice Hall.

Lazarsfeld, P., & Merton, R. (1971). Mass communication, popular taste, and organized social action. In W. Schramm & D. Roberts (Eds.), *Process and effects of mass communication.* Urbana: University of Illinois Press.

Lindberg, B., Hunter, M., & Kruszewski, K. (1998). *Introduction to nursing* (3rd ed.). Philadelphia: Lippincott.

Malone, B. (2001). Nurses in non-nursing leadership positions. In J. Dochterman & H. Grace (Eds.), *Current issues in nursing* (6th ed., pp. 293–298). St. Louis, MO: Mosby.

Mangum, S., Garrison, C., Lind, C., & Hilton, H. (1997). First impressions of the nurse and nursing care. *Journal of Nursing Care Quality, 11*(5), 39–47.

National League for Nursing. (2008, March 3). *Number of nursing school graduates—including ethnic and racial minorities—on the rise but applications to RN programs dip, reflecting impact of tight admissions* (News Release). Retrieved March 4, 2008, from http://www.nln.org/newsreleases/data_release_03032008.htm

Nurses for a Healthier Tomorrow. (2007). Retrieved July 18, 2007, from http://www.nursesource.org/

Pike, A. (2001). Entering collegial relationships. In J. Dochterman & H. Grace (Eds.), *Current issues in nursing* (6th ed., pp. 448–452). St. Louis, MO: Mosby.

Saad, L. (2006, December 14). *Nurses top list of most honest and ethical professions.* Retrieved July 2, 2007, from Gallup Poll Web site: http://www.galluppoll.com/content/?ci=25888&pg=1

Santos, S., & Cox, K. (2002). Generational tension among nurses. *American Journal of Nursing, 102*(1), 11.

Sieber, J. R., Powers, C. A., Baggs, J. R., Knapp, J. M., & Sileo, C. M. (1998). Missing in action: Nurses in the media. *American Journal of Nursing, 98*(12), 55–56.

Siela, D. (2006, December). Managing multigenerational nursing staff. *American Nurse Today,* 47–49.

Smith, M. (1975). *When I say no, I feel guilty.* New York: Bantam.

Stewart, M. (1999). *ANA puts nursing in media spotlight.* Washington, DC: Author.

Stewart, M. (2007). *RN=Real News: Media relations and you.* Retrieved July 3, 2007, from American Nurses Association Web site: http://nursingworld.org/mods/archive/mod230/cernfull.htm

Sullivan, E. J. (2004). *Becoming influential. A guide for nurses.* Upper Saddle River, NJ: Pearson Education.

Sullivan, L., & the Sullivan Commission. (2004). *Missing persons: Minorities in the health professions.* Battle Creek, MI: W. K. Kellogg Foundation.

Tobin, S. (2006, October). How do you look? *American Nurse Today,* 38–39.

Ulrich, B. (2001). Successfully managing multigenerational workforces. *Seminars for Nurse Managers, 9,* 147–153.

U.S. Department of Health and Human Services, Health Resources and Services Administration, Bureau of Health Professions. (2006, June). *The registered nurse population. Findings from the March 2004 national sample survey of registered nurses.* Retrieved June 4, 2007 from http://www.bhpr.hrsa.gov/healthworkforce'rnsurvey04/default.htm

U.S. Department of Labor. Bureau of Labor Statistics. (2006, August 4). *Registered nurses.* Retrieved July 18, 2007, from http://stats.bls.gov/oco.ocos083.htm

Wieck, K., Prydun, M., & Walsh, T. (2002). What the emerging workforce wants in its leaders. *Journal of Nursing Scholarship, 34,* 283–288.

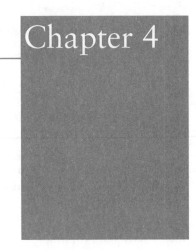

Chapter 4

Nursing Education, Accreditation, and Regulation

CHAPTER OBJECTIVES

At the conclusion of this chapter, the learner will be able to:

- Discuss the differences between nursing education and other types of education.

- Describe the types of nursing programs and degrees.

- Identify the roles of major nursing organizations that have an impact on nursing education.

- Explain requirements and issues related to quality nursing education.

- Discuss the use of distance education in nursing programs.

- Explain the importance of lifelong learning.

- Define certification and credentialing.

- Describe the nursing education accreditation process and its importance.

- Discuss the importance of regulation and its process and critical issues.

CHAPTER OUTLINE

KEY TERMS

- ❏ Accreditation
- ❏ Advanced practice nurse
- ❏ Apprenticeship model
- ❏ Articulation
- ❏ Associate's degree in nursing
- ❏ Baccalaureate degree in nursing
- ❏ Certification
- ❏ Continuing education
- ❏ Credentialing
- ❏ Curriculum
- ❏ Diploma school of nursing
- ❏ Distance education
- ❏ Master's degree in nursing
- ❏ Nurse externship
- ❏ Nurse Practice Act
- ❏ Nurse residency
- ❏ Practicum
- ❏ Preceptor
- ❏ Prescriptive authority
- ❏ Regulation
- ❏ Self-directed learning
- ❏ Standard
- ❏ Training

Introduction

This chapter focuses on three critical concerns in the nursing profession: (1) nursing education, (2) **accreditation** of nursing programs, and (3) regulatory issues such as licensure. These concerns are interrelated because these areas change and require input from the nursing profession. Even after graduation, nurses should be aware of educational issues, such as appropriate and reasonable accreditation of nursing programs, and ensure that regulatory issues support the critical needs of the public for quality health care, and the needs of the profession. Figure 4–1 highlights the components of the education-to-practice process.

Nursing Education

A nursing student might wonder why a nursing textbook has a chapter that includes content about nursing education. By the time a nursing student is reading this textbook, he or she will have selected a nursing program and be in that program. This content is not included in this textbook to help someone decide whether to enter the profession, or which nursing program to attend. Education is a critical component of the nursing profession. Nurses need to understand the structure and process of the profession's education, quality issues, and current issues and trends. Exhibit 4–1 provides an extensive glossary of nursing education terms.

Data indicate that nursing students represent more than half of all healthcare professionals (American Association of Colleges of Nursing [AACN], 2002), and yet in 2006, a total of 32,000 qualified applicants to nursing programs were turned down. However, enrollment in entry-level baccalaureate programs was increasing (AACN, 2007a). The Health Resources and Services Administration (HRSA) indicated that in the next 20 years, the demand for nurses will rise (U.S. Department of Health and Human Services, 2004).

The Health Resources and Services Administration projects that nursing schools must increase the number of graduates by 90 percent in order to adequately address the nursing shortage. With an 18.0 percent increase in graduations from baccalaureate nursing programs this year, schools are falling far short of meeting this target. By the year 2020, HRSA projects that more than one million new

Registered Nurses (RNs) will be needed in the U.S. healthcare system to meet the demand for nursing care. (AACN, 2006a)

Table 4–1 provides data about supply and demand for RNs. Figure 4–2 shows average age and full-time employees by degrees.

Given the critical issues of a growing nursing shortage and the consequent need to attract more students to nursing programs, this section focuses on nursing education to facilitate a better understanding of current and future concerns. The nursing shortage is discussed in more detail in Chapter 14, though it is a recurring issue throughout this textbook.

Nursing Education: This Is Not an English Lit Course!

Nursing education is different—different from other educational programs and courses. Students who enter a college or university nursing program typically have taken a lot of courses in liberal arts and sciences. When they enter a nursing program, they come with certain expectations that are derived from their previous experiences. They expect a didactic course similar to other courses, such as an English literature course. They go to the class, sit there and listen, and then periodically turn in assignments and take exams. Recently, in some cases, students have taken some of these courses online. Nursing courses demand more. More content relies on previous courses and builds to the subsequent ones. The expectation is that students will apply content from previous courses to current courses. Learning becomes more of a continuum, as opposed to neat packages of content that can be filed away when a course ends. Understanding is more important than memorizing (though some memorization is required), and application of information becomes more important in practice and on exams.

In addition, many nursing courses have a clinical or **practicum**, or they may have no didactic

Figure 4–1 From education to practice.

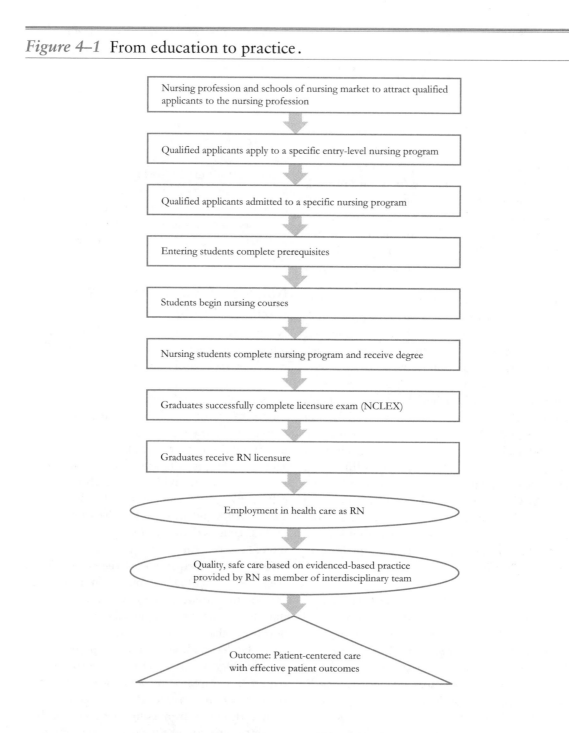

Exhibit 4–1 Definition of Nursing Education Terms

NONBACCALAUREATE PROGRAMS

Licensed practical nursing (LPN or LVN) program: A program that requires at least 1 year of full-time equivalent (FTE) coursework and awards the graduate a diploma or certificate of completion as a LPN/LVN.

LPN (LVN) to associate's degree in nursing (ADN) program: A program that admits licensed practical nurses and awards an associate's degree in nursing at completion.

Associate's degree in nursing (ADN): A program that requires at least 2 academic years of college academic credit and awards an associate's degree in nursing.

BACCAULAREATE PROGRAMS

Generic (basic or entry-level) baccalaureate program: Admits students with no previous nursing education and awards a baccalaureate nursing degree. Program requires at least 4 but not more than 5 academic years of college academic credit.

Accelerated baccalaureate for *nonnursing* college graduates program: Admits students with baccalaureate degrees in other disciplines and no previous nursing education, and awards a baccalaureate nursing degree. Curriculum is designed to be completed in less time than the generic baccalaureate program, usually through a combination of "bridge" or transition courses.

LPN/LVN-to-baccalaureate in nursing program: Admits licensed practical nurses and awards a baccalaureate nursing degree.

RN-to-baccalaureate in nursing (RN baccalaureate; RN completion) program: Admits RNs with associate's degrees or diplomas in nursing and awards a baccalaureate nursing degree.

MASTER'S PROGRAMS

Master of science in nursing (MSN) program: Admits students with baccalaureate nursing degrees and awards a master of science in nursing.

Accelerated baccalaureate-to-master's program: Admits students with baccalaureate nursing degrees and awards a master's in nursing degree. Curriculum is designed to be completed in less time than a traditional master's program, usually through a combination of "bridge" or transition courses, and core courses.

MA in nursing program: Admits students with baccalaureate nursing degrees and awards a master of arts in nursing.

MS with a major in nursing program: Admits students with baccalaureate nursing degrees and awards a master of science with a major in nursing.

Master of nursing (MN) program: Admits students with baccalaureate nursing degrees and awards a master of nursing.

LPN/LVN-to-master's program: Admits RNs without baccalaureate degrees in nursing and awards a master's degree in nursing. Graduates meet requirements for a baccalaureate nursing degree as well.

RN-to-master's program: Admits RNs without baccalaureate degrees in nursing and awards a master's degree in nursing.

Master's for *nonnursing* college graduates (entry-level/second-degree master's) program: Admits students with baccalaureate degrees in other disciplines and no previous nursing education. Program prepares graduates for entry into the profession and awards a master's degree in nursing. Although these programs generally require a baccalaureate degree, a few programs admit students without baccalaureate degrees.

Dual-degree master's programs: Admits RNs with baccalaureate degrees in nursing and awards a master's degree in another field (e.g., master of business administration, master of public health, master of public administration, master of hospital administration, master of divinity, or Juris Doctor).

DOCTORAL PROGRAMS

Doctor of nursing practice (DNP): Admits nurses who want to pursue a doctoral degree that focuses on practice rather than research. This practice-focused doctoral program prepares graduates for the highest level of nursing practice beyond the initial preparation in the discipline and is a terminal degree.

continues

EXHIBIT 4–1 (continued)

Doctoral (research-focused) program: Admits RNs with master's degrees in nursing and awards a doctoral degree. This program prepares students to pursue intellectual inquiry and conduct independent research for the purpose of extending knowledge. In the academic community, the PhD, or doctor of philosophy degree, is the most commonly offered research-focused doctoral degree. However, some schools, for a variety of reasons, may award a doctor of nursing science (DNS or DNSc) as the research-focused doctoral degree.

OTHER PROGRAMS

Clinical nurse specialist (CNS) program: A graduate (master's-level) program in which a defined curriculum includes theory, research, and clinical preparation for competency-based CNS specialty practice.

Nurse practitioner program: A graduate (master's-level) preparation in which a defined curriculum includes theory, research, and clinical preparation for competency-based primary care. Graduates are awarded a master's degree in nursing and are eligible to sit for a national NP certification examination.

Clinical nurse leader program: A graduate (master's-level) program in which a defined curriculum includes leadership content focused on direct patient care.

Postmaster's nurse practitioner program: A formal postgraduate program for the preparation of nurse practitioners that admits registered nurses with master's degrees in nursing. At completion, students are awarded a certificate or other evidence of completion, such as a letter from the program director. Completers are eligible to sit for the national NP examination.

Nurse practitioner: A registered nurse who, through a graduate degree program in nursing, functions in an independent care provider role and addresses the full range of patient/client health problems and needs within an area of specialization.

Nursing students: Students who have been formally accepted into a nursing program regardless of whether they have taken any nursing courses.

Prenursing students: Students who have not been formally accepted into the nursing program.

Source: 2006–2007 Enrollment and Graduations in Baccalaureate and Graduate Programs in Nursing, by American Association of Colleges of Nursing, 2007, Washington, DC: Author.

---

component and be all clinical. A student might think that these courses are equivalent to a chemistry lab, but this is not a fair comparison. A nursing practicum usually covers several hours and in some cases can be 8–12 hours several days a week. Students must prepare for the experience and work these hours as students. Faculty are there to guide student learning, and in some situations, students are assigned to **preceptors,** who are nurses working in the healthcare organization. Students do their clinical work in a variety of clinical settings, such as hospitals, clinics, homes, and community settings. This certainly is not equivalent to a 2-hour chemistry lab

once a week. Some courses use the simulation lab, where students go into a structured learning setting and practice skills and decision making in a simulated situation with faculty guidance. So this is definitely not English Lit! Nursing education is demanding and complex, but how did it get this way, and why is it this way? This section explores the many facets and issues of nursing education, both entry-level education and graduate programs.

STUDENT LEARNING STYLES

As students enter nursing courses, it is helpful for them to consider their own learning styles

Table 4–1 PROJECTED U.S. FTE RN SUPPLY DEMAND AND SHORTAGES

	2000	2005	2010	2015	2020
Supply	1,890,700	1,942,500	1,941,200	1,886,100	1,808,000
Demand	2,001,500	2,161,300	2,347,000	2,569,800	2,824,900
Shortage	(110,800)	(218,800)	(405,800)	(683,700)	(1,016,900)
Supply ÷ Demand	94%	90%	83%	73%	64%
Demand Shortfall	6%	10%	17%	27%	36%

Source: What Is Behind HRSA's Projected Supply, Demand, and Shortage of Registered Nurses? by U.S. Department of Health and Human Services, Health Resources and Services Administration, Bureau of Health Professions, National Center for Health Workforce Analysis, September 2004. Retrieved August 28, 2007, from ftp://ftp.hrsa.gov/bhpr/workforce/behindshortage.pdf

and how their style might or might not be effective. If it is not effective, students may need to consider changes. What does learning style mean? Learning style is a student's preferences for different types of learning and instructional activities. There are a variety of views of these styles. In doing a personal learning style self-assessment, a student might apply Kolb's (1984) learning styles inventory, which was further developed by Honey and Mumford (1986, 1992). Kolb described a continuum of four learning styles: (1) concrete experiences, (2) reflective observation, (3) abstract conceptualization, and (4) active experimentation. No one

Figure 4–2 Average Age and FTEs by Degrees.

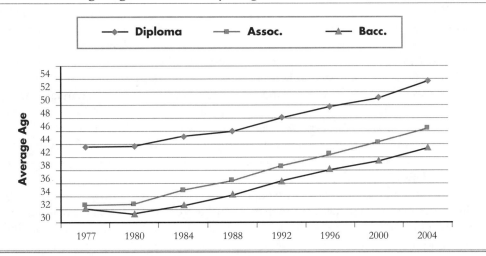

Source: From *The Future of the Nursing Workforce in the United States: Data, Trends and Implications*, by P.I. Buerhaus, D.O. Staiger and D.I. Auerbach, 2009, Sudbury, MA: Jones and Bartlett Publishers. Data from National Sample Survey of Registered Nurses.

person can be placed in only one style, but most people have a predominant style (Kolb, 1984, as cited in Rassool & Rawaf, 2007, pp. 36–37):

1. Divergers: Sensitive, imaginative and people-oriented; often enter professions such as nursing; excel in brainstorming sessions.
2. Assimilators: Less focused on people and more interested in ideas and abstract concepts. Excel in organizing and presenting information; in formal education, prefer reading, lectures, exploring analytical models, and having time to think things through.
3. Convergers: Solve problems and prefer technical tasks; less concerned with people and interpersonal aspects; often choose careers in technology.
4. Accommodators: Excel in concrete experience and active experimentation and prefer to take a practical or experimental approach; attracted to new challenges and experiences; and carry out plans. People-oriented and active learners.

Taking Kolb's proposed styles, the following has been described as a variation.

1. Activists: *Having an experience*; focus on immediate experience; interested in here and now; like to initiate new challenges and be the center of attention.
2. Reflectors: *Reviewing the experience*; observers; prefer to analyze experiences before taking action; good listeners; cautious; tend to adopt low profile.
3. Theorists: *Concluding from experience*; adopt a logical and rational approach to problem-solving but need some structure with a clear purpose or goal; learning weakest when they do not understand the purpose, when activities are less structured, and when feelings are emphasized.

4. Pragmatists: *Planning the next steps*; like to try out new ideas and techniques to see if they work in practice; are practical and down-to-earth; like solving problems and making decisions.

Understanding one's style can help a student when he or she approaches new content, reads assignments, and participates in other learning activities. It can impact how easy or difficult the work may be for the student. Students may need to "stretch"—that is, try to learn or do something that is challenging for them—and they may need to adapt their learning style.

A Brief History of Nursing Education

It is impossible to discuss the history of nursing education without reflecting on the history of the profession and the history of health care. All three are interconnected. Significant professional historical events were discussed in Chapter 1. A key player was Florence Nightingale. She changed not only the practice of nursing but also the **training**, which came to be called education rather than training. Training focuses on fixed habits and skills; uses repetition, authority, and coercion; and emphasizes dependency (Donahue, 1983). Education focuses more on self-discipline, responsibility, accountability, and self-mastery (Donahue, 1983). Up until the time that Nightingale became involved in nursing, there was little, if any, training for the role. Apprenticeship was used to introduce new recruits to nursing, and often it was not done effectively. As nursing changed, so did the need for more information and skills, leading to increasingly structured educational experiences. This did not occur without debate and disagreement regarding the best approach. What did happen, and how does it impact nursing education today?

In 1860, Nightingale established the first school of nursing, St. Thomas, in London, England. She was able to do this because she had received a very good education in the areas of math and science, which was highly unusual for women of her era. With her experience in the Crimean War, she recognized that many soldiers were dying not just because of their wounds but also because of infection and not being placed in the "best light" for healing. Nightingale then devoted her energies to upgrading nursing education; she placed less focus on on-the-job training and more on an educational program of study, creating the training school. This training school and those that quickly followed became a source of cheap labor for hospitals. Students were provided some nursing education, but they also worked long hours in the hospitals and were the largest staff source. The **apprenticeship model**, as it was called, continued, but it became more structured and included a more formal educational component. The educational component was far from ideal, and over time, it expanded and improved. In the same time period, similar programs opened in the United States. These programs were called diploma schools, and the first schools in the United States were Johns Hopkins (Baltimore, Maryland), the New England Hospital for Women and Children (Boston, Massachusetts), Women's Hospital (Philadelphia, Pennsylvania), and Bellevue Hospital (New York City). During this period, Canada developed similar programs.

Hospitals across the country began to open schools as they realized that students could be used as staff in the hospitals. The quality of these schools was variable because there were no **standards** or direction aside from what the individual hospital wanted to do. A few schools recognized early on the need for more content and improved teaching; a few of these schools were creative and formed partnerships with universities so that students could receive some content through an academic institution. Despite these small efforts to improve, the schools continued to be very different, and there were concerns about the quality of nursing education.

In 1918, an important step was taken through an initiative supported by the Rockefeller Foundation to address the issue of the diploma schools. This initiative culminated in the Goldmark report. The key points from this report were (Goldmark, 1923):

- Hospitals controlled the total education hours, with minimal content and, in some cases, no content when that content was needed.
- Sciences, theory, and practice of nursing were often taught by inexperienced instructors with few teaching resources.
- Students were supervised by graduate nurses who had limited experience and limited time to assist the students in their learning.
- Classroom experiences frequently occurred after the students had worked long hours, even during the night.
- Students typically were able to get only the experiences that their hospital provided, with all clinical work taking place in one hospital.

The report had an impact, particularly its key recommendations: (1) separating university schools of nursing from hospitals (not all schools of nursing, only a minority), (2) changing the control of hospital-based programs over to schools of nursing, and (3) requiring a high school diploma for entry into any school of nursing. These were major improvements in nursing education.

Changes were made, but slowly. The National League for Nursing (NLN) started developing and implementing standards for schools, but it took more than 20 years to accomplish this. New schools opened based on the Goldmark recommendations, such as the Yale School of Nursing (New Haven, Connecticut) and Case Western (Cleveland, Ohio).

A second report that had a major impact on improving nursing education was the Brown report (Brown, 1948), which also focused on the quality and structure of nursing education. This report led to the establishment of a formalized process, to be conducted by the NLN, to accredit nursing schools. Accreditation is discussed in more detail in this chapter. This was a critical step toward improving schools of nursing and the practice of nursing because it established standards across schools.

Entry into Practice: A Debate

The challenges in making changes were great when one considers that a very large number of hospitals in communities across the country had diploma schools based on the old model, and these schools were part of, and funded by, the communities. It was not easy to change these schools or to close them without major debate and conflict. These schools constituted the major type of nursing education in the United States through the 1960s and still exist today. The number of diploma schools has decreased primarily because of a critical debate and two decisions made in 1965. The debate focused on what type of education nurses need for entry into practice. The drive to move nursing education into college and university settings was great, but there was also great support to continue with the **diploma schools of nursing**—some of which continue today. In 1965, the NLN and the American Nurses Association (ANA) came out with strong statements endorsing college-based nursing education as the entry point into the profession. The ANA (1965) stated that "minimum preparation for beginning technical (bedside) nursing practice at the present time should be associate degree education in nursing" (p. 107). The situation was very tense. The two largest nursing organizations at the time—one primarily focused on education (NLN) and the other more on practice (ANA)— clearly took a stand. From the 1960s through the 1980s, these organizations tried to alter accredi-

tation, advocated for the closing of diploma programs, and lobbied all levels of government (Leighow, 1996). This was a very emotional issue, and even today it continues to be a tense topic because it has not been resolved. Were changes made? Yes, many:

- The number of diploma schools gradually decreased, *but they still exist*.
- The number of associate degree in nursing (ADN) programs grew. However, there was, and continues to be, concern over the development of a two-level nursing system—ADN and bachelor of science in nursing (BSN)—with one viewed as technical and the other as professional. However, this really has not happened. In fact, ADN programs continue to increase, and there has been no change in licensure for any of the nursing programs. All graduates of diploma programs, associate's degree programs, and baccalaureate programs continue to take the same exam that made nursing the first healthcare profession to have one national exam.
- BSN programs continued to grow, and do so today.

In addition, because of the movement of many nursing schools into the university setting, nursing programs lost their strong connection with hospitals. The nursing education community did want to get away from the control of hospitals, but now nursing educators and students are visitors to hospitals, with little feeling of partnership and connection. This has had an impact on clinical experiences, which will be discussed in this chapter.

Differentiated Nursing Practice

Another issue related to entry-into-practice is differentiated nursing practice. Rick stated that "leaders have yet to fully step up to the plate to determine and articulate what is *really* needed for nursing in the full spectrum of practice environments. Practice settings should offer differentiated nursing roles with distinct *and* complementary responsibilities" (2003, p. 11). What is differentiated practice? First, it is not a new idea; it has been discussed in the literature since the 1990s. Differentiated practice is described as a "philosophy that structures the roles and functions of nurses according to their education, experience, and competence," or "matching the varying needs of clients with the varying abilities of nursing practitioners" (American Organization of Nurse Executives [AONE], 1990, as cited in Hutchins, 1994, p. 52). This is clearly not a new issue, but it is one that still must be resolved.

How does this actually work in practice? Does a clinical setting distinguish between RNs who have a diploma, or ADN or BSN degrees? Does this impact role function and responsibilities? Does the organization even acknowledge degrees on name tags? Most healthcare organizations do note differences when it comes to RNs with graduate degrees but not necessarily to those with a diploma, ADN, or BSN. This approach does not recognize that there are differences in the education for each degree or diploma; this is difficult to resolve because all RNs, regardless of the type and length of their basic nursing education program, take the same licensing exam.

In 1995, a joint report was published by the AACN in collaboration with the AONE, and the National Organization for Associate Degree Nursing (N-OADN). The document described the two roles of the BSN and the ADN graduate (p. 28):

- The BSN is a licensed RN who provides direct care that is based on the nursing process and focused on clients with complex interactions of nursing diagnoses.

Clients include individuals, families, groups, aggregates, and communities in structured and unstructured healthcare settings. The unstructured setting is a geographical or a situational environment that may not have established policies, procedures, and protocols and has the potential for variations requiring independent nursing decisions.

- The ADN is a licensed RN who provides direct care that is based on the nursing process and focused on individual clients who have common, well-defined nursing diagnoses. Consideration is given to the client's relationship within the family. The ADN functions in a structured healthcare setting that is a geographical or situational environment where the policies, procedures, and protocols for provision of healthcare are established. In the structured setting there is recourse to assistance and support from the full scope of nursing expertise.

Despite increased support, such as from the AONE, for making the BSN the entry-level educational requirement, this question continues to be one of the most frustrating issues in the profession and has not been clearly resolved (AACN, 2005a). The AACN believes that "education has a direct impact on the skills and competencies of a nurse clinician. Nurses with a baccalaureate degree are well-prepared to meet the demand placed on today's nurse across a variety of settings and are prized for their critical thinking, leadership, case management, and health promotion skills" (AACN, 2005a, p. 1) What percentage of nurses have a BSN? As of 2005, 43% of the RN workforce have a BSN, 34% have a ADN, and 22% have a diploma, with only 16% of ADN graduates completing a BSN. Today, there is even more evidence to support the value of a BSN. A study by Aiken, Clarke, Cheung, Sloane, and Silber (2003) indicates that there is a "substantial survival advantage" for patients in hospitals with a higher percentage of BSN RNs. Other studies (Estabrooks, Midodzi, Cummings, Ricker, & Giovannetti, 2005) support these outcomes. The long-term impact of these types of studies on the entry into practice is unknown, but there is more evidence now to support the decision made in 1965.

Types of Nursing Programs

Nursing is a profession with a complex education pattern—many different entry-level pathways to licensure, and then many different graduate programs. Exhibit 4–2 and Figure 4–3 describe some data about the number of graduates from the different programs.

Next are descriptions of the major nursing education programs. That there are several entry-level nursing programs complicates the issue and raises concerns about the best way to provide education for nursing students.

DIPLOMA SCHOOLS OF NURSING

Diploma schools of nursing still exist, though many now have partnerships with colleges or universities where students might take some of their courses. Many of these schools have closed, but some have been converted into associate's degree programs. However, there has been an increase in these programs because employers feel that their need for staff nurses is so great, and degree programs are not meeting these needs. New programs are starting, and a new organization, the Association of Diploma Schools of Professional Nursing, represents these schools. Diploma schools are accredited by the NLN. Graduates take the same licensing exam as graduates from all the other types of nursing programs. The nursing **curriculum** is similar; the graduates need the same nursing content for the licensing exam. However, the students typically have fewer prerequisites, particularly in the liberal arts and sciences, though they do have some science content. There is variation in these schools because some students take some of their required courses in local colleges.

ASSOCIATE'S DEGREE IN NURSING

Programs for an **associate's degree in nursing** began when Mildred Montag published a book on the need for a different type of nursing program: a 2-year program that would be established in community colleges (Montag, 1959). At the time that Montag created this proposal,

---

EXHIBIT 4–2 DATA ON THE NUMBER OF GRADUATES PER EDUCATIONAL PROGRAM

- RNs with a diploma as initial preparation: 733,377 (25.2%)
- RNs with an associate's degree as initial preparation: 1,227,256 (42.2%)
- RNs with a baccalaureate degree as initial preparation: 887,223 (30.5%)
- RNs with an MSN or doctoral degree as initial preparation: 15,511 (0.5%)
- RNs with a diploma as highest educational level: 510,209 (17.5%)
- RNs with an associate's degree as highest educational level: 981,238 (33.7%)
- RNs with a baccalaureate degree as highest educational level: 994,240 (34.2%)
- RNs with an MSN or doctoral degree as highest educational level: 377,046 (13.0%)

Source: U.S. Department of Health and Human Services, Health Resources and Services Administration, Bureau of Health Professions, National Center for Health Workforce Analysis. (2004, September). *What Is Behind HRSA's Projected Supply, Demand, and Shortage of Registered Nurses?* Retrieved August 28, 2007, from ftp://ftp.hrsa.gov/bhpr/workforce/behindshortage.pdf

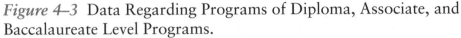

Figure 4–3 Data Regarding Programs of Diploma, Associate, and Baccalaureate Level Programs.

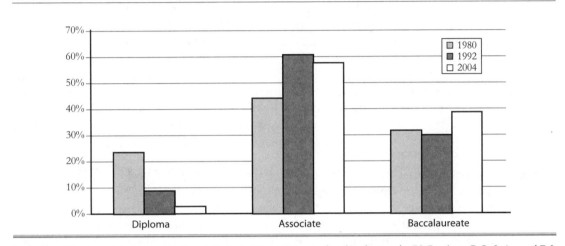

Source: From *The Future of the Nursing Workforce in the United States: Data, Trends and Implications*, by P.I. Buerhaus, D.O. Staiger and D.I. Auerbach, 2009, Sudbury, MA: Jones and Bartlett Publishers. Data from National Sample Survey of Registered Nurses.

there was a shortage of nurses after World War II. Today, some diploma programs that have not closed but that do not want to continue to offer the diploma program have chosen to move to an associate's degree model. For students, ADN programs are cheaper and shorter. The programs are accredited by the NLN. The curriculum includes some liberal arts and sciences at the community college level but really focuses more on technical nursing. Graduates take the same licensing exam as graduates from all other nursing programs.

Recently, there have been a variety of models or opportunities for ADN students and their graduates. Montag envisioned the ADN as a terminal degree; however, this has changed, with a degree being viewed more as part of a career mobility path. The RN-BSN or BSN completion programs that are found throughout the United States are a way for ADN graduates to complete the requirements for a BSN. Typically, these graduates work and then go back to school, often part time, to complete a BSN in

a university-level program. Some prerequisite courses must be taken before these students enter most BSN programs. Additional nursing courses that these students may take are health assessment, community health, leadership and management, research, health policy, and some additional clinical courses, though this is not the major focus of the RN-BSN programs. Content focuses on what they did not cover in their ADN program. Today, many of these RN-BSN programs are offered online, and greater efforts are made to facilitate the transition from the ADN program to the BSN program. The overall goal is to guide all ADN graduates back to school for a BSN, though this has not been accomplished yet.

Another change that has been taking place in the last few years is the development of partnerships with ADN and BSN programs. In these partnerships, the ADN program has a clear relationship with a BSN program. This allows for a seamless transition from one program to the other. Students complete their first 2 years in the ADN program and then complete the last 2 years of the BSN in the partner program. In these types of programs, both the participating ADN and BSN programs collaborate on the curriculum and how to best transition the students. One benefit of this model is that students pay the community college fees, which are less costly than the university fees, for the first 2 years. If there is no BSN program in a community, students can stay within their own community for the first 2 years before transitioning to a BSN program.

BACCALAUREATE DEGREE IN NURSING

The idea for the **baccalaureate degree in nursing** was presented in the Goldmark report, although it took many years for it to gain a hold in nursing education. The earlier programs lasted 5 years, with the first 2 years in liberal arts and sciences, and then 3 years in nursing courses. The programs began to move to a 4-year model, with variations of 2 years in liberal arts and sciences and then 2 years in nursing courses. Some schools introduce students to nursing content during the first 2 years, but typically not a lot. In many colleges of nursing, students are not admitted to the college until they complete the first 2 years, though the students are in the same university. These programs may be accredited by the NLN or through the AACN. (There is more information about accreditation later in the chapter.) BSN graduates take the same licensure exam as all other basic nursing program graduates.

In the 1960s, BSN programs and enrollment grew rapidly. As discussed, the question of the educational level for entry into the profession continues to be unresolved, though since 1965, major nursing organizations have clearly stated that it is the BSN. The RN-BSN programs, which are offered by the BSN programs, have grown in the last few years. A BSN is required for admission to a nursing graduate program. "**Articulation** agreements are important mechanisms that enhance access to baccalaureate level nursing education. These agreements support education mobility and facilitate the seamless transfer of academic credit between associate degree (ADN) and baccalaureate (BSN) nursing programs" (AACN, 2005b, p. 1). These agreements, which may be between individual schools, mandated by state law, or part of statewide articulation plans, facilitate the transfer of credits. This helps students who want to take some courses in an ADN program or who have an ADN degree to enter BSN programs.

ADDITIONAL CLINICAL EXPERIENCES

Students frequently want more clinical experiences in the summer, when many schools of nursing do not offer courses, and they also want to be employed. The nurse externship is a program that offers this for students. Students are also concerned about their first job; they wonder if they are ready. The **nurse residency** program is one way to help with this transition.

Nurse Externships   **Nurse externships** are available in some communities sponsored by hospitals (Beecroft, Kunzman, & Krozek, 2001). These programs are not usually associated with a school of nursing. They are short programs, such as 10 weeks, usually offered in the summer for students who will enter their senior year in the fall. There is great variation in the length of these programs, in what is offered to the student in the program, and in how much support the student receives in the program. The student is employed by the hospital and provided with orientation to the hospital, some content experiences, and precepted and/or mentoring experiences. Students need to investigate the programs and find out what each program offers and whether it meets their needs.

Nurse Residency Programs   Because of the nursing shortage and other job-related issues, such as staff burnout and concern about the level of new graduates' preparation and retention, over the last few years, some hospitals have developed nurse residency programs (Bowles & Candela, 2005; Casey, Fink, Krugman, & Propst, 2004; Halfer & Graf, 2006a, b). The AACN is conducting a pilot program to examine a national accreditation program and is developing standards for nurse residency programs. A nurse residency program is a special program that a nurse applies for after graduation, and it typically (and ideally) lasts a year (Goode & Williams, 2004). This is the nurse's first position as an RN. A nurse resident is employed by the hospital during the residency. The residency helps the new graduate with transition to practice in a structured program that provides content and learning activities, precepted experiences, mentoring, and gradual adjustment to higher levels of responsibility. These are paid positions, and typically the nurse resident must commit to working for the institution for a period of time after the residency. These programs are proving to be helpful to new nurses and are decreasing turnover and improving staff retention. Not all hospitals have residencies, and admission to these programs is competitive. Some residency programs partner with schools of nursing, and this is what the draft of the AACN residency standards recommends (AACN, 2007b). Students who are interested in this type of experience need to investigate these opportunities in their senior year. Additional information about externships and residencies is found in Chapter 14.

MASTER'S DEGREE IN NURSING

Graduate education and the evolution of the **master's degree in nursing** have a long history. Early on, it was called postgraduate education and typically was in areas of public health, teaching, supervision, and some clinical specialties. The first formal graduate program was established in 1899 at Columbia University Teachers College (Donahue, 1983). The NLN supported the establishment of graduate nursing programs, and these programs were developed in great numbers. For example, some of the early programs, such as Yale School of Nursing, admitted students without a BSN but who had a baccalaureate in another major. Today, this is very similar to the accelerated programs in which students with other degrees are admitted to a BSN program that is shorter, covering the same content but in an accelerated approach. These students are typically categorized as graduate students because of their previous degree. However, they must complete BSN work before they can take nursing graduate courses, and in some cases, they are not admitted to the nursing graduate program automatically.

The master's programs in nursing have evolved since the 1950s. A typical length for a master's program is 2 years, and students may attend full time or part time. These programs are accredited by the NLN or AACN and, in some cases, by nursing specialty organizations, as discussed in this chapter. Examples of master's degree programs are:

- Clinical specialty-focused master's: Adult health, psychiatric-mental health, pediatrics, community health, gerontology, and many subspecialty-oriented areas such as neonatal nursing. These master's programs are focused on the functional roles of the **advanced practice nurse** and the clinical nurse specialist.
- Advanced practice nursing (APN): This master's degree can be offered in any clinical area, but typical areas are adult health, pediatrics, family health, women's health, neonatal health, and community health. Graduates take APN exams in their specialty area and must then meet specific

state requirements, such as for **prescriptive authority**, which gives them limited ability to prescribe medications. These nurses usually work in more independent roles. The American Nurses Credentialing Center (ANCC) provides national **certification** for clinical nurse specialists in a variety of areas, as discussed later in this chapter.

- Clinical nurse specialist (CNS): This master's degree can be offered in any clinical area. Specialty exams may also be taken. These nurses usually work in hospital settings (Chapter 15 discusses this role in more depth). The ANCC provides national certification for CNSs in a variety of areas, as discussed later in this chapter. Figure 4–4 shows the clinical tracks comprising the largest percentages of enrollees and graduates in clinical specialist programs.

- Nurse anesthetists: This master's degree is not offered at all colleges of nursing. It takes 2 years to complete and focuses on preparing nurses to deliver anesthesia. This is a highly competitive graduate program. Once certified, the nurse becomes a Certified Registered Nurse Anesthetist. The Association of Nurse Anesthetists handles accreditation of these programs and certification.

- Certified nurse midwife: This master's degree focuses on midwifery—all areas related to pregnancy and delivery, as well as gynecological care of women and family planning. These programs are accredited by the American College of Nurse-Midwives.

- Clinical nurse leader (CNL): This is the newest master's degree (programs have started within the last few years), which prepares nurses for leadership positions that

Figure 4–4 Master's- and post master's clinical nurse specialist specialty areas comprising the largest percentage of enrollees and graduates.

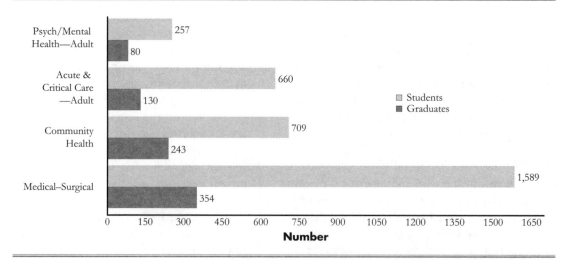

Source: 2006–2007 Enrollment and Graduations in Baccalaureate and Graduate Programs in Nursing, by American Association of Colleges of Nursing, 2007, Washington, DC: Author.

have a direct impact on patient care. "The CNL is a provider and a manager of care at the point of care to individuals and cohorts. The CNL designs, implements, and evaluates patient care by coordinating, delegating and supervising the care provided by the healthcare team, including licensed nurses, technicians, and other health professionals" (AACN, 2007c, p. 6).

- Master's degree in a functional area: This type of master's focuses on the functional areas of administration or education. It was more popular in the past, but with the growing need for nursing faculty, there has been a resurgence of master's degrees in nursing education. In some cases, colleges of nursing are offering certificate programs in nursing education. In these programs, a nurse with a nursing master's degree may take a certain number of credits that focus on nursing education and then receive a certificate of recognition. This provides the nurse with additional background and experience in nursing education.

DOCTORAL DEGREES IN NURSING

The doctoral degree (PhD) in nursing has had a complicated development history. The doctorate of nursing science was first offered in 1960. There were PhD programs in education in nursing as early as 1924, and New York University started the first PhD in nursing in 1953. Today, however, the PhD in nursing is the major emphasis at the post-master's level. Not enough students are entering these programs, and this has had an impact on nursing faculty. Someone with a PhD is not required to teach but is encouraged to do so. Nurses with PhDs usually are involved in research because it is considered a research degree, although a nurse at any level can be involved in research and may or may not teach. Study for a PhD typically takes place after receiving a master's degree in nursing and typi-

cally includes coursework and a research-focused dissertation. This process can take 4–5 years to complete, and much depends on completion of the dissertation. Nurses with PhDs may be called "doctor"; this is not the same as the medical doctor title, but rather the designation or title for their doctoral work in the same way that an English professor with a doctorate is called "Doctor____".

DOCTOR OF NURSING PRACTICE

The doctor of nursing practice (DNP) is the newest nursing degree, with the new degree and role of the CNL entering the profession at about the same time. There was a program similar to the DNP as early as 1979 at Case Western Reserve University (AACN, 2004). The DNP is not a PhD program, though these nurses also say that they can be called "doctor." However, this does not represent the same title as someone with a PhD. The DNP is a practice-focused doctoral degree program. This position has been controversial within nursing and within health care, particularly with physicians. Because this position is new, it is difficult to know what its long-term impact will be on the profession and on health care. The AACN has described the purpose of the DNP as follows:

> *Transforming healthcare delivery recognizes the critical need for clinicians to design, evaluate, and continuously improve the context within which care is delivered. The core function of healthcare is to provide the best possible clinical care to individuals, families and communities. The context within which care is delivered exerts a major impact on the kinds of care that are provided and on the satisfaction and productivity of individual clinicians. Nurses prepared at the doctoral level with a blend of clinical, organizational, economic and leadership skills are most likely to be able to critique nursing and other clinical scientific findings and design programs of*

care delivery that are locally acceptable, economically feasible, and which significantly impact healthcare outcomes. (AACN, 2004, p. 7)

Practice-focused doctoral nursing programs prepare leaders for nursing practice. The DNP is now the terminal practice degree for APN preparation, including, but not limited to, the four current APN roles: CNS, nurse anesthetist, nurse midwife, and nurse practitioner (AACN, 2004). Some of the reasons that the DNP was developed are related to the APN master's degree, which includes a high number of credits and clinical hours, and takes a long time to complete. It was recognized that these students should be getting more for their coursework and effort. Going on to a DNP program allows them to apply some of this credit toward a doctoral-level program. The benefits of practice-focused doctoral programs include (AACN, 2004, pp. 7–8):

- Development of needed advanced competencies for increasingly complex clinical, faculty, and leadership roles
- Enhanced knowledge to improve nursing practice and patient outcomes
- Enhanced leadership skills to strengthen practice and healthcare delivery
- Better match of program requirements and credits and time with the credential earned
- Provision of an advanced educational credential for those who require advanced practice knowledge but do not need or want a strong research focus (e.g., clinical faculty)
- Parity with other health professions, most of which have a doctorate as the credential required for practice
- Enhanced ability to attract individuals to nursing from non-nursing backgrounds
- Increased supply of faculty for clinical instruction
- Improved image of nursing

Because the DNP is a new degree and represents a new nursing role, it is not clear at this time what its impact will be on nursing and on healthcare delivery.

Given the concern about the shortage of nurses, the number of students entering nursing is an issue. Exhibit 4–3 describes some enrollment data, and Table 4–2 shows 5-year trends.

Nursing Education Associations

There are three major nursing education organizations, each with a different program focus. The organizations are the NLN, the AACN, and the N-OADN. The NLN and the AACN are the two major nursing education organizations.

NATIONAL LEAGUE FOR NURSING

The NLN is an older organization than the AACN. It "promotes excellence in nursing education to build a strong and diverse nursing workforce" (NLN, 2007a, p. 2). The NLN's goals for 2007–2012 are (p. 3):

1. Enhance the NLN's national and international impact as the recognized leader in nursing education.
2. Build a diverse, sustainable, member-led organization with the capacity to deliver our mission effectively, efficiently, and in accordance with our values.
3. Be the voice of nurse educators and champion their interests in political, academic, and professional arenas.
4. Promote evidence-based nursing education and the scholarship of teaching.

What is the major difference between the AACN and the NLN? The AACN represents only university-level nursing education programs; for example, it does not represent diploma programs or associate's degree programs. The NLN represents all nursing programs. The NLN accredits nursing programs

---

EXHIBIT 4–3   ENROLLMENT (FALL 2006) AND GRADUATIONS (AUGUST 1, 2005 TO JULY 31, 2006)

- A total of 133,578 students were enrolled in generic (entry-level) baccalaureate nursing education programs. RN-to-baccalaureate enrollment totaled 46,549 (Table 7).
- Enrollment at the master's, doctoral (research-focused), and doctor of nursing practice (DNP) levels totaled 56,028; 3,927; and 862, respectively (Table 7).
- Generic (entry-level) baccalaureate graduates totaled 37,851, and RN-to baccalaureate totaled 13,232. Master's, doctoral (research-focused), and doctor of nursing practice (DNP) levels totaled 13,470; 437; and 74, respectively (Table 7).
- Males accounted for 9.7% of all baccalaureate U.S. resident graduates (generic and RN-to-baccalaureate). The percentage of men graduating from master's, doctoral (research-focused), and doctor of nursing practice (DNP) programs was 9.8, 7.4, and 9.5, in that order (Table 8).
- Almost 35% of undergraduate (24.8%) enrollees and 21.8% of graduate-level enrollees (master's and research-focused doctoral programs) were from racial and ethnic minorities (Table 9).

Source: 2006–2007 Enrollment and Graduations in Baccalaureate and Graduate Programs in Nursing, by American Association of Colleges of Nursing, 2007, Washington, DC: Author.

---

through the National League for Nursing Accrediting Commission, which is also the oldest nursing accrediting commission. Accreditation is discussed in a later section of this chapter. The NLN offers educational opportunities for its members (individual membership and school of nursing membership) and addresses policy and standards issues related to nursing education.

AMERICAN ASSOCIATION OF COLLEGES OF NURSING

The AACN is the national organization that represents university and 4-year programs in

---

Table 4–2 FIVE-YEAR TRENDS IN ENROLLMENTS AND GRADUATIONS BY TYPE OF DEGREE (2002–2006)

| Degree | Students | | Graduates | |
	Average Change per Year*	Significance (*p* value)	Average per Year*	Significance (*p* value)
Generic Bacc.	+10,388	< 0.001	+3,136	0.007
RN-to-Bacc.	+2,920	0.007	+477	0.059
Master's	+4,475	0.002	+679	0.022
Doctoral (Research)	1203	< 0.001	21	0.933

Note: Bold values indicate a statistically significant (p , 0.050) average change per year.
Source: 2006–2007 Enrollment and Graudations in Baccalaureate and Graduate Programs in Nursing, by American Association of Colleges of Nursing, 2007, Washington, DC: Author.

nursing (AACN, 2007a). It has 600 members. Its activities include educational research, government advocacy, data collection, publishing, and initiatives to establish standards for baccalaureate and graduate degree nursing programs, including implementation of the standards. The AACN is also involved in accreditation of nursing programs in university and 4-year programs through its Commission on Collegiate Nursing Education, which is discussed in a later section of this chapter.

NATIONAL ORGANIZATION FOR ASSOCIATE DEGREE NURSING

The N-OADN is the organization that advocates for associate's degree nursing education and practice (N-OADN, 2007). Its major goals are to:

- Maintain eligibility for RN licensure for graduates of ADN programs
- Educate students and promote advanced degree (AD) nursing programs at community colleges nationwide
- Provide a forum for discussion of issues impacting AD education and practice
- Develop partnerships and increase communication with other professional organizations
- Increase public understanding of the role of the associate's degree nurse
- Participate at national and state levels in the formation of healthcare policy
- Facilitate legislative action supportive of the goals of N-OADN

N-OADN began in 1952 when Mildred Montag proposed the ADN—a degree in nursing that was shorter than the BSN (typically a 2-year program) based in a community college. The first programs opened in 1958. As of 2006, there were 940 programs, with over 600 in community colleges (N-OADN, 2006). This organization does not offer accreditation services; accreditation of ADN programs is done through the NLN. Graduates of ADN programs are professional nurses who are (N-OADN, 2006):

- Essential members of the interdisciplinary healthcare team in diverse healthcare settings
- Able to derive strength from their ethnic, cultural, social, economic and gender diversity, thereby enhancing the capacity to respond to the healthcare needs of a diverse nation
- Able to collaborate with all stakeholders for the development of public policy, the delivery of quality outcome-driven healthcare, and to ensure access to healthcare for all individuals
- Caring, competent, and knowledgeable healthcare providers who engage in professional development activities in order to advance safe, effective competent care
- Legally, morally, and ethically accountable

Quality and Excellence in Nursing Education

NURSING EDUCATION STANDARDS

Nursing education standards are developed by the major nursing professional organizations that focus on education: the NLN, AACN, and N-OADN. The accrediting bodies of the NLN and the AACN also set standards. State boards of nursing are also involved. There are also standards that colleges and universities must meet for nonnursing accreditation at the overall college or university level. Standards guide decisions, organizational structure, process, policies and procedures, budgetary decisions, admissions and progress of students, evaluation (program, faculty, and student), curriculum, and other academic issues.

NLN Excellence in Nursing Education Model

Recognition by the NLN as a Center of Excellence (COE) in Nursing Education identifies schools of nursing that demonstrate "sustained, evidence-based, and substantive innovation in the selected area; conduct ongoing research to document the effectiveness of such innovation; set high standards for themselves; and are committed to continuous quality improvement" (NLN, 2007b). These schools make a commitment to pursue excellence in (1) student learning and professional development, (2) development of faculty expertise in pedagogy, or (3) advancing the science of nursing education. This award is given to a school, not a program in a school, for 3 years. After this period, the school must be reviewed again for COE redesignation. This new initiative by NLN is an excellent example of efforts to improve nursing education.

Another new initiative, also by the NLN, to recognize excellence is the Academy of Nursing Education, which inducted its first nurse education fellows in 2007.

The purpose of the Academy of Nursing Education is to foster excellence in nursing education by recognizing and capitalizing on the wisdom of outstanding individuals who have made enduring and substantial contributions to nursing education in one or more areas (teaching/learning innovations, faculty development, research in nursing education, leadership in nursing education, public policy related to nursing education, or collaborative education/practice/community partnerships) and who will continue to provide visionary leadership in nursing education and in the Academy. (NLN, 2007a)

Nurses who are selected as fellows must document distinguished contributions in one or more areas: (1) teaching/learning innovations, (2) faculty development, (3) research in nursing education, (4) leadership in nursing education, (5) public policy related to nursing education, and (6) collaborative education/practice/community partnerships.

Focus on Competencies

The nursing curriculum should identify the competencies expected of students throughout the nursing program. Students need to know what the expected competencies are so they can be active participants in their own learning to reach those competencies. The competencies are used in evaluation and identify the level of learning or performance expected of the student. Nursing is a profession—a practice profession—and thus performance is a critical factor. Competency is the "the application of knowledge and the interpersonal, decision-making, and psychomotor skills expected for the nurse's practice role, within the context of public health, welfare, and safety" (National Council of State Boards of Nursing [NCSBN], 1996a). Competencies should clearly state the parameters related to the behavior or performance. The curriculum should support the development of competencies by providing necessary prerequisite knowledge and learning opportunities to meet the competency. The ultimate goal is a competent RN.

Curriculum

A nursing program's curriculum is the plan that describes the program's philosophy, level, terminal competencies for students (or what they are expected to accomplish by the end of the program), and course content (described in course syllabi). Also specified are the sequence of courses, and a designation of course credits and learning experiences, such as didactic (typically offered in a lecture or seminar setting) and clinical or practicum experiences. In addition, simulation laboratory experiences are used either at the beginning of the curriculum or throughout the curriculum. A nursing curriculum is very important. It tells potential students what they should expect in a program and may influence a student's choice of programs, particularly at the graduate level. It helps orient new students and is important in the accreditation of nursing programs. State boards of nursing review the curricula in their respective states. To keep current, it is important that curricula are reviewed regularly by the faculty and in a manner that allows changes to be made as easily and quickly as possible.

Baccalaureate education is guided by *The Essentials of Baccalaureate Education for Professional Nursing Practice* (AACN, 2008). This document was revised in 2008. A stimulus for this revision is addressing the Institute of Medicine (IOM) core competencies, such as interdisciplinary education, use of informatics, emphasis on patient safety and quality of care, use of evidence-based interventions as cornerstones of care, and recognition of the patient as the center of care. These competencies are discussed in detail in Section III of this book. The following paragraphs provide some history on this change.

The IOM published an important report, *Health Professions Education* (2003) that addressed the need for education in all major health professions to meet several common competencies to improve care. This report was motivated by grave concerns about the quality and safety of care in the United States and the need for nursing education to prepare professionals who provide quality, safe care. "Education for health professions is in need of a major overhaul. Clinical education simply has not kept pace with or been responsive enough to shifting patient demographics and desires, changing health system expectations, evolving practice requirements and staffing arrangements, new information, a focus on improving quality, or new technologies" (IOM, 2001, as cited in IOM, 2003, p. 1)

These competencies are found in the current *Essentials of Baccalaureate Education* (AACN, 2008); however, schools of nursing need to make changes to include the competencies more and, in some cases, to add new content to meet these needs.

Along with the call from the IOM to make major changes in health professions education, there is recognition that nursing education needs improvement and changes to make it more current with practice today. The NLN (2007a) has stated that

> *Student-centered, interactive, and innovative programs and curricula should be designed to promote leadership in students, develop students' thinking skills, reflect new models of learning and practice, effectively integrate technology, promote a lifelong career commitment in students, include intra- and interdisciplinary learning experiences, and prepare students for the roles they will assume.*

Didactic or Theory Content   Nursing curricula may vary as to titles of courses, course descriptions and objectives, sequence, and number of hours of didactic content and clinical experiences, but there are some constants even within these differences. Nursing content needs to include the following broad topical areas:

- Adult health or medical-surgical nursing
- Mental health/psychiatric
- Pediatrics
- Maternal-child (obstetrics, women's health, neonatal care)
- Community health
- Gerontology
- Leadership and management

- Pharmacology
- Health assessment

This content may be provided in clearly defined courses that focus on only one of these topical areas, or integrated with multiple topics. Practica may be incorporated into a course with related didactic content—for example, pediatric content and pediatric clinical, considered one course—or they can be offered as two separate courses, typically in the same semester. Faculty who teach didactic content may or may not teach in the clinical setting.

Practicum or Clinical   The hours for the practica can be highly variable within one school and from school to school (i.e., the number of hours per week and sequence of days, such as practica on Tuesdays and Thursdays from 8 A.M. to 3 P.M.). Many schools are now offering 12-hour clinical sessions. Some schools offer practica in the evenings, at night, and on weekends. It is important for students to understand the time commitment and scheduling, which have a great impact on students' personal lives and employment. In addition, these clinical experiences require preparation time. The types of clinical settings are highly variable and depend on the objectives and what sites are available. Examples of settings are acute care hospitals (all clinical areas); psychiatric hospitals; pediatric hospitals; women's health (may include obstetrics) clinics; community health clinics and other health agencies; home health agencies and patients' homes; hospice centers, including freestanding sites, hospital-based centers, and patients' homes; schools; camps; health-oriented consumer organizations such as the American Diabetes Association; health vans; homeless shelters; doctors' offices; clinics of all types; ambulatory surgical centers; emergency centers; Red Cross centers; businesses with occupational health services; and many more. In some of these sites—for example,

in acute care—faculty remain with the students for the entire rotation time. In others, particularly community health-type settings, faculty visit students at the site because typically only 1–4 students are in each community health site, compared with a larger group (8–10) assigned to a faculty member for hospital experiences. In the hospital setting, the faculty member is typically with the students for the entire rotation. The number of hours per week in clinical experiences increases in a nursing program, with the most hours at the end of the program.

Most schools of nursing use preceptors as part of the nursing curriculum at some time, in both undergraduate and graduate programs. A preceptor is an experienced and competent staff member (RN, or a nurse practitioner or MD for NP students) who has received formal training to function in this role. He or she serves as a role model and a resource for the nursing student and guides learning. The student is assigned to work alongside the preceptor. Faculty provide overall guidance to the preceptor regarding the nature of, and objectives for, the student's learning experiences; monitor the student's progress by meeting with the student and the preceptor; and are on call for communication with the student and preceptor as needed. The preceptor participates in evaluations of the student's progress, along with the student and the faculty member. Preceptors are typically used toward the end of an entry-level nursing program, but some schools use them throughout the program for certain courses. The state board of nursing may dictate how many hours in the total undergraduate nursing program may be devoted to preceptorship experiences. At the graduate level, the number of preceptorship hours is much higher.

Distance Education   **Distance education** has become quite common in nursing education, though not all schools offer courses in this manner. The AACN recognizes distance education as "a set of teaching and/or learning strategies to meet the learning needs of students separate from the traditional classroom and sometimes from traditional roles of faculty (Reinert & Fryback, 1997, as cited in AACN, 1999, p. 1). Distance education technologies have expanded over the last few years as technology develops. Some of the common distance education technologies are e-mail, fax, audiotaped instruction, audiocassette, conference by telephone, CD-ROM, e-mail lists (LISTSERVs), interactive television, desktop video conference, and Internet-based programming. There is no doubt that these methods will continue to expand. The most common and growing method is online courses. Distance education can be configured in several ways:

- Self-study
- Hybrid model—distance education combined with traditional classroom delivery (the most common configuration)
- Faculty-facilitated learning with no classroom activities (the approach that has increased the most)

As stated by the AACN, "When utilizing distance learning methods, a program provides or makes available resources for the students' successful attainment of all program objectives" (2005c, p. 1). For schools to effectively offer courses or entire programs using technologies for distance education, they must ensure that the following are supported:

- Registration
- Library access
- Student affairs support
- Technology support, which is critical and should be available 24/7

Students who participate in distance education must have certain characteristics to be suc-

cessful in this type of educational program. Students need to be responsible for their own learning, with faculty facilitating their learning. Computer competencies are critical for completing coursework and reducing student stress. Students must have required hardware and software. Students who are organized and able to develop and meet a schedule will be able to handle the course requirements. If students are assertive, ask questions, and ask for help, they will be more successful.

Self-directed learning is important for all nursing students because it leads to greater ability to achieve lifelong learning as a professional. What is self-directed learning? There are a variety of definitions, and most are based on Knowles's (1975, p. 18, as cited in O'Shea, 2003, p. 62): "a process in which individuals take the initiative, with or without the help of others, in diagnosing their learning needs, formulating learning goals, identifying human and material resources for learning, choosing and implementing appropriate learning strategies and evaluating learning outcomes." Student-centered learning approaches can assist students—for example, problem-based learning or team-based learning. This type of approach means that the faculty must also change how they teach. Faculty members assume the role of facilitator of learning, which requires a more collaborative relationship between faculty and students. Faculty work with students to develop active participation and goal setting: helping students to work on setting goals, making plans with clear strategies to meet the goals, and encouraging self-assessment. Distance education emphasizes adult teaching and learning principles more than the traditional classroom approach does. These principles were originally described by Knowles (1984) with learners and include:

- Accepting responsibility for collaborating in the planning of their learning experiences

- Setting goals
- Actively participating
- Pacing their own learning
- Participating in monitoring their own progress; self-assessment

The quality of distance education is as important as the quality of traditional classroom courses. Syllabi that describe the course description, objectives, and outcomes should be the same regardless of whether a course is taught using a traditional approach or through distance education. Student evaluation must be built into a distance education course. Schools should ensure that students can provide anonymous evaluations of the course and faculty.

CRITICAL PROBLEMS: FACULTY SHORTAGE AND ACCESS TO CLINICAL EXPERIENCES

Today, the two critical problems that consume a lot of time in nursing education are how to resolve the faculty shortage and finding clinical experiences for students. These are complex problems that require more than one solution, and they have a great impact on the quality of nursing education and student outcomes.

Faculty Shortage

A particular focus on securing and retaining adequate numbers of faculty is essential to ensure that all individuals interested in—and qualified for—nursing school can matriculate in the year they are accepted. Aside from having a limited number of faculty, nursing programs struggle to provide space for clinical laboratories and to secure a sufficient number of clinical training sites at healthcare facilities. (Americans for Nursing Shortage Relief, 2007, p. 2)

A school's faculty should reflect a balance of expert clinicians who can teach, expert researchers and grant writers who can teach, and expert teachers who are pedagogical scholars (NLN, 2007b). Today, schools of nursing, regardless of the type of program, are struggling to meet demand for enrollment because of limited faculty. Schools of nursing are having problems recruiting experienced faculty and faculty new to teaching. This shortage comes at a time when there already is a nursing shortage. Some of the same factors that affect the nursing shortage have an impact on the faculty shortage, such as retirement; this will only increase because a large number of nursing faculty members are approaching retirement age. It is also difficult to attract nurses to teaching because the pay is lower than for nursing practice; for this reason, those with graduate degrees often opt to stay in active practice. Attracting nurses to graduate school is still an issue, particularly at the doctoral level. It is hoped that the DNP will attract more, but these nurses may not be interested in teaching.

In 2002, Congress passed the Nurse Reinvestment Act (P.L. 107-205), which President George W. Bush signed into law. This law includes provisions related to nursing faculty, such as providing loans to nurses who wish to pursue graduate studies with a commitment to teach. Exhibit 4–4 describes this part of the law.

Access to Clinical Experiences   Research reported by the NLN found that in 2005, schools of nursing rejected more than 147,000 qualified applications because of shortages of faculty, classroom space, and clinical placement for students (NLN, 2006). Securing clinical sites to meet course objectives is not easy for any school of nursing. If there are a number of nursing schools in one area, there is also competition for clinical slots. This is particularly pronounced in specialties that have fewer patients and thus tight demand for clinical slots, such as pediatrics, obstetrics, and mental health. Schools of nursing have to be more innovative and

---

Exhibit 4–4 Implications of the Nurse Reinvestment Act P.L. 107-205, 2002, and Nursing Education

SEC. 203. NURSE FACULTY LOAN PROGRAM.
Amends Title VIII of the PHSA by adding a new section:

- **Section 846A** Nurse Faculty Loan Program

Establishes authority for the Secretary, acting through the Administrator of the Health Resources and Services Administration, to enter into agreements with a school of nursing to establish a student loan fund to increase the number of qualified faculty. Agreements include the creation of a student loan fund by the school taking a federal contribution; an amount equal to not less than one-ninth of the federal contribution contributed by the school; and providing for collection of principal, interest and any other earnings on loans made by the fund. The student loan fund may only be used for loans to students and costs of collection of loans and interest.

Students must be pursuing full-time study or, at the discretion of the Secretary, part-time study in an advanced degree program for Advanced Education Nurses as described in Section 811b of the PHSA. A statement of congressional intent clarifies that the student may pursue a master's or doctoral degree. The maximum loan made by the school is $30,000 per student in an academic year.

Students must agree to teach at the school of nursing in exchange for cancellation of up to 85% of their educational loans, plus interest, over a four-year period at a rate of 20% per year for three years and 25% in the final year. Student loans may cover the costs of tuition, fees, books, laboratory expenses, and other reasonable education expenses. An interest rate of 3% for the student pursuing the faculty role begins accruing three months after graduation. If the school of nursing determines that the student will not complete the course of study or serve as a faculty member as required under the agreement, the interest rate on the unpaid balance of the loan will be at the prevailing market rate. The Secretary will pay the school of nursing an amount equal to the proportionate share of the canceled loan. Authorizes "such sums as necessary" for FY 2003 to 2007.

Source: Legislation Nurse Reinvestment Act P.L. 107–205, 2002.

---

recognize that every student may not get the same clinical experiences. There has been increasing use of non–acute care pediatric settings. Some communities do not have pediatric hospitals and may have limited beds assigned to pediatric care. Other sites that might be used are pediatricians' offices, pediatric clinics, schools, daycare centers, and camps. For obstetrics, possible clinical sites are birthing centers, obstetricians' offices, and midwifery practices. Mental health clinicals may take place in clinics, at homeless shelters, in mental health emergency and crisis centers, and at a mental health association site. This difficulty in getting sites has meant that some schools have had to move away from the traditional clinical

hours offered—Monday–Friday during the day. Some schools are recognizing that operating on a 9-month basis with a long summer break affects the availability of clinical experiences. To accommodate the needs of all schools of nursing and the need to increase student enrollment, community-area healthcare providers are working with schools to determine how all these needs can be met effectively.

Clinical Simulation or Laboratory Experiences
Simulation and laboratory experiences have become important teaching methods for developing competencies. NCSBN (2005) defines simulation as "activities that mimic reality of a

clinical environment and are designed to demonstrate procedures, decision making and critical thinking through techniques such as role playing and the use of devices such as interactive videos or mannequins." Simulation helps students feel more confident in a safe setting before caring for patients and can help students to develop teamwork. The simulated environment provides opportunities for teams of nurses or, ideally, interdisciplinary students to work together to solve simulated clinical situations. Students can be evaluated and provided feedback in more structured learning situations. Simulated experiences should be as close to real life as possible, but they are not, of course, totally real. However, this does not mean that these learning situations are not very helpful for student learning.

A simulation lab is expensive to develop and maintain. Students need to respect the equipment and supplies and follow procedures so that costs can be managed. Faculty supervision in the simulation lab can be based on a higher ratio of students to faculty for more cost-effective teaching and learning. With the development of more sophisticated technology, computer simulation can even be incorporated into distance education.

Lifelong Learning for the Professional

Lifelong learning is one of the major characteristics of a professional. This model of learning includes three major components (American Nurses Association, 2000):

1. Academic Education: This component of the model includes courses taken for academic credit—undergraduate and graduate—in an institution of higher learning and may or may not lead to a degree or completion of a certificate program. In this case, these courses are taken after completion of a basic nursing education program.

2. Staff Development: This component of the model involves the systematic process of assessing and developing oneself to enhance performance or professional development—continued competence. Included in staff development are orientation (the process of introducing nursing staff to the organization and position) and in-service educational activities (learning opportunities offered by employers to improve employee performance in assigned functions).

3. **Continuing Education:** This component of the model is systematic professional learning designed to augment knowledge, skills, and attitudes. This section of the chapter includes additional content on continuing education.

Nursing students may wonder why this topic is important to them when they are just now entering nursing education. Lifelong learning begins now, particularly the need to recognize its importance to individual nurses, to the profession, to healthcare organizations, and to patient outcomes. Students often have opportunities to participate in a variety of these learning activities even as students. These activities are excellent opportunities to gain further knowledge and to better understand the importance of lifelong learning. Students will also need to know the requirements for continuing education in the state(s) where they wish to apply for licensure. Lifelong learning must be driven by personal responsibility to improve even with required components. Although professional organizations, regulatory agencies, and employers have an influence on whether nurses participate in lifelong learning, successful lifelong learning is in the hands of the learner, the nurse.

CONTINUING NURSING EDUCATION

In today's challenging healthcare environment, nurses committed to professional continuing education help maintain the standards of nursing practice and improve the health of the public. The American Nurses Association's (ANA) Scope and Standards for Practice for Nursing Professional Development serves as a foundation for the development of the ANCC Commission on Accreditation (COA) criteria. (ANCC, 2007b).

The most common thought is that nurses would naturally want to get more education and stay current, but this is not necessarily the case. Required continuing education (CE) is a great motivator.

CE is required in many states to maintain licensure after initial licensure is received. In these states, the state board of nursing designates how many hours of CE are required for licensure renewal. States vary in terms of what is considered CE—short, structured CE programs, academic courses, attending conferences where educational content is presented, publishing, and so on. Nurses must follow their state's requirements. Another reason for obtaining CE is that it is required for certification, and the amount and type are designated by the certification body.

Sources of CE credit are highly variable. Credit can be obtained, for example, by attending a 1-hour or full-day educational offering, attending part or all of conference, reading an article in a professional journal and then taking an assessment quiz, participating in an online program, and engaging in self-study. Typically a fee is charged unless the costs for the program are covered, such as by a grant to the sponsoring organization. Nurses do need to be careful and make sure that the program's credit is accepted by the organization requiring the CE. Organizations that approve and/or offer CE programs should be accredited programs. The ANCC accredits these programs, and state boards of nursing may have an accrediting process.

Obtaining accreditation is voluntary, but to really get nurses to participate, accreditation is required; nurses want to get CE from accredited programs that are guided by accepted standards. "The accrediting process is intended to strengthen and sustain the quality and integrity of continuing nursing education, making it worthy of public confidence" (ANCC, 2007b). It is assumed that CE has an impact on patient outcomes and quality care, but this is not easy to prove in a consistent manner.

Nurses are responsible for maintaining their own records of CE activities. In states where CE is required for relicensure, nurses may be required to produce documentation of these activities. In addition, nurses need to update their résumés to ensure that learning activities are included. In some cases, employers require documentation. Nurses are usually required to document learning activities on an annual or biannual basis. When nurses select learning programs, they should evaluate the following factors:

- Accreditation of the program
- Number of CE credits and related time commitment
- Schedule and location, including travel issues
- Cost (registration fee, parking and travel, housing and meals)
- Qualifications of faculty
- Whether the program is based on adult learning principles (Is the program designed for the adult learner?)
- Identification of needs (What does the nurse need to gain? What are the personal or professional objectives? Does the course offer content to meet these objectives?)
- The program's learner objectives (Do they correlate with personal professional objectives?)
- Whether the program is based on current and relevant content

- Teaching methods
- Past experiences with the provider of the educational program (Quality programs attract nurses to return for other programs.)

Certification and Credentialing

Certification and **credentialing** are recognition systems to identify whether nurses meet certain requirements or standards. These recognitions may be required or voluntary depending on the circumstances. Credentialing is typically required, and certification is often voluntary. Nurses who have certification or have met credentialing requirements must first be licensed as RNs.

CREDENTIALING

Credentialing is a process that ensures that practitioners are qualified to perform. Typically, it is used by healthcare organizations to check for licensure of healthcare professionals (such as nurses) and to monitor continued licensure. Nurses are required to show their current licensure on an annual basis to their employer, and the employer may then keep a copy of the license. Some states provide access to online checks of licensure status. Education, certification, and maintenance of malpractice insurance also may be reviewed, but this can vary from one healthcare organization to another. The goal is to protect the public by ensuring that specific state requirements are met.

CERTIFICATION

"Certification is a process by which a nongovernmental agency validates, based upon predetermined standards, an individual nurse's qualification and knowledge for practice in a defined functional or clinical area of nursing" (American Association of Critical-Care Nurses Certification Corporation, 2008). Certification is a method of recognizing expertise. This certification is done through an exam, recognition of

completed education, and the description of clinical experience in a designated specialty area covered by the certification. Certification that might be given by a healthcare organization for accomplishing a specific goal, such as cardiopulmonary resuscitation, is not the same type of certification that is awarded after meeting specific professional standards, which includes an exam. This type is a voluntary method in that nurses are not required to have certification, although many employers recognize its importance, and some may require certification for certain positions. This recognition is now available in most specialty areas. For example, the ANCC offers certification in multiple nursing specialties. "More than a quarter million nurses have been certified by ANCC since 1990. More than 75,000 advanced practice nurses are currently certified by ANCC" (ANCC, 2007a). After receiving initial certification, recertification is accomplished through demonstrating ongoing practice and CE. Nurses may be certified in multiple areas as long as they meet the requirements. Cary (2001) identified the benefits of certification (though 25% of survey participants said that they received no benefit from certification):

- Certification recognized or publicized
- Full or partial reimbursement of costs
- Recognized as an expert in the field by colleagues
- Retention in position, one-time bonus
- Eligibility for a higher level position
- Promoted to a higher level position.

Professional certification in nursing is a measure of distinctive nursing practice. The rise in consumerism in the face of a compelling nursing shortage and the profession's movement to elevate nursing as a career option has given prominence to the value of certification in nursing. The value of certification is not only significant for nursing practice rather the focus on professional certification is also essential to meet multiple standards within the American Nurses Credentialing Center's (ANCC's) Magnet Recognition Program for excellence in nursing Services. (American Nurses Credentialing Center, 2004, as stated in Shirey, 2005, p. 245)

The Magnet Recognition Program is described in more detail in Chapter 15. Exhibit 4–5 provides data on AACN certification.

Transforming Nursing Education

In the last 8 years, beginning with the IOM reports (discussed in more detail in Section III) on quality and safety in healthcare delivery, there has been greater urgency to institute changes in nursing education. Porter-O'Grady (2001) identified issues that are important in nursing education as the profession adapts to changing healthcare needs (pp. 184–185):

1. Faculty need to change from being a provider of learning to facilitating learning.
2. Tools of learning are more in the hands of the student, with faculty facilitating the use of these tools.
3. Student's level of maturity, investment, self-direction, and learning skills are critical.
4. There is a need for greater variety of clinical experiences that are not just focused on acute care in the hospital setting.
5. There is a need for greater integration of content.
6. Graduate education needs to integrate several academic areas and pathways.

Nursing students need to be included in the evaluation of nursing education and changes. They can do this by providing course feedback and participating in curriculum committees when requested. Nursing education should

---

EXHIBIT 4–5 AACN CERTIFICATION

Nurse Practitioners
- Acute Care
- Adult
- Adult Psychiatric & Mental Health
- Diabetes Management, Advanced
- Family
- Family Psychiatric & Mental Health
- Gerontological
- Pediatric

Clinical Nurse Specialists
- Diabetes Management, Advanced
- Adult Health (formerly known as Medical-Surgical)
- Adult Psychiatric & Mental Health
- Child/Adolescent Psychiatric & Mental Health
- Gerontological
- Pediatric
- Public/Community Health

Other Advanced-Level Exams
- Diabetes Management, Advanced—Dietician
- Diabetes Management, Advanced—Pharmacist
- Nursing Administration, Advanced

Specialty Certification
- Ambulatory Care Nurse
- Cardiac Vascular Nurse
- Case Management Nurse
- Gerontological Nurse
- Informatics Nurse
- Medical-Surgical Nurse
- Nursing Administration
- Nursing Professional Development
- Pain Management
- Pediatric Nurse
- Psychiatric & Mental Health Nurse

Source: American Nurses Credentialing Center. Retrieved August 28, 2008 from http://www.nursecredentialing.org/cert/eligibility.html

always review content and improve curriculum and must have methods to do this in a timely, effective manner.

> *What is needed by nursing today is to uphold the true spirit of innovation and overhaul traditional pedagogies to reform the way the nursing workforce is educated. This call to action will be accomplished through new pedagogies that are most effective in helping students learn to practice in rapidly-changing environments where short stays in acute care facilities are common and where complex care is being provided in a variety of settings. These new pedagogies must be research-based, pluralistic and responsive to the unpredictable nature of the contemporary healthcare system. (Ben-Zur, Yagi, & Spitzer, 1999, as stated in National League for Nursing, 2003, p. 2)*

Accreditation of Nursing Education Programs

Accreditation is important in evaluating and maintaining effective standards. Potential nursing students may not be as aware of accreditation of the schools they are considering, but they should be. What is accreditation, and why is it important?

Nursing Program Accreditation: What Is It?

Accreditation is a process in which an organization is assessed regarding how it meets established standards. Minimum standards are identified by an accrediting organization, and nursing schools incorporate these standards into their programs. The accrediting organization then reviews the school and its programs. This is supposedly a voluntary process, but in reality it is not; to be effective, a school of nursing must be accredited. Nursing education programs should be accredited by the recognized organizations that provide standards and accreditation for nursing programs. Attending a program that is not accredited can lead to complications in licensure, employment, and opportunities to continue on to graduate programs.

Nursing Program Accreditation: How Does It Work?

What is accreditation, and how does it work? Accreditation is based on minimum standards that schools of nursing must meet to obtain accreditation. The process is complex and takes time. Schools of nursing must pay for the review. Schools may or may not receive accreditation, they may be required to make changes, they may be put on probation, or they may lose accreditation. Accreditation is not a legal requirement, but some states require this type of accreditation from the NLN or ANCC to maintain state accreditation. Some specialty organizations accredit specific graduate programs within a school, such as the American College of Nurse Midwifery and the American Association of Nurse-Anesthetists. A school may choose which organization accredits the program unless mandated by state agency or law. The state board of nursing is involved in this requirement and in the state accreditation process. During the accreditation process, the review team assesses the school's:

- Curriculum
- Structure
- Faculty
- Student outcomes
- Student support
- Admissions process and other academic processes
- Policies and procedures

A critical step in the accreditation process is the on-site survey at the school. Surveyors visit the school and view classes and practica, review documents, meet with school administrative staff, and, if part of a university, meet with university administrative staff. Surveyors also meet with faculty and students. They are typically at the school for several days. Students do have an obligation to participate and provide feedback. The goal is maintenance of minimum standards to ensure an effective learning environment that supports student learning and meets the needs of the profession.

Regulation

How are professional **regulation** and nursing regulation for practice licensure related? Regulation for practice or licensure is clear, though problematic in some cases. This type of regulation is based on laws and regulations and leads to licensure. However, this is different from the professional regulation, in which the profession itself regulates its practice. State boards of nursing are not nursing professional organizations. They are state government agencies, and this can make it difficult to make changes in a state's practice of nursing. Professional organizations do have an impact on practice through the standards they propose and other elements of support and data that they provide. "For effective nursing workforce planning to occur and be sustained, Boards of Nursing must collaborate with nursing education and practice to support the safe and effective evolution of nursing practice" (Damgaard, VanderWoude, & Hegge, 1999, as cited in Loquist, 2002, p. 34).

"In 1950, nursing became the first profession for which the same licensure exam, the State Board Test Pool (now called NCLEX), was used throughout the nation to license nurses. This increased the mobility for the registered nurse and resulted in a significant advantage for the relatively new profession of nursing" (Lundy, 2005, pp. 21–22). The major purpose of regulation is to protect the public, and it is based on the 10th Amendment of the U.S. Constitution, the states' rights amendment. Each state has the right to regulate professional practice, such as nursing practice, within its own state.

In general, the regulatory approach selected should be sufficient to ensure public protection. The following criteria are relevant (NCSBN, 1996b, pp. 8–9):

- *Risk of Harm for the Consumer*—The evaluation of a profession to determine whether unregulated practice endangers the public should focus on recognizable harm. That harm could result from the practices inherent in the nature of the profession, the characteristics of the clients/patients, the settings, supervisory requirements, or a combination of these factors. Licensure is applied to a profession when the incompetent or unethical practice of that profession could cause greater risk of harm to the public unless there is a high level of accountability; and at the other extreme, registration is appropriate for professions where such a high level of accountability is not needed.
- *Skill and Training Needed*—The more highly specialized the services of the professional, the greater the need for an approach that actively inquires about the education and competence of the professional.
- *Level of Autonomy*—Licensure is indicated when the professional uses independent judgment and practices independently with little or no supervision. Registration is appropriate for individuals who do not use independent judgment and practice with supervision.
- *Scope of Practice*—Unless there is a distinguishable scope of practice for the profession that is distinguishable from other professions and definable in enforceable legal terms, there is neither basis nor need

for licensure. This scope may overlap over professions in specific duties, functions, or therapeutic modalities.

- *Consumer Expectation*—Consumers expect that those professions that have a potentially high impact on the consumer, on their physical, mental or economic well-being, are subject to regulatory oversight. The costs of operating regulatory agencies and the restriction of practitioners who do not meet the minimum requirements are justified in order to protect the public from harm.
- *Alternative to Regulation*—There are no alternatives to the selected regulatory approach that would adequately protect the public. It should also be the case that when it is determined that regulation of the profession is required, the least restrictive level of regulation consistent with public protection will be implemented.

The guiding principles of nursing regulation are: (1) protection of the public, (2) competence of all practitioners regulated by the board of nursing, (3) due process and ethical decision making, (4) shared accountability, (5) strategic collaboration, (6) evidence-based regulation, (7) response to the marketplace and healthcare environment, and (8) globalization of nursing (NCSBN, 2007a).

Nurse Practice Acts

Each state has a **nurse practice act** that determines the nature of nursing practice within the state. This is a state law passed by the state legislative body. Nurse practice acts for each state can be found online. Every nurse who has a license should be knowledgeable about his or her nurse practice act, which governs practice in the state in which he or she practices. Typically, nurse practice acts do the following for their state (Masters, 2005, p. 166):

- Define the authority of the board of nursing, its composition, and its powers.
- Define nursing and boundaries of the scope of practice.
- Identify types of licenses and titles.
- State the requirements for licensure.
- Protect titles.
- Identify the grounds for disciplinary action.

The most important function of the nurse practice act is to define the scope of practice for nurses in the state to protect public safety.

State Boards of Nursing

State boards of nursing implement the state's nurse practice act, which is the statutory law governing nursing practice within a state or territory, and recommend state regulations and changes to the act when appropriate. The board is part of state government, though how it fits into a state's governmental organization varies from state to state. RNs serve on state boards of nursing, and they are typically selected by the governor for a specific term of office. Licensed practical nurses (LPNs), laypersons, or consumers (nonnurses) may have representation on the board. The board's primary purpose is to protect the health and safety of the public (citizens of the state). A board of nursing has an executive director who runs the business of the board with staff who work for the board (state). The size of the state has an impact on the size of the board of nursing and its staff. Boards are not only involved in setting standards and licensure of nurses (RNs and LPN/licensed vocational nurses [LVNs]), but they are also responsible for monitoring nursing education (all types of RN and LPN/LVN) programs in the state. The board serves a regulatory function and as such can issue administrative rules or regulations consistent with state law to facilitate the enforcement of the nurse practice act.

The board of nursing in each state also reviews problems with licensure and is the agency that administers disciplinary actions. If a nurse fails to meet certain standards, participates in unacceptable practice, or has problems that interfere with safe practice, and any of these violations are reported to the board, the board can conduct an investigation and review, and determine actions that might need to be taken. Examples of these issues are assaulting or causing harm to a patient; having a problem with illegal drugs or with alcohol (substance abuse); being convicted of, or pleading guilty to, a felony (examples of felonies are murder, robbery, rape, and sexual battery); and having a psychiatric illness that is not being managed and that interferes with safe functioning. A nurse may be reprimanded, be denied a license, have his or her licensure suspended or revoked, or have his or her licensure restricted with stipulations (for example, the nurse must attend an alcohol treatment program). The board must follow strict procedures when taking any action, which must first begin with an official complaint to the board. Anyone can make a complaint to the board—another nurse, another healthcare professional, a healthcare organization, or a consumer. The state nursing practice act identifies the possible reasons for disciplinary action. Boards of nursing publish their disciplinary action decisions because they are part of the public record. When nurses obtain a license in another state, they are asked to report any disciplinary actions that have been taken by another state's board of nursing. Not reporting disciplinary board actions has serious consequences in obtaining (and losing) licensure. A key point is that licensure is a privilege, not a legal right.

The National Council of State Boards of Nursing

The NCSBN is a not-for-profit organization that represents all boards of nursing in the 50 states, the District of Columbia, and four U.S. territories (American Samoa, Guam, Northern Mariana Islands, and the Virgin Islands). Through this organization, all boards of nursing work together on issues related to the regulation of nursing practice that affect public health, safety, and welfare, including the development of licensing examinations in nursing. The NCSBN's functions include (National Council of State Boards of Nursing, 2007b):

- Development of the National Council Licensure Examination (NCLEX)-RN and NCLEX-PN, implementation of testing, and report of results
- Policy analysis and promotion of uniformity in relationship to the regulation of nursing practice
- Dissemination of data related to the licensure of nurses
- Conduction of research pertinent to NCSBN's purpose
- Service as a forum for information exchange for members

Licensure Requirements

Licensure requirements are determined by each state's board of nursing; however, all require passage of the NCLEX-RN, which is a national exam. Other requirements include criminal background checks for initial licensure and continuing education for renewal, which varies from state to state. Many nurses hold licenses in a several states or may be on inactive status in some states. An RN should always maintain one license, even if not practicing, to make it easier to return to practice. Fees are paid for the initial license and for license renewal. States in which a nurse is licensed notify the nurse when the license is up for renewal. It is the nurse's responsibility to complete the required forms and submit payment. Examples of licensure requirements and renewal requirements, which vary from state to state, are:

- Fee (always required, though the amount varies and is dependent on active or inactive licensure status)
- Passage of NCLEX (required for first licensure and then covered for renewals or change of license)
- Continuing education credits within a specified time period (varies from state to state)
- Criminal background check (required)
- Active employment for a specific number of hours within a specified time period (varies from state to state)
- Number of hours of professional nursing activities (varies from state to state)

Ultimately, each RN is responsible for maintaining competency for safe practice. Any person who practices nursing without a valid license commits a minor misdemeanor. If licensed in one state, the nurse can typically do the following in another state in which he or she is not licensed:

- Consult
- Teach as guest lecturer
- Conduct evaluation of care as part of an accreditation process

NCLEX

The NCLEX is developed and administered through the National Council of State Boards of Nursing (NCSBN, 2007b). There are two forms of the exam—NCLEX-RN for RN licensure, and NCLEX-PN for practical nurse licensure.

Entry into the practice of nursing in the United States and its territories is regulated by the licensing authorities within each jurisdiction. To ensure public protection, each jurisdiction requires a candidate for licensure to pass an examination that measures the competencies needed to perform safely and effectively as a newly licensed, entry-level registered nurse. (NCSBN, 2007b)

The examination is offered online. Most of the questions are written at the cognitive levels of application or higher, requiring the candidate to use problem-solving skills to select the best answer. The exam is a computerized adaptive test (CAT). In this type of exam, the computer adjusts questions to the individual candidate so that the exam is then highly individualized, offering challenging questions that are not too easy or too difficult. The NCLEX-RN has a range of questions from 75 to 265. The exam ends when the computer determines with 95% certainty that the person's ability is either below or above the passing standard. The exam can also end when the time runs out or there are no more questions. Because of these factors, candidates do not all have the same number of questions. The exam includes the following types of questions:

- Multiple-response items; candidate required to select one or more responses
- Fill-in-the-blank items; candidate required to type in numbers in a calculation item
- Hot spot items; candidate identifies an area on a picture or graphic
- Chart/exhibit format; candidate presented with a problem and then must read information in a chart/exhibit to answer the question
- Drag-and-drop item; candidate ranks orders or moves options to provide correct answer

The NCLEX may be repeated. Most schools of nursing provide some type of preparation (for example, throughout the nursing program, or near the end). Prep programs that charge a fee are available to students, and many publications to assist with preparation may be purchased. The exam preparation takes place every day in the nursing programs—in courses and in clinical practice.

How Does the Process Work? Students are asked by their school to complete an application for NCLEX in the final semester before graduation. This application is sent to the state board of nursing in the state where the student is seeking licensure. After a student completes the nursing program, the school must verify that the student has graduated. At this point, the student becomes an official NCLEX candidate. He or she will receive an Authorization to Test (ATT), and exam instructions and information about scheduling the exam. The ATT is the nursing graduate's "pass" to take the exam, so it is important to keep it. Students then schedule their own exam within their given time frame. The student goes to the designated exam site on the scheduled date for the computerized exam. Candidates are fingerprinted and photographed to ensure security for the exam. Testing sites are available in every state, and a candidate may take the exam in any state. Licensure, however, is awarded by the state in which the candidate has applied for licensure. An exam session lasts a maximum of 6 hours, but because of the CAT method, the amount of time that an individual candidate takes on the exam varies; that time does not affect passing or failing. Every candidate must answer a minimum of 75 questions. This means that the exam is completed when *one* of the following occurs: (1) results measure a level of competency above or below the standard, and a minimum of 75 questions have been answered, (2) the candidate completes the maximum number of 265 questions, or (3) the candidate has used the maximum time of 6 hours. Candidates are provided an orientation and a brief practice session prior to taking the exam. Passing scores are the same for every state and set by the NCSBN. Candidates are usually informed of their results within 3–4 weeks; the result is pass or fail, with no specific score provided. Schools of nursing receive composites of student results.

CRITICAL CURRENT AND FUTURE REGULATION ISSUES

Compact Licensure In recent years, there has been a growing need to find licensure methods that address the following situations: A nurse lives in one state but works in an adjacent state; a nurse works for a managed care company in several states; and a nurse works in telehealth, by which care might be provided via technology in more than one state. To address these issues, the NCSBN created a new model for licensure called mutual recognition, or compact licensure.

The mutual recognition model of nurse licensure allows a nurse to have one license (in his or her state of residency) and to practice in other states (both physical and electronic), subject to each state's practice law and regulation. Under mutual recognition, a nurse may practice across state lines unless otherwise restricted. (NCSBN, 2007c)

Each state in a mutual recognition compact must enact legislation or regulation authorizing the nurse licensure compact and also adopt administrative rules and regulations for implementation of the compact. Each compact state also appoints a nurse licensure compact administrator to facilitate the exchange of information between the states that relates to compact nurse licensure and regulation.

Although the 15 states that have adopted the model have not demonstrated that the model has increased their ability to recruit additional nurses into their states, it does facilitate the interstate practice of nursing for traveling nurses. Nurses licensed by mutual recognition are required to abide by the laws of the state in which practice occurs. This places additional responsibility on employers to provide adequate orientation and training for the job. (Loquist, 2002, p. 38)

Some states have decided that this model is unconstitutional in their states because it delegates authority for licensure decisions to other states.

Recently, the same type of licensure questions related to advanced practice nurses have arisen. In 2002, the NCSBN Delegate Assembly approved the adoption of model language for a licensure compact for advanced practice registered nurses (APRNs). Only those states that have adopted the RN and LPN/LVN Nurse Licensure Compact may implement a compact for APRNs. From 2004 to 2007, three states passed legislation: Utah, Iowa, and Texas. These states are now working on the implementation regulations because this must be done prior to implementation of the compact. The APRN compact offers states the mechanism for mutually recognizing APRN licenses and authority to practice (NCSBN, 2007d).

Mandatory Overtime   A critical concern in practice today is requiring nurses to work overtime. Employers make this decision, and it is called mandatory overtime. This policy impacts the quality and safety of care and has affected staff satisfaction and burnout. This critical topic will be discussed further in Chapter 14. Boards of nursing in some states are beginning to work with their state legislators to end mandatory overtime (Loquist, 2002).

Although legislative and regulatory responses have provided nurses with additional support for creating safer work environments, each of these legislative responses has a significant effect on

the numbers and types of nursing personnel that will be required for care delivery systems in the future as well as the cost of care. Clearly, there is concern at the state and national levels regarding the impact that fewer caregivers will have on the health and safety of patients. (Loquist, p. 37)

As students and new graduates interview for their first positions, they should ask about mandatory overtime if they are not in a state that has a law to protect them from it. Research is now being done regarding sleep deprivation and its connection to the rising number of medical errors (Girard, 2003; Manfredini, Boari, & Manfredini, 2006; Montgomery, 2007; Sigurdson & Ayas, 2007). This area of research is fairly new, and researchers will need to continue to provide concrete evidence of the links among sleep deprivation, long work hours, and medical errors. Certainly, the aviation industry has cut back the number of hours that flight crews can work without sleep. It is highly likely that this will occur in health care as well.

Foreign Nursing Graduates: Entrance to Practice in the United States   The number of nurses from other countries coming to the United States to work and/or study has increased. Some nurses want to work here only temporarily, and some want to stay permanently. This movement of nurses internationally typically increases during a shortage, and today, there is a worldwide shortage and a lot of nursing migration, which will be discussed more in Chapter 14 (International Centre on Nurse Migration, 2007).

The NCSBN recently passed a new position statement regarding international nurse immigration, reaffirming that foreign-educated nurses need to comply with standards of approved or comparable education, hold a verified valid and unencumbered state license, and be proficient in their written and spoken English language skills. There still is the ethical question of "poaching" nurses from one country to another that results in the reduction of a scarce national resource in this worldwide shortage. (NCSBN, 2001, as cited in Loquist, 2002, p. 37)

What do these nurses have to do to meet practice requirements in the United States? The Commission on Graduates of Foreign Nursing Schools (CGFNS) is an organization that assists these nurses in evaluating their credentials and verifies their education, registration, and licensure (CGFNS, 2007). This is an internationally recognized immigration-neutral nonprofit organization that protects the public by ensuring that these nurses are eligible and qualified to meet U.S. licensure and immigration requirements. These nurses must also take the Test of English as Foreign Language to ensure that their English language ability is at an acceptable level. This also applies to students who want to enter U.S. nursing programs. A nurse who is licensed in another country must also successfully complete the NCLEX and meet the state licensure requirements where he or she will practice. If the nurse is going into a nursing program as a graduate student, he or she would need to get a U.S. license for clinical work that would be done as part of the educational program. This is not required for a prelicensure program in nursing.

Global Regulatory Issues   With the development of the Internet, telehealth and global migration have been forcing nursing to confront change related to interstate nursing practice. Globalization has had a similar impact on migration (Fernandez & Hebert, 2004). This migration phenomenon supports the need for an international credentialing of immigrant nurses to ensure public safety as defined by the International Council of Nurses (Schaefer, 1990).

New models for practice will continue to emerge to manage change, care, and plan for the future. Electronic technologies provide an opportunity to develop a new identity for nursing practice. New regulatory requirements will emerge to meet the need of practitioners to ensure public safety. As a new paradigm for ensuring competencies and self-regulation in a global market evolves, the need to explore global licensure will emerge. The future belongs to those who will accept the challenge to make a difference in a global marketplace and take the necessary risks to make things happen. (Fernandez & Hebert, 2004, p. 132)

The Global Alliance for Nursing Education is a new nursing organization that focuses on getting nurse educators from around the world to work together to develop and facilitate nursing education and research in order to improve care globally (AACN, 2006b). These new efforts to recognize the need for international standards in nursing education and regulation represent a significant step; nursing has moved from a focus on individual hospitals, to the state level, to the national level, and now globally.

Conclusion

This chapter has described critical issues related to nursing education, accreditation of nursing education programs, and regulation and nursing practice. All these elements interact to better ensure quality, safe patient care, from education to practice.

CHAPTER HIGHLIGHTS

1. The evolution of nursing education influences how nursing is taught.

2. Different levels of nursing education have different competencies and expectations, yet all levels take the same licensure examination.
3. Accreditation of nursing programs ensures quality education.
4. Licensure and the regulation of nursing practice also set standards and rules about nursing education.

Linking to the Internet

- American Association of Colleges of Nursing (AACN)
  http://www.aacn.nche.edu
- National League for Nursing (NLN)
  http://www.nln.org
- National Council of State Boards of Nursing (NCSBN)
  http://www.ncsbn.org

- American Nurses Association (ANA)
  http://nursingworld.org
- Commission on Graduates of Foreign Nursing Schools (CGFNS)
  http://www.cgfns.org
- National Association of Clinical Nurse Specialists (NACNS)
  http://www.nacns.org
- American Association of Nurse Anesthetists (AANA)
  http://www.aana.com/
- American College of Nurse Midwives
  http://www.midwife.org
- American Academy of Nurse Practitioners (AANP)
  http://www.aanp.org

DISCUSSION QUESTIONS

1. Why do you think it is important that nursing now emphasizes education over training? Consider Donahue's definitions for education and training found in the chapter.
2. Compare and contrast the types of entry programs in nursing: diploma, ADN, BSN, and accelerated or second-degree program.
3. Select one of the following graduate nursing programs (master's—any type; doctoral; and DNP) and find, through the Internet, two different universities that offer the program. Compare and contrast admission requirements and the curricula.
4. Visit the NCLEX Web site (https://www.ncsbn.org/1200.htm). Review the "Candidates" section and describe the exam process and what happens on exam day. Go to https://www.ncsbn.org/1287.htm and review the current NCLEX-RN Detailed Test Plan for candidates. What type of information is included in the plan? How might this information help you, now and closer to the time when you take the NCLEX?
5. Does your state participate in the Nurse Licensure Compact? Visit https://www.ncsbn.org/158.htm to find out. Why might this be important to you when you become licensed in your state after graduation?

CRITICAL THINKING ACTIVITIES

1. Conduct a debate in class with one other classmate. Take the side of no specific level of entry-into-practice, with the other classmate supporting the BSN as the entry-into-practice. The class should then vote on the side that presents the best support for one of the perspectives.
2. Conduct a debate in class with one other classmate. Take the side supporting the PhD in nursing, with the other classmate supporting the DNP. The class should then vote on the side that presents the best support for one of the perspectives. You will need to research your issue and present a substantiated rationale for your side of the issue.
3. Consider the learning styles described in this chapter. Where do you fit in? Why do you think the style(s) apply to you? What impact do you think the style(s) you identified will have on your own learning in the nursing program? Are there changes you need to work on?
4. Review your school's philosophy and curriculum. What are the key themes in this information? Do you think that the themes and content are relevant to nursing practice, and if so, why? Do you think anything important is missing, and if so, what is it?

CASE STUDIES

1. Read this article: "The Johns Hopkins Training School for Nurses: A Tale of Vision, Labor, and Futility," by M. Ramos, 1997, *Nursing History Review, 2*, pp. 23–48. This article provides an account of the struggle of one diploma school's efforts to change from a diploma school model to a university-based model.

Case Questions

1. What was the early history of the school?
2. How did this history impact the desire to change?
3. What role did physicians and funding play?
4. What other factors influenced the process?
5. What was the final result?
6. Given what you have learned in this chapter, how does this example relate to the chapter's content?

2. Read this article: "Backrubs vs. Bach. Nursing and the Entry-Into-Practice Debate: 1946–1986,"

by S. Leighow, 1996, *Nursing History Review, 4*, pp. 3–17. This article discusses the critical issue of entry-into-practice.

Case Questions

1. What is the historical setting of the initial part of the debate?
2. What roles did nursing organizations play in the debate? Do you think that the debate would have progressed if there had been no organized nursing organizations? If not, why?
3. What happened in the area of college education and nursing?
4. Review Table 4-1 in this chapter for data from 2000–2020. What is the current status of the number of students enrolled in each of the three programs (diploma, ADN, and BSN)? Search for the data on the Internet.
5. What were the critical issues in the debate? Take each issue and provide your opinion on the issue.

WORDS OF WISDOM

Joy R. O'Rourke, BSN, RN
Norman, Oklahoma

Nursing school taught me essential clinical skills to care for clients as an LPN. At this level of education, we are taught "how" to give quality health care. I decided to continue my education in an LPN-BSN program to learn in more depth about "why" things are done a certain way. I was delighted to learn this program focuses on holistic care as well as the leadership skills needed to work effectively as a team. It is imperative to function as a team when caring for members of the community. The healthcare field is constantly changing. We as nurses must strive to reach our full potential to keep up with these changes. Nursing is an exciting and rewarding field with new things to learn every day.

Sherri Jones, LPN
New Directions/Geriatric Psych Unit, McCurtain Memorial Hospital, Idabel, Oklahoma; student in LPN-to-BSN program

My Journey from LPN to BSN: During LPN school, I felt at times if I could just survive the year, that was as far as I cared to excel in my nursing education. After my first year working as an LPN on a medical/surgical unit, I realized the importance of continuing to the RN level, but uncertain whether or not to go for my AD or BSN. The University of Oklahoma College of Nursing LPN-BSN program allows me to obtain my BSN in about the same time frame as the local associate's program. I believe the more credentialed a nurse is, the more employable he/she is, and the more amplified your voice becomes when areas in the workplace perhaps need to be changed/modified. It was not an easy decision because most LPNs choose the local ADN program, and I was intimidated about stepping out on my own

(it did not help the fact that a local college counselor tried to discourage me and told me "You're flying by the seat of your pants."). Thanks to her kind words and some encouragement from another LPN in this program, my decision was made, and I have absolutely loved the LPN-BSN program. The most awesome thing about being a nurse is the fact that going to work does not feel like a burden but more like a privilege that has been entrusted to me. The only down side to nursing is the nursing shortage, which can affect quality of time spent in patient care.

Julia Jackson, MSN, RN, CNL
Clinical Nurse III, Women's and Infants' Services, Saint Francis Hospital, Tulsa, Oklahoma; Legal Nurse Consultant, Best and Sharp, Inc., Tulsa, Oklahoma

Tulsa Saint Francis Hospital has not yet utilized the "role" of CNL; however, it changes nothing in my mind regarding my practice. Pay for performance and care maintenance programs will continue to push the CNL role. It is my hope other nurses will choose this education track regardless of their institution's view on the ability to create and pay a position.

Being educated as a Clinical Nurse Leader has cemented my model for nursing practice and professional leadership. Having gained insight for the value that all members of the global healthcare team bring to the patient care picture allows me to maintain clinical objectivity, more appropriately utilize system resources, all while keeping the patient as the center focus of my practice. Being a Clinical Nurse Leader is more than a role, it's a mindset.

Lessons Learned the Hard Way
Francene Weatherby, PhD, RNC
Professor
The University of Oklahoma College of Nursing

Member of the Oklahoma Board of Nursing

1. The license belongs to me (the nurse) to safeguard . . . *not* to the doctor or the supervisor or the RN.

   I've learned that this is a difficult concept for some people to acknowledge. New graduates, those individuals who are quick to try to shift responsibility to others and those individuals who don't think critically but simply react reflexively to an "order," have particular difficulty with this idea.

   Example: A new nurse practitioner, educated in Texas, took her first position in a hospital in Oklahoma. She was told by a physician that she did not need a DEA number for prescribing narcotics. Since he was her supervising physician, he said his DEA number would "cover" her. She didn't bother to check Oklahoma law regarding prescriptive authority. This nurse was required to take a course in nursing jurisprudence, a course in critical thinking, a course in roles and responsibilities in prescribing controlled and dangerous substances, pay a fine, and received a reprimand in her file at the Board of Nursing.

2. Use equipment as the manufacturer intended it to be used.

   "Necessity is the mother invention" is a great saying if you're out of buttermilk for your cake and substitute whole milk with a little vinegar because you have both of these on hand. "Invention" is not always good in a hospital setting.

   Example: A nurse mistakenly attached a nasogastric tube feeding of Crucial to a patient's triple lumen peripherally inserted central venous catheter. When the supervisor asked how this could possibly happen when tube feeding tubing is specifically designed *not* to fit into vascular tubing, three important errors were discovered: (1) The nurse was hanging a feeding prepared by a second nurse. The second nurse could not find

any tube feeding tubing, so to save time and avoid delaying the patient's feeding, she substituted IV tubing in the tube feeding setup. (2) The first nurse did not know what Crucial was. (3) The first nurse did not check the orders or ask for clarification, but simply went in and attached the tubing to patient. Thereafter, the patient died.

3. The function of the board of nursing is to protect the public, *not* to protect the nurse.

   This is perhaps one of the most difficult lessons a nurse who is serving on the board of nursing has to learn. Too often after hearing a case, the "nurse's cap" takes over and the board member begins to rationalize the nurse's actions . . . maybe the shift was extremely busy, maybe there were lots of new admissions that night, maybe the staffing was short, or maybe there were two critical patients down the hall. We're all too familiar with the many possibilities. But the bottom line is that each and every patient deserves and must be assured of receiving the best possible nursing care. This is one of the major criteria of a profession . . . that the members regulate their own. The public trusts us to carry out this monitoring and take corrective actions when patient safety is violated. I don't think all nurses really appreciate this fact.

   Example: A nurse was caring for a patient with diabetes in a long-term care facility. She obtained finger stick blood sugar reading as follows: 8:30 P.M. = 35; 8:45 P.M. = 39; 9:15 P.M. = 42. At 9:30 P.M., she reported the patient's status to one of the oncoming nurses. At 10:30 P.M., the blood sugar reading was 39. An ambulance was called, the nursing director was notified, and the patient was taken to the hospital and later died of hypoglycemic shock. The nurse responded that the wrong time was noted on the chart because the clock on the wall was one hour off. She indicated she had given the patient orange juice and sugar but didn't have the patient's chart with her, so she didn't write it down. The nurse surrendered her license and received a fine.

4. It's great to be a patient advocate, but advocacy has to be done according to protocol.

There's a right way to do things, and there's a wrong way to do things. All nursing students learn early in the nursing school days that an important role of the nurse is to be a patient advocate. No nurse would deny this critical role. However, *how* to go about being an advocate is not often made clear. It's important to remember that there is a chain of command in reporting to follow, and there are facility policies and procedures to which the nurse must adhere or go through the proper steps to change. In an effort to take action as quickly as possible on the patient's behalf, these steps are often brushed aside for the nobler goal. When something goes wrong in the process, the nurse often finds herself "out on a limb" with no legal defense.

Example: A nurse working in a nursing home discovered gross neglect regarding wound care a particular patient was receiving. She discussed this situation with her supervisor, who commented that he remembered a similar case when he was in nursing school. The solution in that case had been to irrigate the decubitus ulcer with hydrogen peroxide (a wound care practice no longer recommended).

After 2 days off, the nurse returned on the night shift to find the patient decubitus in even worse shape. She decided to irrigate the ulcer with hydrogen peroxide without a physician order and in the process found bits of old dressing deep within the wound. Outraged with this discovery, the nurse first called the physician to report the situation. Receiving no response from the doctor, she next called the patient's family and told them they needed to have the patient transferred to another facility "right away." The daughter of the patient had the patient transferred in the middle of the night. The next morning, the physician was very disturbed the patient had been transferred and filed a complaint with the facility against the nurse for failing to follow facility protocol regarding patient transfer.

The facts and circumstances in all the previous examples have been changed and do not reflect exact cases heard by the board. Every case must be examined to determine what, if any, violation of the Nursing Practice Act occurred and what discipline should or should not be imposed.

References

Aiken, L., Clarke, S., Cheung, R., Sloane, D., & Silber, J. (2003). Educational levels of hospital nurses and surgical patient mortality. *Journal of the American Medical Association, 290,* 1617–1623.

American Association of Colleges of Nursing. (2008). The essentials of baccalaureate education for professional nursing practice. Retrieved August 30, 2008, from http://www.aacn.nche.edu/Education/pdf/BaccEssentials98.pdf

American Association of Colleges of Nursing. (1999). *Distance technology in nursing education.* Retrieved February 24, 2007, from http://www.aacn.nche.edu/Publications/WhitePapers/whitepaper.htm

American Association of Colleges of Nursing. (2002). *Your nursing career: A look at the facts.* Retrieved July 18, 2007, from http://www.aacn.nche.edu/education/Career.htm

American Association of Colleges of Nursing. (2004). AACN Position Statement on the Practice Doctorate in Nursing. Retrieved August 30, 2008, from http://www.aacn.nche.edu/DNP/DNPPosition Statement.htm

American Association of Colleges of Nursing. (2005a, May 6). AACN *applauds decision of the AONE board to move registered nurse education to the baccalaureate level* (Press Release). Washington, DC: Author.

American Association of Colleges of Nursing. (2005b). *Fact sheet: Articulation agreements among nursing education programs.* Washington, DC: Author.

American Association of Colleges of Nursing. (2005c). *Alliance for nursing accreditation statement on distance education policies.* Retrieved August 30, 2008, from http://www.aacn.nche.edu/education/disstate.htm

American Association of Colleges of Nursing. (2006a). *Student enrollment rises in U.S. nursing colleges and universities for the 6th consecutive year* (Press Release). Retrieved August 28, 2007, from http://www.aacn.nche.edu/Media/NewsReleases/06Survey.htm

American Association of College of Nursing. (2006b). *Academic leaders form new global alliance on nursing education to focus on improving patient care worldwide* (Press Release). Retrieved September 5, 2007, from http://www.aacn.nche.edu/Media/NewsReleases/2005/GANE.htm

American Association of Colleges of Nursing. (2007a). Retrieved March 16, 2007, from http://www.aacn.nche.edu

American Association of Colleges of Nursing. (2007b). AACN/UHC Nurse Residency Programs. Retrieved August 30, 2008 from http://www.aacn.nche.edu/Education/nurseresidency.htm

American Association of Colleges of Nursing. (2007c). *White paper on the education and role of the clinical nurse leader.* Washington, DC: Author.

American Association of Colleges of Nursing, American Organization of Nurse Executives, & National Organization for Associate Degree Nursing. (1995). *A model for differentiated nursing practice.* Washington, DC: Authors.

American Association of Critical-Care Nurses. (2008). Retrieved August 28, 2007, from http://www.aacn.org/DM/MainPages/CertificationHome.aspx

American Nurses Association. (1965). Education for nursing. *American Journal of Nursing, 65*(12), 107–108.

American Nurses Association. (2000). *Scope and standards of practice for nursing professional development.* Washington, DC: Author.

American Nurses Credentialing Center. (2004). *Magnet recognition program recognizing excellence in nursing service: Application manual 2005.* Washington, DC: Author.

American Nurses Credentialing Center. (2007a). Retrieved August 28, 2007, from http://www.nursecredentialing.org/cert/index.htm

American Nurses Credentialing Center. (2007b). Retrieved September 1, 2007, from http://www.nursecredentialing.org

American Organization of Nurse Executives. (1990). *Current issues and perspectives of differentiated practice.* Chicago: American Hospital Association.

Americans for Nursing Shortage Relief. (2007) *Assuring quality healthcare for the United States: Building and sustaining an infrastructure of qualified nurses for the nation* (Consensus Document). Arlington, VA.

Beecroft, P., Kunzman, L., & Krozek, C. (2001). RN internship: Outcomes of a one-year pilot program. *Journal of Nursing Administration, 31*(12), 575–582.

Ben-Zur, H., Yagi, D., & Spitzer, A. (1999). Evaluation of an innovative curriculum: Nursing education in the next century. *Journal of Advanced Nursing, 30,* 1432–1531.

Bowles, C., & Candela, L. (2005). First job experiences of recent RN graduates. *Journal of Nursing Administration, 35*(3), 130–137.

Brown, E. (1948). *Nursing for the future: A report prepared for the National Nursing Council.* New York: Russell Sage Foundation.

Cary, A. (2001). Certified registered nurses. Results of the study of the certified workforce. *American Journal of Nursing, 10*(1), 44–52.

Casey, K., Fink, R., Krugman, M., & Propst, J. (2004). The graduate nurse experience. *Journal of Nursing Administration, 34*(6), 303–311.

Commission on Graduates of Foreign Nursing Schools. (2007). Retrieved August 27, 2007, from http://www.cgfns.org/

Damgaard, G., VanderWoude, D., & Hegge, M. (1999). Perspectives from the prairie: The relationship between nursing regulation and South Dakota Nursing Workforce Development. *Journal of Nursing Administration, 29*(11), 7–9, 14.

Donahue, M. (1983). Isabel Maitland Stewart's philosophy of education. *Nursing Research, 32,* 140–146.

Estabrooks, C., Midodzi, W., Cummings, G., Ricker, K., & Giovannetti, P. (2005). The impact of hospital nursing characteristics on 30-day mortality. *Nursing Research, 54*(2), 74–84.

Fernandez, R., & Hebert, G. (2004). Global licensure. New modalities of treatment and care require the development of new structures and systems to access care. *Nursing Administration Quarterly, 28,* 129–132.

Girard, N. J. (2003). Lack of sleep another safety risk factor-Editorial-medical errors. *AORN Journal, 78,* 553–556.

Goldmark, J. (1923). *Nursing and nursing education in the United States.* New York: Macmillan.

Goode, C., & Williams, C. (2004). Post-baccalaureate nurse residency program. *Journal of Nursing Administration, 34*(2), 71–77.

Halfer, D., & Graf, E. (2006a). Graduate nurse experience. *Journal of Nursing Administration, 34*(6), 303–311.

Halfer, D., & Graf, E. (2006b). Graduate nurse perceptions of the work experience. *Nursing Economics, 24,* 150–155.

Honey, P., & Mumford, A. (1986). *The manual of learning styles*. Maidenhead, England: Peter Honey.

Honey, P., & Mumford, A. (1992). *The manual of learning styles* (3rd ed.). Maidenhead, England: Peter Honey.

Hutchins, G. (1994). Differentiated interdisciplinary practice. *Journal of Nursing Administration, 24*(6), 52–58.

Institute of Medicine. (2001). *Crossing the quality chasm: A new health system for the 21st century*. Washington, DC: Author.

Institute of Medicine. (2003). *Health professions education: A bridge to quality*. Washington, DC: Author.

International Centre on Nurse Migration. (2007). Retrieved August 28, 2007, from http://www.intlnursemigration.org/

Knowles, M. (1975). *Self-directed learning: A guide for learners and teachers*. Chicago: Follett.

Knowles, M. (1984). *Andagogy in action*. San Francisco: Jossey-Bass.

Kolb, D. (1984). *Experiential learning: Experience as the source of learning and development*. Toronto, ON: Prentice Hall.

Leighow, S. (1996). Backrubs vs. Bach. Nursing and the entry-into-practice debate: 1946–1986. *Nursing History Review, 4*, 3–17.

Long, K. (2003). *The Institute of Medicine Report: Health Professions Education: A Bridge to Quality. Policy, Politics, and Nursing Practice, 4*, 259–262.

Loquist, R. (2002). State boards of nursing respond to the nurse shortage. *Nursing Administration Quarterly, 26*(4), 33–39.

Lundy, K. (2005). A history of healthcare and nursing. In K. Masters (Ed.), *Role development in professional nursing practice* (Ch. 1). Sudbury, MA: Jones and Bartlett.

Manfredini, R., Boari, B., & Manfredini, F. (2006). Adverse events secondary to mistakes, excessive work hours, and sleep deprivation. *Archives of Internal Medicine, 166*, 1422–1433.

Masters, K. (2005). *Role development in professional nursing practice*. Sudbury, MA: Jones and Bartlett.

Montag, M. (1959). *Community college education for nursing: An experiment in technical education for nursing*. New York: McGraw-Hill.

Montgomery, V. L. (2007). Effect of fatigue, workload, and environment on patient safety in the pediatric intensive care unit. *Pediatric Critical Care Medicine, 8*(Suppl. 2): S11–16.

National Council of State Boards of Nursing. (1996a). Retrieved September 8, 2008, from https://www.ncsbn.org

National Council of State Boards of Nursing. (1996b). *Why regulation paper: Public protection or professional self-*

preservation? Retrieved September 8, 2007, from https://www.ncsbn.org/why_regulation_paper.pdf

National Council of State Boards of Nursing. (2001). *Position Statement: International Nurse Immigration*. Chicago: Author.

National Council of State Boards of Nursing. (2005). *Position paper: Clinical instruction in prelicensure nursing programs*. Retrieved November 17, 2008, from http:www.ncsbn.org/pdfs/Final_Clinical_Instr_Pre_Nsg_programs.pdf

National Council of State Boards of Nursing. (2007a). *Guiding principles of nursing regulation*. Retrieved September 8, 2007, from https://www.ncsbn.org/Guiding_Principles.pdf

National Council of State Boards of Nursing. (2007b). *Boards of nursing*. Retrieved September 6, 2007, from http://www.ncsbn.org/boards.htm

National Council of State Boards of Nursing. (2007c). *NCLEX examinations*. Retrieved September 5, 2007, from https://www.ncsbn.org/nclex.htm

National Council of State Boards of Nursing. (2007d). *National licensure compact (NLC)*. Retrieved September 5, 2007, from https://www.ncsbn.org/nlc.htm

National League for Nursing. (2003). *Position statement: Innovation in nursing education: A call to reform*. New York: Author.

National League for Nursing. (2006). *Despite encouraging trends suggested by the NLN's comprehensive survey of all nursing programs, large numbers of qualified applicants continue to be turned down*. Retrieved June 3, 2007, from http://www.nln.org/newsreleases/nedsdec05.pdf

National League for Nursing. (2007a). The National League for Nursing strategic plan for 2007–2012. *The NLN Report, 1*(Summer), 1–12.

National League for Nursing. (2007b). *Academy of nursing education*. Retrieved September 1, 2007, from http://www.nln.org/excellence/academy/index.htm

National Organization for Associate Degree Nursing. (2006). *Position Statement of Associate Degree Nursing*. Retrieved September 5, 2008, from https://www.noadn.org/component/option,com_docman/Itemid,0/task,doc_view/gid,16/

National Organization for Associate Degree Nursing. (2007). Retrieved September 5, 2007, from http://www.noadn.org/all.php?l=&w=1280

O'Shea, E. (2003). Self-directed learning in nurse education: A review of the literature. *Journal of Advanced Nursing, 43*(1), 62–70.

Porter-O'Grady, T. (2001). Profound change: 21st century nursing. *Nursing Outlook, 49*, 182–186.

Rassool, G., & Rawaf, S. (2007). Learning style preference of undergraduate nursing students. *Nursing Standard, 32*(21), 35–41.

Reinert, B., & Fryback, P. (1997). Distance learning and nursing education. *Journal of Nursing Education, 36*(9), 421.

Rick, C. (2003). AONE's leadership exchange: Differentiated practice. Get beyond the fear factor. *Nursing Management, 34*(1), 11.

Schaefer B. (1990). International credentials review: crucial and complex. *Nursing Healthcare, 11*, 431–432.

Shirey, M. (2005). Celebrating certification in nursing. Forces of magnetism in action. *Nursing Administration Quarterly, 29*, 245–253.

Sigurdson, K., & Ayas, N.T. (2007). The public health and safety consequences of sleep disorders. *Canadian Journal of Physiology and Pharmacology, 85*, 179–183.

U.S. Department of Health and Human Services, Health Resources and Services Administration, Bureau of Health Professions, National Center for Health Workforce Analysis. (2004, September). *What is behind HRSA's projected supply, demand, and shortage of registered nurses?* Retrieved August 28, 2007, from ftp://ftp.hrsa.gov/bhpr/workforce/behindshortage.pdf

U.S. Department of Health and Human Services. (2006, April). Nursing resources. Retrieved August 30, 2008 from http://bhpr.hrsa.gov/nursing/

The Healthcare Context

Section II sets the stage for the student. What is the healthcare environment in which the student now enters? It is complex. Chapter 5 introduces the topics of health policy and political action, and how they relate to the nursing profession. Chapter 6 moves to the related topics of ethics and legal issues that impact practice. With this background, Chapter 7 begins a more in-depth discussion of health promotion, disease prevention, and illness—all part of the continuum of care. The last chapter in this section, Chapter 8, examines one healthcare organization, the acute care hospital, in depth as an exemplar of how healthcare organizations function and how nurses are involved in these organizations.

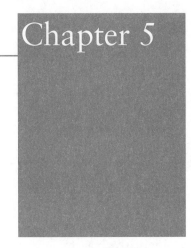

Chapter 5

Health Policy and Political Action: Critical Actions for Nurses

CHAPTER OUTLINE

DISCUSSION QUESTIONS
CRITICAL THINKING ACTIVITIES
CASE STUDY
WORDS OF WISDOM
REFERENCES

KEY TERMS

- ❏ Executive branch
- ❏ Judicial branch
- ❏ Legislative branch
- ❏ Lobbying
- ❏ Lobbyist
- ❏ Policy

- ❏ Political Action Committee (PAC)
- ❏ Politics
- ❏ Private Policy
- ❏ Public Health Act (1944)
- ❏ Public policy
- ❏ Social Security Act (1935)

Introduction

The focus of the second section of this textbook is the healthcare context. The present chapter begins this section by introducing content about health **policy** and the political process. Both have a major impact on nurses, nursing care, and healthcare delivery. When nurses participate in the policy process, they are acting as advocates for patients.

> *Nurses are well aware that today's healthcare system is in trouble and in need of change. The experiences of many nurses practicing in the real world of healthcare are motivating them to take on some form of an advocacy role in order to influence change in policies, laws, or regulations that govern the larger healthcare system. This type of advocacy necessitates stepping beyond their own practice setting and into the less familiar world of policy and **politics**, a world in which many nurses do not feel prepared to participate effectively. (Abood, 2007, p. 3)*

Importance of Health Policy and Political Action

Why is it important for nurses to have knowledge about health policy? Every day, healthcare delivery is impacted by health policy, such as through reimbursement, through decisions made about how and where care might be provided and to whom, or through decisions about whether someone receives care when it is needed. Understanding healthcare policy requires the nurse to step back and see a broader picture while understanding how it impacts individual care. Political action plays a role in recognizing the need for health policy, in the development of policy, and in the implementation of policy, including financing policy decisions. Nurses offer the following to health policy-making:

- Expertise
- Understanding of consumer needs
- Experience with assisting consumers in making healthcare decisions

- A link to healthcare professionals and organizations
- Understanding of the healthcare system
- Understanding of interdisciplinary care

Definitions

What does policy mean? A policy is a course of action that affects a large number of people and is stimulated by a specific need to achieve certain outcomes. The best approach to understanding health policy is to describe the difference between **public policy** and **private policy**. A public policy is "policy made at the legislative, executive, and **judicial branches** of federal, state, and local levels of government that affects individual and institutional behaviors under the government's respective jurisdiction. Public policy includes all policies that come from government at all levels" (Magill, 1984, as cited in Block, 2008, p. 7). Policy is a method for finding solutions to problems, but not all solutions are policies. Many solutions have nothing to do with government. There are two main types of public policies: (1) regulatory policies (e.g., registered nurse (RN) licensure that regulates practice) and (2) allocative policies, which involve money distribution. Allocative policies provide benefits for some at the expense of others to ensure that certain public objectives are met. Often the decision relates to funding certain healthcare programs but not others. Health policy is policy that focuses on health and health-related issues. Examples of policies that have had national impact are those prohibiting smoking in public places (initiated through the **legislative branch**) and abortion rulings made by the U.S. Supreme Court (initiated through the judicial branch). Private policy is made by nongovernmental organizations. This chapter focuses on public policy related to health because this is the most important type of health policy. Health policies include (Longest, 1998, as cited in Block, 2008, p. 6):

- Health-related decisions made by legislators that then become laws
- Rules/regulations designed to implement legislation/laws or that are used to operate government and its health-related programs
- Judicial decisions related to health that have an impact on how healthcare is delivered, reimbursed, etc.

Policy planning is developing a plan to change the value system or laws and regulations. This is broad health planning because it typically impacts a large portion of the population.

Policy: Relevance to the Nation's Health and to Nursing

Policy has an impact on all aspects of health and healthcare delivery, such as how care is delivered, who receives care, the types of services received, reimbursement, and the types of providers and organizations that provide health care. Policy impacts nursing in similar areas, as shown in Figure 5–1.

Each of these areas relates to individual nurses and to the profession. *Roles and standards* are found in state laws and rules/regulations. Boards of nursing and each state's Nurse Practice Act impact professional expectations and what a nurse does. *Federal laws and rules/regulations* related to Medicare and Medicaid address issues such as reimbursement for nurse practitioners (NPs). How *nursing care* is provided and what care is provided are influenced by Medicare, Medicaid, nurse practice acts, and other laws and rules/regulations made by federal, state, and local governments. *Health* is influenced by federal policy decisions related to Medicare reimbursement for preventive services, the Department of Health and Human Services (DHHS), and its agencies rules and regulations. An agency for which rules and regulations are very important is the Food and Drug

Figure 5–1   Healthcare policy: Impact on healthcare and nursing.

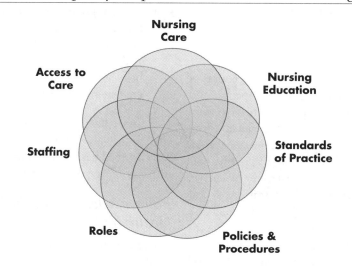

Administration because of the agency's drug approval process. *Staffing levels* may be determined by state laws, such as those passed in California and other states limiting or eliminating mandatory overtime. *Access to care* is often impacted by policy, particularly that related to reimbursement, and what services can be provided and by whom. This is particularly relevant to Medicare, Medicaid, and state employee health insurance. Organizations have *policies and procedures,* and often these are influenced by public policy. This type of policy is discussed further in Chapter 12 as a part of quality improvement. Public policy has an impact on *nursing education* through laws and rules/regulations—for example, funding for faculty and scholarships, funding to develop or expand schools of nursing and their programs, evaluation standards through state boards of nursing, and much more. *Nursing research* is also impacted by policy; funding for research primarily comes through government sources, and legislation designates funding for government research.

Nurses are experts in health care, and because of this, they can contribute to the healthcare policy-making process. Nurses' expertise and knowledge about health and healthcare delivery are important resources for policy makers. Nurses also have long served as consumer advocates for their patients and patients' families. Advocacy means to speak for, or be persuasive for, another's needs. This does not mean that the nurse takes over for the patient. When nurses are involved in policy development, they are acting as advocates. Nurses get involved in policy as individuals and as representatives of the nursing profession, such as by representing a nursing organization. Both of these forms of advocacy are examples of nursing leadership. Collaboration is very important for effective policy development and implementation. The goal with health policy should be better health care for citizens. When nurses are advocating for professional issues such as pay, work schedules, the need for more nurses, and so forth, they are also impacting healthcare delivery. If there are not enough nurses because pay is low, then care is compromised. If there are not enough nurses because few are entering the profession, or schools do not have the funds to increase enrollment, this compromises care. In other cases, nurses advocate directly for healthcare delivery issues, such as reimbursement for hospice care, or through supporting mental health parity legislation to improve access to care for people with serious mental illness.

General Descriptors of U.S. Health Policy

U.S. health policy can be described by the following long-standing characteristics, which have an impact on the types of policies that are enacted and the effectiveness of the policies (Shi & Singh, 1998). Whereas many countries have a universal healthcare system, the United States does not. The private sector is the dominant player in the U.S. system. The issue of a universal right to health care has been a contentious one for some time. Government does play an important role in the U.S. healthcare system, but it is not the major role as is the case with a universal system. This is mostly due to Americans' view that the government's role should be limited. The second characteristic is the approach taken to healthcare policy, which has been, and continues to be, fragmented and incremental. This approach does not look at the whole system and how its components work or do not work together effectively; parts are not connected to constitute a whole. Coordination between state and federal policies, and even between the branches of the government, is also limited. A wide array of reimbursement sources complicate the system further (reimbursement is discussed in Chapter 8). The third characteristic is the role of the states. States have a significant role in policy, and health policies vary from state to state. In some cases, there is a shared role with the federal government—for example, the Medicaid program. The last important characteristic is the role of the President (**executive branch** of government), which can be significant. How does the President influence healthcare policy? An example is President Clinton and his initiative to review the safety and quality of health care in the United States. He established a commission to start this process. This commission no longer exists, but it set the direction for extensive reviews and recommendations that have been identified in the last decade through the Institute of Medicine (IOM; this is discussed in Chapter 12). Clinton also pushed to get the Health Insurance Portability and Accountability Act (HIPAA) and the State Children's Health Insurance Program (S-CHIP) passed. Both laws resulted from the work of this healthcare commission. The work of this commission was to be part of a major healthcare reform initiative that did not succeed at the time of the Clinton administration. Its goal was to make major changes in healthcare reimbursement, but this did not happen. Some significant policies did come from these efforts, such as the two mentioned laws and the IOM quality initiative.

Some legislative efforts are diluted over time or cancelled. The most recent example is S-CHIP. In 2007, Congress tried to expand this program, but it was vetoed by President George W. Bush. So, 10 years after this legislation was passed, the program has weakened. S-CHIP was established to provide states with matching funds from the federal government to allow states to extend health insurance to children from families with incomes too high to meet Medicaid criteria but not high enough to purchase health insurance. Matching funds is one method used by the government to fund programs. This method means that the federal government pays for half, and the states pay for the other half (or some other configuration of sharing costs). Medicaid is funded with matching funds, whereas Medicare is funded only by the federal government. Why did the issue of S-CHIP come up again when there was already a program? The legislation was expiring, which opened it up for cancellation, or renewal with or without changes. S-CHIP has been an effective program; it has provided reimbursement for needed care for many children, improved access to care and preventive care, and improved the health status of children. Congress and the administration were in disagreement over expansion and funding of the program. This is a example of how legislation can get passed, but it can be vetoed by the administration.

Examples of Critical Healthcare Policy Issues

Many healthcare policy issues are of concern to local communities, states, and the federal government, some of which are indentified in Exhibit 5–1.

This exhibit highlights a long list of issues. Some of these issues are of particular current concern to nurses, nursing, and healthcare delivery in general. How policy is developed, or whether

policy related to each of these issues is developed at all, may vary. Examining some of these issues in more depth provides a better understanding of the complexity of health policy issues.

- Nursing Shortage and Staffing
  The nursing shortage, which is discussed in more detail in Chapter 14, impacts care delivery through a lack of the right number and type of nurses for care needs and not having enough faculty to provide the education needed to increase the number of graduates. This issue has led to policy decisions. A major policy decision and related legislation addressing the shortage is the Nurse Reinvestment Act of 2002. What does this law do? It establishes (1) nurse scholarships, (2) nurse retention and patient safety enhancement grants, (3) comprehensive geriatric training grants for nurses, (4) a faculty loan cancellation program, (5) a career ladder grant program, and (6) public service announcements to advertise and promote the nursing profession and to educate the public about nursing careers. This is a significant law that has an impact on a broad range of nursing education and

---

Exhibit 5–1 Potential Policy Issues

- Access to Care
- Acute and Chronic Illness
- Aging
- Changing Practice Patterns and the Physician
- Diversity in Healthcare Workforce
- Disparities in Health Care
- Advanced Practice Nursing
- Diagnosis-Related Groups
- Healthcare Consumerism
- Healthcare Commercialization and Industrial Complex
- Healthcare Role Changes
- Immigration: Impact on Care and Providers

- International Health Issues
- Managed Care
- Mental Health Parity
- Minority Health
- Move from Acute Care to Ambulatory Care
- Nursing Education
- Poverty and Health
- Public Health
- Quality Safe Care
- Reimbursement
- Restructuring and Reengineering
- Uninsured and underinsured

practice issues. It all flows from the concern about the nursing shortage.

Numerous professional nursing associations supported the Nurse Reinvestment Act and it received additional support from other professional bodies, including the American Hospital Association, the American Medical Association, the American College of Physicians, and the American Society of Internal Medicine. On February 18, 2003, both chambers of Congress passed the $397.4 billion FY 2003 Omnibus Appropriations bill and thus the Nurse Reinvestment Act (PL 107-205) was enacted and funded. The FY 2003 appropriations amounted to $113 million, a $20 million increase over FY 2002. These state and federal initiatives indicate that professional organizations, health care institutions, and other experts have succeeded in alerting policy makers to the problems associated with a shortage of a skilled nursing workforce. If forecasts of a massive gap between the supply and demand for nurses in the future are correct, however, it is likely that the scope and scale of initiatives—particularly, the level of financial resources from public and private sources—will need to be significantly expanded to reverse current trends. (KaiserEDU.org, 2005)

As policy makers debate the issues related to the nursing shortage, discussion will likely focus on several key issues (KaiserEDU.org, 2005):

1. How and why is this current nursing shortage different from previous shortages? Do the policy options address the current problems or are they responding to historical problems?
2. How does the nursing shortage affect the quality of care for patients?
3. Is assuring an adequate nurse workforce a federal responsibility? What is the correlation, if any, between the availability of nurses in the health workforce and the nature and funding of federal discretionary nursing programs?
4. What other federal policies affect the demand for and supply of nurses?
5. What is the nature of states' "safe staffing" legislation? Why are states addressing the nursing shortage this way? Does this policy have potential unintended consequences? Will an inability to find enough qualified RNs force hospitals to eliminate beds and reduce access to care?
6. Do state nursing policies affect the supply of nurses from state to state? If so, how?

Another issue related to the nursing shortage is mandatory overtime, also discussed in Chapter 14. Federal legislation was introduced in the House of Representatives to limit the amount of overtime that healthcare facilities are permitted to mandate to 12 hours per workday, or 60 hours per week. This bill applied only to RNs and licensed practical nurses. This law was not meant to prevent employees from working voluntary time. Mandatory overtime would be permitted in the case of a declared emergency or unforeseeable catastrophic event. Vacancies that arise as the result of chronic short staffing or a labor dispute are not considered emergencies or unforeseeable catastrophic events. This act covered acute care hospitals, psychiatric hospitals, long-term care facilities, medical units in the Department of Corrections, and all other facilities licensed by the Department of Health. The bill was not passed in the Senate, but many states are now passing similar legislation applicable only to those states.

- Cost of Health Care
  The cost of health care in the United States is on a steady rise. There is no doubt that there are better drugs, treatment, and

technology today to improve health and meet treatment needs for many problems; however, these new preventive and treatment interventions have increased costs. Defensive medicine, in which the physician and other healthcare providers order tests and procedures to protect themselves from lawsuits, increases costs. Insurance coverage has expanded, and beneficiaries of coverage expect to get care when they feel they need it. Cost containment and cost-effectiveness have become increasingly important. Health policy often focuses on reimbursement, control of costs, and greater control of provider decisions to reduce costs. The latter has not been popular with consumers/patients. A critical issue is whether the United States should move to a universal healthcare system. Coffey (2001) discussed universal health coverage and identified five reasons that this should be of interest to nurses: (1) Insuring everyone under one national health program would spread the insurance risk over the entire population; (2) the cost of prescription drugs would decrease; (3) billions of dollars in administrative costs would be saved; (4) "competition" could focus on quality, safety, and patient satisfaction; and (5) resources would be redirected toward patients. This healthcare policy issue was a major one in the 2008 presidential campaign. Chapter 8 discusses costs of care in more detail.

- Healthcare Quality and Safety
  This is the "hot" issue today in health care and is discussed in detail in Chapter 12. Following President Clinton's establishment of the Advisory Commission on Consumer Protection and Quality in Healthcare (1996–1998), a whole area of policy development was opened up: How can healthcare quality and safety be improved? What needs to be done to accomplish this?

This led to federal government's request for the IOM to further assess health care in the United States, resulting in major reports and recommendations related to quality and safety, and other important topics. Chapters 9–13 include content on these reports and their implications for nursing and healthcare delivery.

- Disparities in Health Care
  The IOM reports on diversity in health care and disparities, and the Sullivan report on healthcare workforce diversity (IOM, 2002; 2004; Sullivan, 2004) opened up this critical policy concern. Nurses need more knowledge about culture and health needs, health literacy, and how different diverse groups respond to care (IOM, 2002, 2004). How does this impact health policy? Does it mean that certain groups may not get the same services (disparities)? If so, what needs to change? Chapter 9 discusses this topic in more detail.

- Consumers
  There is increasing interest in the role of consumers in health care. Today, consumersare more informed about health and healthcare services. A recent example of a law that focuses on health is HIPAA. The major content of this law really addresses the issue of "carrying" health insurance from one employer to another, but it also includes expectations regarding privacy of patient information. This is now the content most commonly considered by healthcare providers in daily practice. Chapter 9 discusses consumers in more detail.

- Commercialization of Health Care
  As will be discussed in Chapter 8, the organization of healthcare delivery systems has been changing into a multi-pronged system. These multiple organizations generally form a corporate model. Such corporations may exist in a local community,

statewide, or even nationally. Some of the large healthcare corporations also have hospitals in other countries. This change has impacted policy, particularly that related to financing health care and quality concerns.

- Reimbursement for Nursing Care
  Reimbursement of nursing care must be viewed from two perspectives. The first is how to reimburse for inpatient nursing care, and there has not been much progress in this area. Hospitals still do not clearly identify the specific costs of nursing care in a manner that directly impacts reimbursement. The second view involves reimbursement for specific individual provider services instead of reimbursement for an organization provider, such as a hospital. Physicians are reimbursed for their services. There have been major changes in how NPs are reimbursed. This is improving but must improve further. An example in nursing might be to ask, If an NP provides care in a clinic or his or her private practice, how is he or she reimbursed for the care? Will the patient's health insurance pay for these services? Some services are covered by federal government plans, but there is great variation in reimbursement from nongovernment plans. Chapter 8 includes content on reimbursement.

- Immigration and the Nursing Workforce
  Chapter 14 includes content on immigration of nurses to the United States and the impact of this on international healthcare delivery; however, it needs to be recognized as an important policy issue as yet unresolved. Important issues are regulatory (visas to enter the United States and work; licensure), level of language expertise, quality of education, orientation and training needs, and whether immigration of RNs should be limited. Some of the issues need

to be addressed by laws, rules and regulations related to laws, and state boards of nursing.

These examples of policy issues related to nursing are not the only healthcare policy issues, but they illustrate the types that can be considered health policy issues.

In 2005, the American Nurses Association (ANA) published a revision of its *Health Care Agenda*. The agenda highlighted the problem with the healthcare system as one of a "patchwork approach" to healthcare reform and to policy development. The system is fragmented and expensive, and this has not changed over the last few decades. The agenda states,

> ANA *remains committed to the principle that all persons are entitled to ready access to affordable, quality health care services. Nursing, as the pivotal health care profession, is well positioned to advocate on behalf of and in concert with individuals, families and communities who are in desperate need of a well financed, functional and coordinated health care system that provides safe, quality care. Indeed, all of us stand to benefit from such a system. Accessible, affordable, and quality health care will positively contribute to our individual health, the strength of society, our national well-being, and overall productivity.* (p. 4)

Access to care means that care should be affordable for, available to, and acceptable to a great variety of patients. Quality of care is still a problem (as will be discussed more in Chapter 12), as is safety. The ANA supports the recommendations of the IOM *Quality Chasm* series, which is discussed in more detail in Chapters 9–13. All care should be safe, effective, timely, patient centered, efficient, and equitable. "ANA believes that the development and implementation of health policies that reflect these aims, and are based on effectiveness and outcomes research, will ultimately save money" (American Nurses Association, 2005, p. 7). The agenda also addresses the critical issue of the workforce and the need for an "adequate supply of well-educated, well-distributed, and well utilized registered nurses" (American Nurses Association, 2005, p. 10). The agenda concludes,

> *The need for fundamental reform of the U.S. health care system is more necessary today than in 1991 (date of previous ANA agenda). Bold action is called for to create a healthcare system that is responsive to the needs of consumers and provides equal access to safe, high-quality care for every citizen and resident in a cost-effective manner. Working together—policy makers, industry leaders, providers, and consumers—we can build an affordable health care system that meets the needs of everyone. (p. 12)*

The ANA agenda is an example of how a professional organization speaks for the profession, delineates issues that need to be addressed through policies, commits to collaborating with others to accomplish this, and advocates for patients.

The Policy-Making Process

Health policy is developed at the local, state, and federal levels of government, but the two most common levels are state and federal. At the state level, the typical broad focus areas are public health and safety (e.g., immunization, water safety, and so forth); care for those who cannot afford it; purchasing care through state insurance, such as for state employees; regulation (e.g., RN licensure); and resource allocation (e.g., funding for care services). At the federal level, there are many different needs and policy makers. The focus areas are much the same as at the state level but apply to the nation.

Federal legislation is an important source of health policy. The two laws that have had the most impact on U.S. health care are the **Social Security Act** of 1935 and the **Public Health Act** of 1944. Both have had amendments over the years. Why are these laws so important? The Social Security Act established the Medicare and Medicaid programs, two major reimbursement programs. These laws also provided funding for nursing education through amendments to the law. The Public Health Act consolidated all existing (1944) public health legislation into one law, and it too has had amendments. Some of the programs and issues addressed in this law are health services for migratory workers; National Institutes of Health; nurse training acts; prevention and primary care services; rural health clinics; communicable disease control; family planning services; and more. An amendment to this law established *Healthy People* in 2000 and its subsequent extension.

The policy-making process is described in Figure 5–2. The first step is to recognize that an issue might require a policy. The recognition of the need for a policy can come from a variety of sources: professional organizations, consumers/citizens, government agencies, and lawmakers. The second step is not to develop a policy but first to learn more about the issue. There may not be a need for a policy. There may be, and often is, disagreement about the need, and then how to resolve it if there is a need. Information data are collected to get a clearer perspective on the issue. This information may come from experts, consumers, professionals, relevant literature (such as professional literature), and research. Using this information, policy makers identify possible solutions. They should not consider just one solution because only under rare circumstances is only one solution possible. During this process, policy makers consider the costs and benefits of each of the solutions. Costs are more than financial; a cost might be that some people will not receive a service, whereas

Figure 5–2 The policy-making process.

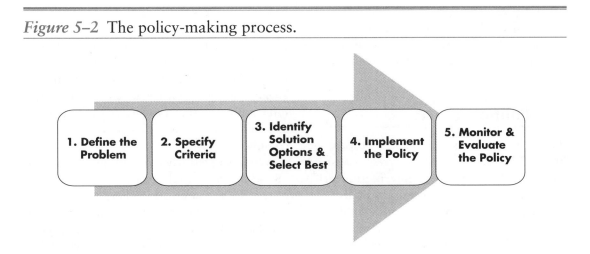

others will. What impact will this have on both groups? After the cost-benefit analysis is done, a solution is selected, and the policy is developed. It is at this time that implementation begins, though how a policy might be implemented must be considered as the solution is selected and policy developed. It may be that implementation is very complex, and this will impact the policy. For example, if a policy decision was made that all U.S. citizens should receive healthcare insurance, the policy statement is very simple; however, when implementation is considered, this is very complex. How would this be done? Who would administer it? What funds would be used to pay for this system? What would happen to current employer coverage? Would all services be provided? How much decision-making power would the consumer have? How would providers be paid, and which providers would be paid? Many more questions could be asked. Policy development must include an implementation plan. Implementation of policy is influenced by social, economic, legal, and ethical forces. The best policy can fail if the implementation plan is not reasonable and feasible. As will be discussed in the next section on the political process, the policy often is legislation (law). The next step is implementing the policy, which is largely determined by the rules and regulations.

Coalition building is important in gaining support for a new policy. As will be discussed in the next section on the political process, gaining support is important in getting laws passed. Regarding a healthcare issue, some groups that might be included in coalition building are healthcare providers (medical doctors, nurses, pharmacists, and so on); healthcare organizations, particularly hospitals; professional organizations (e.g., the ANA, the American Medical Association, the American Hospital Association, the Joint Commission, the American Association of Colleges of Nursing (AACN), the National League for Nursing (NLN), and many others); state organizations; elected officials; business leaders; third-party payers; and pharmaceutical industry representatives. Members of a coalition in support of a policy may offer funding to support the effort, act as expert witnesses, develop written information to support the policy, and work to get others to support the policy; some, such as lawmakers, may be in a position to actually vote on the policy. After a policy is approved and implemented, it should be monitored and its outcomes evaluated. This may lead to future changes or to the determination that a policy is not effective. The process may then begin again.

The Political Process

Politics is "the process of influencing the authoritative allocation of scarce resources" (Kalisch & Kalisch, 1982, p. 31). Typically, nurses participate in the policy-making process by using or participating in the political process. Public policy should meet the needs of the public, but it is more complex than this. Politics influences policy development and implementation, and sometimes politics interferes with the effectiveness of policy development and implementation. Political feasibility must be considered because this can be the difference between a successful policy and an unsuccessful policy. Political support, usually from multiple groups, is critical. Most major policy changes or new policies are made through the legislative process. This process can be correlated with the policy-making process.

Steps 1–4 are similar in the legislative process. Once the policy is developed in the form of a proposed law, the legislative process merges with the policy-making process. The legislative process varies from state to state, but all states have a legislative process that is similar to the federal process. When a bill is written and then introduced in Congress, it is given a number with either H.R. (House of Representatives) or S. (Senate; Hart & Jackson, 2000). The bill is then assigned to a committee or subcommittee by the leadership of the Senate or House, depending on where the bill begins its long process to approval through a final vote. At this point in the committee, the bill may actually "die," meaning that nothing is done with it. If,

however, there is some support for the bill, the committee or the subcommittee will assess the content. This might include holding hearings on the bill for extensive discussion, often with witnesses. Amendments may be added. If the bill began in a subcommittee, it can be sent on to a full committee, then progress to the full House or Senate. If it began in a committee, it may go straight to the full House or Senate.

What happens when the bill gets to the full House or Senate? In the House, the bill first goes to the Rules Committee. There, decisions are made about debate on the bill, such as the length of debate. These decisions can have an impact on the successful passage of the bill. The Senate does not have a rules committee, and senators can add amendments and filibuster, or delay a vote on the bill. There is more flexibility in the Senate than in the House. The leaders in the Senate (Majority Leader) and the House Leader have a lot of power over the legislative process. Can a bill be passed only in the House or only in the Senate and still become law? No, it must be passed by both. Sometimes a bill is introduced at the same time in the House and the Senate, allowing the approval process to continue in both simultaneously. Decisions may need to be made about differences in the two bills. If this is the case, a conference committee composed of both representatives and senators work to accomplish this. The altered bill must then go back for a vote in the House and in the Senate. If both the House and Senate pass the bill, it must go to the President for signature. At this time, the bill moves from the legislative branch of government to the executive branch. Figure 5–3 identifies the branches of government.

The President has 10 days to decide to sign the bill into law. If the President waits longer than 10 days or the Congress is no longer in session, the bill automatically becomes law as if the President had signed it. The President,

Figure 5–3 The branches of the federal government in the United States.

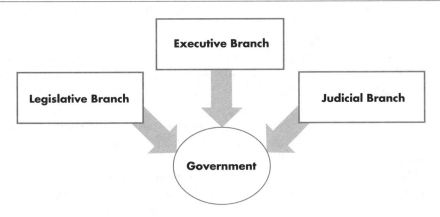

however, may choose not to sign a bill. If this is the case, the Congress may decide not to pursue the bill any further, or the Congress could decide to bring the bill back for another vote to try to override the President's veto. This may or may not be successful and is a highly political situation. If there are a sufficient number of votes, the bill could become law or die. If the President signs the bill or if the Congress overrides a presidential veto, the bill goes to the regulatory agency that would have jurisdiction over that particular type of law. For example, a health law would typically go to the DHHS. If it dealt with Medicare, it would go to the Centers for Medicare & Medicaid Services (CMS), an agency within the DHHS. It is at this point that a very important step in the process occurs: Rules are written for the law that specifically state how the law will be implemented. This can make a significant difference in the effectiveness of the law. At specific steps in the regulatory development process, the public, including healthcare professionals, can participate by providing input. It is important that this input be given. Once the final rules are approved, the law is imple-

mented. There may be a date that the law ends, or "sunsets." If so, the law may expire, or it may be reintroduced into the legislative process.

What is the connection between policy development and politics? A policy is not accepted by all, and efforts may be made to defeat a policy. Because of the various viewpoints on the same issue, there are competing interests (Abood, 2007). There are also partisan issues, Democrat and Republican, that can impact the policy. "Decision-makers rely mainly on the political process as a way to find a course of action that is acceptable to the various individuals with conflicting proposals, demands, and values. . . . Throughout our daily lives, politics determines who gets what, when, and how" (Abood, p. 3).

Nurses' Role in the Political Process: Impact on Healthcare Policy

Nurses bring a unique perspective to healthcare policy development because of their education training, professional values and ethics, advocacy skills, and experiential background. Significant progress has occurred over the years toward advancing nursing's presence, role, and influence in the development of healthcare policy. However, more nurses need to learn how to identify issues strategically; work with decision makers; understand who holds the power in the workplace, communities, state and federal level organizations; and understand who controls the resources for healthcare services. (Ferguson, 2001, p. 546)

Nurses have expertise; understand consumer needs, the healthcare system, and interdisciplinary care; and have an appreciation of the care process. Though nursing has gained political power, it is still weaker than it should be. Given the number of nurses, the nursing profession should have more power. Each nurse is a potential voter, and this means potential influence over who will be elected and over legislative decisions. However, nursing as a profession has struggled with organizing. This has diluted the value of the number of nurses in the United States. Nursing has had serious problems defining itself. The use of multiple entry levels, licensure issues, and multiple titles confuses the public and other healthcare professionals. Policy makers do not understand the roles and titles, and this makes it difficult for nurses to speak with one voice.

Nurses need to develop political competence. What is political competence? It involves the ability to use opportunities: networking, highlighting nursing expertise, using powerful persuasion, demonstrating a commitment to working with others, thinking strategically, and persevering. Political competence means being aware of the rules of the game and recognizing that the other side needs something. Sometimes giving up one viewpoint or action may lead to more effective results. Collective strength can be powerful, so finding partners makes a difference. Network to find those partners. Sometimes they may be found in the least likely groups. A pol-

icy is a tool for change, and nurses are very adept at working with change. This should help nurses develop political competence. "Successful advocacy depends on having the power, the will, the time, and the energy, along with the political skills needed to 'play the game' in the legislative area" (Abood, 2007, p. 3). How can nurses make an impact on healthcare policy?

GETTING INTO THE POLITICAL SYSTEM AND MAKING IT WORK FOR NURSING

Lobbying   **Lobbying** is a critical part of the U.S. political process, and nurses are involved in lobbying. A **lobbyist** is a person who represents a specific interest or interest group that tries to influence policy-making. The first amendment to the U.S. Constitution gives citizens the right to lobby—to assemble and to petition the government for redress of grievances. Lobbyists try to influence not only legislators, the decision makers, but also public opinion. Lobbyists often use coalitions and work with other interest groups to gain more support for a specific interest. Lobbyists particularly want to make contact with legislative staff. The legislative staff play a major role in getting data about an issue; formulating solutions that may become bills and, if passed, laws; and communicating with elected representatives, their bosses, to accept a particular approach or solution. Nurses who visit state and federal representatives typically meet with legislative staff. Professional organizations hire staff to be lobbyists at the state and federal levels. The ANA, the NLN, the AACN, and other nursing organizations have lobbyists in Washington, D.C. Box 5–1 identifies the federal government agencies monitored by the ANA.

COMMITTEES

At both the state and federal levels of government, the legislative branches are highly depen-

---

BOX 5–1 IMPORTANT FEDERAL GOVERNMENT DEPARTMENTS AND AGENCIES

- Agency for Healthcare Research and Quality (AHRQ), http://www.ahrq.gov/
- Center for Medicare and Medicaid Services (CMS), http://www.cms.hhs.gov/
- Centers for Disease Control and Prevention (CDC), http://www.cdc.gov/
- U.S. Consumer Product Safety Commission (CPSC), http://www.cpsc.gov/
- U.S. Department of Health and Human Services (DHHS), http://www.hhs.gov/
- U.S. Food and Drug Administration (FDA), http://www.fda.gov/
- National Institute for Occupational Safety and Health (NIOSH), http://www.cdc.gov/NIOSH/
- National Institutes of Health (NIH), http://www.nih.gov/
- Occupational Safety and Health Administration (OSHA), http://www.osha.gov/
- Department of Veterans Affairs (VA), http://www.va.gov/

---

dent on committees. Legislative work mainly occurs within committees. There are committees on both sides of the legislative body, the House and the Senate. Review the healthcare-related committees in the U.S. Congress identified in Exhibit 5–2.

Within the House and the Senate, committees have representatives from both major parties, Democrat and Republican. The party with the majority in the House and in the Senate

decides who will chair committees and who will serve on each committee. To effectively influence legislation, it is important to understand which committee will be involved in the legislation and who is on that committee. What are the chair's and the committee members' views on the issue? How can they be persuaded? Knowing this information can help in the development of a more effective strategy to influence the course of policy or to prevent it from progressing.

EXHIBIT 5–2 U.S. CONGRESSIONAL COMMITTEES WITH JURISDICTION OVER HEALTH MATTERS

U.S. House of Representatives
- House Appropriations Committee
- House Commerce Committee
- House Commerce Committee Subcommittee on Health and Environment
- House Ways and Means Committee
- House Ways and Means Committee Subcommittee on Health

U.S. Senate
- Senate Appropriations Committee
- Health, Education, Labor and Pensions Committee
- Health, Education, Labor and Pensions Committee Subcommittee on Public Health
- Senate Finance Committee
- Senate Finance Committee Subcommittee on Health Care

Political Action Committee Political Action Committees (PACs) are very important in the political process. A PAC is a private group, whose size can vary, that works to get someone elected or defeated. PACs represent a specific issue or group. The Federal Election Campaign Act covers PACs and defines a PAC as an organization that receives contributions or makes expenditures of $1,000 for the purpose of influencing an election. Other rules about PAC operations are also identified. Why would nurses need to know about PACs? Nursing has PACs, such as the ANA PAC. The ANA considers political action to be a core mission activity, and the PAC is critical to success on the Hill (Congress; Conant & Jackson, 2007). The PAC is a form of political advocacy that focuses on supporting candidates who support nursing issues. The PAC endorses candidates, makes minimal campaign donations, and campaigns for candidates; the decision to support a candidate is not based on the candidate's party, but rather on whether the candidate supports issues important to nursing. In the end, this empowers members: nurses. Its overall goal is to improve the healthcare system in the United States. Any nurse can join this PAC by making a contribution to it. Nurses work in the PAC to get the desired results.

Working to Get the Message Across: Grassroots Advocacy Many nurses work directly to communicate with legislators about specific issues of concern. How do they do this? One method is through written communication. In the past, this was primarily done through letter writing, but now it is easier, and preferred by legislators, to use e-mail. It is more efficient, and nurses can respond quickly to a call to communicate their views. This call may come through a nursing organization, through a personal recognition that something is going on that impacts health care and nursing, or through a colleague. In this written communication, it is important to state what the issue is, provide the bill number (if related to a pending bill), succinctly state one's position, and provide a brief rationale. The letter or e-mail should include one's full name, credentials, and contact information. To be more effective, the best contact is the nurse's elected representatives. Another method of communication is to call elected representatives' offices. Before the call, prepare a brief statement that should address the specific issue. A third method is to visit elected representatives' offices. This could be an elected official's local office, or his or her office in the state capitol or in Washington, D.C. As mentioned earlier, the nurse probably will meet with the legislative staff, preferably staff who are responsible for health issues. This is not a step down, because staff members really play a major role in the process. Make an appointment if possible and be on time. The meeting may be short or long. Be engaging, and let the staff or representative/senator know what you do as a nurse, where you work, and your nursing and healthcare concerns. Be prepared about the topic but also the activities of the representative—his or her legislation and interests. Give specifics and stories that support facts, and avoid generalities. Come prepared with facts and present them concisely. Give some useful information. Following up is important; send a thank-you note with a reminder of the discussion. All these examples demonstrate leadership by the nurses who participate in these efforts to advocate for health care. Exhibit 5–3 identifies some grassroots tips.

Nursing organizations are involved in policy development through lobbying, through members and officers serving as expert witnesses to government groups and agencies, and through publishing information about issues in both professional and lay literature. Nurses may also be interviewed by radio and television journalists.

Exhibit 5–3 Grassroots Tips

Letter or E-Mail Communication with Legislators or Staff
- Make sure your topic is clear.
- Do not assume anything.
- Get the facts.
- Be brief and concise.
- Find a local focus.
- Make it personal.
- Identify that you are a nurse and include your credentials. For example, "I am a nurse who works at Hospital Y in Middletown, Missouri."
- Include your contact information.

Phone Calls to Legislators or Staff
- Where can you find the telephone numbers?
  State: Call the state legislative body, get a directory, or visit your state government's Web site
  Federal: Call (202) 224-3121, or visit Web sites (http://www.house.gov, http://www.senate.gov)
- Prepare what you will say before you call; consider the comments made about written communication.
- Be sure to communicate up front what you are calling about.

Visiting Members of Congress or State Legislature
- You can visit when a representative is in the home district.
- You can visit the state capitol or Washington, D.C.
- You should make an appointment.
- Follow all guides mentioned for other methods of contact. Time will be short, so you need to be prepared.
- Do not be disappointed if you meet with a staff person. Staff are very important and give the representative the information to make decisions and in some cases are very involved in the decision making.
- Be ready to answer questions; prepare for this possibility.
- Be on time, but you may have to wait.
- Dress professionally.
- Enjoy yourself and be proud that you are a professional and an expert.

These activities place nurses directly in the policy-making process and also improve nurses' public image as experts and consumer advocates. The ANA recently began a new initiative related to policy (Patton, 2007). Throughout the year, the ANA holds several conferences that focus on a specific policy issue. The purposes of these conferences are to increase nurses' participation at the policy-making table, disseminate information, and educate nurses about policy-making. The first policy conference was held in June 2007, and its focus was Nursing Care in Life, Death, and Disaster (related to the Hurricane Katrina disaster). Rebecca Patton, president of the ANA, stated, "With your input, ANA will develop guidance dedicated to reconciling the professional, legal, and regulatory conflicts that can occur during such difficult times" (p. 22). To increase its ability to influence policy, the ANA invited representatives from the Centers for Disease Control and Prevention, Public Health Emergency Preparedness (agency of the DHHS), the U.S. Public Health Service, the National Bioterrorism Hospital Preparedness program, and the Agency for Healthcare Research and Quality, all of whom attended. This is an example of professional organization and power in numbers; the ANA demonstrated expertise and leadership, advocacy for the good of consumers, and collaboration and strategic thinking.

Nurses in Government Nurses are elected to government positions at the local, state, and federal levels. They also serve as staff in health-related government agencies. Nurses who serve in these government positions use their nursing expertise, and this provides many opportunities for nurses to be more be visible at all levels of the government—legislative, administrative, and judicial. However, there needs to be greater representation of nurses in these positions. There are opportunities for nurses to gain some experience in the area of government practice. There are fellowships, many of which are short term, at the federal and state levels that provide opportunities for nurses to learn more about politics and the legislative process and to interact with people who work in government. This is a great way to learn more about health policy. Graduate programs that focus on health policy provide formal academic experiences that can lead to a career in the health policy field. Running for office at any level requires political support, finances, and guidance from those experienced in the world of politics and campaigning. It does take time to build up support for a campaign. There are also positions for nurses at all levels of government. These positions provide great opportunities to use nursing expertise and to participate in health policy development and implementation.

Conclusion

Nurses can and do play a critical role in policy-making at the local, state, and federal levels of government. Through this role, they demonstrate leadership, expertise, advocacy, and the ability to collaborate with others to meet identified outcomes. Sometimes nurses are successful in getting the policy that they feel is needed for patients and for nursing, and sometimes they are not. The key to policy-making is to come back and try again, but first to learn from the previous experience to improve the effort.

CHAPTER HIGHLIGHTS

1. Healthcare policy directly impacts nurses and nursing.
2. Nurses participate in policy-making by sharing their expertise, serving on policy-making committees, working with consumers to get their needs known, and serving in elected offices.
3. A policy is a course of action that affects a large number of people and that is stimulated by a specific need to achieve certain outcomes.
4. Policies are associated with roles and standards; specific laws and related programs such as Medicare and Medicaid; delineation of reimbursement requirements for services; staffing levels; access to care; policies and procedures; and nursing education.
5. Critical healthcare policy issues relevant to nursing are the nursing shortage and staffing, the cost of health care, healthcare quality and safety, disparities in health care, consumer issues, commercialization of health care, reimbursement for nursing care, and immigration and the nursing workforce.
6. The policy-making process and the political process are connected, and it is important that nurses understand these processes in their advocacy efforts on behalf of consumers and for better health care.

7. Methods that nurses use when involved in the policy-making and political processes are lobbying, interacting with legislative committees, serving on PACs, participating in grassroots advocacy, working with elected officials who are nurses, and serving as elected officials themselves.

Linking to the Internet

- American Nurses Association (ANA): Health Care Policy
  http://www.nursingworld.org/MainMenu Categories/HealthcareandPolicyIssues.aspx
- American Nurses Association (ANA): Federal Government Affairs
  http://www.nursingworld.org/MainMenu Categories/ANAPoliticalPower/Federal.aspx
- National League for Nursing (NLN): Government Affairs
  http://www.nln.org/governmentaffairs/ index.htm
- Kaiser Foundation: Health Policy Facts
  http://facts.kff.org
- National Council of State Boards of Nursing (NCSBN): Government Relations & Policy
  https://www.ncsbn.org/government.htm
- Association of Women's Health, Obstetric and Neonatal Nurses (AWOHNN): Health Policy & Legislation
  http://www.awhonn.org/awhonn/content .do;jsessionid=428BB2815133ED9028C4 3C99945E3B41?name=05_HealthPolicyL egislation/05_HealthPolicyLegislation_ landing.htm
- National Association of Pediatric Nurse Practitioners (NAPNAP): Advocacy
  http://www.napnap.org/index.cfm?page=11
- American Association of Psychiatric Nurses (APNA): Government Affairs
  http://www.napnap.org/index.cfm?page=11
- Association of periOperative Registered Nurses (AORN): Public Policy
  http://www.aorn.org/PublicPolicy/

DISCUSSION QUESTIONS

1. Why is policy important to nursing?
2. Describe the relationship between the policy-making process and the political process.
3. Discuss the roles of nurses in the policy-making process.
4. Why is advocacy a critical part of policy-making?
5. Describe the political process.
6. Discuss the methods that nurses use to get involved in the policy-making process and the political process.

CRITICAL THINKING ACTIVITIES

1. Select one of the following topics and search the Internet to learn more about the issue. Why would this issue be of interest to nursing? Why would this be a healthcare policy issue? Has anything been done to initiate legislation on this issue? Teams of students can work on an issue and then share their work.
   a. Rural health care
   b. Health professions education
   c. Mental health parity
   d. Aging and long-term care
   e. Healthcare unions
   f. Home care
   g. Emergency room diversions
2. Would you feel comfortable lobbying for a nursing issue? Why or why not?
3. Visit http://rnaction.org/politicalpower/home.tcl and open the Political Action section of the American Nurses Association Web site (tab at the top of the screen).
   a. Click on Federal Legislation and review the current bills that ANA is focusing on. Select one bill and review information on that bill. Why is this bill important? What impact might it have on nursing and on health care? Do you think it will pass? Why or why not? What would you say to a legislative staff member to try to persuade staff to support the bill?
   b. Click on the Capital Update. Review the current issue. What are the current issues discussed? Explore one of them.
4. Visit http://www.nursingworld.org/MainMenuCategories/ANAPoliticalPower.aspx and open the Health Care Policy section of the ANA Web site (tab at top of the screen). The pull-down screen has several subtopics. Select one to review. What can you learn about that topic? What are your views on the topic?
5. Form a debate team that will address the following question: How would you support or not support universal health care in the United States? The team should base its viewpoint on facts and relevant resources. Present the debate in class or online. Viewers (students who are not on the debate team) should vote for the viewpoint that they think is most persuasive.
6. In 2006, Vermont initiated major changes in its state healthcare system. This is an example of a complex policy initiative. Review a fact sheet about this change (http://www.kff.org/uninsured/upload/7723.pdf). What is your opinion of this system? What is the comprehensive healthcare reform legislation? Describe the use of information technology in the program. How is chronic care management part of the funding? How is the program funded? What do you think are the pros and cons to this type of statewide program?
7. Visit the U.S. House of Representatives (http://www.house.gov) and U.S. Senate (http://www.senate.gov) Web sites and see if you can find which representatives and senators are RNs. Explore their Web sites and learn about the legislation that they have sponsored.

CASE STUDY

A nurse works in community health in a very large neighborhood of mostly African Americans and Hispanics. The socioeconomic level is low, with most people eligible for or covered by Medicaid and Medicare. The nurse is concerned about the level of care that community members' children receive. Clinic services are inadequate, and the clinics that are available are open during hours that are often difficult for working parents. The teens in the area are involved in a lot of drug activity and have little to do after school. The community has one urban high school, one middle school, and one elementary school. There are two small daycare centers for preschool run by the city. The nurse is motivated to tackle some of these problems, but she is not sure how to go about it.

Case Questions

1. Do these problems have health policy relevance? Why or why not?
2. What steps do you think the nurse should take in light of what you have learned about health policy in this chapter? Be specific regarding stakeholders, strategies, and political issues to consider.

WORDS OF WISDOM

Jennie Chin Hansen, MS, RN, FAAN; President, AARP; Senior Fellow, the Center for the Health Professions, University of California, San Francisco; and Part time faculty, San Francisco State University School of Nursing

Jennie Chin Hansen represents a nurse who recognizes the importance of health policy and the nurse's role in it. She was elected by the American Association of Retired Persons (AARP) Board to serve as AARP president for the 2008–2010 biennium. In addition, Ms. Hansen serves on the Governance Committee. She has previously chaired the AARP Foundation Board and served on the AARP Services Board.

She transitioned to teaching in 2005 after nearly 25 years as executive director of On Lok, Inc., a nonprofit family of organizations in San Francisco that provide integrated and comprehensive primary and long-term care and community-based services. On Lok was the prototype for the Program of All-Inclusive Care for the Elderly, which was signed into federal legislation in 1997, making this Medicare/Medicaid program available to all 50 states.

Ms. Hansen serves in various leadership roles, including as commissioner of the Medicare Payment Advisory Commission and board member of the National Academy of Social Insurance and of the Robert Wood Johnson Executive Nurse Fellows Program. She is also on the boards of Lumetra (California's Quality Improvement Organization) and the California Regional Health Information Organization. Ms. Hansen serves as a national juror for the Purpose Prize, sponsored by Civic Ventures. She is a past president of the American Society on Aging.

Among Ms. Hansen's awards are the 2005 CMS Administrator's Achievement Award, the 2002 Gerontological Society of America's Maxwell Pollack Award for Productive Living, and the 2000 Women's Healthcare Executive Woman of the Year of Northern California, and she was the 1997 "Women Who Could Be President" Honoree from the League of Women Voters of San Francisco. She is a fellow in the American Academy of Nursing, and she has received several alumni awards from the University of California, San Francisco, and Boston College, including an honorary doctorate from Boston College in 2008.

These are her Words of Wisdom:

> *We start our care in nursing focusing on a safe, evidence-based, and compassionate commitment to the patient and family. This is at the core of our professional practice. Over time, though, we learn through our experience how important critical systems thinking and cultural anthropology is for nurses to incorporate in order to assure we deliver on the goal of the best and most appropriate care for individual patients and society at large. We have an opportunity and obligation to contribute to the development, implementation, and evaluation of safe systems and cultures of caring and competence. We are fortunate to have the framing of issues and suggested tools that come from the rigorous work of the IOM studies. As the largest and most trusted health professional workforce in America, we have a wonderful chance to make a great and significant difference to health care in our country.*

Student Perspective
Evan Skinner, Senior, the University of Oklahoma College of Nursing

Globalization, advances in technology, and labor standards are representatives of a dynamic landscape in which we all live. The constant modification of our world forces humans to struggle to maintain balance. Nurses are not exempt from the shifting sands of change; we are subject to the turbulent uncertainties of life, and we must competently encounter each challenge and adapt. Therefore, it is incumbent upon nurses to adopt what the military refers to as "situational awareness." This means that one is to remain vigilant and be knowledgeable of current events. Of that which we must be observant, legislative actions take priority. It is vital that nurses become politically active in order to promote and preserve the integrity and legacy of the profession of nursing. Alterations in public policy have the potential for profound impact upon our scope of practice, opportunity for advancement, and work schedules. Awareness and activism within the political realm permit the informed nurse to protect the foundation of our profession against insult and promote its prosperity. Political activism, then, should not be considered merely an additional chore, but a duty.

References

Abood, S. (2007). Influencing healthcare in the legislative arena. *The Online Journal of Issues in Nursing, 12*(1), 3.

American Nurses Association. (2005). *ANA's Health Care Agenda-2005.* Silver Spring, MD: Author.

Block, L. (2008). Health policy: What it is and how it works. In C. Harrington & C. Estes (Eds.), *Health policy* (5th ed., pp. 4–14). Sudbury, MA: Jones and Bartlett.

Coffey, J. (2001). Universal health coverage. *American Journal of Nursing, 101*(2), 11.

Conant, R., & Jackson, C. (2007, March). Brief overview of ANA political action committee. *American Nurse Today,* p. 24.

Ferguson, S. (2001). An activist looks at nursing's role in health policy development. *Journal of Obstetric, Gynecologic, and Neonatal Nursing, 30,* 546–551.

Hart, S., & Jackson, N. (2000). Primer on policy: The legislative process at the federal level. In C. Harrington & C. Estes (Eds.), *Health policy* (5th ed., pp. 27–29). Sudbury, MA: Jones and Bartlett.

Institute of Medicine. (2002). *Unequal treatment: Confronting racial and ethnic disparities in health care.* Washington, DC: National Academies Press.

Institute of Medicine. (2004). *Health literacy: A prescription to end confusion.* Washington, DC: National Academies Press.

KaiserEDU.org. (2005). *Addressing the nursing shortage: Background brief*. Retrieved December 13, 2007, from http://www.kaiseredu.org/topics_im.asp?imID= 1&parentID=61&id=138

Kalisch, B. J., & Kalisch, P. (1982). *Politics of nursing*. Philadelphia: Lippincott.

Patton, R. (2007, March). From your ANA President: Taking a seat at ANA's policy-making table. *American Nurse Today*, p. 22.

Shi, L., & Singh, D. (1998). *Delivering health care in America*. Gaithersburg, MD: Aspen.

Sullivan, L., & Commission on Diversity in the Healthcare Workforce. (2004). *Missing persons: Minorities in the health professions. A report of the Sullivan Commission on diversity in the healthcare workforce*. Retrieved December 13, 2007, from http://www.aacn .nche.edu/Media/pdf/SullivanReport.pdf

Ethics and
Legal Issues

CHAPTER OBJECTIVES

At the conclusion of this chapter, the learner will be able to:

- Apply ethical principles.
- Describe ethical decision making.
- Discuss the importance of ethics to the nursing profession and its professional recognition.
- Summarize current ethical issues.

- Define major legal terms.
- Discuss the relevance of legal issues to nursing practice.
- Explain how malpractice relates to nursing practice.
- Discuss examples of ethical and legal issues.

CHAPTER OUTLINE

INTRODUCTION
ETHICS AND ETHICAL PRINCIPLES
Definitions
Ethical Principles
Ethical Decision Making
Professional Ethics and Nursing Practice
Current Ethical Issues
Organizational Ethics
LEGAL ISSUES: AN OVERVIEW
Critical Terminology
Malpractice: Why Should This Concern You?
CRITICAL ETHICAL AND LEGAL PATIENT-ORIENTED ISSUES

KEY TERMS

❏ Advance directives
❏ Breach of duty
❏ Confidentiality
❏ Do-not-resuscitate
❏ Ethical decision making
❏ Ethical principles
❏ Ethics
❏ Informed consent

❏ Legal issues
❏ Living will
❏ Malpractice
❏ Medical power of attorney
❏ Negligence
❏ Organizational ethics
❏ Power of attorney
❏ Professional ethics

Introduction

The content in this chapter addresses **ethics** and **legal issues**. in nursing. As a profession, nursing has ethical responsibilities. In the practice of nursing, legal issues arise that every nurse needs to understand, and he or she must take appropriate steps as required to address them. Ethics and legal issues involve professionalism, health policy, reimbursement issues, and the organizations that provide health care.

Ethics and Ethical Principles

Definitions

The first question that could be asked in this type of content is, What is ethics? It is easy to confuse ethics with morals. Morals refer to an individual's code of acceptable behavior, and they shape one's values according to cultural influences. Ethics refers to a standardized code or guide to behaviors. Morals are learned through growth and development, whereas ethics typically is learned through a more organized system, such as a standardized ethics code developed by a professional group. Ethics deals with the rightness and wrongness of behavior. Bioethics relates to decisions and behavior related to life and death issues. The latter sometimes come into conflict with a patient's morals, values, and ethics and a nurse's morals, values, and ethics. There may also be conflict between a nurse and an organization's approach to morals, values, and ethics.

Ethical Principles

Four **ethical principles** are used in nursing. These are highlighted in Figure 6–1.

Ethics is a difficult area, and these principles help guide nurses when confronted with ethical issues. Throughout this chapter, the term *patient* will be used, but in the case of a minor or a person who is under legal guardianship or **power of attorney**, *the patient* will refer to the family or guardian.

- *Autonomy* focuses on the patient's right to make decisions about matters that impact the patient. This means that if the patient wants to be involved in the treatment decisions, he or she makes the final decisions about treatment. To do this, patients need open information, and this ties in with **informed consent**. The nurse's role is to provide information or ensure that the patient is informed by others, such as the physician, and then support the patient's decision. Supporting the patient's decision is not always easy because the nurse may think that the patient is making the wrong decision. It is not the role of the nurse to argue with the patient, but rather to be the patient's advocate, respecting his or her choice. The nurse can discuss the decision and ensure that the patient recognizes the potential consequences of decisions.
- *Beneficence* relates to doing something good and caring for the patient; this is more than physical care, but also involves awareness of the patient's situation and needs. In the case of nurses, this also means doing no harm and safeguarding the patient, or *nonmaleficence*.
- *Justice* is about treating people fairly—for example, regarding which patients receive treatment and which might not. There are more concerns about justice in health care today because of problems with disparity (e.g., some people are not getting care when they need it). This is discussed more in Chapter 9.
- The fourth principle is *veracity*, or truth. For example, what information is the patient given during the informed consent process? Trust plays a major role in this principle. Veracity can be a difficult principle to apply because sometimes a family member may request that the patient not be fully informed. Some believe that if another principle is involved, it might be considered first. For example, if it is believed that the truth would cause more harm, does beneficence outweigh justice? In any ethical dilemma, it is important to remember that no two situations are the same.

Other principles have been suggested that are applicable to today's healthcare delivery system. These are advocacy, caring, stewardship (manage-

Figure 6–1 Ethical decision-making principles.

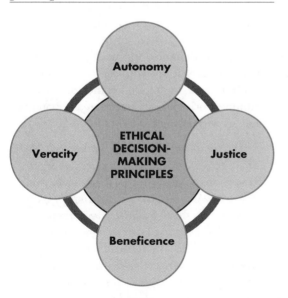

ment of finite resources), respect, honesty, and **confidentiality** (Koloroutis & Thorstenson, 1999).

Ethical Decision Making

Ethical decision making is about ethical dilemmas. An ethical dilemma occurs when a person is forced to choose between two or more alternatives, none of which is ideal. Typically, strong emotions are tied to the issue and alternative solutions. There is no way to say that one is better than the other. What are the roles and responsibilities of a nurse regarding an ethical dilemma and decision making? First, the nurse needs to be involved. If the issue does not concern the nurse, he or she should not step in. The next step is to get facts—assessment. What are the medical facts, including information about treatment? What are the psychosocial facts? What does the patient want? What values are involved, and what is the conflict? Getting this information requires talking to others: the patient, family and significant others, and other healthcare providers. A nurse does not make decisions for the patient, nor does the nurse make these decisions alone; he or she is part of a treatment team. Sometimes it is the nurse who thinks that the treatment team does not recognize that there is an ethical dilemma; in this case, the nurse identifies this to the team. After the assessment is concluded, the information is used to develop a plan to address the dilemma. This requires looking at the choices, goals, and who is involved. Options need to be prioritized. Key to all this is patient involvement if he or she is able and willing. The decision must be one that the patient can accept. During implementation, the nurse must be the patient's advocate even if the nurse does not agree with the patient's final decision.

Professional Ethics and Nursing Practice

Professional ethics are a part of any occupation, and in nursing, it is part of daily practice. Benner has described seven moral skills for nurses (2000, p. 7):

1. Relational skills in meeting the other in his or her particularity, drawing on life-manifestations of trust, mercy, and openness of speech
2. Perceptiveness, e.g., recognizing when a moral principle such as justice is at stake
3. Skilled know-how that allows for ethical comportment and action in particular encounters in a timely manner
4. Moral deliberation and communication skills that allow for justifications of and experiential learning about actions and decisions
5. An understanding of the goals or ends of nursing practice
6. Participation in a practice community that allows for character development to actualize and extend good nursing practice
7. The capacity to love ourselves and our neighbors, and the capacity to be loved

These views by Benner may be difficult to grasp or even may not be accepted by some. Understanding of, and experience with, practice are critical for a greater appreciation of these moral skills. Benner does include the nursing practice skills that one thinks of as "nursing"—communication, need for outcomes, and need for community orientation. But there are potential problems with Benner's view of ethical expertise.

One must question how meaningful, let alone, helpful, it is to conceptualize nursing as fundamentally moral work. Where is the purpose in reclassifying activities such as pain management, the shift to palliative care at the end-of-life, and family care as moral as opposed to clinical skills? When the capacity of the system to provide nurses to deliver care is seriously under threat, how helpful is it to cast nursing as essentially "good" work and to assign the better

Ethics and Ethical Principles 199

or more expert nurse to the higher moral ground?
(Nelson, 2006, p. 84)

It is not easy to find the right perspective of ethics in professional roles and in the care provided. Each nurse works to find this and how it meshes with his or her personal views. This is the potential dilemma between the nurse's view of ethical behavior and the patient's.

American Nurses Association Code of Ethics

Professional organizations such as the American Nurses Association (ANA) and many of the specialty groups set forth a "code" to follow along with interpretative statements to help a nurse understand the intent of the guiding principle. The ANA *Code of Ethics for Nurses with Interpretive Statements* (2001) is the primary source or guide for nurses when ethical issues are encountered. There have been several editions of the code to ensure that the content and expectations are current with practice and healthcare issues.

> *Individuals who become nurses are expected not only to adhere to the ideals and moral norms of the profession but also to embrace them as part of what it means to be a nurse. The ethical tradition of nursing is self-reflective, enduring, and distinctive. A code of ethics makes explicit the primary goals, values, and obligations of the profession. (American Nurses Association, 2001, p. 5)*

Obtaining a registered nurse (RN) license and entering the profession requires that nurses meet the professional roles and responsibilities. Ethics is a part of this. Self-reflection, or the ability to look at a variety of possibilities and consider pros and cons, is also important. This is part of critical thinking and is particularly important when there does not seem to be one "right" answer, which is frequently the case when an ethical dilemma is experienced. The ANA *Code of Ethics* is described in Exhibit 6–1.

Reporting Incompetent, Unethical, or Illegal Practices

Each nurse has a responsibility to report incompetent, unethical, or illegal practices to the nurse's state board of nursing (American Nurses Association, 1994a). However, others can also report nurses, such as employers, consumers, and family members. Each state's nurse practice act serves as the guide for the nurses in the state. It should be familiar to all licensed nurses. Nurse practice acts vary from state to state because each act is considered part of a state's law and is not administered at the federal level. State boards have specific processes and procedures that must be followed regarding complaints and how they are handled. The source of a complaint remains private. This confidentiality is to protect the person who reports the complaint and also to eliminate fear of reprisal that would limit reporting of complaints. What types of complaints might come to the board? Some of the common complaints involve using illicit drugs or alcohol while practicing, stealing drugs from the healthcare organization, committing a serious error that might demonstrate incompetence, and falsifying records. It is important to remember that a complaint or an initiative by the board to investigate a nurse does not mean that the nurse is "guilty." A legal process must be followed that gives the nurse rights to defend himself or herself. Any nurse who has a complaint or a chance of a complaint should consult an attorney, and not the attorney who represents the nurse's employer; the nurse should have a personal attorney. Dealing with disciplinary actions is a major responsibility of boards of nursing, and this issue takes time to address in board meetings. The media, legislators, and policy makers are interested in disciplinary actions that the boards take. A board of nursing has to find a balance between protecting the public and protecting the individual nurse's right to practice.

EXHIBIT 6–1 ANA CODE OF ETHICS FOR NURSES

1. The nurse, in all professional relationships, practices with compassion and respect for the inherent dignity, worth, and uniqueness of every individual, unrestricted by considerations of social or economic status, personal attributes, or the nature of health problems.
2. The nurse's primary commitment is to the patient, whether an individual, family, group, or community.
3. The nurse promotes, advocates for, and strives to protect the health, safety, and rights of the patient.
4. The nurse is responsible and accountable for individual nursing practice and determines the appropriate delegation of tasks consistent with the nurse's obligation to provide optimum patient care.
5. The nurse owes the same duties to self as to others, including the responsibility to preserve integrity and safety, to maintain competence, and to continue personal and professional growth.
6. The nurse participates in establishing, maintaining, and improving health care environments and conditions of employment conducive to the provision of quality health care and consistent with the values of the profession through individual and collective action.
7. The nurse participates in the advancement of the profession through contributions to practice, education, administration, and knowledge development.
8. The nurse collaborates with other health professionals and the public in promoting community, national, and international efforts to meet health needs.
9. The profession of nursing, as represented by associations and their members, is responsible for articulating nursing values, for maintaining the integrity of the profession and its practice, and for shaping social policy.

Source: From *Code of Ethics for Nurses with Interpretive Statements*, by the American Nurses Association, 2001, Silver Spring, MD: American Nurses Publishing. Copyright © 2001 by the American Nurses Association, Retrieved August 31, 2008, from http:/nursingworld.org/ethics/code/protected_nwcoe813.htm

---

An action that a board can take for some situations, such as drug abuse, involves the use of alternative programs. These programs are not treatment programs. However, they do offer nurses who meet specified criteria to maintain their licensure and practice if they enter a nondisciplinary program that provides identification and treatment support, if they agree to monitoring upon return to practice, and if they submit to regular drug testing. Alternative programs are not treatment programs; they are monitoring programs. The risk of public knowledge about a drug problem may compel a nurse to accept the alternative program. Compliance with treatment and aftercare recommendations is required. Return to practice or continuation of practice is not guaranteed, and the nurse is carefully monitored to ensure public safety.

Current Ethical Issues

RATIONING CARE: WHO CAN ACCESS CARE WHEN NEEDED

Does the United States ration care? Yes, it does, though not formally. Rationing is the systematic allocation of resources, typically limited resources. In this case, the limited resources are funds to pay for care. Some people receive care, and others do not; some insurers cover some care and not other care, depending on certain criteria. There are other forms of rationing. Organ transplantation is a form of rationing—both allocation of funds to perform transplants, and allocation of limited organs. Patients are put into a database to receive organ donations, and the order in which patients may receive a transplant is dependent on specified criteria. Oregon developed a rationing system for Medicaid by identifying the types of treatment that it would cover, but this approach has not been successful. This is an example of a situation in which the ethical principle of justice might be applied, because rationing, or allocation of resources, is related to equity. It appears to be more acceptable to say "resource allocation" than rationing, but in the end, resource allocating and rationing are similar.

HEALTHCARE FRAUD AND ABUSE

Healthcare fraud and abuse are not so uncommon. *Fraud* is a legal term that means a person deliberately deceived another for personal gain. Fraud has a nonlegal definition too, but the focus here is on fraud that involves breaking the law. How does this happen in health care? Usually it involves money and reimbursement. For example, a patient is charged for care that he or she did not receive or is charged more than the usual fee. In the 1990s, the federal government investigated and revealed major fraud and abuse in the third-party payer system. This fraud represented a loss of $100 billion (U.S. House of Representatives, 1994). Fraud involves physicians, phar-

macists, medical equipment companies, and healthcare organizations. Exhibit 6–2 identifies examples of Medicaid fraud schemes. Areas of health care that have experienced the most fraud are psychiatric care, home care, long-term care, and large corporate healthcare organizations.

ETHICS AND RESEARCH

Research is an area with complex concerns about ethics and legal issues. Research has a history of ethical problems. Some key examples of situations in which research participants were abused are the Nazi medical experiments in World War II; the Tuskegee Syphilis Study, in which African-American men with syphilis were not treated so that researchers could observe the course of the disease (1932–1972); and the Willowbrook Study, in which residents of an institution for mentally retarded children were deliberately infected with hepatitis (mid-1950s to the early 1970s). These major abuses led to reforms and the creation of legal guidelines in the late 1970s that must be followed. The Belmont Report (National Commission for the Protection of Human Subjects of Biomedical and Behavioral Research, 1978) identified the key concerns and

---

EXHIBIT 6–2 EXAMPLES OF MEDICAID FRAUD SCHEMES

- Billing for "phantom patients" who did not really receive services
- Billing for medical services or goods that were not provided
- Billing for old items as if they were new
- Billing for more hours than there are in a day
- Billing for tests that the patient did not need
- Paying a "kickback" in exchange for a referral for medical services or goods
- Charging Medicaid for personal expenses that have nothing to do with caring for a Medicaid client
- Overcharging for healthcare services or goods that were provided
- Concealing ownership in a related company
- Using false credentials
- Double-billing for healthcare services or goods that were provided

Source: Department of Health and Human Services, Centers for Medicare and Medicaid Services. Retrieved December 19, 2007, from http://www.cms.hhs.gov/FraudAbuseforConsumers/04_Rip_Offs_Schemes.asp#TopOfPage

the need for greater attention to ethical principles in conducting and reporting research.

Participation in research must include informed consent, and there are rules regarding how this consent must be obtained. Some of the information that must be revealed is:

- The nature and purpose of an intervention; potential risks, discomforts, and benefits to the patient; alternative treatments
- Compensation if injury occurs
- Compensation for participating
- A clear statement that the participant may withdraw at any time without any negative impact on the patient

The National Institutes of Health provides information about this consent. The Institutional Review Board (IRB) is an organization's committee or department that ensures that the process meets ethical and legal requirements in protecting participants in biomedical or behavioral research. Hospitals, universities, and other organizations that conduct research have IRBs. The following passage describes the differences between practice and research because they can be confused in healthcare delivery (U.S. Department of Health and Human Services, 1993):

> *While recognizing that the distinction between research and therapy is often blurred,* practice *is described as interventions that are designed solely to enhance the well-being of an individual patient or client and that have a reasonable expectation of success. The purpose of medical or behavioral practice is to provide diagnosis, preventive treatment, or therapy to particular individuals. The Commission distinguishes* research *as designating an activity designed to test a hypothesis, permit conclusions to be drawn, and thereby to develop or contribute to generalizable knowledge (expressed, for example, in theories, principles, and statements of relationships).*

> *Research is usually described in a formal protocol that sets forth an objective and a set of procedures designed to reach that objective. The Report recognizes that "experimental" procedures do not necessarily constitute research, and that research and practice may occur simultaneously. It suggests that the safety and effectiveness of such "experimental" procedures should be investigated early, and that institutional oversight mechanisms, such as medical practice committees, can ensure that this need is met by requiring that "major innovation{s} be incorporated into a formal research project."*

The risks that research subjects may be exposed to have been classified as physical, psychological, social, and economic (Levine, 1986, p. 42; U.S. Department of Health and Human Services, 1993).

- **Physical Harms.** Medical research often involves exposure to minor pain, discomfort, or injury from invasive medical procedures or harm from possible side effects of drugs. All of these should be considered "risks" for purposes of IRB review. Some of the adverse effects that result from medical procedures or drugs can be permanent, but most are transient. Procedures commonly used in medical research usually result in no more than minor discomfort (*e.g.*, temporary dizziness, the pain associated with venipuncture). Some medical research is designed only to measure more carefully the effects of therapeutic or diagnostic procedures applied in the course of caring for an illness. This research may not involve any significant risks beyond those presented by medically indicated interventions. Research designed to evaluate new drugs or procedures may present more than minimal risk, and sometimes can cause serious or disabling injuries.

- **Psychological Harms**. Participation in research may result in undesired changes in thought processes and emotion (*e.g.*, episodes of depression, confusion, or hallucination resulting from drugs, feelings of stress, guilt, and loss of self-esteem). These changes may be transitory, recurrent, or permanent. Most psychological risks are minimal or transitory, but IRBs should be aware that some research has the potential for causing serious psychological harm. Stress and feelings of guilt or embarrassment may occur simply from thinking or talking about one's own behavior or attitudes on sensitive topics such as drug use, sexual preferences, selfishness, and violence. These feelings may be aroused when the subject is being interviewed or filling out a questionnaire. Stress may also be induced when the researchers manipulate the subjects' environment—as when "emergencies" or fake "assaults" are staged to observe how passersby respond. More frequently, however, IRBs will confront the possibility of psychological harm when reviewing behavioral research that involves an element of deception, particularly if the deception includes false feedback to the subjects about their own performance. Invasion of privacy is a risk of a somewhat different character. In the research context, it usually involves either covert observation or "participant" observation of behavior that the subjects consider private. "The IRB must make two determinations: (1) Is the invasion of privacy involved acceptable in light of the subjects' reasonable expectations of privacy in the situation under study? and (2) Is the research question of sufficient importance to justify the intrusion? The IRB should also consider whether the research design could be modified so that the study can be conducted without invading the privacy of the subjects.

  Breach of confidentiality is sometimes confused with invasion of privacy, but it is really a different problem. Invasion of privacy concerns access to a person's body or behavior without consent; breach of confidentiality concerns safeguarding information that has been given voluntarily by one person to another. Some research requires the use of a sub-ject's hospital, school, or employment records. Access to such records for legitimate research purposes is generally acceptable, as long as the researcher protects the confidentiality of that information. The IRB must be aware, however, that a breach of confidentiality may result in psychological harm to individuals (in the form of embarrassment, guilt, stress, and so forth) or in social harm (see below).

- **Social and Economic Harms**. Some invasions of privacy and breaches of confidentiality may result in embarrassment within one's business or social group, loss of employment, or criminal prosecution. Areas of particular sensitivity are information regarding alcohol or drug abuse, mental illness, illegal activities, and sexual behavior. Some social and behavioral research may yield information about individuals that could "label" or "stigmatize" the subjects (e.g., as actual or potential delinquents or schizophrenics). Confidentiality safeguards must be strong in these instances. The fact that a person has participated in human immunodeficiency virus-related drug trials or has been hospitalized for treatment of mental illness could adversely affect present or future employment, eligibility for insurance, political campaigns, and standing in the community. A researcher's plans to contact these individuals for follow-up studies should be reviewed with care.

Participation in research may result in additional actual costs to individuals. Any anticipated costs to research participants should be described to prospective subjects during the consent process.

See Exhibit 6–3, which is an excerpt from the Belmont Report's introduction.

Why should nurses be concerned about these issues? First, nurses conduct research, and they must follow the same rules as anyone else who uses human subjects or even animal subjects. Second, nurses assist in data collection and work in areas where research is ongoing. In these situations, the nurse must continue to act as the patient advocate and ensure that the patient's rights are upheld. Knowledge and application of the ethical principles related to research need to

---

EXHIBIT 6–3 THE BELMONT REPORT

On September 30, 1978, the National Commission for the Protection of Human Subjects of Biomedical and Behavioral Research submitted its report entitled "The Belmont Report: Ethical Principles and Guidelines for the Protection of Human Subjects of Research." The Report, named after the Belmont Conference Center at the Smithsonian Institution where the discussions which resulted in its formulation were begun, sets forth the basic ethical principles underlying the acceptable conduct of research involving human subjects. Those principles, **respect for persons**, **beneficence**, and **justice**, are now accepted as the three quintessential requirements for the ethical conduct of research involving human subjects.

- *Respect for persons* involves recognition of the personal dignity and autonomy of individuals, and special protection of those persons with diminished autonomy.
- *Beneficence* entails an obligation to protect persons from harm by maximizing anticipated benefits and minimizing possible risks of harm.
- *Justice* requires that the benefits and burdens of research be distributed fairly.

The Report also describes how these principles apply to the conduct of research. Specifically, the principle of respect for persons underlies the need to obtain informed consent; the principle of *beneficence* underlies the need to engage in a risk/benefit analysis and to minimize risks; and the principle of *justice* requires that subjects be fairly selected. As was mandated by the congressional charge to the Commission, the Report also provides a distinction between "practice" and "research." The text of the *Belmont Report* is thus divided into two sections: (1) boundaries between practice and research; and (2) basic ethical principles. The full text of the *Belmont Report*, which describes each of the three principles and its application, is provided in the Guidebook in Appendix 6; a summary follows.

Boundaries Between Practice and Research

While recognizing that the distinction between research and therapy is often blurred, *practice* is described as "interventions that are designed solely to enhance the well-being of an individual patient or client and that have a reasonable expectation of success. The purpose of medical or behavioral practice is to provide diagnosis, preventive treatment, or therapy to particular individuals." The Commission distinguishes *research* as designat[ing] an activity designed to test an hypothesis, permit conclusions to be drawn, and thereby to develop or contribute to generalizable knowledge (expressed, for example, in theories, principles, and statements of relationships). Research is usually described in a formal protocol that sets forth an objective and a set of procedures designed to reach that objective. "The Report recognizes that "experimental" procedures do not necessarily constitute research, and that research and practice may occur simultaneously. It suggests that the safety and effectiveness of such "experimental" procedures should be investigated early, and that institutional oversight mechanisms, such as medical practice committees, can ensure that this need is met by requiring that "major innovation[s] be incorporated into a formal research project."

Applying the Ethical Principles

Respect for Persons. Required by the moral principle of respect for persons (*see* definition, above), **informed consent** contains three elements: information, comprehension, and voluntariness. First, subjects must be given sufficient information on which to decide whether or not to participate, including the research procedure(s), their purposes, risks and anticipated benefits, alternative procedures (where therapy is involved), and a statement offering the subject the opportunity to ask questions and to withdraw at any time from the research. Responding to the question of what constitutes adequate information, the Report suggests that a "reasonable volunteer" standard be used: "the extent and nature of information should be such that persons, knowing that the procedure is neither necessary for their care nor perhaps fully understood, can decide whether they wish to participate in the furthering of knowledge. Even when some direct benefit to them is anticipated, the subjects should understand clearly the range of risk and the voluntary nature of participation." Incomplete disclosure is justified only if it is clear that: (1) the goals of the research cannot be accomplished if full disclosure is made; (2) the undisclosed risks are minimal; and (3) when appropriate, subjects will be debriefed and provided the research results.

Second, subjects must be able to comprehend the information that is given to them. The presentation of information must be adapted to the subject's capacity to understand it; testing to ensure that subjects have understood may be warranted. Where persons with limited ability to comprehend are involved, they should be given the opportunity to choose whether or not to participate (to the extent they are able to do so), and their objections should not be overridden, unless the research entails providing them a therapy unavailable outside of the context of research. [*See* discussions on this issue in other sections of the Guidebook, including Chapter 6, "Special Classes of Subjects."] Each such class of persons should be considered on its own terms (*e.g.*, minors, persons with impaired mental capacities, the terminally ill, and the comatose). Respect for persons requires that the permission of third persons also be given in order to further protect them from harm.

Finally, consent to participate must be voluntarily given. The conditions under which an agreement to participate is made must be free from coercion and undue influence. IRBs should be especially sensitive to these factors when particularly vulnerable subjects are involved.

Beneficence. Closely related to the principle of beneficence (*see* definition, above), **risk/benefit assessments** "are concerned with the probabilities and magnitudes of possible harms and anticipated benefits." The Report breaks consideration of these issues down into defining the nature and scope of the risks and benefits, and systematically assessing the risks and benefits. All possible harms, not just physical or psychological pain or injury, should be considered. The principle of beneficence requires both protecting individual subjects against risk of harm and consideration of not only the benefits for the individual, but also the societal benefits that might be gained from the research.

In determining whether the balance of risks and benefits results in a favorable ratio, the decision should be based on thorough assessment of information with respect to all aspects of the research and systematic consideration of alternatives. The Report recommends close communication between the IRB and the investigator and IRB insistence upon precise answers to direct questions. The IRB should: (1) determine the "validity of the presuppositions of the research;" (2) distinguish the "nature, probability and magnitude of risk...with as much clarity as possible;" and (3) "determine whether the investigator's estimates of the probability of harm or benefits are reasonable, as judged by known facts or other available studies."

Five basic principles or rules apply when making the risk/benefit assessment: (1) "brutal or inhumane treatment of human subjects is never morally justified;" (2) risks should be minimized, including the avoidance of using

continues

EXHIBIT 6–3   (continued)

---

human subjects if at all possible; (3) IRBs must be scrupulous in insisting upon sufficient justification for research involving "significant risk of serious impairment" (e.g., direct benefit to the subject or "manifest voluntariness of the participation"); (4) the appropriateness of involving vulnerable populations must be demonstrated; and (5) the proposed informed consent process must thoroughly and completely disclose relevant risks and benefits.

Justice. The principle of justice mandates that the **selection of research subjects** must be the result of fair selection procedures and must also result in fair selection outcomes. The "justness" of subject selection relates both to the subject as an individual and to the subject as a member of social, racial, sexual, or ethnic groups.

   With respect to their status as individuals, subjects should not be selected either because they are favored by the researcher or because they are held in disdain (*e.g.*, involving "undesirable" persons in risky research). Further, "social justice" indicates an "order of preference in the selection of classes of subjects (*e.g.*, adults before children) and that some classes of potential subjects (*e.g.*, the institutionalized mentally infirm or prisoners) may be involved as research subjects, if at all, only on certain conditions."

   Investigators, institutions, or IRBs may consider principles of distributive justice relevant to determining the appropriateness of proposed methods of selecting research subjects that may result in unjust distributions of the burdens and benefits of research. Such considerations may be appropriate to avoid the injustice that "arises from social, racial, sexual, and cultural biases institutionalized in society."

   Subjects should not be selected simply because they are readily available in settings where research is conducted, or because they are "easy to manipulate as a result of their illness or socioeconomic condition." Care should be taken to avoid overburdening institutionalized persons who "are already burdened in many ways by their infirmities and environments." Nontherapeutic research that involves risk should use other, less burdened populations, unless the research "directly relate[s] to the specific conditions of the class involved."

Source: Institutional Review Board Guidebook, by Department of Health and Human Services. Retrieved December 23, 2007 from http://www.hhs.gov/ohrp/irb/irb_guidebook.htm

---

be part of practice when nurses are directly or indirectly involved in research. Exhibit 6–4 identifies key points of the *Code of Federal Regulations* related to research.

Organizational Ethics

In the past 10–20 years, there have been serious breaches of **organizational ethics**. A major stimulus to address this problem occurred in 1994, when it was recognized that the federal government lost 10% of the total healthcare expenditures because of fraud, which was equivalent to $100 billion (U.S. House of Representatives, 1994). Because of increasing corporate healthcare fraud and abuse of patients, the Centers for Medicare and Medicaid Services, through legislation, now requires any healthcare organization that is reimbursed through Medicare or Medicaid meet certain compliance conditions to better ensure organizational ethics. It is a rare that a hospital does not receive this type of reimbursement to cover care provided to Medicare or Medicaid enrollees, so this really does have an impact on the majority of hospitals. Organizations must identify a compliance officer who audits and monitors actions taken to detect, correct, and prevent fraud. Staff must be informed regarding how to report concerns related to ethical behavior and potential fraud, and provided education about these critical issues. Why has the federal government established these requirements? The government certainly does not want patients abused; in addition, the government is concerned about the

---

EXHIBIT 6–4 CODE OF FEDERAL REGULATIONS

1. Risks to subjects are minimized.
2. The risks to subjects are reasonable in relation to anticipated benefits.
3. The selection of subjects is equitable.
4. Informed consent must be sought from potential subjects or their legal guardians.
5. Informed consent must be properly documented.
6. When appropriate, research plans monitor data collection to ensure subject safety.
7. When appropriate, privacy of subjects and confidentiality of data are maintained.
8. Safeguards must be in place when subjects are vulnerable to coercion.

Source: From *Evidence-Based Practice for Nurses: Appraisal and Applications of Research*, by N.A. Schmidt and J.M. Brown, 2009, Sudbury, MA: Jones and Bartlett Publishers. Data adapted from National Cancer Institute (n.d.)

---

major loss of funds that have occurred because of fraud, such as paying for care that was not given, paying more than the typical rate, paying for patients who did not receive care, and so forth.

Whistle-blowing can be part of fraud and abuse situations. This action occurs when a person who works for an organization that is committing fraud and abuse reports these activities to legal authorities, sharing extensive information that would be difficult for the authorities to obtain on their own. Whistle-blowers are protected by a very old law, the False Claims Act, which was passed during the Civil War and amended in 1982 to further protect whistle-blowers. Whistle-blowers are protected from being sued and from loss of job for reporting the organization or staff within the organization. If the federal government pursues the case and recovers funds, the whistle-blower is given a portion of the funds. Anyone can be a whistle-blower, but he or she must have information that could not be obtained otherwise or information that was not public knowledge (such as that reported in a newspaper). This action is very difficult and complicated.

Legal Issues: An Overview

Legal issues are a part of each nurse's practice. Licensure itself is a legal issue that is imple-

mented through the legal system. The nurse practice act in each state is state law. Legal concerns are also directly related to practice. Following are some examples:

- When the nurse administers a narcotic medication, specific procedures must be followed to ensure that the medication is received only by the patient per physician order; the drug is "counted" to make sure the amounts are correct. If there are errors, it could mean that a criminal act occurred—someone took the drug with no right to do this.
- Restraining a patient without a physician's order can be assault and battery.
- Falsifying medical records can lead to legal consequences.
- Accessing an electronic medical record for a patient who is not in a specific nurse's care can be questioned.
- Inadequate supervision of patients that leads to falls or a suicide can have legal consequences.

Critical Terminology

The following content defines critical legal terms that a nurse may encounter.

- *Assault*—The threat or use of force on another that causes that person to feel reasonable apprehension about imminent harmful or offensive contact. An example is threatening to medicate a patient if he or she does not comply with treatment. This type of threat is not uncommon in behavioral or psychiatric care but should never be done.

- *Battery*—The actual intentional striking of someone, with intent to harm, or in a "rude and insolent manner" even if the injury is slight. An example of battery is conducting a procedure, such as starting an intravenous line, without asking the patient. If this is an emergency situation and the patient's life is at risk, or there is risk of serious damage and the patient is not able to provide consent, this would not be battery.

- *Civil law*—One of two prominent legal systems; the law of private rights.

- *Criminal law*—Those statutes that deal with crimes against the public and members of the public, with penalties and all the procedures connected with charging, trying, sentencing, and imprisoning defendants convicted of crimes.

- *Doctrine of res ipsa loquitur*—A doctrine of law that one is presumed to be negligent if he, she, or it had exclusive control of whatever caused the injury, even though there is no specific evidence of an act of **negligence**, and without negligence, the accident would not have happened.

- *Emancipation*—A child is a minor, and therefore under the control of his or her parent(s)/guardian(s), until he or she attains the age of majority (18 years), at which point he or she is an adult. In special circumstances, a minor can be freed from control by his or her guardian and given the rights of an adult before turning 18. In most states, the three circumstances under which a minor becomes emancipated are

(1) enlisting in the military (which requires parent/guardian consent), (2) marrying (requires parent/guardian consent), or (3) obtaining a court order from a judge (parent/guardian consent not required). A minor can also petition the court for this status if financial independence can be proven and the parents or guardian agree. An emancipated minor is legally able to do everything an adult can do, with the exception of actions that are specifically prohibited if one has not reached the age of 18 (such as buying tobacco). From a healthcare perspective, emancipated minors can sue and be sued in their own name, enter into contracts, and seek or decline medical care.

- *Expert witness*—A person with specific expertise and knowledge who can provide testimony to prove the standard of care. A nurse may serve as an expert witness for nursing care but not for medical care issues. Typically, the nurse is also a specialist in the specific area of care being addressed in the legal case. For example, for a case involving the death of a newborn in a neonatal intensive care unit, the expert witness would be a neonatal nurse.

- *False imprisonment*—When a person is confined against his or her will. This can happen in health care—for example, when a patient wants to leave the hospital and is retained (an exception is when a patient is legally committed for medical reasons); when a patient is threatened or his or her clothes are taken away to prevent him or her from leaving; or when restraints are used without written consent or a sufficient emergency reason.

- *Good Samaritan laws*—Laws that protect a healthcare professional from being sued as a result of providing emergency care outside a healthcare setting. The provider must provide the care in the same manner that an ordinary, reasonable, and prudent professional would in similar circumstances, including following practice standards. An example is a nurse stopping on the highway to assist an accident victim and following the expected standard for providing care to a person with a severe burn to maintain respiratory status under emergency conditions.

- *Malpractice*—An act or continuing conduct of a professional that does not meet the standard of professional competence and results in provable damages to his or her patient.
- *Negligence*—Failure to exercise the care toward others that a reasonable or prudent person would under the circumstances; an unintentional tort.
- *Proximate cause*—A cause that is legally sufficient to result in liability.
- *Respondent superior*—A principal (employer) responsible for the actions of his, her, or its agent (employee) in the "course of employment." This doctrine allows someone—for example, a patient—to sue the employee who is accused of making an error that resulted in harm. The patient also may sue the employer, the hospital, because the employer is responsible for supervising the staff member. For example, a nurse administers the wrong medication, and the patient experiences complications. The nurse can be sued for the action, and the hospital also can be sued for not providing the appropriate education regarding medications and medication administration, for not ensuring that the nurse received the education, and/or for not providing proper supervision. Typically, in legal actions such as these, multiple persons and organizations may be sued.
- *Standards of practice*—Minimum guidelines identified by the profession (local,

state, national) and healthcare organization policies and procedures. Expert opinion, literature, and research also may be used as standards. Standards are used in legal situations to assess negligence malpractice actions. (Standards were discussed in Chapter 1 and are discussed in more detail in Chapter 12 in relation to quality improvement.)

- *Statutory law*—The body of law derived from statutes rather than constitutions or judicial decisions.
- *Tort*—A civil wrong for which a remedy may be obtained in the form of damages. An example of tort that is most relevant to nurses and other healthcare providers is negligence, an unintentional tort.

Malpractice: Why Should This Concern You?

Negligence does occur in nursing. Examples include medication errors, failing to prevent falls, not adequately providing for patient access to a call light when he or she needs help, a lack of assessment of risk for falls, and not instituting appropriate interventions. Another example would be failure to communicate information that impacts care, which encompasses situations such as not documenting care provided or response to care; not contacting the physician with information that would inform him or her of the need for change in treatment; and failing to document lack of monitoring, changes in status, assessment of wound sites or skin status, or malfunctioning intravenous equipment. Negligence also includes inadequate patient teaching, inadequate monitoring and maintenance of medical equipment, lack of identification of an allergy or not following known information about allergies, failure to obtain informed consent, and failure to report another staff member to supervisory staff for negligence or problems with practice. All these examples can lead to malpractice suits.

Malpractice is an act or continuing conduct of a professional that does not meet the standard of professional competence and results in provable damages to his or her client or patient. Anyone can sue if an attorney can be found to support the suit; however, winning a lawsuit is not so easy. To be successful with a malpractice lawsuit, all of the following criteria have to be met.

1. The nurse (as person being sued) must have a duty to the patient or a patient–nurse professional relationship. The nurse must have provided care to the patient or been involved in his or her care.

2. The duty must have been breached. This is called negligence, or the failure to exercise the care toward others that a reasonable or prudent person would under the circumstances. How is this proved? Any of the following could be used: a nurse practice act, professional standards, healthcare organization policies and procedures, expert witnesses (RNs), accreditation and licensure standards, professional literature, and research.

3. The **breach of duty** must be the proximate (foreseeable) cause, or the cause that is legally sufficient to result in liability-harm to the patient. There must be evidence that the breach of duty (what the nurse is accused of having done or not done based on what a reasonable or prudent person would do given the circumstances, such as what other nurses would have done in a similar situation) led directly to the harm that the patient is claiming. There might be other causes of the harm that the patient experienced that have nothing do with the breach of duty.

4. Damages or injury to the patient must have occurred. What were the damages or injury? Are they temporary or permanent? What impact do they have on the patient's life? These questions and many more will be asked about the damages and injury. If the lawsuit is won, this information is also used to assist in determining the amount of damages that will be awarded, though the plaintiff (person suing) will identify an amount when the suit is brought.

Malpractice elements are illustrated in Figure 6–2.

The plaintiff's attorney must prove that each of these elements exists before the judge or the jury agrees that all elements are present and that the plaintiff should be awarded damages. The nurse's attorney will defend the nurse by proving that one or more elements do not exist. If just one element does not exist, malpractice cannot be proved.

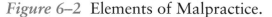

Figure 6–2 Elements of Malpractice.

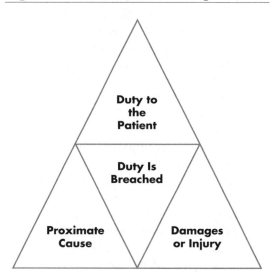

Malpractice lawsuits have become very expensive and have had an impact on practice and cost of care. This is particularly true for medical malpractice. The cases are very expensive to conduct, and awards are very high. This has led to "defensive medicine," in which physicians use excessive diagnostic testing and other procedures to protect them. This approach increases the costs of care and in some situations can increase patient risk if testing or procedures are invasive. Medical malpractice insurance is expensive, and this also increases medical costs because physicians and healthcare organizations that must carry this insurance will cover their costs through patient service charges.

There are pros and cons to nurses carrying professional liability insurance. These policies are not expensive for nurses, and the nurse needs to be clear about what the policy offers. A question could be asked as to why nurses would be sued when typically they do not have high levels of personal funds; however, they are sued. Often the nurse is included in a group that is being sued— for example, the physician(s); the hospital; and specific staff in the hospital (or other type of healthcare organization), to include the nurse(s); and others. When a nurse is sued, he or she should not rely on his or her employer's attorneys. The nurse needs an attorney who represents only the interests of the nurse. Professional liability insurance covers fees for this service. As soon as a nurse learns of a possible suit, he or she should contact an attorney for advice. If the nurse has liability insurance, he or she would contact the insurer for legal advice, and the insurer may assign an attorney to the case. In addition, the nurse should recognize that after the conclusion of a lawsuit in which the nurse and the nurse's employer were sued, the employer may then sue the nurse to reclaim damages. Nurses must make informed decisions about whether they would rather have an institution's attorney defend them or one that is covered under their own policy. In some instances,

if the nurse has a personal attorney/malpractice policy, the institutional legal team will not assist the nurse. There are also differences in the types of malpractice insurance that can be obtained. Two of the common types are (1) *claims-made* coverage, which covers only those incidences that occur and that are reported during the policy's effective period, and (2) *occurrence* coverage, which provides protection for an incident that took place while the policy was in effect even if the claim was not filed until after the policy terminated. When accepting a job, the nurse must explore the various pros and cons of carrying personal professional malpractice/liability insurance. Where does this leave students? Students are responsible for their own actions and can be liable. Students are not practicing under the license of their faculty (Guido, 2001). Because of this, students must never accept assignments or do procedures for which they are not prepared. It is also critical that students discuss these situations with faculty rather than taking them on without guidance.

Critical Ethical and Legal Patient-Oriented Issues

Confidentiality and Informed Consent

Confidentiality is an issue that is relevant to practice every day. Nurses have the responsibility to keep patient information confidential except as is required to communicate in the care process and with team members. It is important to remember that patient information should not be discussed in public areas (e.g., elevators, cafeteria, hallways) or any place where the information may be overheard by persons who have no right to hear the information. Nurses will encounter patients who are part of the nurse's personal life; however, the nurse must remember that what is known about the patient is private. Nurses who work in the community and make phone calls to and about patients using mobile phones in public places can easily forget that their conversations can be overheard. The Health Insurance Portability and Accountability Act (HIPAA, 1996) has had a major impact on information technology and patient information. Nurses are required to follow this law to protect patient privacy. Patients are informed about HIPAA when they enter a hospital or other type of healthcare facility for care.

Another legal concern related to confidentiality is consent. Consent occurs when the patient agrees to treatment, and it may be given orally or written. Whenever possible, consent should be informed consent. The patient's physician or other independent healthcare practitioner is required by law to explain or disclose information about the medical problem and treatment or procedure so that the patient can have informed choice. The patient has the right to refuse. Lack of informed consent puts the practitioner at risk for negligence. How does this apply to nurses? A nurse practitioner (NP) does have to get informed consent for treatment and procedures. The nurse who is not an NP does not have to get informed consent for every nursing intervention. The nurse would not be the staff member to obtain patient consent for treatment or procedures. In some cases, the nurse may ask a patient to sign a written consent form, but in doing so, it is assumed that the patient's physician has explained the information to the patient. If the patient indicates that this has not occurred, the nurse must talk with the physician and cannot have the patient sign the form until the patient and the physician have discussed the specific treatment or procedure. If a nurse is directly involved in getting the informed consent, he or she is at risk for negligence. A second type of consent is consent implied by law. This consent is applicable only in emergency situations, when a patient may not be able to give informed consent. Healthcare providers can provide care if the patient's life is at risk or if major damage or injury to the patient is likely. In this case, the assumption is that the patient would most likely give consent if he or she could, based on what a reasonable person would do. Nurses who work in the emergency department encounter this type of consent situation.

Advance Directives, Living Wills, Medical Power of Attorney, and Do-Not-Resuscitate

Advance directives are now part of the healthcare system. This is a legal document that allows a person to describe his or her medical care preferences. Often these documents describe the person's wishes related to his or her end-of-life needs ahead of time. This is called a **living will**. Patients have the right to develop this plan, and healthcare providers must follow it. Interventions that are typically covered are (1) use of life-sustaining equipment, such as a ventilator, respirator, or dialysis, (2) artificial hydration and nutrition (tube feeding), (3) "do-not-resuscitate" (DNR) or "allow a natural death" (AND) orders, (4) withholding of food and fluids, (5), palliative care, and (6) organ or tissue donation. The DNR, or the AND directive is either a form of advance directive or may be part of an extensive advance directive. This order means that there should be no resuscitation if the patient's condition indicates need for resuscitation. A physician may write a DNR/AND order without an advance directive, but the physician must follow hospital policy and procedures. It is highly advisable that this be discussed with the patient, if he or she is able to comprehend, and with family. The nurse may be present for this discussion but would not make this type of decision. If there are concerns about how it is handled, the nurse should consult with his or her supervisor, and if the organization has an ethics committee, the nurse may consult with the committee. End-of-life issues are never simple.

A **medical power of attorney** (POA) may be designated by the individual in the advance directives. Another name for this is durable power of attorney for health care, or a healthcare agent or proxy. This person is given the right by the individual to speak for the person if he or she cannot do so in matters related to health care. If a person does not designate a medical POA and the person is married, the spouse can make the decisions. If there is no spouse, the decision would be made by adult children or parents. A person should speak with the person who will be his or her medical POA about preferred types of care and how aggressive that care should be. The proxy or agent is not forced to follow instructions if they are not written in a legal document, so the person should trust that the proxy or agent will follow the guide discussed.

> *The decision not to receive "aggressive medical treatment" is not the same as withholding all medical care. A patient can still receive antibiotics, nutrition, pain medication, radiation therapy, and other interventions when the goal of treatment becomes comfort rather than cure. This is called palliative care, and its primary focus is helping the patient remain as comfortable as possible. Patients can change their minds and ask to resume more aggressive treatment. If the type of treatment a patient would like to receive changes, however, it is important to be aware that such a decision may raise insurance issues that will need to be explored with the patient's healthcare plan. Any changes in the type of treatment a patient wants to receive should be reflected in the patient's living will. (National Cancer Institute, 2000)*

Organ Transplantation

Organ transplantation is a form of resource allocation. Specific criteria are developed for each type of organ donation, and potential recipients are categorized according to the criteria to determine who might receive a donation and in what order.

Organ transplantation registries are a critical component of the process. However, it is not always so clear as to who should get a transplant. Many factors are considered—such as age, other illnesses, what the person might be able to contribute, whether the person is single or married, whether the person has children, comorbidities (other illnesses) such as substance abuse, and his or her ability to comply with follow-up treatment—and some of these complicate the decision-making process. Transplantations are expensive and may not be covered, or only partially covered, by health insurance. The patient will need lifetime specialized care, which is also costly. The other aspect of transplantation is organ donation, which must occur first. Some people designate their willingness to be organ donors while they are healthy—for example, on their driver's license. However, when the time comes to actually implement the request, family members may be reluctant. And then there are the many patients who have not identified themselves as organ donors when healthy, and then something happens that makes them eligible to be organ donors. This situation is even more complex, ethically and procedurally. Healthcare providers do ask for organ donations, and hospitals have policies and procedures that describe what needs to be done. It is still difficult to approach a family member, say that a loved one is no longer able to sustain himself or herself, and ask for an organ donation at the same time. With organ donations and transplants, time is a critical element to maintain organ viability. Nurses do not ask for the donation but may assist the physician in this most difficult discussion. Later, family members or the patient (if responsive) may want to discuss it further with the nurse.

Assisted Suicide

Assisted suicide is a complex ethical and legal issue, but the nurse's role is very clear: The nurse cannot participate in helping a person end his or her life. Only one state has a law that protects healthcare providers who participate in this process: Oregon passed a law in 1997, the Death with Dignity Act, which allows terminally ill citizens of Oregon to end their lives through voluntary self-administration of lethal medications prescribed by a physician for this purpose. The law describes who can be involved and the procedure or steps that must be taken. Two physicians must be involved in the decision. Countries other than the United States allow assisted suicides. "The American Nurses Association (ANA) believes that the nurse should not participate in assisted sui-cide. Such an act is in violation of the *Code of Ethics for Nurses with Interpretive Statements* [American Nurses Association, 1994b] and the ethical traditions of the profession. Nurses, individually and collectively, have an obligation to provide comprehensive and compassionate end-of-life care which includes the promotion of comfort and the relief of pain, and at times, foregoing life-sustaining treatments" (American Nurses Association, 1994c).

Conclusion

This chapter presented introductory information about the ethical and legal issues in nursing. Nurses deal daily with ethical concerns about their patients and encounter numerous legal issues that could lead to potential legal concerns. A professional cannot avoid either ethics or legal issues in his or her practice. A nurse cares for patients, families, and communities, and in doing so must consider how the care impacts the feelings and rights of others. From the time a nurse receives licensure, he or she operates under a legal system through the Nurse Practice Act and other laws and regulations.

CHAPTER HIGHLIGHTS

1. Ethics is concerned with a code of behaviors, whereas bioethics relates to life and death decisions.

2. Ethical dilemmas arise when there is conflict between a nurse's, profession's, organization's, or patient's "code" for decision making.

3. Principles of ethical behavior fall into four areas: autonomy, beneficence, justice, and veracity.

4. Benner (2000) outlined moral skills as a part of a nurse's toolkit to guide ethical behavior.

5. A professional code of ethics guides disciplines and is generally set at the national level.

6. State boards of nursing outline the expectations of nurses within their jurisdiction.

7. Reporting unethical, immoral, and unsafe actions is part of a nurse's ethical responsibility to protect the public from harm.

8. Some of the ethical issues in today's healthcare delivery involve scarcity of resources and resource allocation, or rationing of services.

9. Healthcare fraud and abuse involve deliberate deceptive activities to garner funds.

10. Research activities require stringent considerations of ethical principles, such as protection of the public from physical, psychological, social, and economic harm, and informed consent for the research protocol offered in language that is understandable to the research subject.

11. An emancipated minor is one who is afforded all the rights of an adult unless expressly prohibited by state or federal law.

12. Organizational ethics refers to an institution's ethical expectations of itself as an organization and its employees, and the patient's rights.

13. Malpractice and negligence charges can be filed against a nurse. The nurse must understand both of these concepts.

14. A nurse must consider the pros and cons of, and the differences in, institutional and personal professional liability insurance coverage.

Linking to the Internet

- Department of Health and Human Services Office for Human Research Protections http://www.hhs.gov/ohrp/irb/irb_guidebook.htm
- U.S. National Institutes of Health, National Cancer Institute: Introduction to Clinical Trials http://www.cancer.gov/clinicaltrials/learning
- American Association of Legal Nurse Consultants http://www.aalnc.org/
- American Nurses Association: Ethics and Standards http://www.nursingworld.org/MainMenu Categories/ThePracticeofProfessional Nursing/EthicsStandards.aspx

---

DISCUSSION QUESTIONS

1. Describe malpractice and how it applies to nursing care.
2. What is the Institutional Review Board?
3. Explain the "harms" that the Institutional Review Boards are concerned with in research.
4. How does ethical decision making apply to nursing students?
5. Explain how the profession of nursing incorporates ethics into practice and the profession.
6. Discuss one example of an ethical issue and how the ethical principles apply to this issue.

CRITICAL THINKING ACTIVITIES

1. Compare and contrast the description of the ethical principles found in the Belmont Report with ethical principles applied to practice.
2. Visit your state board of nursing Web site and find information about making complaints to the board. Review the information. What do you think about it?
3. Visit https://www.ncsbn.org/912.htm, the National Council of State Boards of Nursing, and select one of the topics under Discipline. Summarize the topic and discuss why it is relevant to you now as a student, and why it would be relevant to you as a nurse.
4. Select one of the following topics: confidentiality and informed consent; advance directives; living wills; DNR; or organ donation. Explain what it is in language that consumers could understand. What makes the issue you selected an ethical and legal issue?

CASE STUDY

A 5-day-old premature baby was viewed to require a blood transfusion because of increasing anemia. The parents were Jehovah's witnesses and did not wish to have blood or blood products given to the baby. A court order had been obtained the day before with the parents' knowledge, and blood had been given. However, the physician on call this particular night did not want to obtain the court's consent because it had been granted before. The blood was ordered, and the nurse was asked to hang the blood. The nurse refused for ethical and legal reasons.

Case Questions

1. What would be the ethical and legal reasons that the nurse would refuse to follow the physician's orders?
2. What should the nurse do (i.e., steps the nurse should take)?
3. How do you think the nurse should respond to the parents?

WORDS OF WISDOM

Pamela Holtzclaw Williams JD, MS, RN University of Washington School of Nursing 2006 Biobehavioral Nursing Research Fellow

A competent nurse applies ethical values in all nursing practices; the need for application does not simply kick in only when there are controversies, conflicts, or disagreements regarding what is right or wrong. Ethical values are learned norms of professional behavior applicable in all nursing roles and activities. These values must be cultured and prioritized, of course, in classwork, but especially in applied reality settings such as student clinicals. After formal education, graduation, and immersion in the clinical setting, the new nurse benefits from reinforcement of these values through continuing education formats. Employers and nursing professional organizations should strive to provide ethics mentorship for nurses as a worthwhile goal.

References

American Nurses Association. (1994a). *Guidelines on reporting incompetent, unethical or illegal practice.* Silver Spring, MD: Author.

American Nurses Association. (1994b). *Code for nurses with interpretive statements.* Silver Spring, MD: Author.

American Nurses Association. (1994c). Position statement: Assisted suicide. Silver Spring, MD: Author.

American Nurses Association. (2001). *Code for nurses with interpretive statements.* Silver Spring, MD: Author.

Benner, P. (2000). The roles of embodiment, emotion, and lifeworld for rationality and agency in nursing practice. *Nursing Philosophy*, 1(1), 5–19.

Guido, G. (2001). *Legal and ethical issues in nursing.* Upper Saddle River, NJ: Prentice Hall.

Health Care Portability and Accountability Act of 1996 (HIPAA), Pub. L. No. 104-191, 110 Stat. 1998 (1996).

Koloroutis, M., & Thorstenson, T. (1999). An ethics framework for organizational change. *Nursing Administrative Quarterly*, 23(2), 9–18.

Levine, R. (1986). *Ethics and regulation of clinical research* (2nd ed.). Baltimore: Urban and Schwarzenberg.

National Cancer Institute. (2000). *Fact sheet: Advance directives.* Retrieved December 18, 2007, from http://www.cancer.gov/cancertopics/factsheet/support/advance-directives

National Commission for the Protection of Human Subjects of Biomedical and Behavioral Research.

(1978). *The Belmont Report: Ethical principles and guidelines for the protection of human subjects of research.* Washington, DC: Author.

Nelson, S. (2006) Ethical expertise and the problem of the good nurse. In S. Nelson & S. Gordon (Eds.), *The complexities of care* (pp. 69–87). Ithaca, NY: Cornell University Press.

U.S. Department of Health and Human Services. (1993). *Protecting human research subjects: Institutional Review Board guidebook.* Retrieved December 23, 2007, from http://www.hhs.gov/ohrp/irb/irb_guidebook.htm

U.S. House of Representatives. (1994, July 19.) *Deceit that sickens America: Healthcare fraud and its innocent victims. Hearings before the Subcommittee on Crime and Criminal Justice of the Committee on the Judiciary House of Representatives, one hundred and third Congress, second session.* Washington, DC: U.S. Government Printing Office.

Chapter 7

Health Promotion, Disease Prevention, and Illness: A Continuum of Care

CHAPTER OUTLINE

KEY TERMS

- Acute care
- Case management
- Continuum of care
- Collaboration
- Coordination
- Coping
- Extended care
- Health
- Health prevention
- Health promotion
- *Healthy People 2010*

- Home care
- Hospice
- Illness
- Long-term care
- Occupational health care
- Palliative care
- Rehabilitation
- Resilience
- Stress
- Stress management

Introduction

This chapter focuses on an introduction to the **continuum of care** and how care is delivered in a variety of settings to different types of patients. Nursing programs provide clinical experience for students in many of the settings and situations discussed in this chapter. Where do patients receive care? Who are the patients? How are **health** and **illness** viewed by patients and by nurses, and what impact does this view have on healthcare delivery? Nurses need an understanding of these critical issues.

Continuum of Care: An Overview

The continuum of care is an important concept in nursing, though it is not always directly mentioned. This section of the chapter discusses the concepts of the continuum of care and continuity of care, and their implications for nursing care and to health care in general.

Description: Continuum of Care and Continuity of Care

Continuum of Care

The Joint Commission (2004) defined the continuum of care as "matching an individual's ongoing needs with the appropriate level and type of medical, psychological, health, or social care or service within an organization or across multiple organizations" (p. 317). The goal of the continuum is to decrease fragmented care and costs. The continuum includes **health promotion**, disease and illness prevention, ambulatory care, **acute care**, tertiary care, home health care, **long-term care**, and **hospice** and **palliative care**. In the current healthcare delivery system, patients receive care in a variety of settings from a variety of healthcare providers, and they move back and forth along the continuum. The continuum is a view of health care that describes a range of services and care settings that a patient might receive at different stages of health and illness.

Continuity of Care

"Continuity of care is the degree to which a series of discrete events is experienced as coherent and connected and consistent with the patient's medical needs and personal context" (Haggerty, Reid, Freeman, Starfield, Adair, & McKendry, 2003, p. 1219). This definition was developed after a multidisciplinary review of continuity of care literature to determine how different healthcare professionals viewed the concept. It was also noted that continuity of care is different from other views of care because it focuses on care over time and on individual patients. The review also identified three types of continuity of care. Each is emphasized at different times and is dependent on the care setting.

1. *Informational continuity*—Information is very important in health care, across the continuum of care and with continuity of care. This type of continuity focuses on information that is needed to link care from one provider and setting to another. This information includes medical information and the patient's preferences, values, and context.

2. *Management continuity*—When patients have complex and chronic problems, management of several providers becomes critical to ensure that all providers are aware of what each is doing and are working toward the same outcomes. This requires sharing information and plans and being flexible to ensure quality, safe care. A common problem that occurs in these situations is that one provider does not know what the other provider has prescribed.

Often a home health nurse discovers this when he or she reviews all the medications a patient is taking that were prescribed by different physicians. Serious medication errors can result from this problem.

3. *Relational continuity*—This type of continuity concerns the needs of patients to build relationships with providers, particularly a primary care provider. The primary care provider often serves as the entry point into the healthcare system and should coordinate the patient's overall care and make referrals to specialists when necessary. This was the goal of the primary care provider position when it was designed by managed care, but it has not been all that successful for all patients. This type of continuity emphasizes the need for providers to be familiar with the patient and the patient's history so that when he or she becomes ill, there is someone who has a relationship with the patient and who has past medical information.

Nurses are very involved in continuity of care because of their emphasis on the need to transfer and coordinate care over time and their focus on consistency of care. Typically, this is done through discharge planning.

> *Staff nurses feel responsible for their patients to get well, recover, or return to baseline prior to hospital discharge; yet in the new reality, patients' recovery may involve several settings across the continuum of care. Staff nurses must create fluid nursing environments and provide the appropriate nursing activities at the right time along this continuum, even if it requires discarding traditional care regimens they believe are fundamental.* (Dingel-Stewart & LaCosta, 2004, p. 214)

Access to Care

Access to care is, of course, the first step in receiving care, and it is not a simple process for many people; for some, there are major barriers. One typically thinks of access as the ability to physically get somewhere, but access to care involves many factors:

- The ability to pay for care or to have care paid for
- Transportation to get to care
- Hours of operation at the clinical site
- Waiting time to get an appointment, and long waits at the time of appointment to see a physician or another healthcare provider
- The ability to get an appointment
- Availability of type of healthcare provider needed
- Ability of the patient and provider to communicate and make use of accommodations for language, hearing, and sight
- Timeliness of laboratory tests
- Handicap provisions at the healthcare site
- Childcare provisions to go to the appointment
- Cultural barriers
- Inadequate information or lack of information
- Lack of provider time (rushed)
- Preexisting conditions that do not allow for reimbursement
- Insurer not covering care
- Provider not accepting patient's insurance coverage

With this many factors involved, access is a complex issue. It has a major impact on the continuum of care. Can the patient get the care that is needed when it is needed? When patients experience barriers to access, they may neglect routine care and put off getting care when it is needed. These patients may then need more serious care and use the safety net, which are services that cover patients who cannot pay for care or who have other access barrier problems. Some examples are free clinics, academic medical centers, and emergency rooms. This type of care may (or may not) meet the patient's immediate need, but it does not support an effective continuum of care, and continuity of care is often neglected. These patients get lost in the system, and the outcomes are not positive. ***Healthy People 2010*** includes a goal (Goal 2) that focuses on this concern (U.S. Department of Health and Human Services, 2000).

Goal 2: Eliminate health disparitites

Objectives Related to Access to Care (or Goal 2) are:

1-1   Increase the proportion of persons with health insurance.

1-4.a Increase the proportion of persons who have a specific source of ongoing care

One approach to improving access to healthcare services is to offer comprehensive and wraparound services. Comprehensive services are best described as "one-stop shopping," in that the patient can go to one place and receive multiple services. These services are typically offered in convenient locations such as neighborhoods, schools, or work sites. Health promotion and illness prevention can also be built in to these services. Wraparound services can be combined with comprehensive services when the healthcare sites also offer social and economic services, recognizing that social and economic problems have a major impact on a person's health and access to services needed. These wraparound services might include access to a social worker who can help with getting food and housing, with job issues, and with reimbursement for health care.

Individual, Family, and Community Health

The usual assumption is to consider the patient to be an individual, and most patients are individuals. However, there are other views of who

the "patient" is. The family, the community, and specific populations are viewed as "patients."

A family is defined as "two or more individuals who depend on one another for emotional, physical, and/or financial support. Members of a family are self-defined" (Kaakinen, Hanson, & Birenbaum, 2006, p. 322). Functional families are considered healthy families in which there is a state of bio/psycho/socio/cultural/spiritual well-being. A healthy family provides autonomy and is responsive to individual members within the family. Dysfunctional families have poor communication and relationships with one another and do not provide support to members. Nurses work with families in many ways along the continuum of care. The family itself may be the "patient," or the nurse may be involved with a family because of one family member's illness.

Family members may also be caregivers. A caregiver is someone who provides care to another. This is a nonprofessional healthcare provider. Serving as a caregiver long-term for a family member can lead to psychological, physical, social, and financial problems for the caregiver. The majority of caregivers are women; men are more likely to be cared for by their wives than vice versa because men have a shorter life expectancy (Schumacher, Beck, & Marren, 2006). This is something that the nurse needs to assess periodically to ensure that the caregiver, and thus the family, receives the support needed. Primary caregivers provide the majority of daily aspects of care, and secondary caregivers help with intermittent activities (shopping, transportation, home repairs, getting bills paid, emergency support, and so on). Both types of caregiving can put a strain on the caregiver, but primary caregivers are at greater risk.

The community can also be viewed as the patient or client. A community is defined as "people and the relationships that emerge among them as they develop and use in common some agencies and institutions and share a physical environment" (Williams, 2006, p. 3). Nursing offers services in communities as part of community health. Nurses may focus on an entire community, or a population that lives in the community. For the community, a nurse may be involved in managing clinics that are located in the community or in developing a disaster plan for the community. The nurse may focus on a population, which is "a collection of people who share one or more personal or environmental characteristics" (Williams, p. 4). Examples of populations within a community are children, the elderly, those with a chronic illness, and the homeless. A nurse might work in school health, assess needs of the elderly in the home, develop programs to screen for diabetes in people in the community who might be at risk, or manage a clinic for the homeless. There are many ways that a nurse might work with different populations within a community.

Across the Life Span

Patients may enter the healthcare system for a variety of needs and services, and they may enter at any point in the life span. This span includes:

- Conception to birth
- Infancy
- Childhood
- Adolescence
- Young adulthood
- Adulthood
- Maturity/older adulthood
- Death

Each of these periods of the life span includes specific health concerns and needs, as well as potential disease and illness risks. In addition, social and psychological risks impact health and wellness. These include situations such as the death of a loved one, change in or loss of a job, beginning school, moving, marriage, birth of a child, divorce, the need to care for a family member who is ill, and other stressful situations. The federal government collects data about health and illness across the life span. Table 7–1 shows data about the leading causes of death. The critical thinking activities include one centered on health status.

Healthy People

Healthy People 2010 (U.S. Department of Health and Human Services, 2000) is a national prevention initiative that focuses on improving the health of Americans by providing a comprehensive set of disease prevention and health promotion goals and objectives with target dates. These goals and objectives are used by the U.S. Department of Health and Human Services and other health agencies (federal, state, and local) to develop programs that promote health and the prevention of disease and illness and that are used to evaluate outcomes. The ultimate measure of success of this health improvement initiative is the health status of the target population. There have been three editions of *Healthy People* (1979, 1990, and 2000). The Department of Health and Human Services is approaching the end of the 2000 edition, which ends in 2010. What are the major goals that should be reached by 2010? *Healthy People 2010* identifies two broad goals, along with 467 objectives in 28 focus areas. Each edition of *Healthy People* has built on data and outcomes from previous editions. The two major goals that should be reached by 2010 are:

1. *Increase quality and years of healthy life.* This goal focuses on life expectancy, quality of life, and achieving a longer and healthier life.
2. *Eliminate health disparities.* This goal focuses on a variety of factors that have an impact on health disparities, such as gender, race and ethnicity, income and education, dis-

Table 7–1 Leading Causes of Death 2005

Rank	Cause of death based on ICD-10, 1992)	Number	% of total deaths	2005 crude death rate	Age-adjusted death rate 2005	Percent change 2004 to 2005	Ratio Male to Female	Ratio Black to White	Ratio Hispanic to non-Hispanic White
	All causes	2,448,017	100.00	825.9	798.8	-0.2	1.4	1.3	0.7
1	Diseases of heart	652,091	26.6	220.0	211.1	-2.7	1.5	1.3	0.7
2	Malignant neoplasms	559,312	22.8	188.7	183.8	-1.1	1.4	1.2	0.7
3	Cerebrovascular disease	143,579	5.9	48.4	46.6	-6.8	1.0	1.5	0.8
4	Chronic lower respiratory diseases	130,933	5.3	44.2	43.2	5.1	1.3	0.7	0.4
5	Accidents (unintentional injuries)	117,809	4.8	39.7	39.1	3.7	2.2	1.0	0.8
6	Diabetes mellitus	75,119	3.1	25.3	24.6	0.4	1.3	2.1	1.6
7	Alzheimer's disease	71,599	2.9	24.2	22.9	5.0	0.7	0.8	0.6
8	Influenza & pneumonia	63,001	2.6	21.3	20.3	2.5	1.3	1.1	0.8
9	Nephritis, nephritic syndrome & nephrosis	43,901	1.8	14.8	14.3	0.7	1.4	2.3	0.9
10	Septicemia	34,136	1.4	11.5	11.2	0.0	1.2	2.2	0.8
11	Intentional self-harm (suicide)	32,637	1.3	11.0	10.9	0.0	4.1	0.4	0.4
12	Chronic liver disease & cirrhosis	27,530	1.1	9.3	9.0	0.0	2.1	0.8	1.6
13	Essential (primary) hypertension & hypertensive renal disease	24,902	1.0	8.4	8.0	3.9	1.0	2.6	1.0
14	Parkinson's disease	19,544	0.8	6.6	6.4	4.9	2.2	0.4	0.6
15	Assault (homicide)	18,124	0.7	6.1	6.1	3.4	3.8	5.7	2.8
...	All other causes (residual)	433,800	17.7	146.4	...	...	...	...	...

Source: National Vital Statistics Report. Volume 56, Number 10, April 24, 2008. Retrieved May 28, 2008 from the National Center for Health Statistics Web site: http://www.cdc.gov/nchs/products/pubs/pubd/nvsr/nvsr.htm#vol56

ability, geographic location, and sexual orientation to achieve equity.

Healthy People defines the key terms in these goals. *Life expectancy* is the average number of years that people born in a given year are expected to live based on a set of age-specific death rates. As of 2000, the average life expectancy at birth is nearly 77 years (U.S. Department of Health and Human Services, 2000). The United States does not have the highest life expectancy. *Quality of life* reflects a sense of happiness and satisfaction with personal lives and environment. Health-related quality of life reflects a personal sense of physical and mental health and the ability to react to factors in the physical and social environments. To determine quality of life, persons are asked to identify, from their personal perspectives, the number of healthy days that they have experienced in the year, and how many healthy years. The goal is that with increased life expectancy and quality of life, individuals will achieve longer and healthier lives.

Health disparity has become even more important in last 5 years; the Institute of Medicine (IOM) has issued reports with supporting data demonstrating that the U.S. healthcare system has severe problems with health disparities (IOM, 2002). A health disparity is an inequality or gap that exists between two or more groups. Health disparities are believed to be the result of the complex interaction of personal, societal, and environmental factors (U.S. Department of Health and Human Services, 2000). Figure 7–1 illustrates the concept of *Healthy People*. The figure emphasizes the structure of *Healthy People* by beginning with the goals and objectives.

These goals and objectives then influence the determinants of health. The determinants of health care are:

- *Biology*: The individual's genetic makeup, family history, and physical and mental health problems acquired during life.
- *Behaviors*: Individual responses or reactions to internal stimuli and external conditions.
- *Social environment*: Interactions with family, friends, coworkers, and others in the community.
- *Physical environment*: That which can be seen, touched, heard, smelled, and tasted; physical environment can harm a person and community but can also promote health (providing exercise areas, controlling pollution).
- *Policies and interventions*: Can impact health, for example, health promotion campaigns, laws controlling the sale of cigarettes.

The determinants of health interact with one another. They need to be monitored and evaluated to improve health status of individuals and communities. According to *Healthy People*, health status is determined by measuring birth and death rates, life expectancy, quality of life, morbidity from specific diseases, risk factors, use of ambulatory care and inpatient care, accessibility of health providers and facilities, financing of health care, health insurance coverage, and other factors. Access to health care is critical. This is a complex area, and all of this impacts the health status of individuals and communities. An example is that the leading cause of death in the United States is not the result of one cause or behavior, but multiple ones: injury, violence, and other factors in the environment, and the unavailability or inaccessibility of quality health services (U.S. Department of Health and Human Services, 2000).

Both *Healthy People* and the IOM (2003) reports on priority areas identified critical focus areas for healthcare improvement. The IOM priority areas are viewed from the continuum of care perspective across the life span. Exhibit 7–1 identifies the crit-

Figure 7–1 Healthy people in healthy communities: A systematic approach to health improvement.

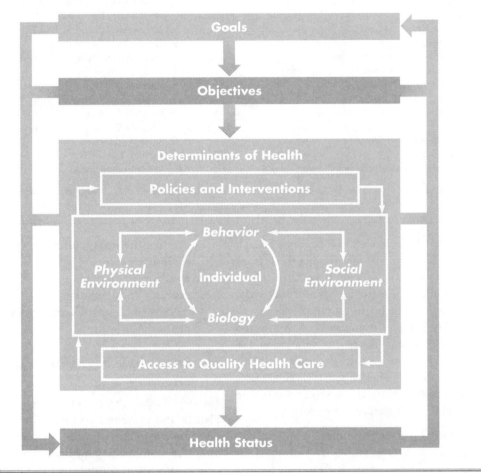

Source: Healthy People 2010 (2nd ed.), by U.S. Department of Health and Human Services, 2000. Washington, DC: U.S. Government Printing Office. http://www.healthypeople.gov

ical focus areas from *Healthy People 2010*, and Exhibit 7–2 identifies the IOM priority areas.

These two lists are similar. The priority areas identified by the IOM are periodically reviewed and altered based on health needs and outcome data. Why is this information important? It can guide healthcare providers in identifying areas

that need careful consideration in monitoring and improving care. These are the areas that require improvement because care is not meeting positive outcomes for patients.

The *Healthy People 2010* Leading Health Indicators are being used to measure the health of the nation over the 10-year period that con-

---

EXHIBIT 7–1 HEALTHY PEOPLE 2010 FOCUS AREAS

1. Access to Quality Health Services	15. Injury and Violence Prevention
2. Arthritis, Osteoporosis, and Chronic Back Conditions	16. Maternal, Infant, and Child Health
3. Cancer	17. Medical Product Safety
4. Chronic Kidney Disease	18. Mental Health and Mental Disorders
5. Diabetes	19. Nutrition and Overweight
6. Disability and Secondary Conditions	20. Occupational Safety and Health
7. Educational and Community-Based Programs	21. Oral Health
8. Environmental Health	22. Physical Activity and Fitness
9. Family Planning	23. Public Health Infrastructure
10. Food Safety	24. Respiratory Diseases
11. Health Communication	25. Sexually Transmitted Diseases
12. Heart Disease and Stroke	26. Substance Abuse
13. HIV	27. Tobacco Use
14. Immunization and Infectious Diseases	28. Vision and Hearing

Source: *Healthy People 2010* (2nd ed.), by U.S. Department of Health and Human Services (2000). Washington, DC: U.S. Government Printing Office.

---

cludes in 2010. Each of the 10 Leading Health Indicators has one or more objectives from *Healthy People 2010* associated with it. These indicators reflect the major health concerns in the United States at the beginning of the 21st century. The Leading Health Indicators were selected on the basis of their ability to motivate action, the availability of data to measure progress, and their importance as public health issues (U.S. Department of Health and Human Services, 2000). The Leading Health Indicators focus on:

- **Physical Activity:** Promote regular physical activity.
- **Overweight and Obesity:** Promote healthier weight and good nutrition.
- **Tobacco Use:** Prevent and reduce tobacco use.
- **Substance Abuse:** Prevent and reduce substance abuse.
- **Responsible Sexual Behavior:** Promote responsible sexual behavior.
- **Mental Health:** Promote mental health and well-being.
- **Injury and Violence:** Promote safety and reduce violence.

- **Environmental Quality:** Promote healthy environments.
- **Immunization:** Prevent infectious disease through immunization.
- **Access to Health Care:** Increase access to quality health care.

Healthy People in Healthy Communities

Healthy People 2010 (U.S. Department of Health and Human Services, 2000) considers not only the health of individuals and families but also community health. The initiative defines a healthy community as a community that embraces the belief that health is more than merely an absence of disease; a healthy community includes those elements that enable people to maintain a high quality of life and productivity. What are some characteristics of a healthy community? It is safe; it provides both treatment and prevention services to all community members; it has the infrastructure (roads, schools, playgrounds, and other services) to meet needs; and it has a safe, healthy environment (regarding issues of pol-

---

EXHIBIT 7–2 INSTITUTE OF MEDICINE PRIORITY AREAS FOR NATIONAL ACTION

- Care Coordination
- Self-Management/Health Literacy
- Asthma—appropriate treatment for persons with mild/moderate persistent asthma
- Cancer Screening—evidence-based, with a focus on colorectal and cervical cancer
- Children with Special Needs—who are at increased risk for chronic physical, developmental, and behavioral conditions
- Diabetes—focus on appropriate management of early disease
- End-of-Life with advanced organ system failure—focus on congestive heart failure and chronic obstructive pulmonary disease
- Frailty Associated with Old Age—preventing falls and pressure ulcers, maximizing function, and developing advanced care plans
- Hypertension—focus on appropriate treatment of early disease
- Immunization—children and adults
- Ischemic Heart Disease—prevention, reduction of recurring events, and optimization of functional capacity
- Major Depression—screening and treatment
- Medical Management—preventing medication errors and overuse of antibiotics
- Nosocomial Infections—prevention and surveillance
- Pain Control in Advanced Cancer
- Pregnancy and Childbirth—appropriate prenatal and intrapartum care
- Severe and Persistent Mental Illness—focus on treatment in the public sector
- Stroke—early treatment in the public sector
- Tobacco Dependence Treatment in Adults
- Obesity

Source: From *Priority Areas for National Action: Transforming Healthcare Quality* (p. 3), by Institute of Medicine, 2003, Washington, DC: National Academies Press. Copyright © 2003 by the Institute of Medicine. Reprinted with permission.

---

lution, for example). *Healthy People 2010* provides a guide for communities to assess their health (community, families, and individuals) and compare it with others. It also recommends interventions that can be used to improve the health of the community and all its members.

How might a population go about developing a healthy community? One method recommended through *Healthy People* is MAP-IT, which is an approach to working with the community and planning what needs to be done to improve the community's health:

- Mobilize individuals and organizations that care about the health of your community into a coalition.

- Assess the areas of greatest need in your community, as well as the resources and other strengths that you can tap into to address those areas.
- Plan your approach: Start with a vision of where you want to be as a community; then add strategies and action steps to help you achieve that vision.
- Implement your plan using concrete action steps that can be monitored and that will make a difference.
- Track your progress over time.

Through MAP-IT, communities can begin to meet *Healthy People* goals and objectives.

Healthy People 2010 not only provides a 10-year plan to improve healthcare in the United

States but also monitors progress periodically to determine if the goals and objectives are being met. Data about current outcomes can be found on the *Healthy People* Web site (http://www .healthypeople.gov). When the 10-year time period is completed, all outcomes will be evaluated, and this information and data will be used to develop the goals and objectives for the next 10 years.

Important Concepts

Health and Illness

Health and *wellness* are terms that tend to be used interchangeably. But what does *health* mean? There is no simple response to this question. A simple definition, though not complete, is to be structurally and functionally whole. Absence of this state is illness. The World Health Organization (WHO) defines health as "a state of complete well-being, physical, social, and mental, and not merely the absence of disease or infirmity" (WHO, 2007a). This is a common definition that is often quoted.

WHO addresses health and illness from the global perspective. The principles found in its constitution are (WHO, 2006):

- Health is not merely the absence of disease or infirmity.
- The enjoyment of the highest attainable standard of health is one of the fundamental rights of every human being without distinction of race, religion, political belief, economic or social condition.
- The health of all peoples is fundamental to the attainment of peace and security and is dependent upon the fullest cooperation of individuals and states.
- The achievement of any state in the promotion and protection of health is of value to all.

- Unequal development in different countries in the promotion of health and control of disease, especially communicable disease, is a common danger.
- Healthy development of the child is of basic importance; the ability to live harmoniously in a changing total environment is essential to such development.
- The extension to all peoples of the benefits of medical, psychological, and related knowledge is essential to the fullest attainment of health.
- Informed opinion and active cooperation on the part of the public are of the utmost importance in the improvement of the health of the people.
- Governments have a responsibility for the health of their peoples that can be fulfilled only by the provision of adequate health and social measures.

Effective definitions of health should be applicable to all—to those who are well; to those with illness or disease that can be treated; and to those with acquired or genetic impairments that result in a chronic disease or disability. The definition has to be applied to individuals, communities, and nations (Robert Wood Johnson Foundation [RWJF], 2000). The determinants of health or factors that have an impact on health are physical, mental, social, and spiritual. **Stress** and socioeconomic factors are also very important because they can have an impact. Stress can lead to health problems or can have an impact on current health status; for example, a patient with a cardiac problem can experience more symptoms when experiencing high levels of stress. Patients who have socioeconomic problems may not have an adequate diet because of lack of money, or they may experience sleep problems because they work two jobs.

Disease and *illness* are terms that are often used interchangeably. Disease is an indication of a physiological dysfunction or pathological reaction. Other terms related to health and illness are *episodic* and *distributive* care. "Episodic care refers to the curative and restorative aspects of practice, or secondary and tertiary prevention" (Pizzuti, 2006, p. 594). "Distributive care refers to health maintenance and disease prevention or primary prevention" (p. 594). A nurse in a clinic changing a dressing on a patient who has a leg ulcer is an example of episodic care; during the visit, the nurse provides information about weight reduction, which is an example of distributive care.

Life expectancy for Americans has reached an all-time high, according to the latest U.S. mortality statistics released by the Centers for Disease Control and Prevention (CDC). The report, "Deaths: Preliminary Data for 2003," prepared by CDC's National Center for Health Statistics, shows life expectancy at 77.6 years in 2003, up from 77.3 in 2002. The gap between male and female life expectancy closed from 5.4 years in 2002 to 5.3 years in 2003, continuing a trend toward narrowing since the peak gap of 7.8 years in 1979. Record-high life expectancies were found for White males (75.4 years) and Black males (69.2 males), and for White females (80.5 years) and Black females (76.1 years) (CDC, 2005).

Public health plays a critical role in improving and maintaining health of individuals, families, and communities. The goal of public health is to secure health and promote wellness (RWJF, 2000). There is a great need to address multiple complex health problems in communities, such as violence, including domestic, child, and elder abuse; substance abuse and alcohol dependency; tobacco use; injuries; automobile accidents; environmental factors such as air and water quality; food safety and consequent health issues; and communicable diseases. Public health has recently become important, with the increasing concern about disaster management and terror-

ism. Communities need to develop effective plans to provide healthcare services in major crisis situations. All these concerns require more than just care for individuals who are experiencing these problems. Public health is based on three functions:

1. Assessment: Assess and diagnose the status of the community's health and identify the needs for services using epidemiology, surveillance, research, and evaluation.
2. Policy development: These problems require changes in laws, programs for prevention and treatment, and reimbursement for these services. There is a great need for strategic plans and interventions, and appropriate evaluation of outcomes need to be developed through the government and its agencies at all levels (local, state, and federal).
3. Assurance: Ensure universal access to care when it is needed and to health promotion and prevention of disease and illness through community-wide health services.

Patient as Focus of Care and Member of the Healthcare Team

The patient is the focus of care. Much more will be discussed about the patient, or consumer of care, in Chapter 9, but it is important to recognize the role of the patient in this discussion. Patients should be viewed as members of the healthcare team and should be involved in decision making about their own care. Patient-centered care means that the patient is the center of that care—receiving the care—and must be involved in care decisions.

The Curative Model

The curative model has long been viewed as the best approach to health; however, this model has recently come under criticism (RWJF, 2000).

Yes, cure is a good goal, but is this a view that really can be applied to the complex area of health? There are other important goals, as noted by the RWJF:

- Restoring functional capacity
- Relieving suffering
- Preventing illness, injury, and untimely death
- Promoting health
- Caring for those who cannot be cured

These additional goals expand what can be done to help those who need it. Cure is not always possible, and with the increase of chronic illness and the growing elderly population, cure is becoming less important from the patient's daily perspective. The curative model focuses more on the biological approach that forms a hierarchical system of decision making, with physicians making diagnoses. Nursing is more involved in additional functions, though the nurse certainly participates in providing care that is directed at cure, such as surgery to repair a fractured hip. The hip can be repaired, but the patient typically has other needs after this surgery that are tied to the additional functions. The patient will need help gaining functional capacity, and he or she may never regain full capacity. The patient may need help promoting health if the cause of the fracture was osteoporosis (e.g., lifestyle changes related to diet, vitamins, and exercise).

Stress, Coping, Adaptation, and Resilience

Stress is a complex experience, felt internally, that makes the person feel a loss or threat of a loss. Stress is present in all parts of life, and it plays a role in health and illness. The most effective intervention for stress is **stress management**. Eliminating stress completely is not possible, but helping individuals, families, vulnerable populations, and communities better

cope with stress is an important goal in improving health and developing health-promoting behaviors. Effective **coping** can reduce the negative impact of stress and, in many cases, prevent the person from experiencing stress. This might be done through identifying stressors or stimuli that cause a person to experience stress; stressors can be biological, sociological, psychological, spiritual, or environmental. Self-assessment to determine the stressors goes a long way to improving coping. Stress management interventions might include relaxation techniques, humor, better sleep, healthy diet, exercise, music, and use of assertiveness. Not all persons who experience stress experience negative outcomes. **Resilience**, or the ability to cope with stress, is an important factor. Adaptation to situations is also important. Stress was discussed in Chapter 1 as it relates to students, but the same principles apply to anyone, including patients.

Along the Continuum of Care

Disease Prevention and Health Promotion

Disease prevention and health promotion can be easily confused, but they are different and related. One schema for understanding health promotion and prevention was developed by Leavell and Clark (1965):

1. Health promotion (primary prevention)
2. Specific protection (primary prevention)
3. Early diagnosis and treatment (secondary prevention)
4. Disability limitation (secondary prevention)
5. Restoration and **rehabilitation** (tertiary prevention)

HEALTH PREVENTION

Health prevention means to try and stop the development of disease, but it also includes treatment to prevent disease from progressing further and leading to complications. The major levels of prevention are primary, secondary, and tertiary. *Primary prevention* includes interventions that are used to maintain health and are used before illness occurs. Health promotion is a critical component of primary prevention. Examples are teaching people about healthy diets before they become obese, and encouraging adequate exercise (education about health and healthy lifestyles is an important intervention at this level). *Secondary prevention* occurs after disease has begun but before symptoms are evident, and it focuses on preventing further complications. Examples are breast cancer screening using mammography, and blood pressure screening to identify hypertension. *Tertiary prevention* occurs when there is disability and the need to maintain or, if possible, improve functioning. Examples would be teaching a person with diabetes how to administer insulin and manage the disease, or referring a stroke patient for rehabilitation.

HEALTH PROMOTION

Health promotion focuses on changing lifestyle to maximize health and is an important part of primary prevention. This is very difficult to accomplish for most people. In 2006, the National Prevention Summit addressed disease prevention, health preparedness, and health promotion and featured innovative programs that are making a difference in communities across the country to build a healthier country (Office of Disease Prevention and Health Promotion, 2006). These programs focused on healthy lifestyle choices—eating a nutritious diet, being physically active, making healthy choices, and getting preventive screenings—to help prevent major health threats and burdens such as obesity, diabetes, asthma, cancer, heart disease, and stroke. One special emphasis in 2006 was the prevention of childhood overweight and obesity, which

have become major problems and can lead to long-term chronic illnesses such as diabetes. Another emphasis was on preparing for public health emergencies, such as avian influenza, and this preparation continues.

Many models describe how health promotion might be effective. Pender's Health Promotion Model (Pender, 1982; Pender, 1996, as cited in Pender, Murdaugh, & Parsons, 2006) is a nursing model that has been used in many studies about health promotion. It is a model that does not include fear or threat as a motivator to make people change their behaviors, and it is one that can be used across the life span. What is included in this model of health promotion?

- Individual characteristics and experiences:
- Emphasizes that each person is unique.

These aspects of health promotion have an impact on health and must be considered.

- *Prior related behavior*: The frequency of the same or similar behavior in the past is the best predictor of behavior.
- *Personal factors*: Biological (examples: age, weight, pubertal status, strength), psychological (examples: self-esteem, coping style, self-motivation), and sociocultural (examples: race, ethnicity, education, socioeconomic status) factors that influence the cognitions, affects, and health behavior that is the focus.
- *Behavior-specific cognitions and affect*: These are very important because nursing interventions can make a difference, and this can move the person toward health-promoting behaviors.
- *Perceived benefits of action*: Whether a person will be active in participating in changing behavior is highly dependent on whether the person sees any benefit in doing so— perceived benefits. It is important to determine whether perceived barriers are real. If

perceived barriers to success are felt by the person, it is much more difficult for that person to change his or her behavior to a health-promoting behavior.

- *Perceived self-efficacy*: Self-efficacy relates to whether the person feels that he or she can do what he or she will need to do. It does not mean that the person has the competency to do this, but centers on whether the person feels that he or she could actually do what needs to be done.

- *Activity-related affect*: Emotions tied to actions are important to recognize. What these emotions are can determine whether a person repeats a behavior. Did the person feel good about what he or she did? Did it make the person anxious?

- *Interpersonal influences*: Each person is influenced by others—family, friends, coworkers, peers, healthcare providers, and so on. This influence—what it might be and how it might be felt—may or may not be reality based, but it still can influence a person's behavior and his or her ability to change to health-promoting behavior.

- *Situational influences*: A situation or context can influence a person's behavior. If a person smokes and is told that all smoking must take place outside the building in a designated area regardless of the weather, this situation or context may influence a change in behavior.

- *Commitment to a plan of action*: Is the person committed to a specific plan to change to health-promoting behavior? Commitment is not enough; strategies must be laid out to reach outcomes.

- *Immediate competing demands and preferences*: What might interfere with the person changing to health-promoting behavior? Will the family be supportive? Are there other actions that must take precedence (for example, work over exercise)? Each person

has alternative behaviors that compete with what he or she needs to do to move to a healthier lifestyle.

- *Health-promoting behavior*: This is the outcome, and from this, the person reaches positive health outcomes.

Occupational Health Care

Occupational health care may seem a strange topic, but it is an active setting for health promotion, disease and illness prevention, and treatment, and it also involves looking at risks of illness and injury due to the work environment. Providing these services at the work site makes it easier for the employee to obtain the services with less concern about getting to appointments during work hours. Many employers have found it to be beneficial to them to provide these services on-site for employees, often reducing potential health risks and providing prompt treatment. All of this can reduce employer health insurance costs. Employers may provide a variety of health promotion and prevention services, such as exercise classes or even gym access, stress management resources and classes, diet and weight-loss classes, smoke cessation programs, immunizations, weight management services, and other types of opportunities for employees to maintain a healthy lifestyle. Employers may also consider factors such as the food served in the cafeteria, environmental health issues, walking areas for employees during breaks, equipment to prevent back injuries, and so on.

Illness: Acute and Chronic

Acute illness is typically self-limiting and occurs in a short period of time. Cure is the focus for care. Some of the care for acute illness takes place in the hospital, commonly referred to as the acute care setting, but today, more care is taking place in the home or community through primary care and ambulatory services. Examples of acute illness are an infectious disease such as the flu or pneumonia, a broken leg, appendicitis, urinary tract infection, and many others.

Chronic illness is a serious problem in the United States and worldwide. It can be difficult for a healthcare provider to understand the need for a change in perspective when caring for patients with chronic illnesses if he or she more commonly cares for patients with sudden-onset illnesses or with injuries for which the cure model is the focus. Chronic illnesses are illnesses for which there is no effective cure, and treatment focuses on control of symptoms, support, psychosocial issues, and, if possible, prevention of deterioration. Examples of chronic diseases are heart disease, diabetes, stroke, hypertension, rheumatoid arthritis, obesity, and even cancer (many people with cancer are surviving and now must live with long-term effects of the cancer and/or the treatment). Worldwide, "out of the 35 million people who died from chronic disease in 2005, half were under 70 and half were women" (World Health Organization, 2007a). Eliopoulos (2001) identified key goals for chronic care:

- Maintain or improve self-care capacity
- Manage the disease effectively
- Boost the body's healing abilities
- Prevent complications
- Delay deterioration and decline
- Achieve highest possible quality of life
- Die with comfort, peace, and dignity

Chronic care is discussed in more detail in Chapter 9.

Home Health Care

Care provided in the home has increased in the United States. Patients are being discharged earlier and earlier from the hospital because of managed care and efforts to control costs. Many patients are not fully recovered or ready to care for themselves. **Home care** provides healthcare services in the home. These services can vary as to the amount of time that the care provider is in the home, the number of visits per week, and for how many weeks or months. In addition, there is variation in the type of healthcare provider needed: a home health aide who provides activities of daily living services (bathing, ambulation, simple care, light housekeeping, food preparation); a registered nurse who assesses the patient, develops the care plan, monitors progress, assesses the home environment for safety, and provides more complex care; a physical therapist who helps the patient with exercises to gain strength; or a social worker who assists with obtaining other services that the patient may need such, as Meals on Wheels, payment for healthcare services, and so on. Telehealth is used in some home care situations; health information is sent from one site to another by electronic communication. (See more on this topic in Chapter 13.) With the growing number of persons with chronic illness and the aging population, it is expected that home health care will continue to grow.

Rehabilitation

Rehabilitation is part of tertiary prevention. The goal of rehabilitation interventions is to attain and retain the best possible level of functioning for a person who has an illness or disability that is permanent and irreversible. Rehabilitation can take place in the hospital, in an **extended care** or long-term care facility, in an ambulatory care facility, or in the home. Rehabilitation therapists assist the patient. The nurse may be the healthcare provider who identifies the need for rehabilitation, or he or she may be involved by following the rehabilitation plan. A patient may require a specialized therapist, such as a physical therapist, an occupational therapist, a speech-language pathologist, or a vocational therapist. Patients may need to learn how to complete daily-living activities, such as taking care of personal hygiene and dressing; ambulating safely with or without assistive devices such as a walker, cane, or wheelchair; learning basic life skills, such as cooking or driving with a disability; and learning new job skills. Some patients may recover more fully than others. Examples of patients who may require rehabilitation are those who have suffered a stroke, a major automobile accident, severe burns, or a work-related accident, such as a serious fall or damage from equipment.

Extended Care, Long-Term Care, and Elder Care

The population is aging, and the need for services to meet this population is growing. Gerontological nursing is an important specialty that focuses on care of the elder population in all settings; however, the most important extended care settings involve skilled nursing, or intermediate care and long-term care in which patients can receive a range of services, from housing, meals, and activities to routine personal care, rehabilitation, and specialized treatment. There is great need within the community for more elder-care services, such as adult day care (a facility where elders may go during the day for socializing and activities), home health, and retirement and assistive-living facilities (these can vary from single rooms to independent living situations with support services as needed). These patients can experience health problems in all body systems and psychologically. They also experience social problems, with loss of spouse and friends and lessened ability to be mobile, and they may be isolated. Financial problems are not uncommon, which impact food, housing, and access to medical care.

Hospice and Palliative Care

Hospice care is a philosophy of care for the terminally ill that involves supporting the quality of life as long as possible. It is not a place, though it can be—for example, a freestanding building in which hospice services are provided. Hospice care can also be provided in the patient's home or in a special unit of an acute care hospital. This philosophy of care includes active participation of the patient and family in all care decisions. Staff are specially trained to support the patient and family during the critical last stages. Palliative care focuses on alleviating symptoms and meeting the special needs of the terminally ill patient and the family. The hospice is the organization or system in which palliative care is provided. A place designated for patients to come and receive palliative care may be referred to as a hospice, or care providers may provide palliative care at the patient's home.

Case Management

Case management is a system that aims to get the right services to the patient at the right time and avoid fragmented and unnecessary care that can be costly. It facilitates effective care delivery and outcomes for patients. Case management requires **collaboration** or cooperative effort among healthcare providers and other sources of resources that the patient may require. **Coordination** is required to organize care so that it is available when needed. Communication is also critical because the case manager must work with many people to get the care required. Case managers frequently do all their work on the telephone and never actually see the patient or family. They are typically employees of an insurance company, a government agency, or a healthcare organization, particularly acute care settings (hospitals). Because one of their concerns is cost-effective care delivery, they have to know something about reimbursement and how to manage the care services in a manner that controls costs. Case managers who may be nurses or social workers work directly with patients (clients) and their families to assess needs, direct the patient to care when needed, and monitor progress. Case management is a growing area of care delivery that has proved to be effective in helping patients get the care they need in a healthcare system that is complex and confusing.

Genetics: Rapid Change With Major Impact

The Human Genome Project (HGP) was funded by the U.S. Department of Energy and the National Institutes of Health. It was begun in 1990 and completed in 2003. The project focused on mapping all the loci of the 20,000–25,000 genes that make up the human body. The implications of this project are many. We have learned that the interaction of the genetic make-up of an individual and the environment (genomics) often determines whether the person will be healthy or ill for the majority of his or her life. The benefits of this research are listed as:

- *Improved diagnosis of disease*
- *Earlier detection of genetic predispositions to disease*
- *Rational drug design*
- *Gene therapy and control systems for drugs*
- *Pharmacogenomics "custom drugs"* (Human Genome Project, 2007)

When this information is used with the Family History Tool to gather information about diseases in the family, a very thorough risk assessment can be completed (U.S. Department of Health and Human Services, 2007). If this risk assessment is used in health promotion, the health professional can explain to patients and families not only their risk of a disease due to their genetic profile but also the interactions with the environment?genomic risk. With the knowledge of how a person's genes interact with drugs, better pain medications that are designed for that individual are possible–pharmacogenomics. We now have the ability to "fix" a bad

gene because we know the location. The technology to diagnose even prenatally is possible, giving us the tools to allow a fetus to continue to grow normally instead of having major anomalies at birth. The possibilities are endless for disease prevention and management. Type II diabetes treatment has changed in the last few years because of knowledge of the role that genes play in diabetes ("Researchers Locate Type II Diabetes Gene," 2004). This change in disease management will continue. We are just at the beginning of a new frontier of nursing care. The essentials for genetics competencies have been written and are in the process of being introduced into nursing curricula (Consensus Panel, 2006). These are just as critical as the other competencies regarding nursing process that lead to better patient outcomes and safe care.

Complementary and Alternative Therapies or Integrative Medicine

The National Center for Complementary and Alternative Medicine (NCCAM; 2007) describes complementary and alternative medicine (CAM) as a group of diverse medical and healthcare systems, practices, and products that are not presently considered part of conventional medicine. Conventional medicine is medicine as practiced by holders of medical doctor or doctor of osteopathy degrees and by their allied health professionals, such as physical therapists, psychologists, and registered nurses. Some health care providers practice both CAM and conventional medicine. Although some scientific evidence exists regarding some CAM therapies, for most, there are key questions that have yet to be answered through well-designed scientific studies—questions such as whether these therapies are safe and whether they work for the diseases or medical conditions for which they are used. The list of what is considered CAM changes continually as therapies that are proved to be safe and effective are adopted by conventional health care and as new approaches to health care emerge.

Many of these interventions are not new, but their use has come more into mainstream use. However, many of these CAM interventions still have a long way to go to be part of conventional medicine. Examples of these interventions are acupuncture, acupressure, massage, light energy, botanical treatment, reiki, tai chi, and the use of a variety of herbs and so forth, such as garlic, shark cartilage, and ginseng. With the creation of the NCCAM, there is now an organized system for clinical trials using CAM to gather data about their use and outcomes. Nurses provide some CAM interventions in their practice, and some insurers cover these services. As more data are obtained to support their efficacy, there will probably be more inclusion of these interventions in care, and they will gain greater reimbursement coverage.

Vulnerable Populations

A vulnerable population is a group of persons who are at risk for developing health problems. They need careful assessment and monitoring to identify problems early so that complications can be prevented. Typically, complex factors increase their risk, such as economic, ethnic, social, and communication factors. They may have problems related to diet, housing, safety, and transportation, and they may have problems accessing care when they need it. What are some of the vulnerable populations? They are children, the elderly, people with chronic illness, immigrants, illegal aliens, migrant workers, people who live in rural areas, homeless people, the seriously mentally ill, victims of abuse and violence, preg-

nant adolescents, and people who are human immunodeficiency virus positive. Poverty is an important concern with many of these populations. Poverty guidelines are determined by the federal government based on the income of a family of a specific size. This amount changes annually. Poverty guidelines are important because financial eligibility for certain federal programs is based on poverty levels; to receive services, a person must not have an income higher than the poverty level.

Global Healthcare Concerns and International Nursing

The WHO is the major international health organization. Its major goals focus on (1) development to decrease poverty, (2) fostering health security, for example, deceasing infectious diseases and epidemics, (3) strengthening the health systems needed for people to provide health care, (4) using research, evidence-based practice, and information to support care decisions, (5) building partnerships to ensure stronger care systems, and (5) improving performance (WHO, 2007b).

> *In September 2000, leaders from 189 nations agreed on a vision for the future: a world with less poverty, hunger and disease, greater survival prospects for mothers and their infants, better educated children, equal opportunities for women, and a healthier environment; a world in which developed and developing countries worked in partnership for the betterment of all. This vision took the shape of eight Millennium Development Goals, which provide a framework for development planning for countries around the world, and time-bound targets by which progress can be measured. (WHO, 2007a)*

Exhibit 7–3 describes the Millennium Development Goals. The WHO Constitution

---

EXHIBIT 7–3 WORLD HEALTH ORGANIZATION MILLENNIUM DEVELOPMENT GOALS

Millennium Development Goals (MDGs)	
Goals and Targets (from the Millennium Declaration)	Indicators for monitoring progress
Goal 1: Eradicate extreme poverty and hunger	
Target 1: Halve, between 1990 and 2015, the proportion of people whose income is less than one dollar a day	1. Proportion of population below $1 (PPP) per day[1] 2. Poverty gap ratio [incidence $\times$ depth of poverty] 3. Share of poorest quintile in national consumption
Target 2: Halve, between 1990 and 2015, the proportion of people who suffer from hunger	4. Prevalence of underweight children under five years of age 5. Proportion of population below minimum level of dietary energy consumption
Goal 2: Achieve universal primary education	
Target 3: Ensure that, by 2015, children everywhere, boys and girls alike, will be able to complete a full course of primary schooling	6. Net enrollment ratio in primary education 7. Proportion of pupils starting grade 1 who reach grade 5[2] 8. Literacy rate of 15-24 year-olds
Goal 3: Promote gender equality and empower women	
Target 4: Eliminate gender disparity in primary and secondary education, preferably by 2005, and in all levels of education no later than 2015	9. Ratios of girls to boys in primary, secondary and tertiary education 10. Ratio of literate women to men, 15-24 years old 11. Share of women in wage employment in the non-agricultural sector 12. Proportion of seats held by women in national parliament
Goal 4: Reduce child mortality	
Target 5: Reduce by two-thirds, between 1990 and 2015, the under-five mortality rate	13. Under-five mortality rate 14. Infant mortality rate 15. Proportion of 1 year-old children immunised against measles
Goal 5: Improve maternal health	
Target 6: Reduce by three-quarters, between 1990 and 2015, the maternal mortality ratio	16. Maternal mortality ratio 17. Proportion of births attended by skilled health personnel
Goal 6: Combat HIV/AIDS, malaria and other diseases	
Target 7: Have halted by 2015 and begun to reverse the spread of HIV/AIDS	18. HIV prevalence among pregnant women aged 15-24 years

continues

EXHIBIT 7–3 (continued)

	19. Condom use rate of the contraceptive prevalence rate[3]
	  19a. Condom use at last high-risk sex
	  19b. Percentage of population aged 15–24 years with comprehensive correct knowledge of HIV/AIDS[4]
	  19c. Contraceptive prevalence rate
	20. Ratio of school attendance of orphans to school attendance of non-orphans aged 10-14 years

Target 8: Have halted by 2015 and begun to reverse the incidence of malaria and other major diseases	21. Prevalence and death rates associated with malaria 22. Proportion of population in malaria-risk areas using effective malaria prevention and treatment measures[5] 23. Prevalence and death rates associated with tuberculosis 24. Proportion of tuberculosis cases detected and cured under directly observed treatment short course DOTS (Internationally recommended TB control strategy)

Goal 7: Ensure environmental sustainability

Target 9: Integrate the principles of sustainable development into country policies and pro-grammes and reverse the loss of environmental resources	25. Proportion of land area covered by forest 26. Ratio of area protected to maintain biological diversity to surface area 27. Energy use (kg oil equivalent) per \$1 GDP (PPP) 28. Carbon dioxide emissions per capita and consumption of ozone-depleting CFCs (ODP tons) 29. Proportion of population using solid fuels
Target 10: Halve, by 2015, the proportion of peo-ple without sustainable access to safe drinking water and basic sanitation	30. Proportion of population with sustainable access to an improved water source, urban and rural 31. Proportion of population with access to improved sanitation, urban and rural
Target 11: By 2020, to have achieved a significant improvement in the lives of at least 100 million slum dwellers	32. Proportion of households with access to secure tenure

Goal 8: Develop a global partnership for development

Target 12: Develop further an open, rule-based, predictable, non-discriminatory trading and financial system	*Some of the indicators listed below are monitored separately for the least developed countries (LDCs), Africa, landlocked developing countries and small island developing States.*

Includes a commitment to good governance, development and poverty reduction – both nationally and internationally

Target 13: Address the special needs of the least developed countries

Includes: tariff and quota free access for the least developed countries' exports; enhanced programme of debt relief for heavily indebted poor countries (HIPC) and cancellation of official bilateral debt; and more generous ODA for countries committed to poverty reduction

Target 14: Address the special needs of land-locked developing countries and small island developing States (through the Programme of Action for the Sustainable Development of Small Island Developing States and the outcome of the twenty-second special session of the General Assembly)

Target 15: Deal comprehensively with the debt problems of developing countries through national and international measures in order to make debt sustainable in the long term

Official development assistance (ODA)

33. Net ODA, total and to the least developed countries, as percentage of OECD/DAC donors' gross national income
34. Proportion of total bilateral, sector-allocable ODA of OECD/DAC donors to basic social services (basic education, primary health care, nutrition, safe water and sanitation)
35. Proportion of bilateral official development assistance of OECD/DAC donors that is untied
36. ODA received in landlocked developing countries as a proportion of their gross national incomes
37. ODA received in small island developing States as a proportion of their gross national incomes

Market access

38. Proportion of total developed country imports (by value and excluding arms) from developing countries and least developed countries, admitted free of duty
39. Average tariffs imposed by developed countries on agricultural products and textiles and clothing from developing countries
40. Agricultural support estimate for OECD countries as a percentage of their gross domestic product
41. Proportion of ODA provided to help build trade capacity

Debt sustainability

42. Total number of countries that have reached their HIPC decision points and number that have reached their HIPC completion points (cumulative)
43. Debt relief committed under HIPC Initiative
44. Debt service as a percentage of exports of goods and services

Target 16: In cooperation with developing countries, develop and implement strategies for decent and productive work for youth

45. Unemployment rate of young people aged 15–24 years, each sex and total[6]

Target 17: In cooperation with pharmaceutical companies, provide access to affordable essential drugs in developing countries

46. Proportion of population with access to affordable essential drugs on a sustainable basis

Target 18: In cooperation with the private sector, make available the benefits of new technologies, especially information and communications

47. Telephone lines and cellular subscribers per 100 population
48. Personal computers in use per 100 population Internet users per 100 population

continues

EXHIBIT 7–3 (continued)

The Millennium Development Goals and targets come from the Millennium Declaration, signed by 189 countries, including 147 heads of State and Government, in September 2000 (http://www.un.org/millennium/declaration/ares552e.htm). The goals and targets are interrelated and should be seen as a whole. They represent a partnership between the developed countries and the developing countries "to create an environment—at the national and global levels alike—which is conducive to development and the elimination of poverty".

Source: *Official List of MDG Indicators*, by the World Health Organization, 2007. Retrieved October 4, 2007 from http://millenniumindicators.un.org/unsd/mdg/Host.aspx?Content=Indicators/OfficialList.htm

[1]Note: Goals, targets and indicators effective 8 September 2003. For monitoring country poverty trends, indicators based on national poverty lines should be used, where available.

[2]An alternative indicator under development is "primary completion rate".

[3]Amongst contraceptive methods, only condoms are effective in preventing HIV transmission. Since the condom use rate is only measured among women in union, it is supplemented by an indicator on condom use in high-risk situations (indicator 19a) and an indicator on HIV/AIDS knowledge (indicator 19b). Indicator 19c (contraceptive prevalence rate) is also useful in tracking progress in other health, gender and poverty goals.

[4]This indicator is defined as the percentage of population aged 15-24 who correctly identify the two major ways of preventing the sexual transmission of HIV (using condoms and limiting sex to one faithful, uninfected partner), who reject the two most common local misconceptions about HIV transmission, and who know that a healthy-looking person can transmit HIV. However, since there are currently not a sufficient number of surveys to be able to calculate the indicator as defined above, UNICEF, in collaboration with UNAIDS and WHO, produced two proxy indicators that represent two components of the actual indicator. They are the following: a) percentage of women and men 15-24 who know that a person can protect herself/himself from HIV infection by "consistent use of condom"; b) percentage of women and men 15-24 who know a healthy-looking person can transmit HIV.

[5]Prevention to be measured by the percentage of children under 5 sleeping under insecticide-treated bednets; treatment to be measured by percentage of children under 5 who are appropriately treated.

[6]An improved measure of the target for future years is under development by the International Labour Organization.

---

reads, "the enjoyment of the highest attainable standard of health is one of the fundamental rights of every human being" (WHO, 2007a).

The International Council of Nurses (ICN) plays a role in global health by providing a voice for nursing throughout the world. Its stated mission is

> *to lead our societies toward better health. Working together within ICN, we harness the knowledge and enthusiasm of the entire nursing profession to promote healthy lifestyles, healthy workplaces, and healthy communities. We foster the health of our societies as well as individuals by supporting strategies of sustainable development that mitigate poverty, pollution,*

and other underlying causes of illness. (ICN, 1998)

Both this organization and the WHO focus on the health of individuals, families, and communities.

Conclusion

This chapter presented content related to the continuum of care across the life span. Concepts related to health and illness were highlighted to provide a framework in which health care is delivered to facilitate a better understanding of what patients experience. The continuum of care covers all aspects of health and wellness, and delivery of healthcare services to those who experience illness or injury.

CHAPTER HIGHLIGHTS

1. The focus of health care is changing to patient-focused care, with the patient in the key decision-making position.
2. Stress, coping, and resilience have an impact on health promotion, disease prevention, and illness.
3. Continuum of care means that nursing care must be provided in the home, community, and acute care settings.
4. The critical elements of the continuum of care are health, disease prevention, health promotion, occupational health care, illness (acute and chronic), home healthcare rehabilitation, extended care, long-term care, elder care, hospice and palliative care, and case management.
5. *Healthy People 2010,* coupled with the Institute of Medicine reports, requires health professionals to understand the concepts of patient safety, quality of care, health outcomes, and health indices, as well as to address health disparities in everyday care.
6. The Institute of Medicine has identified the priority areas of care that require more intensive monitoring regarding outcomes and quality. These areas will change as care is improved to meet outcomes.
7. The HGP has changed our knowledge of disease risk factors, identification, and management. It also has brought about recognition of the role that genomics plays in disease prevention, health promotion, and care management.
8. Complementary and alternative therapies are growing but are not yet part of mainstream treatment methods.
9. Vulnerable populations are groups of people who are at risk for developing health problems. Examples include children, the elderly, people with chronic illnesses, the homeless, and others.
10. The World Health Organization focuses its attention on global health issues.

Linking to the Internet

- *Healthy People 2010* Progress Reviews
  http://www.healthypeople.gov/data/PROGRVW/
- Be a Healthy Person
  http://www.healthypeople.gov/BeHealthy/
- Consumer e-Health Tools
  http://www.health.gov/communication/ehealth/ehealthTools/default.htm
- HealthierUS.gov
  http://www.healthierus.gov/index.html
- World Health Organization
  http://www.who.org
- Department of Health and Human Services Poverty Guidelines, Research, and Measurements
  http://aspe.hhs.gov/poverty/

DISCUSSION QUESTIONS

1. What are the differences and similarities between the *Healthy People 2010* indicators and the Millennium Development Goals?
2. Discuss the various views of health and illness presented in this chapter. Compare with your own perspective of health and illness.
3. Compare and contrast the three levels of prevention.
4. How does the life span impact the continuum of care?
5. What is the relationship between the continuum of care and continuity of care?

CRITICAL THINKING ACTIVITIES

1. Go to the *Take the first step to PREVENTION* page at the Centers of Disease Control Web site (http://wonder.cdc.gov/data2010/HU.htm). Search for your state and the most current data. Select a specific health indicator, and look at the national data and then those from your own state. How do they compare? Search for data for a specific population.
2. Visit the National Center for Health Statistics Web site (http://www.cdc.gov/nchs/) Search for current data related to births/natality, infant health, child health, adolescent health, men's health, women's health, and older people's health.
3. Visit these World Health Organization sites:
   http://www.who.int/whosis/database/life_tables/life_tables.cfm
   http://www.who.int/healthinfo/morttables/en/index.html
   http://www.who.int/healthinfo/bodestimates/en/index.html
   What can you learn about global life expectancy, mortality, and the burden of disease? How does the United States compare with other countries?
4. The WHO Constitution states that "the enjoyment of the highest attainable standard of health is one of the fundamental rights of every human being." Debate this view, with half of the team agreeing with this statement and half not agreeing.
5. Select one of the vulnerable populations and apply the content about health and illness to that population, discussing issues that would have an impact on health and illness.

CASE STUDY

You are a member of an interdisciplinary team in your state's rural area. The team is looking into improving the health status of the community. The community has a high rate of cancer (particularly breast and lung), accidents (farm related), alcohol abuse, particularly among teens, and obesity (adults, but with increasing weight gain in children). The interdisciplinary team is composed of two reg-istered nurses (one who works in the local hospital, and you, the only school nurse in the area), one physician in private practice, the hospital administrator, the mayor of the largest town in the area, and a clergyman.

Case Question

1. Describe how you think the team should approach these problems based on what you have learned in this chapter.

WORDS OF WISDOM

Edith Neusner, BSN, RN, BC
Greater Cincinnati Behavioral Health
Services, Cincinnati, Ohio

My current semiretirement nursing job is my all-time favorite. I work for a nonprofit community-based mental health agency that provides interdisciplinary support to 3,000 adults who have long-term major mental health diagnoses. I provide support to clients who need education and help managing their symptoms and medications. Many clients have chronic medical illness and challenges, such as diabetes, hypertension, and vision deficits, and they need support to promote self-management of those problems as well. It is easy to form a bond with these men and women, who have not had easy lives—they appreciate a friendly greeting by name, concern about their family relationships, or even a Happy Birthday post-it. Every day is different, and every interaction makes a difference to someone. As nurses, we have a huge array of career choices, in setting, focus, and location. I have worked in two hospitals, a university, a state college, and a camp. Additionally, I taught childbirth education and nurse aide training, and I served on a committee of a state nursing organization. There is always something new to learn and do, and never a boring workday.

Catherine Strunk, BSN, RN
Research Nurse III, Surviving the Teens
Program Director and Educator
Division of Psychiatry, Cincinnati
Children's Hospital

I began my nursing career in 1979 after graduating from a hospital school of nursing. After working 6 long weeks of night shifts with mostly geriatric patients at the hospital where I graduated, however, I realized my niche was really working with children. I was then hired to work on the orthopedic floor at our local children's hospital and remained there for 14 years until the unit finally closed due to a decreasing number of admissions related to more outpatient surgical procedures being performed. I was devastated having to be separated from my long-time coworkers and leave a unit I called "home" and an area in which I had an expertise. While there, however, I developed skills not only as an orthopedic nurse, but also in attending to the psychosocial needs of children and their families, which is especially important in pediatric nursing.

I was then placed on a general medical unit and worked there per diem for 2 years until transferring to the new adolescent psychiatric unit as it was being prepared to open. Although this was a totally new experience for me, I welcomed the opportunity to once again develop skills on a specialty unit. I worked there for

5 years, which prepared me for my present position at Children's Hospital. A new position was then posted for a psychiatric nurse with at least 5 years of experience to start a suicide prevention program in high schools. The position was being funded by a grant, which was only for a 3-year period.

Although this position offered no job security, I took a risk, leaving my area of comfort, and applied for the position and was immediately hired. It is now 7 years later, and the program has grown beyond anyone's expectations. I named the program Surviving the Teens® in 2004 and have completely developed and instituted a 4-day curriculum in more than 34 high schools, teaching approximately 30,000 teenagers about stressors, coping, depression, and suicide prevention. I have also developed the content for the Surviving the Teens program Web pages, a program for parents, and do teacher training. This program is now getting media attention, and I am continuing to develop and expand the program while collaborating with other professionals. Through this process, I have learned that a nurse can not only accomplish whatever he or she sets her mind on, but can venture beyond what is imagined.

Tina M. Marrelli, MSN, MA, RN
President, Marrelli and Associates, Inc.
Editor, Home Healthcare Nurse
news@marrelli.com;
http://www.marrelli.com

The patient's home can be, and should be, the healthcare setting of choice for numerous reasons. Some of the easy-to-understand reasons include lower costs, the general absence of causative virulent agents that can be found within hospital walls, patient choice, and the patient being a true equal partner in care and care planning. A more important reason might be the safety considerations of being in one's own home—because there is only one patient, there is less room for medication or other treatment errors being provided to the wrong patient. However, the most important reasons for home being the best site for care comes from patients and families themselves. This includes such seemingly simple things as no one (e.g., as opposed to the hospital or nursing home) telling patients what to wear (e.g., a hospital gown), the age of their visitors, what time to eat, the times visitors may visit, and numerous other reasons. When you add the fact that particularly older adult patients know their environment the best, that situation further supports safety as patients know every inch of their house, what they can (or cannot) navigate safely, and how things "work" for themselves and their families. It is not surprising that patients who had no history of mentation problems, falls, and other safety concerns at home experience these problems in an inpatient setting but do not experience these problematic symptoms when within the confines of their own home space.

There is no better place for health education and promotion to occur—the education/intervention is one-to-one, truly individualized, families/friends are involved, and the patient is in charge. The nurse and other team members are truly guests in any patient's home, and this dynamic alone provides a special situation that I believe further enhances the therapeutic relationship.

References

Centers for Disease Control. (2005, February 28). *Fact Sheet: Life expectancy hits record high.* Washington, DC: U.S. Department of Health and Human Services, Centers for Disease Control. Retrieved October 1, 2007, from http://www.cdc.gov

Consensus Panel. (2006). *Essential nursing competencies curricula guidelines for genetics and genomics.* Retrieved August 31, 2008, from http://www.nursingworld.org/ MainMenuCategories/ThePracticeofProfessional Nursing/EthicsStandards/CEHR/Genetics_1/ CompetenciesandCurriculaforGeneticsandGenomics/ EssentialNursingCompetenciesandCurriculaGuidelines forGeneticsandGenomics.aspx

Dingel-Stewart, S., & LaCosta, J. (2004). Light at the end of the tunnel. A vision for an empowered nursing profession across the continuum of care. *Nursing Administration Quarterly, 28,* 212–216.

Eliopoulos, C. (2001). *Gerontological nursing.* Philadelphia: Lippincott.

Haggerty, J., Reid, R. J., Freeman, G. K., Starfield, B. H., Adair, C. E., & McKendry, R. (2003). Continuity of care: A multidisciplinary review. *British Medical Journal, 327,* 1219–1221.

Human Genome Project. (2007). *Potential benefits of Human Genome Project Research.* Retrieved October 7, 2007, from http://www.ornl.gov/sci/techresources/ Human_Genome/project/benefits.shtml

Institute of Medicine. (2002). *Unequal treatment: Confronting racial and ethnic disparities in health.* Washington, DC: National Academies Press.

Institute of Medicine. (2003). *Priority areas for national action: Transforming healthcare quality.* Washington, DC: National Academies Press.

International Council of Nurses. (1998). *ICN's vision for the future of nursing.* Retrieved October 4, 2007, from http://www.icn.ch/visionstatement.htm

Joint Commission on Accreditation of Healthcare Organizations. (2004). *Hospital accreditation standards.* Oakbrook Terrace, IL: Author.

Kaakinen, J., Hanson, M., & Birenbaum, L. (2006). Family development and family nursing assessment. In M. Stanhope & J. Lancaster (Eds.), *Foundations of nursing in the community* (pp. 321–340). St. Louis, MO: Mosby.

Leavell, H., & Clark, A. (1965). *Preventive medicine for doctors in the community.* New York: McGraw-Hill.

National Center for Complementary and Alternative Medicine. (2007). Retrieved October 5, 2007, from http://nccam.nih.gov/

Office of Disease Prevention and Health Promotion, U.S. Department of Health and Human Services. (2001). *Healthy people in healthy communities.* Retrieved October 1, 2007, from http://www.healthypeople.gov/ Publications/HealthyCommunities2001/default.htm

Office of Disease Prevention and Health Promotion. (2006). *National Prevention Summit: Prevention, preparedness, and promotion.* Retrieved October 1, 2007, from http://www.healthierus.gov/steps/summit.html

Pender, N. (1982). *Health promotion in nursing practice.* Norwalk, CT: Appleton and Lange.

Pender, N., Murdaugh, C., & Parsons, M. (2006). *Health promotion in nursing practice.* Upper Saddle River, NJ: Pearson Education.

Pizzuti, D. (2006). The nurse in home health and hospice. In M. Stanhope & J. Lancaster (Eds.), *Foundations of nursing in the community* (pp. 587–609). St. Louis, MO: Mosby.

Researchers locate Type II Diabetes gene. Associated Press. (2004). Retrieved October 7, 2007, from http://www.msnbc.msn.com/id/6339987/

Robert Wood Johnson Foundation. (2000). *Definition of healthcare.* Retrieved August 31, 2008, from www.rwjf.org/reports/grr/036111.htm

Schumacher, K., Beck, C., & Marren, J. (2006). *American Journal of Nursing, 106*(8), 40–48.

U.S. Department of Health and Human Services. (2000). *Healthy People 2010: Understanding and improving health* (2nd ed.). Washington, DC: U.S. Government Printing Office.

U.S. Department of Health and Human Services. (2007). *U.S. Surgeon General's Family Initiative.* Retrieved October 7, 2007, from http://www.hhs.gov/ familyhistory/

Williams, C. (2006). Community-oriented nursing and community-based nursing. In M. Stanhope & J. Lancaster (Eds.), *Foundations of nursing in the community* (pp. 3–16). St. Louis, MO: Mosby.

World Health Organization. (2006). *WHO Constitution.* Retrieved October 4, 2007 from http://www.who .int/governance/eb/constitution/en/index.html

World Health Organization. (2007a). Retrieved October 4, 2007, from http://www.who.org

World Health Organization. (2007b). *Millennium development goals indicators.* Retrieved October 4, 2007, from http://millenniumindicators.un.org/unsd/mdg/Default .aspx

Chapter 8

The Healthcare Delivery System: Focus on Acute Care

CHAPTER OBJECTIVES

At the conclusion of this chapter, the learner will be able to:

- Discuss the corporatization of health care by comparing and contrasting for-profit and not-for-profit systems.
- Define the structure and process of an organization.
- Identify the types of hospital classifications.
- Identify the typical departments in a hospital and their services.
- Describe the healthcare provider team and its relationship to nursing.

- Discuss critical elements related to healthcare financial issues and reimbursement.
- Explain the importance of organizational culture.
- Discuss examples of changes in the healthcare delivery system.
- Describe how nursing fits into the overall hospital organization and how it functions.
- Explain how shared governance may empower nurses.

CHAPTER OUTLINE

KEY TERMS

- ❏ Annual limit
- ❏ Copayment
- ❏ Corporatization
- ❏ Deductible
- ❏ Empower
- ❏ For-profit
- ❏ Managed care
- ❏ Medicaid

- ❏ Medicare
- ❏ Not-for-profit
- ❏ Organizational culture
- ❏ Process
- ❏ Reimbursement
- ❏ Shared governance
- ❏ Structure

Introduction

Healthcare delivery is a complex process and system. The total system includes a variety of types of healthcare provider organizations, such as acute care organizations (hospitals), ambulatory care centers (clinics), private provider offices, community health facilities, home care agencies, hospice agencies, extended care facilities, and so on. Many of these were mentioned in Chapter 7. This chapter focuses on the largest type of healthcare organization: the acute care hospital. This does not mean that the others are not important; however, students typically spend more of their clinical time in hospitals. Many of the organizational elements of a hospital are similar to those of other healthcare organizations but may vary depending on the organization and purpose. The content in this chapter explores current issues related to hospitals, hospital organization and function, and the hospital provider team, and provides an introduction to healthcare financial issues and nursing organization and functions within the hospital.

Many factors impact hospitals, leading them to change their services, collaborate with others in their communities, realign their organization with other organizations, close because of financial issues, and so forth. What are some of the factors that influence hospitals today?

- Increase in healthcare costs
- Shortage of healthcare staff (nurses and other providers)
- Increased number of uninsured and underinsured who cannot pay for care
- Compromised access to care for some individuals, leading to disparities in healthcare services
- Improved technology that can improve care but that may be costly and require special staff training; may not be accessible to those who cannot pay
- Growing diversity in patients (consumers) and workforce—for example, the need for interpreter services and greater representation of ethnic groups in the healthcare workforce
- Increasing consumerism—more knowledgeable patients who demand more information and participation
- Hospital mergers and closings, altering access to services
- Shifting of beds and changing number of beds; changing specialty services (e.g., increasing the number of intensive care beds or eliminating obstetrical services)
- Changes in patient demographics that require reassessment of services and how

services are provided (e.g., increasing services for the elderly, immigrants, and single parents; expanding clinic hours to facilitate access; and so on)

Examples of key influences on health care are highlighted in Figure 8–1. Box 8–1 identifies examples of organizations that influence healthcare delivery.

Corporatization of Health Care: How Did We Get Here?

Using the term ***corporatization*** or *business* in association with a hospital may seem strange; however, health care is a business—a very large business. It provides services to most of the population at some time during a person's life. Hospitals have a very large employee pool and provide jobs for many people—both professionals and nonprofessionals—and represent one of the largest employment sectors. Within a community, healthcare organizations usually own or lease a large amount of property, purchase a great amount of supplies and equipment, have a large number of employees, and pay taxes, bringing income to the community. Typically, healthcare leaders hold significant positions in the business community. Health care consumes the largest amount of federal and state dollars through healthcare **reimbursement** programs such as **Medicare** and **Medicaid**.

For-Profit and Not-for-Profit: What Does This Mean?

The terms *for-profit* and *not-for-profit* can be confusing. The first critical point is that every hospital needs to make a profit, which means to have money left over after expenses are paid. The distinguishing characteristic between for-profit and not-for-profit is what is done with that profit. The assumption by most is that all

Figure 8–1 Influences on healthcare delivery.

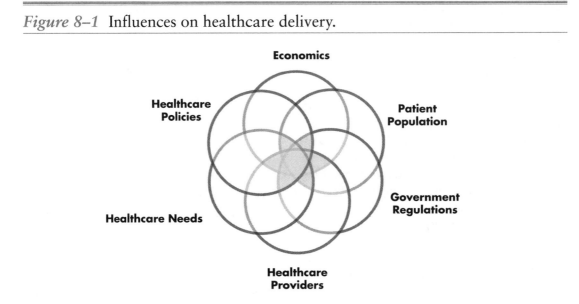

hospitals are not-for-profit, but this really has been changing. Many large healthcare organizations are for-profit corporations. Some of their profit must go to their stockholders/shareholders or to their owners. However, even for-profits must reinvest money into the hospital for maintenance, to expand buildings, to develop new services, and to purchase equipment, supplies,

---

BOX 8–1 EXAMPLES OF ORGANIZATIONS IMPORTANT TO THE HEALTHCARE DELIVERY SYSTEM

- National Association of Children's Hospitals and Related Institutions (NACHRI), http://www.childrens hospitals.net/AM/Template.cfm?Section=Homepage&Template=/customSource/homepage/homepage.cfm
- American Academy of Hospice and Palliative Medicine (AAHPM), http://www.aahpm.org/
- American Association of Homes and Services for the Aging (AAHSA), http://www2.aahsa.org/
- American Association of Retired Persons (AARP), http://www.aarp.org/
- American Health Care Association (AHCA), http://www.ahcancal.org/Pages/Default.aspx
- American Hospital Association (AHA), http://www.aha.org/aha/about/
- American Nurses Association (ANA), http://www.nursingworld.org/
- Nursing Specialty Organizations, http://www.nursingcenter.com/library/JournalArticle.asp?Article_ID=623779
- American Public Health Association (APHA), http://www.apha.org/
- Arthritis Foundation (AF), http://www.arthritis.org/
- American Diabetes Association (ADA), http://www.diabetes.org/home.jsp
- The Joint Commission http://www.jointcommission.org/
- National Association of Public Hospitals (NAPH), http://www.naph.org/
- National Committee on Quality Assurance (NCQA), http://web.ncqa.org/
- National Health Council (NHC), http://nationalhealthcouncil.org

and so on. Not-for-profits do not have stock-holders/shareholders, but these hospitals still need to make a profit for the same reasons that for-profits need a profit.

Why should nurses want to know if the hospital they work for is for-profit or not-for-profit? This information can help one to understand why and how decisions are made. For example, if a not-for-profit is burdened with a high number of nonpaying patients, the hospital may eventually spend more than it is making and thus be "in the red" as debt increases. When this happens, the hospital may cut staff, limit new equipment purchases, fail to maintain equipment ineffectively, attempt to reconfigure services to attract paying patients, and make many other changes to improve the hospital's financial condition. A for-profit healthcare organization must always have funds to pay stockholders or owners, and this can have an impact on the availability of money for other purposes that affect nurses and nursing.

The Healthcare Organization

Hospitals are one type of healthcare organization, and the largest. Other types of healthcare organizations are identified in Exhibit 8–1. All healthcare organizations can be described by their structure and process, and staff and organizational culture. Although the majority of RNs work in hospitals, many work in other healthcare organizations, and the percentage working in hospitals has decreased. Table 8–1 provides some data on employment settings.

This section of the chapter focuses on the acute care hospital as an example of a healthcare organization. How hospitals are organized does vary, but there are some standard types of organizations. In the past, it was more common to have a single hospital operating as a single organization. Now, more hospitals have formed complex organizations of multiple hospitals and, in some cases, these systems also include other healthcare entities such as home care agencies, rehabilitation centers, long-term care facilities, freestanding ambulatory care centers, and so on. Why has this occurred? Most of the reasons are related to financial issues and the survival of the organization—to keep patients in the system, increase services, and expand the continuum of care. Some communities have seen multiple changes in their hospitals, with hospitals switching systems or trying to go it alone. The critical message is that hospitals are changing their organization, and it is not clear what the future holds. Small hospitals with 100 beds or fewer and hospitals in rural areas are particularly vulnerable. They have difficulty filling beds and thus lose revenues (money coming in). In addition, they must keep costly equipment current, purchase new equipment, and maintain equipment and the physical facility. These

---

EXHIBIT 8–1 TYPES OF HEALTHCARE ORGANIZATIONS

- Substance Abuse Treatment Centers (inpatient and outpatient)
- School Health Clinics
- Diagnostic Centers
- Ambulatory Care Surgical Centers
- Dental Offices and Clinics
- Long-Term Care Facilities
- Skilled Nursing Facilities
- Occupational Health Clinics
- Acute Care Hospitals
- Physician Offices
- Advanced Practice Nurses Practice Sites
- Specialty Hospitals (e.g., pediatric)
- Long-Term Care Hospitals (e.g., psychiatric)
- Urgent Care Centers
- Home Health Agencies
- Hospice Care
- Ambulatory Care/Clinics

Table 8–1 Employment Settings of RNs over Time, Selected Years

	1980 % of		1992 % of		2004 % of	
	FTE RNs	Workforce	FTE RNs	Workforce	FTE RNs	Workforce
Hospital Care	713,242	67.5%	1,066,263	67.4%	1,195,498	58.6%
Physician and Clinical Services	76,402	7.2%	118,157	7.5%	233,636	11.4%
Home Health Care	16,033	1.5%	79,476	5.0%	96,818	4.7%
Nursing Home Care	80,313	7.6%	110,782	7.0%	131,518	6.4%
Public Health	58,199	5.5%	76,414	4.8%	133,173	6.5%
Nursing Education	37,081	3.5%	28,125	1.8%	50,558	2.5%
School Settings	30,148	2.9%	33,936	2.1%	53,942	2.6%
Industry/Occupational Settings	26,098	2.5%	17,143	1.1%	60,091	2.9%
Government and Other Settings	18,699	1.8%	50,875	3.2%	85,969	4.2%

Source: From *The Future of the Nursing Workforce in the United States: Data, Trends and Implications*, by P.I. Buerhaus, D.O. Staiger and D.I. Auerbach, 2009, Sudbury, MA: Jones and Bartlett Publishers. Data from National Sample Survey of Registered Nurses.

vulnerable hospitals also have problems recruiting registered nurses (RNs) given the shortage; many RNs prefer to work in urban centers and in large, up-to-date hospitals. Schools of nursing in states with large rural areas are increasingly partnering with rural hospitals to improve enrollment from these areas. These partnerships provide courses and clinical experiences in rural healthcare settings and use distance education to facilitate the programs.

Structure and Process

One way to describe a hospital is to consider its **structure** and **process**. A hospital's structure is based on how the organization is configured, and the best source for a view of a hospital's structure is its organizational chart. Figure 8–2 is an example of a hospital organizational chart.

The chart displays the components of the hospital. The structure can be described as vertical. The chart identifies whom staff report to, or rather, who is a staff member's manager or supervisor. Organizations that focus more on this type of structure tend to be bureaucratic and highly centralized, and decisions are made by key persons in the organization. Characteristics of bureaucratic organizations are:

1. Division of labor: descriptions of jobs that include clearly defined tasks
2. Defined hierarchy: clear description of the reporting relationships
3. Detailed rules and regulations: greater emphasis on policies and procedures; expectation that these will be followed and will guide decision making
4. Impersonal relationships: expectation that staff will do their jobs and that supervisors will ensure that jobs are done as expected

This bureaucratic organization is less common today; however, many hospitals still operate as bureaucratic organizations, emphasizing a vertical structure that includes these elements, but are less rigid. Line authority, or chain of command, is very important in that each staff member knows whom to report to, and it is

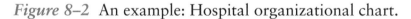

Figure 8–2 An example: Hospital organizational chart.

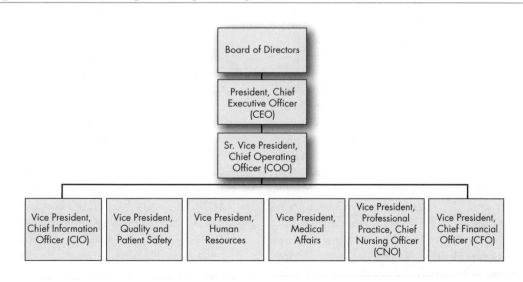

expected that this will be followed. A *true* bureaucratic organization does not expect or want much staff input regarding decisions.

Horizontal structure is decentralized, and emphasis is placed on departments or divisions; decisions are made closer to the staff who do the work. Departments or divisions are focused on special functions such as the nursing, laboratory, or dietary departments. Each of these focuses on a function—nursing care, laboratory tests, and nutrition and patient food services. This is called departmentalization. Structure includes the span of control, or the number of staff managed by each supervisor or manager. The more staff a manager supervises, the more complex that supervision becomes. The matrix organization structure is newer and less clear than the traditional bureaucratic organization that is centered on departments. In a matrix organization, staff might be part of a functional department, such as nursing services, but if the nurse works in behavioral health, he or she is also considered a staff member in the behavioral health services/department. This type of organization is considered "flatter" because decisions do not flow from the top down.

Hospitals typically use hierarchy management levels. The top level is the board of trustees or board of directors. This board typically includes members of the community and community leaders who are not directly involved in health care. The board is responsible for developing the overall direction of the hospital and ensuring that the goals of the organization are met. The chief executive officer (CEO) or president is hired by the board and reports to the board. The CEO then hires the other major leaders for the hospital, such as the chief financial officer and the nursing leader. The nursing leader may be the chief nursing executive (CNE), the chief nursing officer (CNO) or, in some cases, the vice president for nursing or patient services. This latter title may reflect oversight of other disciplines or ancillary services, such as occupational therapy, physical therapy, or nutrition. Often the board approves these hires. Because the board has ultimate responsibility for the budget, it has significant influence over matters that impact nurses, such as staffing and other resources important to nursing.

Process, the other dimension of organizations, focuses on how the organization functions. How would a staff member gain an understanding of a hospital's process? The hospital's vision, mission statement, and goals are a good place to begin to find out what is important to the organization and how the hospital describes itself and its functioning. Other sources of information relevant to process include policies and procedures, communication systems and expectations, decision-making processes, delegation, implementation of coordination (teams), and evaluation methods (quality improvement). Additional content on these topics is found in Section III in this textbook. The key question is, how does the work get done?

Classification of Hospitals

Hospitals can be classified using a variety of descriptors. The following are some of these descriptors:

- *Ownership*: Is the hospital for-profit (investor owned), not-for-profit, part of a corporate system, faith based, or government (state, federal)? The common government hospitals are the Veterans Administration (VA), military hospitals, state mental health hospitals, the National Institutes of Mental Health Clinical Center, and Indian Health Service hospitals.
- *Public access*: How much access does the general community have to the hospital's services? Is it a community or private hospital?
- *Number of beds*: Bed size, or the number of beds from hospital to hospital, can vary widely.

- *Licensure*: Licensure of hospitals is done by each state's health department, which ensures that hospitals meet certain state standards. Licensure and accreditation are not the same. Licensure comes from a government agency. Accreditation is a process to determine if a hospital meets certain minimal standards; the process is voluntary and is provided by a nongovernment organization. Chapter 12 discusses accreditation in relationship to quality. For hospitals to receive Medicare and Medicaid reimbursement—and this is an important source of income—they must be certified, or given authority by the Centers for Medicare and Medicaid Services (CMS), to provide services to Medicare and Medicaid recipients. Meeting all these requirements and participating in the surveys take staff time, which is costly, but it is very important for the financial status of an institution. In addition, hospitals that do not meet these requirements cannot be used as sites for clinical practice for healthcare professional students (nursing, medicine, and others).
- *Teaching*: A hospital is classified as a teaching hospital if it offers residency programs for physicians. The expansion of nurse residency programs may also become a method for classifying hospitals in the future, though this is unknown at this time.
- *Length-of-stay*: Length-of-stay (LOS) refers to how long patients typically stay in a hospital, and this is a range, or average LOS. Fewer than 30 days is referred to as short stay, and more than 30 days is long term. LOS has been decreasing in the last 15 years because of decreasing reimbursement of hospital care and a greater push to provide more healthcare services outside the hospital.
- *Multihospital system*: In the last 20 years, there has been a growth in large hospital systems that are really multiple hospitals;

these often include other types of provider organization services, such as hospice care, home care, long-term care, and others. This partnering provides the hospitals with a continuum of services, from acute care to longer term needs for their patients. In a sense, the system does not lose the patient; the patient just goes on to a different part of the system for additional care needs and may return for other services if needs change. For example, a patient has been in a hospital intensive care unit (ICU) for complications related to chronic obstructive pulmonary disorder. The patient returns home after discharge and receives home care. One week after discharge, the home care nurse assesses the patient and decides that he may need to be rehospitalized. The patient has pneumonia and is admitted back to the hospital.

Typical Departments in a Hospital

As was discussed in relation to the structure of organizations, hospitals are made up of departments. This structure has existed for a long time. Students need to be familiar with these departments because nurses interact with all of them at some point in their practice, and they need to know how to coordinate care using services from a variety of departments. What are some of the departments found in an acute care hospital? (Titles may vary from hospital to hospital, but the functions are typical and part of daily hospital operations.)

- *Administration*: This is the leadership for the hospital, the central decision-making source—for example, the CEO or administrator, assistant administrators, financial services and budget staff, and often the CNO, CNE, or vice president for nursing or patient services.
- *Nursing*: This is the largest department in terms of employee numbers. Often it is

called patient services, which is a newer title used in the last 15–20 years. This does not mean that patients receive only nursing care; many other departments are directly involved in patient care, such as laboratory, dietetic services, respiratory services, pharmacy, and others. However, nursing services is the 24-7 coordinator of patient care and provides the larger percentage of direct care to patients.

- *Medical Staff*: Physicians who practice in a hospital, if not part of a training program such as a residency or fellowship, must be members of the medical staff. Their credentials are reviewed, and they are given admitting privileges. This is done to ensure that standards are met. A director or chief of medical staff leads the medical staff.

- *Admission and Discharge*: This department manages all aspects of admission and discharge for patients, including paperwork, reimbursement, patient room assignments, and, in some cases, assignment of physicians. Case management may be part of this department or part of patient services.

- *Medical Records*: Documentation is a critical part of all aspects of care. This department provides oversight of documentation, whether hard copy documentation or information in a computerized system. It is a complex function and one that requires nursing input to ensure that nursing documentation needs are recognized and information is included.

- *Information Management:* This department ensures that required information is collected, analyzed, monitored, and summarized. It is directly related to medical records and documentation.

- *Infection Control*: This function has become increasingly important with the greater need to provide services that decrease infection risk. Nurses are very active staff members in this department; they develop policies and procedures, monitor infection rates, and train staff.

- *Evidence-Based Practice*: This department is one of the newest in hospitals, and not all hospitals have them. Some hospitals are incorporating the management of evidence-based practice (EBP)—medicine and nursing—into other departments, such as EBP for nursing. This department may be in nursing or patient services, quality improvement, or evidence-based medicine related to medical staff organization. EBP is one of the core competencies discussed in more detail in Chapter 11.

- *In-Service or Staff Development*: This is the department that implements orientation and education for staff.

- *Environmental Services* (housekeeping): Staff from this department interact with nurses in the patient care areas to ensure that areas are clean for patients.

Other departments focus on specific health needs, such as pharmacy, respiratory therapy, clinical laboratory, infusion therapy, occupational therapy, radiology, physical therapy, and social services. Nurses get involved in all these services. Hospitals are typically organized around clinical areas (units, services and in some cases, departments) such as medicine, surgery, intensive care (medical ICU, surgical ICU, cardiac care unit [CCU], neonatal ICU), post-anesthesia unit, labor and delivery, postpartum, nursery, gynecology, pediatrics, emergency, urgent care, psychiatric or behavioral health, ambulatory care, ambulatory care surgery, and dialysis. Clinical areas may also be specific to a specialty, such as medical units for post-CCU, referred to as step-down units, and oncology or surgical units that focus on orthopedics, urology, and so on.

Healthcare Providers: Who Is on the Team?

The hospital healthcare team is composed of a variety of healthcare providers, both professional and nonprofessional. All are important in the care process. In addition, many other staff are critical to the overall operation of a hospital, such as office support staff, dietary staff, housekeeping staff, facilities management and maintenance staff, transportation staff, medical records staff, communications (information technology) staff, equipment maintenance and repair staff, and many others. For the purposes of this textbook, the focus is on the staff who provide care, either direct care or indirect care, to a patient. A staff member who provides direct care, such as a nurse, comes in contact with the patient. An indirect care provider might be someone who works in the lab to complete a lab test, but he or she may never actually see the patient. However, the work done in the lab is very important to the patient's care. The group of providers who provide care to a patient is referred to as a team. They have a common purpose: providing patient care. Chapter 10 discusses teams in more detail; interdisciplinary teamwork is one of the five core competencies for all healthcare professionals. Nurses work with other nursing staff (RNs, licensed vocational nurses [LVNs]/licensed practical nurses [LPNs], and assistants on teams) to provide care; however, today, there is greater emphasis on the need for interdisciplinary or interprofessional teams in which nurses collaborate and coordinate with members of multiple disciplines, such as physicians, pharmacists, social workers, and many more members as described next.

Who might be on the healthcare team, and what are their main functions? The following are some of the major team members. Not all patients require services from all these healthcare professionals. Services are based on individual patient needs.

- *Registered Nurses* (RNs): Nurses are the backbone of any acute care hospital. They work in a great variety of positions and departments, not just the nursing department. Nurses also work in medical records, quality improvement, infusion therapy, case management, staff development, radiology, and ambulatory care, among other departments. Some nurses are in management positions and may not provide direct care.
- *Nurse Practitioner*: A nurse practitioner (NP) is an RN with a master's degree in a specialty; he or she can provide some services independently of physician orders, such as prescribing certain medications and treatment procedures. NPs may work in clinics but typically do not work in acute care units, though this is changing. In some states, NPs may have admitting privileges along with their prescriptive authority (i.e., the right to prescribe medication).
- *Clinical Nurse Specialist*: A clinical nurse specialist (CNS) is an RN with a master's degree. He or she is prepared to provide care in acute care settings and guides the care provided by other RNs. Examples of CNS specialties are cardiac care and behavioral health (psychiatry). This advanced practice nurse may have prescriptive authority, and if so, usually only for specific types of medications. Typically, CNSs do not prescribe medications as often as NPs.
- *Clinical Nurse Leader*: The clinical nurse leader (CNL) is a new position. This nurse has a master's degree and is a "provider and a manager of care at the point of care to individuals and cohorts. The CNL designs, implements, and evaluates client care by

coordinating, delegating and supervising the care provided by the healthcare team, including licensed nurses, technicians, and other health professionals" (American Association of Colleges of Nursing, 2007, p. 6).

- *Nurse Midwife*: A nurse midwife (NM) has a master's degree and is prepared to provide women's health services and services to obstetrical patients. In some states, NMs may have admitting privileges. Their scope of practice may be regulated under either the medical or nursing practice act, depending on the state. These nurses are certified and referred to as CNMs.

- *Nurse Anesthetist*: A nurse anesthetist (NA) has a master's degree and is prepared to provide services to those patients requiring anesthesia. These nurses are usually referred to as CRNAs because they are certified registered nurse anesthetists.

- *Physician* (MD): An MD has a medical degree and typically has a specialty such as surgery, medicine, pediatrics, or obstetrics and gynecology, and he or she may even have a subspecialty. For example, a physician with a specialty in internal medicine may subspecialize in rheumatology, dermatology, oncology, or neurology. A surgeon may specialize in orthopedics, oncology (and even more specialized in breast surgery), and so on. In a teaching hospital, which has medical students and residents, the typical team includes faculty/attending, chief resident, residents, interns, and medical students.

- *Licensed Practical/Vocational Nurse*: An LPN/LVN is a member of the nursing staff who has completed a 1-year nursing program that specifically trained him or her to be an LPN/LVN and to take the LPN/LVN licensing exam. These nurses are supervised by RNs and are important team members. The state board of nursing determines what care they may provide. It is important for RNs to know what LPNs/LVNs are allowed to do and to provide supervision for this care. RNs can delegate to LPNs/LVNs but not the reverse. Delegation is discussed in Chapter 10.

- *Occupational Therapist* (OT): OTs are not present in every hospital, but they provide important services for patients with rehabilitation needs due to impaired functioning, such as stroke patients or patients who have experienced a serious automobile accident. Another type of therapist that might be used, especially for stroke patients, is a speech-language pathologist. These types of therapists are found commonly in rehabilitation services but can be provided in all types of settings, such as in hospitals, in long-term care facilities, and in home care.

- *Patient Care Assistants* or *Nursing Assistants*: Patient care assistants or certified nursing assistants may have a variety of titles. They are nonprofessional staff who have a short training period (typically a few months) to provide direct care, such as activities of daily living (bathing, vital signs, and so on). They are supervised by RNs and are important members of the team.

- *Pharmacist*: The pharmacist has completed professional education and ensures that pharmaceutical care is appropriate for patient needs. With the growing concern about medication errors, pharmacists are important members of the team, and nurses should work closely with them. Some hospitals have a centralized department, with all pharmaceutical services coming from a central unit. Others have moved to include pharmacists as direct team members on units, providing an invaluable service at the point-of-care.

- *Physical Therapist*: Physical therapists provide musculoskeletal care to patients, such as assisting with teaching stroke patients how to walk, to use crutches, or to use other assistive devices, and helping design exercises to ensure or increase mobility.
- *Registered Dietitian* (RD): Dietitians work with patients to help resolve dietary and nutritional needs. Nurses work with them as patient dietary needs are identified.
- *Respiratory Therapist*: Respiratory therapists (RTs) provide care to patients who have a variety of respiratory problems. RTs are trained to provide specific types of treatments, such as oxygen therapy, inhalation therapy, intermittent positive pressure ventilators, and artificial mechanical ventilators. RTs come to the patient's bedside for these treatments, and some RTs may be assigned to work solely in intensive care units, where there is great need for these treatments. RTs are also part of the team that responds to codes when patients experience cardiac or respiratory arrests.
- *Social Worker*: Social workers (SWs) have professional degrees and assist patients and their families with such issues as reimbursement, discharge concerns, housing, transportation, and other social services. Nurses work with SWs to identify patient issues that need to be resolved in order to decrease stress on patients and families. An SW may serve as a case manager, but many case managers are RNs.

One of the newest members of the healthcare team is the hospitalist, or the intensivist. This position usually is an MD, though some NPs and CNS-Bs hold this position in some hospitals. The hospitalist is a generalist MD who covers patients as the primary provider while the patient is in the hospital, and he or she coordinates the care. The patient's primary provider outside the hospital is not involved in the inpatient care, and the patient returns to that provider after discharge. This reduces the time that the primary care provider (PCP) (internist, family practitioner, pediatrician) has to devote to inpatient care. Thus, the PCP has more time to focus on the outpatient needs of his or her patients. In addition, the hospitalist is more current with acute care and the treatment required. The intensivist is similar to the hospitalist, but this MD focuses on care of patients in intensive care, which is a more specialized area of care. These two positions were developed to increase coordination and continuity of care. Both of these providers are paid by the hospital as hospital employees. A major disadvantage of this model of medical care is that the patient has no relationship with the hospitalist or the intensivist prior to hospitalization and will not have any contact with him or her after hospitalization. Patients may complain about this to nurses and may actually turn to nurses for advice because they often develop a stronger relationship with the people who care for them 24-7. Exhibit 8–2 identifies some of the benefits of using hospitalists and intensivists.

Healthcare Financial Issues

Healthcare financial issues can be viewed from three perspectives. The first is the micro view, which focuses on a specific healthcare organization and its budget. Nurses are not usually involved in the development of budgets unless they are in a management position; however, it is important for nurses to understand what a

---

Exhibit 8–2 Benefits of Hospitalists/Intensivists

Benefits for the patient due to expertise of the hospitalist/intensivists

- Clear and timely explanations about care
- Rapid access to physician to solve patient needs 24 hours a day
- Rapid physician response to emergencies
- Continued access to other specialists as needed
- Reduction in the length-of-stay
- Decreased utilization of resources, improving resources management
- Enhanced coordination with other participants in an integrated delivery model
- Reduced risk of untoward events

Benefits to the patient's personal physician

- Enhanced economic security
- Referral to specialists remains unchanged
- Enhanced productivity/revenue gain for group practice
- Improved clinical outcomes
- Enhanced training programs

Benefits to care providers on the hospital team, including nurses

- Increased communication and coordination among the care team
- Cost containment by control of formulary, procedures, and purchased goods
- Shared responsibility for outcomes
- Consistent approach to care with immediate response
- Improved access to physicians

Benefits to the hospital and payers

- Reduction in the variability of care
- Reduction in the length-of-stay
- Decreased utilization of resources
- Enhanced coordination with all other participants of an integrated delivery model
- Reduced risk of liability

Source: Adapted from "The Hospitalist: The New Addition to the Inpatient Management Team," by B. Noyes and S. Healy, 1999, *Journal of Nursing Administration*, 29(2), pp. 21–24. Reprinted with permission.

---

budget is and why it is important. The second perspective is the macro view, or the status of healthcare finances viewed from a national or a state perspective. The third perspective focuses on payment of care or reimbursement.

The Nation's Health Care: Financial Status (Macro View)

The United States as a nation spends a lot of money on health care. Reimbursement issues, which are discussed in a later section of this chapter, play a major role in the status of health care and coverage of these expenses. Figure 8–3 describes the nation's healthcare dollar: How much is spent on different categories of services, and where does the money come from for these services?

Figure 8–4 describes the actual and projected national Medicare healthcare expenditures for specific years. Are these expenditures changing? Yes they are, and they are increasing.

Figure 8–3 The nation's healthcare dollar.

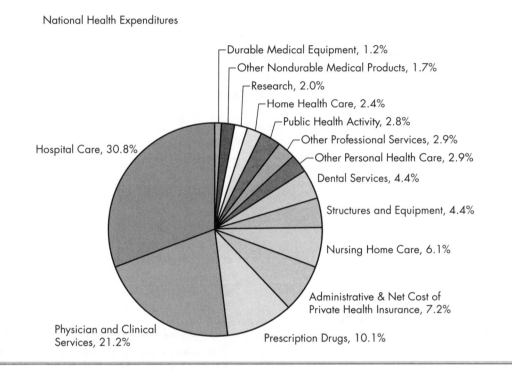

National Health Expenditures

Durable Medical Equipment, 1.2%
Other Nondurable Medical Products, 1.7%
Research, 2.0%
Home Health Care, 2.4%
Public Health Activity, 2.8%
Other Professional Services, 2.9%
Other Personal Health Care, 2.9%
Dental Services, 4.4%
Structures and Equipment, 4.4%
Nursing Home Care, 6.1%
Administrative & Net Cost of Private Health Insurance, 7.2%
Prescription Drugs, 10.1%
Physician and Clinical Services, 21.2%
Hospital Care, 30.8%

Source: From *The Future of the Nursing Workforce in the United States: Data, Trends and Implications*, by P.I. Buerhaus, D.O. Staiger and D.I. Auerbach, 2009, Sudbury, MA: Jones and Bartlett Publishers. Data from National Health Expenditures, Centers for Medicare and Medicaid Services.

The Individual Healthcare Organization and Its Financial Needs (Micro View)

The hospital budget is used by every hospital to manage its financial issues. The budget is prepared for a specific time period, such as a year. In addition, a longer term plan covering several years is prepared, though this often must be adjusted because of changes in the organization's financial status. The budget describes the expected expenses, such as staff salaries and benefits, equipment, supplies, utilities, pharmaceutical needs, facility maintenance, dietary needs, administrative services, staff education, legal fees, parking and security, and so on. The budget also describes the projected revenues, or money coming into the organization. It is very important that nursing management participate in the budget process because the budget has a major impact on nurses and nursing care. The final approval of the budget is made by the board of directors. After a budget is approved and implemented, it is important that budgetary data are monitored on a regular basis and that this information is shared with all managers. This monitoring is done to better ensure that the budget goals are met and to facilitate early recognition of budget issues that may require adjustment.

Figure 8–4 Overall Medicare spending: 1980 actual through 2016 projected.

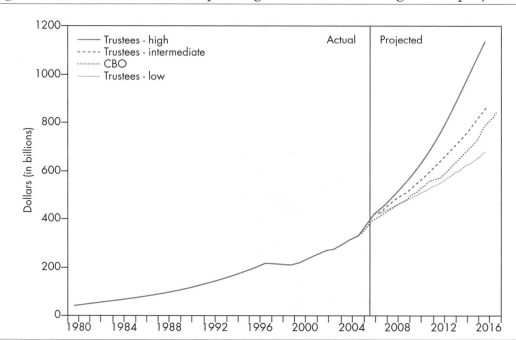

Note: CBO (Congressional Budget Office). All data are nominal, gross program outlays (mandatory plus administrative expenses) by calendar year.

Source: Medicare Trustees Report 2007. CBO March 2007 baseline.

Reimbursement: Who Pays for Health Care?

Reimbursement is a critical topic in healthcare, and it is complex. It represents the third perspective of healthcare financial issues. Nursing students may wonder why this topic is relevant to them or even to nurses in general. Basically, reimbursement pays the patient's bill for services provided, and reimbursement in turn covers costs of care, such as staff salaries and benefits; drugs; medical supplies; physician fees; facility maintenance and upgrades; equipment; general supplies; and much more. The health-

care delivery system is long past focusing on charity care.

Hospitals that do not bring in enough money to pay their bills are said to be operating "in the red," and this is not a good position for a hospital to be in. It means that the hospital cannot pay all its bills. Most hospitals are operating in the red, but how far in the red the hospital is can make the difference between modernizing or filling staff positions, and not—and whether the hospital "keeps open for business." Some hospitals in this country have closed. Particularly hard-hit are hospitals in rural areas and small hospitals that are not able to compete for patients. This has a major impact on access to care. Some patients may not have a local hospital for needed services, or even for emergency services. Some people may have to travel long distances for obstetrical care or specialized care for children (pediatrics, neonatal care for newborns), mental health services, oncology (diagnosis and treatment), complex surgical procedures, and many other services.

The United States is experiencing a serious crisis in its safety net hospitals. These are public hospitals that serve the populations who have limited or no resources to pay for services. This does not mean that these hospitals do not or could not serve patients with excellent reimbursement; however, it is typically the case that the majority of their patients do not have sufficient reimbursement. The patients are also more complex; many are vulnerable and have had limited preventive care. Some have chronic medical conditions that have not been treated. Other complications include socioeconomic problems, language issues, and immigrant status, all of which contribute to the need for complex healthcare treatment.

> *Though Grady Memorial Hospital (Atlanta, Georgia) is among the distressed of the country's 1,300 public hospitals, others have faced similar challenges in recent years, including those in Miami, Memphis, and Chicago. . . . There are 300 fewer public hospitals today than 15 years ago, with hospitals having closed in Los Angeles, Washington, St. Louis, and Milwaukee. . . . A third of the hospital's patients, including those treated as outpatients, are uninsured, among them a rapidly growing group of immigrants . . . the National Association of Public Hospitals says its members account for 2 percent of all hospitals, but provide 25 percent of the nation's uncompensated care. (Dewan & Sack, 2008, p. A18)*

It is clear that the safety net hospital system is not operating effectively and cannot meet the complex needs of vulnerable populations today.

It is important for nurses to understand basic information about reimbursement. Patients today frequently worry about payment for care. Questions that arise are: Do patients have insurance coverage? How much of their care will be covered by insurance, and will they get the treatment they need from the providers they prefer? Experiencing an illness is difficult for any patient and his or her family, and to add worry about payment for services to this stress can have an impact on a patient's health as well as his or her response to the health problem. This stress can impact whether patients can follow treatment recommendations. Can the patient afford the medications, or would the costs compromise his or her ability to buy food or pay rent? Can the patient afford to take a bus or taxicab to a doctor's appointment? Can the patient afford to take off work for an appointment? None of this is simple.

THE THIRD-PARTY PAYER SYSTEM

The U.S. healthcare delivery system is funded primarily through a third-party payer system (insurance), with healthcare services paid by someone other than the patient. Examples of third-party payers are Blue Cross, Humana, Medicaid, and Medicare. The patient pays for part of the care, but the payment for most patients goes through another party, the insurer (the third-party payer). Typically, the patient or enrollee in the insurance policy covers the enrollee as part of a group, which is the most likely through the enrollee's employer healthcare policies. An individual can also buy insurance to cover himself or herself, but this is expensive and not as common. Typically, these persons do not have access to employer healthcare insurance (e.g., someone who is self-employed).

Fee-for-service is the most common reimbursement model in the United States. In this model, physicians or other providers, such as hospitals, bill separately for each patient encounter or service that they provide rather than receiving a salary or a set payment per patient enrolled. The third-party payer actually pays the bills, but the enrollee usually has some payment responsibilities that vary from one policy to another. This is a complex area, so nurses, as consumers of health care and as healthcare providers, need to understand the basics. Enrollees (patients) may pay any or all of the following:

- **Deductible:** This is the part of the bill that the patient must pay before the insurer will pay the bill for the services. After the patient pays that amount due per year, no further deductible is paid by the patient for that year.
- **Copayment**/coinsurance: This is the fixed amount that a patient may be required to pay per service (MD visit, lab test, prescription, and so on). This is typically a small amount; for example, $10 per physician visit.

Both the deductible and the copayment represent the patient's out-of-pocket expenses each year, in addition to the annual fee that the employee pays for the coverage. Employers also pay a portion of the annual insurance fee. Fees vary from policy to policy and from one employer to another. There is no requirement in the United States that every employer provide healthcare insurance coverage.

Annual limits are also important. This means that enrollees have a defined amount that they would have to pay—a maximum amount—and after that level is reached, they no longer have to contribute to the payment. For example, the employee or enrollee has bills of over $5,000, and the annual limit is $5,000. This enrollee or patient would not have to pay any more for care that year after paying $5,000; thereafter, the patient is 100% covered for care. Employees may include their families on their employer insurance coverage. Typically, employees have to pay more per year for family insurance, and there may be different requirements for the family (e.g., a higher annual limit). Another critical element of reimbursement is a preexisting condition. This is a medical condition that a person has developed before he or she applies for a particular health insurance policy; this condition could affect the person's (enrollee or employee) ability to get coverage or how much the enrollee has to pay for it. What is considered a preexisting condition varies from one policy to another, but it is important for the enrollee to understand what these are because it can have a major impact on the costs to the enrollee. Table 8–2 describes expenditures from the perspective of out-of-pocket expenses, private insurance, and public reimbursement.

Managed Care

Managed care has been in existence since the 1920s, but it has become more common since the 1980s. Today, it is an integral part of the reimbursement system. What is managed care? This is a method used to reimburse or pay for healthcare services, but it includes more than just payment. This reimbursement method also controls the delivery services—for example, by identifying the type of provider that may be seen, even to the extent of identifying specific names of providers; controlling how many physician visits or how many days a patient may stay in the hospital; and identifying the types of medications that may be prescribed. Managed care organizations may also monitor providers to ensure that the providers are staying within certain ranges regarding type of procedure, lab tests, medications, and so on. If the providers do not meet

Table 8–2 An Example of Out-of-Pocket Expenses

Physician's charge for GYN visit	$150
Insurer's charge for GYN visit (amount insurer will pay)	$100
Patient's copayment of 30% ($100 × .30)	$30
Uncovered part of the bill; must be paid by patient ($150 – $100)	$50
Copayment ($30) + uncovered portion ($50)	$80

these criteria, they may be denied payment. Most consumers think of health maintenance organizations (HMOs) as managed care, and they are. There are, however, many other forms of managed care. Another common model is the preferred provider organization (PPO), in which the enrollee is given a list of providers, and to receive reimbursement of services, the enrollee must use a provider on this identified list. In an HMO, an enrollee typically has less choice about providers. Traditional third-party insurance focuses only on payment for services and is not involved in the services aspect as managed care has been.

Government Reimbursement of Healthcare Services

State and federal governments cover a large portion of the healthcare costs in the United States, but there is no universal coverage, meaning that not all citizens have healthcare coverage. The United States is one of the few industrialized countries that do not have universal coverage. There are several types of government-sponsored reimbursement.

The largest programs are Medicare and Medicaid, which are managed by the CMS, Department of Health and Human Services. Medicare was established in 1965 by Title XVIII, amendment to the Social Security Act. Medicare is the federal health insurance program for people aged 65 and older, persons with disabilities, and people with end-stage renal disease. Medicare had about 41 million beneficiaries in 2003, and this number increases each year. The need for Medicare coverage is growing because of the increase in the population over age 65. Medicare covers hospital services (Part A) and physician and outpatient care (Part B), and it offers coverage for prescriptions. Enrollees have to pay a portion of costs for Part B and prescriptions. Medicare does not pay for long-term care but does cover some skilled nursing and home health care for specific conditions. The CMS sets standards and monitors Medicare services and payment. Many patients in acute care today are covered by Medicare. It is a very important part of the U.S. healthcare delivery system that supports older citizens and other identified populations; however, there is concern about financing this program in the future because of the increase in the number of citizens who will be 65 and older.

Medicaid, established in 1965 by Title XIX of the Social Security Act, is the federal/state program for certain categories of low-income people. Medicaid covers health and long-term care services for over 51 million Americans, including children, the aged, the blind, disabled persons, and people who are eligible to receive federally assisted income maintenance payments, and this number is increasing. This program is funded by both federal funds and state funds, but each state sets its own guidelines and administers the state's Medicaid program. The Federal Poverty Guidelines, the annual income level for poverty defined by the federal government, are important in identifying people who meet coverage criteria for Medicaid reimbursement. Table 8–3 describes the poverty guidelines for 2007.

What does Medicaid cover? Services include inpatient care (excluding psychiatric or behavioral health); outpatient care with certain stipulations; laboratory and radiology services; care provided by certified pediatric and family nurse practitioners when licensed to practice under state law; nursing facility services (long-term care) for beneficiaries aged 21 and older; early and periodic screening, diagnosis, and treatment for children under 21; family planning services and supplies; physician services; medical and surgical dentist services; home health for beneficiaries who are entitled to nursing facility services under the state's Medicaid plan; NM services;

pregnancy-related services and services for other conditions that might complicate pregnancy; and 60-days postpartum pregnancy-related services. There is a second group of eligible persons: the medically needy. These are persons who have too much money (which may be in savings) to be eligible categorically for Medicaid but require extensive care that would consume all their resources. Each state must include the following in this group: pregnant women through a 60-day postpartum period; children under the age of 18; certain newborns for 1 year; and certain protected blind persons. States may add others to this list. The federal government requires that each state cover, at a minimum, persons who qualify for Aid to Families with Dependent Children; all needy children under 21; those who qualify for Old-Age Assistance; those who qualify for Aid to the Blind; persons who are permanently or totally disabled; and those over 65 who are on welfare.

The government also reimburses care through the military, the VA, the Federal Employees

Table 8–3 2007 HEALTH AND HUMAN SERVICES POVERTY GUIDELINES

Persons in Family or Household	48 Contiguous States and D.C.	Alaska	Hawaii
1	$10,210	$12,770	$11,750
2	13,690	17,120	15,750
3	17,170	21,470	19,750
4	20,650	25,820	23,750
5	24,130	30,170	27,750
6	27,610	34,520	31,750
7	31,090	38,870	35,750
8	34,570	43,220	39,750
For each additional person, add	3,480	4,350	4,000

Source: Federal Register, Vol. 72, No. 15, January 24, 2007, pp. 3147–3148.

Health Benefit Program (FEHBP), and state insurance programs for state employees.

- Military health care: In this system, the government not only pays for the care but also is the provider of the care through military hospitals and other healthcare services. The military also covers care of dependents whose care may or may not be provided at a military facility.
- U.S. Department of Veterans Affairs: The VA provides services to veterans at VA facilities and covers the cost of these services. VA hospitals are found across the country and provide acute care; ambulatory care; pharmaceutical, rehabilitation, and specialty services; and, in some cases, care at long-term care facilities.
- Federal Employees Health Benefit Program: This reimbursement for federal employees is mandated by law. Over 10 million federal employees, retirees, and their dependents are covered. Enrollees choose from a variety of healthcare insurance plans as part of the FEHBP benefit program. This is just a reimbursement program; it is not involved in the actual delivery of services.
- State insurance programs: States offer health insurance to their state employees. Typically, the state government is the largest employer in a state and thus the state's largest insurer. State employees choose from a variety of plans and contribute to the coverage in the same way that non–state employees pay into their employer health programs.

The Uninsured and the Underinsured

The United States has experienced a growing number of people who are not insured or who are underinsured (i.e., they do not have enough insurance coverage to pay for their needs). The federal government estimates that during 2006, 47 million individuals lacked health insurance coverage of any kind. Other research indicates that tens of millions more Americans go without health coverage for shorter periods. Data about this problem include the following (Cover the Uninsured, 2007; Reuters Health Information, 2007):

- Recent U.S. Census Bureau data show that the problem of the uninsured continued in 2006. According to figures released in August 2007, 47 million people—15.8% of the total U.S. population—were uninsured in 2006, up slightly from 15.3% in the previous year (2005).
- The percentage of the uninsured non-elderly population has climbed steadily, from 15.2% in 1994 to 17.2% in 2005.
- In 2006, the number of people with employer health insurance decreased by 2.3 million.
- Nearly 60% of children are covered by their parents' employer coverage. In 2006, 3.4 million fewer children had these benefits than in 2003.
- Thirty-eight states had significant decreases in employer benefits for people younger than 65.

The uninsured and underinsured are in great need of healthcare services—preventive, ongoing, acute, and chronic care. They have complex needs related to housing, finances, food, transportation, and education. Discharge planning to meet these needs should include a thorough assessment of the patient's needs at home and a plan to ensure that patients receive the care they need posthospitalization. The example of Grady Memorial Hospital discussed earlier in the chapter demonstrates how these complex and vulnerable populations in need of care are at serious risk for not being able to access the care they need, and in some cases, can no longer access care when needed.

Organizational Culture

Typically, *culture* refers to an individual person's culture, the culture of a group in a country, or a country's culture, but there is also **organizational culture**. What does this mean? Curtin (2001) described organizational culture in this way:

> *There is in each institution an implicit, invisible, intrinsic, informal, and yet instantly recognizable* welenschaung *that is best described as "corporate culture." Like most important things, it is difficult to define or even describe. It is not "corporate climate," "organizational climate," or "corporate identity." The corporate culture embodies the organizational values that implicitly and explicitly specify norms, shape attitudes, and guide the behaviors of the members of the organization. (p. 219)*

Organizational culture has an impact on nursing. First, the overall healthcare organization has a culture. Nursing within an organization also has a culture; the nursing department and even separate divisions or units can have different cultures. New staff members need to get to know the culture of the organizations that they are considering for employment. Students may be able to identify cultural issues in the units where they have practicum.

Two major terms are used to describe organizational culture: *dissonant* and *consonant*. Hospital leaders need to be aware of the state of the organization's culture. A dissonant culture means that the organization is not functioning effectively. Characteristics of these organizations are (Jones & Redman, 2000, p. 605):

- Unclear individual staff and department expectations (*Staff do not know what they*

should be doing and how they should be working.)
- Lack of consistent measurement of quality of service (*Data from quality assessment lead to improvement, but a dysfunctional organization is not as interested in improvement.*)
- Organized to serve the staff (providers of care) instead of serving the consumers (patients) (*Consumers are less important, and thus services will not focus on consumer needs.*)
- Limited concern for employee welfare (*Employees are seen as workers and not valued.*)
- Limited education and training of staff (*Educated staff members lead to better care and improvement, but the dysfunctional organization is not interested in improvement and better patient outcomes or has difficulty providing education that is of benefit to the staff.*)
- Frequent disagreements among staff that relate to control (turf battles) (*This indicates a high stress level among staff and thus impacts effective functioning.*)
- Lack of patient involvement in decision making (*Lack of interest in consumers impacts the type of product produced or the care provided.*)
- Limited recognition of staff accomplishment. (*Organization does not value staff.*)

The goal is to develop and maintain a consonant culture, or a functional and effective organization—one that would do the opposite of each of the characteristics of a dissonant organization.

People like to work in organizations that are effective, creative, and productive. How does an organization attain these characteristics? First, the hospital's formal framework lays the groundwork for this type of effective workplace. This includes the hospital's structure, chain of command, rules and regulations, and policies and procedures. The hospital's vision and mission statements are important. The vision statement describes the hospital's values and its view of the future, and it provides direction for the organization. The mission statement describes the hospital's purpose. Another way of understanding mission and vision: The mission describes the current state of the organization, and the vision is what the organization aspires to be. Hospitals also identify goals and objectives that flow from the vision and mission statements. All these are part of the organization's process and are very important to the organization's culture. The vision, mission, goals, and objectives should not be filed away, but rather implemented in the hospital's process and in its structure.

What aspects of a hospital organization should be assessed when determining its culture? It is not always easy to describe an organization's culture. The first response to an organization's culture is a gut feeling that a person has when he or she enters the hospital and observes its physical appearance, how staff respond, the ease of finding one's way around, services set up for the consumer, and so on. The following are other considerations.

- The organization's structure and process
- Communication (types, effectiveness, who is included in communication, level of secrecy, information overload, timeliness of communication, and so on)
- Acceptance of new staff (who become members of the organization)
- Willingness of staff to listen to new ideas
- Inclusion of staff in decision making
- Morale
- Vacancies and turnover
- Acceptance of students (all types of healthcare professions)
- Patients feeling positive about their care experiences
- Visitors feeling welcomed

Nurses usually know which hospitals are functional (consonant) organizations in the communities in which they live and practice. They share this information with colleagues, and this can have an impact on recruitment of new staff.

Chapter 9 includes information about diversity in health care; however, it needs to be noted here that workforce diversity and patient diversity impact the hospital's culture. The organization's culture is affected by all the people who work in the organization and all the people who interact with the organization, such as the patients and their families. Workforce diversity has become a critical issue in health care. There is need for greater diversity in all healthcare professions. Labor laws affect this diversity. Title VII of the Civil Rights Act of 1964 and Executive Order 11246 prohibit employer discrimination on the basis of race, color, religion, sex, or national origin. The Americans with Disabilities Act of 1990 prohibits discrimination due to disability, including mental illness, if the person can complete the job requirements. These are all federal laws and are applied to any hospital that receives federal funds such as Medicare or Medicaid reimbursement. This really means nearly all hospitals, because few do not provide services to patients covered by these two payment systems. Language is also an issue that will be discussed further in Chapter 9. Hospitals need to have access to interpreters to communicate with patients if staff cannot do so.

Another view of the hospital's culture is critical to its effectiveness and has become more recognized in the last 10 years: Is the environment a healing environment? This is just as difficult to define or describe as organizational culture. Some of the issues considered when assessing the environment are (1) the privacy provided, (2) air quality, (3) noise levels, (4) views from windows, and (5) visual characteristics. The needs of patients can vary and thus impact the type of healing environment needed. The elderly may require more safety measures to prevent falls, but if this is done by constraining patients, the person's view of the environment may be impacted. Constraining a patient may prevent injury, but he or she may feel "imprisoned." The elderly often have problems hearing and can tolerate more noise. Others may not be able to tolerate a lot of noise and may complain that they cannot sleep in the hospital. As described in Chapter 1, Nightingale's view of care was associated with healing and the patient's need for fresh air, cleanliness, quiet, diet, and light. Other aspects of a healing environment include what the site looks like—use of color, sameness or variety, sense of warmth in furnishings, type of artwork on the walls, and so on. Some colors are more peaceful than others. Is the architecture patient centered? Planetree is a nonprofit organization concerned with the environmental impact of the delivery system on health care. It is one example of a model of healing in health care. The focus in this model is on body, mind, and spirit, with active patient and family involvement. Hospitals that meet specific criteria can be designated as Planetree Hospitals. This patient-centered healing environment model emphasizes the principles found in Exhibit 8–3.

Changes in Healthcare Delivery

Historically, hospitals have experienced much change. In earlier chapters, it was noted that hospitals had a significant role to play in nursing education, but their most important new role is the provision of healthcare services to their communities. What has been the history of hospitals? The reengineering of health care, or the redesigning of how care is provided and how the organization functions, has led to major changes in organizations. Many healthcare organizations have undergone some level of reengineering in the last decade. This might include remodeling, restructuring, developing new services, and improving processes and systems, or perhaps decreasing services. A major response to the shortage of healthcare workers has been to redesign how work is done and by whom. If

---

EXHIBIT 8–3 PLANETREE COMPONENTS

Human Interactions
Planetree is about human beings caring for and serving other human beings. This involves not only the provision of nurturing, compassionate, personalized care to patients and families, but just as important, how staff care for themselves and each other; and, how organizations create cultures which support and nurture their staffs. Experiential staff retreats sensitize staff to the anatomy of a hospital experience from the patient's perspective and better enable them to holistically serve the patient. Healing partnerships between patients, family members and caregivers are encouraged by a care model which enables patients to be active participants in their health care.

Architectural & Interior Design Conducive to Health & Healing
Planetree firmly believes that the physical environment is vital to the healing process of the patient. Facility design should include efficient layouts which support patient dignity and personhood. Domestic aesthetics, art and warm home-like, non-institutional designs which value humans, not just technology, are emphasized. Architectural barriers which inhibit patient control and privacy as well as interfere with family participation are removed. Awareness of the symbolic messages communicated by design is essential.

   Designing and maintaining an uncluttered environment encourages patient mobility and a sense of "safe shelter." The design of a Planetree facility provides patients and families with spaces for both solitude and social activities, and includes libraries, kitchens, lounges, activity rooms, chapels, and gardens. Comfortable space and accommodations are provided for families to stay overnight. Healing gardens, fountains, fish tanks and waterfalls are provided to connect patients, families and staff with the relaxing, invigorating, healing, and meditative aspects of nature.

It is just as essential to create healing environments for the staff as it is for patients. Physicians, nurses and ancillary staff are very much affected by their working environment. It is very hard to help patients heal and recover in inhospitable, cold and impersonal spaces. Lounges and sacred space for staff are an important component in the creation of a healing environment.

The Importance of the Nutritional and Nurturing Aspects of Food

Nutrition is recognized as an integral part of health and healing essential not only for good health, but as a source of pleasure, comfort and familiarity. With all the scientific data demonstrating the role of nutrition in health and disease, health care facilities have a responsibility to be role models for delicious, healthy eating. This can be accomplished by making low-fat entree selections available in the cafeteria, as well as healthy choices in vending machines. Kitchens on the floor encourage families to prepare favorite foods or meals for their loved ones. They also serve as gathering places, much as they do in our homes, for patients and families, and thus help create spontaneous support groups.

Cooking demonstrations and classes are provided by nutritionists and volunteers. Nutrition education focuses on not only the patient's current illness but on healthy living for the whole family. Volunteer bakers bake breads, muffins and cookies to provide "aromatherapy," and to create a nurturing environment.

Empowering Patients Through Information and Education

Planetree's patient-centered model of care and consumer-sensitive healing approach is an idea whose time has truly come. In this era of health care consumerism, there is a rapidly expanding mass of educated and empowered consumers demanding more involvement in their health care. Planetree's model delivers!

The Model's emphasis on patient and family education is carried out through such strategies as customized information packets, collaborative care conferences and patient pathways. The open chart policy enables patients to read and write in their medical records. In the self-medication program patients who are able can keep their medications at the bedside and assume responsibility for their administration.

Planetree recognizes that the experience of illness has the potential to transform the patient. It can be a time of great personal growth for the patient as life goals and values are reevaluated, priorities are clarified, and inner resources are discovered. A variety of educational materials are made available to the patient, the family and the community through consumer-friendly health resource centers and satellite centers. The Planetree Classification System aids those in search of information as they review broad collections of medical texts and journals. Video and audio tapes, computer services and much more, support patients' increasing hunger for information about their health and medical care.

The Importance of Family, Friends, and Social Support

Social support has been shown to be vital to good health. An increasing number of medical and social researchers are finding that anything that promotes a sense of love and intimacy, connection and community is healing. Planetree supports and encourages involvement of family and significant others whenever possible. The Care Partner Program provides education and training to assist family participation in the care of patients while hospitalized and at home after discharge. As part of the health care team, significant others can make a valuable contribution to the quality of the patient's hospital experience. Volunteer care partners are available for those patients who are alone. One such program, the volunteer hand holding program, trains volunteers to accompany patients having minor surgery into the operating room to provide emotional support. Another element of the Planetree Model which assists families in being involved is unrestricted visiting hours, even in the ICU.

continues

EXHIBIT 8–3 (continued)

Spirituality: The Importance of Inner Resources

Planetree recognizes the vital role of spirituality in healing the whole person. Supporting patients, families and staff in connecting with their own inner resources creates a more healing environment. Chapels, gardens and meditation rooms provide opportunities for reflection and prayer, and Chaplains are seen as vital members of the health care team.

The Importance of Human Touch

Touch is an essential way of communicating caring and is unfortunately often omitted from the clinical setting. Therapeutic full body or chair massage is available for patients, families and staff. Internship programs for massage therapists and training for volunteers to give hand and foot rubs are also available and help keep costs minimal. Families, as part of the Care Partner Program, can also be taught to give massages to loved ones while in the hospital and at home. Nurses, doctors and other staff find chair massage focusing on the neck, shoulders and back, a useful way to relieve stress and re-energize.

Healing Arts: Nutrition for the Soul

Music, storytellers, clowns, and funny movies create an atmosphere of serenity and playfulness in the Planetree Model. Artwork in patient rooms, treatment areas and on art carts adds to the ambiance. Volunteers work with patients who would like to create their own art, while involvement from artists, musicians, poets and story tellers from the local community helps to expand the boundaries of the health care facility.

Complementary Therapies

Complementary and alternative medical (CAM) therapy use and expenditures have increased substantially in the last decade. All data confirm this trend among consumers will continue to grow in the coming years. Some individuals choose these therapies because of dissatisfaction with conventional therapies, while others do so because they have found these health care alternatives to be more congruent with their own beliefs, values and philosophical orientations toward health and life. In either case, it is important to realize a growing number of patients are desiring treatment options which are more natural, less toxic, less invasive and holistic, to complement more conventional medical approaches.

Aromatherapy's calming effect on agitated patients is now being used during MRIs and with geropsychiatric patients. Pet therapy has also been successfully implemented in Planetree hospitals. A number of studies have shown that pets can have beneficial effects on health, including a lowered blood pressure, mood elevation and enhanced social interaction.

To meet the growing consumer demand for CAM therapies, Planetree affiliates have instituted heart disease reversal programs, mind/body medicine interventions such as meditation and healing guided imagery, therapeutic massage, therapeutic touch, Reiki, acupuncture, Tai Chi and yoga.

Healthy Communities

Expanding the boundaries of health care. Working with schools, senior centers, churches and other community partners, organizations are redefining health care to include the health and wellness of the larger community.

Source: Planetree Web site: http://www.planetree.org/about/components.htm Reprinted with permission.

---

there are not enough providers, the organization needs to consider how people are working and how work can be improved to be more effective. As hospitals change, many factors influence the need for change and how it occurs. Some of these factors were highlighted in Figure 8-1, presented at the beginning of this chapter.

Change is inevitable in any organization today, particularly in health care. Science and knowledge have driven some of this change, but there are other factors. Change is a process that is driven by forces that motivate a person or an organization to consider what needs altering. The key is to be clear about this and to understand the "why" before taking the next steps. It is also important to consider if staff are ready for the change. Staff can act as barriers to, or facilitators of, change. Staff members are typically tired of changes and feel that there are too many. They often also feel left out of the decision process that leads to changes. They then become critical of the change and feel limited, or they feel no commitment to the change. This becomes a major barrier. For example, if the staff do not understand the need behind a decision to change a form in the medical record, it is more difficult to train them in the use of the form, and it may be difficult to get them to use the form correctly. The complexity of the change and how frequently changes are made can lead to overload for staff. The goal is to have staff behind the change and committed to it; they will then be facilitators of change. Understanding resistance to change can help in preparing for the change and in developing any training that might be required. When changes are planned within a hospital, planners need to consider the impact that the change may have on policies and procedures; accreditation and regulation requirements; financial issues; the structure of the organization; how staff do their work; patients, visitors, and students (e.g., nursing, medical, other); and much more. The change process includes:

1. Identifying the issue or problem/need for change and factors that influence the need for change.
2. Gathering information to better understand the need and possible solutions.
3. Identifying barriers to and support for the change.
4. Identifying solutions in order to solve a problem or improve (change).

5. Deciding which solution to implement.
6. Preparing staff for the change (informing them of the change, the reasons for the change, what the change will be, and the timeline; training staff if needed).
7. Implementing the change (solution).
8. Evaluating the results (including staff feedback).
9. Determining any adjustments that are needed. Ideally, relevant staff need to be included early in the process to enhance staff commitment.

Healthcare Reform

In the last decade, there have been attempts to reform the healthcare delivery system. Most of these efforts have failed. This failure was typically caused by political issues. Healthcare delivery is a critical political issue because it impacts taxes and is a very expensive business. The 2008 presidential election brought healthcare reform to the forefront again. As was true with other efforts, nursing organizations got involved and spoke out about proposed changes. It is very important that nursing do this because healthcare reform will definitely have an impact on nursing.

Despite 15 years of incremental, market-based approaches to reform healthcare payment and delivery systems in the United States, systemic transformation remains elusive. The healthcare system continues to be inequitable, fragmented, ineffective, costly and often fraught with errors. American Nurses Association (ANA) embraces an ongoing commitment to the principle that all persons are entitled to affordable, readily accessible, high quality healthcare services. ANA has pursued this mission through an integrated series of public and private sector advocacy and education efforts using, as its foundation, the tenets of ANA's Healthcare Agenda 2005, ANA's current policy statement on the subject. (ANA, 2007a)

What are some of the changes that the health-care delivery system is experiencing? *Nurses are in new roles.* Some of these new roles have been discussed in Chapter 4 and will be further discussed later in this textbook. They include advanced NPs, NMs, CNLs, and CNS-Bs. How they are used in hospitals varies. In some cases, nurses with these advanced degrees receive admitting privileges, meaning that they can admit their patients to the hospital from private practice or clinics. This is not the norm, but it does occur.

Emergency services have been experiencing changes because of problems with how they are used by patients. Some patients use the emergency department (ED) as their private physician, coming in for services that are not acute or of an emergency nature. This has a major impact on the flow of patients into and out of the ED. This can cause a backup, making it difficult to admit more patients for emergency services. In some cases, this may result in the temporary diversion of patients to other EDs. Another type of problem occurs when patients are not discharged in a timely manner from inpatient units, and beds are full. ED patients who need to be admitted for inpatient treatment must wait in the ED, sometimes for days.

The increased number of patients who cannot pay for services and have no insurance coverage causes major financial problems for hospitals. In some situations, this may lead to the closing of beds (decreasing size of hospital), termination of staff, and, in extreme cases, the closing of hospitals. Patient access to care has become a major problem in some communities. Access is more than just the ability to get an appointment; it involves the availability of services at times convenient for the patient (time of day and day of week), transportation to and from the care facility, reimbursement for care, and receiving the right type of care, such as from a specialist.

Patient education is an important part of nursing care. It is important in helping patients and their families cope with illness and any long-term care issues. With the increase in the number of persons with chronic illnesses, patient education is even more important. However, with the rapid turnover in patients in hospitals as LOSs decrease, there is less time to teach patients what they need to know. Nurses need to develop new methods to better ensure quality, timely patient education.

The Nursing Organization Within the Hospital

RNs are members of the nation's largest healthcare profession, and they practice wherever people need nursing care. Common care sites are hospitals, homes, schools, workplaces, and community centers, and less common areas include children's camps and homeless shelters. Over 2.4 million of the nation's 2.9 million RNs were employed in 2004, about one quarter of them on a part-time basis (ANA, 2007b). About 56% of nurses currently work in hospitals. The median salary of a staff nurse working full time in a hospital in 2005 was $56,880 (ANA, 2007b). Examples of other settings in which nurses practice are community/public health facilities (14.9%), ambulatory care facilities (11.5%), nursing homes (6.3%), and in nursing education (2.6%). As mentioned in Chapter 4 and discussed in greater detail in Chapter 14, there is a serious shortage throughout nursing, and this includes nursing faculty.

Nurses play critical roles in a variety of healthcare settings, which is explored throughout this text; in this chapter, the focus is on hospitals as one example of a healthcare organization. Nursing services may be organized differently in hospitals. The traditional nursing organization, still the most common type, is a nursing department, as illustrated in Figure 8–5.

Nursing staff (RNs, LPNs/LVNs, patient care assistants) are all part of the nursing department, which often includes unit support staff or a unit clerk as well. The title for the unit clerk position varies, but this is the person(s) who helps with administrative issues such as records, supplies, reception at the central desk area, and so on.

Figure 8–5 An example: Nursing department organizational chart.

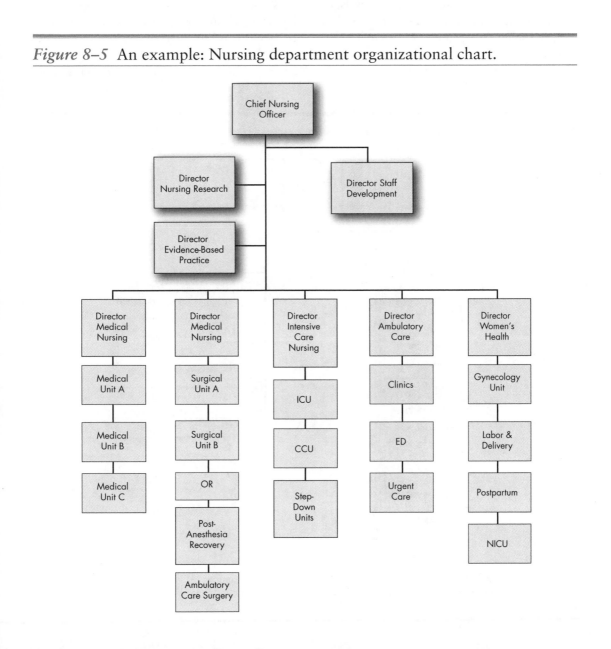

The second and newer organization model is a patient services department. In this case, the department focuses on the function of patient services, not just nursing. This department includes nursing but also might include other patient care services such as medical records, respiratory therapy, infusion therapy, infection control, and so on. The configuration varies widely from one hospital to another. Figure 8–6 shows an example of this organization.

Who leads in these two department models? An RN is the designated leader. An RN must be the leader of nursing services to meet The Joint Commission standards. The Joint Commission is discussed in more detail in Chapter 12. The nurse leader title has changed over time. Director of nursing (DON) was the common title, and it is still used today. The traditional DON just focused on nursing and had little, if any, input into the functioning of the hospital as

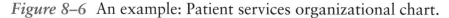

Figure 8–6 An example: Patient services organizational chart.

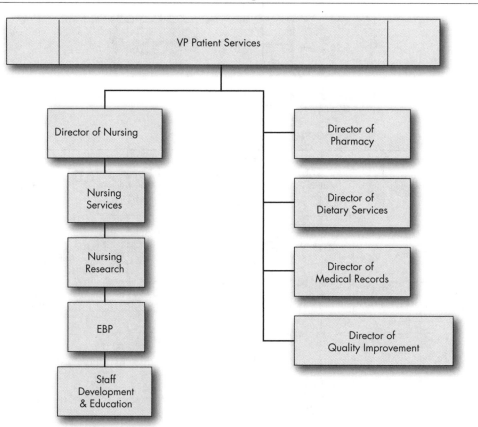

Each service area has additional details about components within it. For example, for Nursing Services, the description of unit organization in Figure 8–8 would be added. Staff Development and Education would include a director, instructors, and secretarial support.

a whole and no input into the budget. Today, even if the nurse leader is called a DON, he or she has much more input into all aspects of the hospital. This was an important change. Given that nurses represent the largest proportion of hospital staff and provide most of the direct care, it is critical that nurses are represented by a nurse leader who is recognized in the organization as an important leader, and who can participate in major decision making. In the 1970s and 1980s, DONs began to get more power, and their title began to change to vice president (VP) for nursing or patient services in recognition of their organization leadership role, but the focus was still on nursing. At this time, increasing numbers of nursing leaders began to complete graduate degrees. It was recognized that they were running large, complex departments that represented a significant portion of the overall hospital budget. Gradually, the VP of nursing entered into the budget process as an equal partner. The next change involved the VP of patient services, in which the nurse leader was responsible for more than just nursing. This was a major shift, but the idea that a nurse could manage other healthcare disciplines changed slowly. As is true for all such information about hospitals, there is great variation from one hospital to another. The size of the hospital has an impact on how the nursing services are organized. More nurses today are also taking positions in hospital administration that are not related to just nursing; a nurse could be the chief operating officer or CEO. This is a major shift, and there are not many nurses in these positions. Today, any nurse who serves in a nursing leadership position in a healthcare organization needs to be competent in administrative responsibilities such as planning, budgeting, staffing, communicating, coordinating, and public speaking. He or she must also have the ability to involve others in decision making and teamwork and have the ability to

work with other healthcare professionals. What does a nursing department look like?

The nursing organization or department includes nursing management staff. There are three levels of management.

1. *Upper level*: Responsible for establishing goals, objectives, and strategic plans for the organization. The DON, VP of nursing, or VP of patient services positions are in upper-level management.
2. *Middle level*: Supervise first-level managers. For example, there may be directors of specific types of services—director of women's health, director of surgical services, director of behavioral health, and so on. These directors supervise multiple units that have a common function, such as women's health (e.g., gynecology, obstetrics).
3. *First level*: Managers who provide the day-to-day or operational direction for the nursing service and units. This group is composed of supervisors or managers. Titles for these managers vary. Some examples are nurse manager, head nurse (not used much today), nursing unit manager, and nursing or nurse coordinator. They are critical to the effectiveness of any hospital because they ensure the daily functioning of patient care areas, quality and safety, staffing, budget implementation and use of resources, staff issues and morale, teamwork, coordination, and communication. They work with multiple disciplines to ensure that patients get the care they need. Nurse managers do not typically provide direct care. They need to be competent in communication, coordination, directing staff, performance evaluation, group management, effective use of teams, budgeting, planning, mentoring staff, delegation, problem-solving, and evaluating outcomes.

Effective nurse managers are able to listen, control their emotions, and use analytical thinking. They have good clinical judgment, can persuade others, are flexible, are outcome-oriented, and have self-confidence. Qualifications for nurse managers can vary, though they should ideally have, at a minimum, a bachelor of science degree in nursing. A master's degree provides additional background for this very demanding position. This type of position requires nursing experience. New graduates should not hold management positions. The majority of nurses in a hospital do not hold formal management positions. As new graduates transition to professional practice, they become more involved in the unit where they work. They learn about how the unit runs, what information is needed, quality and safety issues, staffing, and participation in committees.

The nurse manager is very important to the unit's culture. How the nurse manager leads and manages can make the difference in whether a unit is an open and comfortable place to work, or one that is oppressive, with dissatisfied staff. Nurse managers need to have continuing staff development to improve their leadership and management competencies. Many nurse managers have been promoted to this position without sufficient experience and management training. This makes it difficult for the nurse manager to be effective and has an impact on the unit and its work. Figure 8–7 describes an example of an individual nursing unit.

Leadership and management are concepts that are often confused. Organizations need both leaders and managers, and they may be the same people. Leaders who are involved with strategic planning and vision use the change process carefully to improve the organization and its functions. Managers are in a formal position; their focus is on managing or maintaining the equilibrium, or getting the work done. Leaders provide broad guidance and direction.

In today's increasingly less hierarchical and more lateral organization structures, leadership is not about position of authority, as much as it is a role of influence. Staff nurses can and must lead through teamwork, through the development of better practices, through the development of centrality in communication networks, and in contributing to the strategic management of units and departments. The leadership role and tasks are pivotal, not peripheral, to the success of the healthcare facilities. (Ferguson & Brindle, 2000, p. 5)

A leader does not have to be in a formal management position, though many are. All nurses need to develop leadership competencies because they serve as leaders in the healthcare process and in the management of patient care. Leaders ask questions, provide inspiration to others, take risks, challenge others, and view change as opportunity. This is best described as transformational leadership. "The transforming leader looks for potential motives in followers, seeks to satisfy the needs and engages the full person of the followers. The result of transforming leadership is a relationship of mutual stimulation and elevation that converts followers into leaders and leaders into moral agents" (Curtin, 2001, p. 227). Transformational leaders are also concerned with operational issues—making sure the work is done effectively—but they are also involved in the "bigger picture" to improve the organization. Managers focus on the key management functions of planning, organizing, leading, and controlling. Today, managers are also changing how they approach their jobs. Some of the newer

Figure 8–7 An example: Medical nursing unit organizational chart.

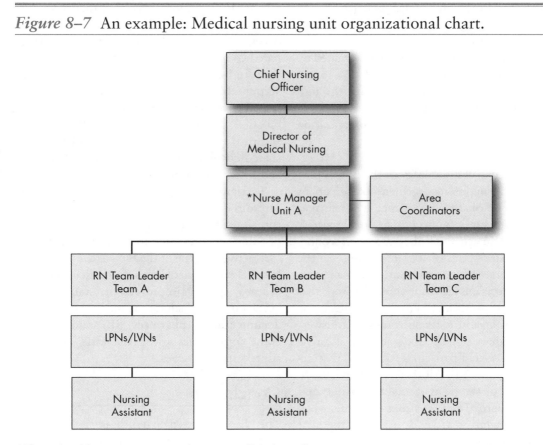

*Alternative titles: nurse manager, unit manager, clinical coordinator.

skills needed for managers are the ability to (Porter-O'Grady, 1999, p. 40):

- Change focus from process to outcomes
- Align role to information infrastructure rather than functional performance
- Focus on team results rather than individual events
- Facilitate resources that then direct work
- Develop staff self-direction rather than giving direction
- Focus on obtaining value rather than simply finding costs

- Focus on consumer-driven structure rather than provider-based system
- Construct horizontal relationships rather than maintain vertical control

Shared Governance: Empowering Nursing Staff

Shared governance is a process that "legitimizes nurses' decision-making control over professional practice" (Hess, 1995, p. 14). Through shared governance, nurses in an organization can:

1. Control their professional practice
2. Influence organizational resources that support practice
3. Gain formal authority, which is granted by the organization
4. Participate in decision making through committee structure
5. Access information about the organization
6. Set goals and negotiate conflict

In this type of organization, the nurses play an active role in the "management" of the patient care services. Shared governance is a management model, but it is also a professional practice model and an accountability model. Accountability and responsibility are shared by the nurses. Nurses have the authority to make sure the right decisions are made about the work that they do. *Accountability* means that the nurse accepts responsibility for outcomes or is answerable for what is done. *Responsibility* is to be "entrusted with a particular function" (Ritter-Teitel, 2002, p. 34). All these are connected to autonomy, or the right to make decisions and control actions. The best situation occurs when the nurse who provides care is also the staff member who works to resolve issues to ensure that patient outcomes are met at the point-of-care, limiting the number or layers of staff who must be involved. Shared governance is dependent on effective collaboration, communication, and teamwork and spreads departmental and organizational decision making over a large number of staff. This approach, however, does not mean that managers do not have to meet their managerial responsibilities or that all decisions are made by the staff. It is not helpful if decision making is blocked by the process (i.e., too much time taken). Shared governance is not easy to develop, and it can become a barrier. It takes time to be effective. Neither staff nor leaders/managers should assume that the approach

relieves leaders and managers of their responsibility to do their jobs. Decision making is more decentralized and takes place through a designated committee or council structure, but both staff and managers have responsibilities and accountability. Typically, hospitals that have a shared governance model find that staff are more satisfied, and turnover is lower. Staff like working in the organization. Not all hospitals use shared governance, and how it is implemented and its effectiveness can vary widely.

Participation in nursing committees and interdisciplinary committees provides opportunities for nurses to be directly involved in decision making and to have an impact on care delivery. Some of the typical committees in hospitals are those that focus on policies and procedures, quality improvement, staffing, staff development and education, medical records and documentation, pharmacy, EBP, and research. Some committees are special task forces that address specific issues.

Conclusion

This chapter focused on healthcare organizations, with acute care hospitals as the major example of a healthcare organization. Understanding how hospitals are structured and their processes (functions) helps the nurse practice in this setting. The departments and team members play important roles in how the organization functions. The healthcare system has been undergoing many changes, and this will continue. Nurses are very much involved in these changes and should participate in the change process. Financing healthcare is a challenge because it is expensive, and there are a variety of approaches to covering these costs through reimbursement. Reimbursement impacts nursing care. Related questions are, for example: (1) Are there enough nursing staff? (2) Are there support services for nurses so

Figure 8–8 A need to change health-

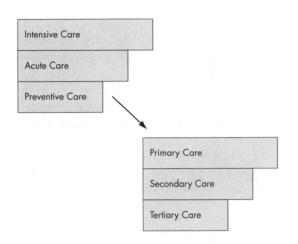

that they are free to provide care? (3) Are the most up-to-date supplies and equipment available? (4) Is there an efficient computerized documentation system? (5) Is orientation sufficient for new staff? (6) Do nursing staff receive the training they need? (7) Are nurse managers provided with effective training and education?

Greater emphasis has been placed on shared governance because of the need for greater input from nurses regarding the hospital decision-making process. Though this chapter focuses on acute care hospitals, the United States has been moving toward changes in healthcare priorities that impact the healthcare setting as described in Figure 8–8.

CHAPTER HIGHLIGHTS

1. Healthcare delivery is a complex process and system that includes multiple delivery sites: acute care organizations (hospitals), ambulatory care clinics, private provider offices, community health facil-

ities, home care agencies, hospice agencies, extended care facilities, and so on.

2. Hospitals are impacted by many factors that cause changes in their services and in how they collaborate with others, realign their organization with the external environment, or even close because of financial issues.

3. Health care is a business; it provides services to the population.

4. Healthcare entities may be for-profit or not-for-profit depending on what they do with their revenues.

5. Healthcare organizations may differ depending on their structure and process. For example, a bureaucratic structure receives little input from staff in determining decision-making processes.

6. Horizontal structure is decentralized, with an emphasis on departments or divisions; decisions are made closer to the staff who do the work.

7. The matrix organization structure is newer and less clear than the traditional bureaucratic organization centered on departments. A matrix organization is "flatter" (i.e., decisions do not flow from the top down).

8. The process of an organization focuses on how it functions.

9. Classification of hospitals varies greatly and may reflect a hospital's mission of teaching or research, for example. Hospitals may be public or private.

10. The hospital healthcare team is composed of a variety of healthcare providers, both professional and nonprofessional.

11. Hospitalists and intensivists are generally physicians who specialize in acute in-hospital care, though some hospitals use CNSs and advanced practice nurses in these roles.

12. Healthcare finances can be viewed from a micro, macro, or reimbursement perspective.

13. Managed care is a method used to reimburse or pay for healthcare services, but it includes more than just payment; this method controls the delivery services.

14. Medicare was established in 1965 by Title XVIII, amendment to the Social Security Act. Medicare is the federal health insurance program for people aged 65 and older, persons with disabilities, and people with end-stage renal disease.

15. Medicaid, established in 1965 by Title XIX of the Social Security Act, is the federal–state program for certain categories of low-income people and includes children, the disabled, blind persons, and so forth.

16. The numbers of uninsured and underinsured individuals are growing. The federal government estimates that 47 million individuals lacked health insurance coverage of any kind during 2006.

17. The organizational culture reflects the mission, core values, and vision of the entity.

18. Healthcare delivery systems are now also being viewed as a healing environment.

19. Healthcare delivery has been reorganized or redesigned for many reasons. One of the major reasons has been the shortage of healthcare workers. How work is done, and by whom, has had to change in the face of this shortage.

20. Healthcare reform has been undertaken for a variety of reasons, not the least of which are access and health disparities issues.

21. Nursing within an organization is a critical component of healthcare delivery and is an essential ingredient in patient satisfaction.

22. Shared governance models of decision making **empower** nurses and give them a voice in their organizations.

Linking to the Internet

- American Hospital Association
  http://www.aha.org
- The Joint Commission
  http://www.jointcommission.org
- Centers for Medicare and Medicare Services
  http://www.cms.hhs.gov
- Planetree Healing Environments
  http://www.planetree.org

DISCUSSION QUESTIONS

1. What is the difference between organizational structure and process? Identify examples for each.
2. If you were not a nursing student, what other healthcare team member would you want to be and why?
3. Compare and contrast the three types of financial issues—macro, micro, and reimbursement—related to health care.
4. Describe how nursing services might be organized in a hospital, their key roles, and their relationship to other departments.
5. What does organizational culture mean, and why is it important?
6. What is your opinion of the health environment model? How do you think the designation of a Planetree hospital might impact nursing care?
7. How does shared governance increase nurse participation in decision making and empower nurses?

CRITICAL THINKING ACTIVITIES

1. What is your reaction to the topic of the corporatization of health care?
2. Search the Internet for a hospital Web site. See if you can find information on its vision, mission, goals, and objectives. Many hospital Web sites include this information. After you find an example, review the information. How would you see this information as applying to nursing?
3. Visit the Web site for the American Hospital Association (AHA) (http://www.aha.org/aha/about/). What is the AHA? Click on Issues and select one issue to explore. What have you learned about the issue? Groups of students should select a different issue to review and then share what they learned. Consider the implications for nursing.
4. Search the Internet for information about one type of healthcare team member to learn more about the profession.
5. Describe the culture of a clinical unit in which you are getting clinical experiences. Write down your description and then discuss your views with your classmates in groups of four. How are they similar, and how are they different? Did you notice the culture soon after being on the unit, or did it take some time? Is the culture one that would encourage you to work there? Why or why not? How would you describe the culture of your school of nursing?
6. Visit the Cover the Uninsured Web site (http://covertheuninsured.org/states/) and find your state. What can you learn about the uninsured and underinsured in your state?
7. Visit the consumer site for Medicare (http://medicare.gov). If you were a consumer, how helpful would this site be? What information can you find? Click on Compare Hospitals in Your Area and review those hospitals from the perspective of a consumer who is 70 years old and needs to have a hip replacement. Then find out what preventive services are covered by Medicare. Visit http://www.cms.hhs.gov/center/ombudsman.asp and find out what the ombudsman does.

CASE STUDY

Ms. Jones is a nurse consultant who works for a large healthcare organization. As part of her benefits package, she can select either a PPO or an HMO. The premiums on these two options are different, and the HMO has a lower cost. She opts to elect the HMO as her provider. Shortly after selecting this option, Ms. Jones becomes ill while traveling. She requires medical assistance and must be seen by a physician. This problem does not require a hospitalization but does require two physician visits within 24 hours. She is informed that because she opted for HMO coverage, these visits are considered out of network; if she had selected the PPO, the physician visits still would still have been out of network but the costs would have been lower. This case highlights the need for consumers to understand their healthcare options in light of their lifestyles.

Case Questions

1. What is the difference between a PPO and an HMO? What type of health insurance do you have?
2. What does your health insurance cover?
3. What would you have to do if you were in the same situation as Ms. Jones?
4. How might universal health insurance solve Ms. Jones's problem?

WORDS OF WISDOM

Kendra Coleman, BSN, RN
Graduate Student, University of Oklahoma
College of Nursing
Nurse Manager, Labor & Delivery, St. John
Medical Center, Tulsa, Oklahoma

Making the transition into management has definitely been a challenge. I have asked myself on more than one occasion, "Why did I want to get into management?" Then I would remind myself that my number one goal was to support the nursing staff and empower them to practice excellent nursing without the intimidation of physicians. On the other hand, I had to show the physicians that we appreciate their business and wanted to do what was in the best interest of the patients. What I quickly learned was I must always be armed with the latest research to support our practice and display the recommendations of our professional organization as well as the board of nursing.

I was placed in a unique situation in that the previous manager stepped down to be a floor nurse on the unit (I was now her manager), and I had previously worked on this particular floor.

So I knew most of the staff, but it was very important for me to connect with my team members and for them to see me in my new role. Over the first month, I sat down with each employee and laid out my expectations. This was very important for them to know that I had the same conversation with each person, and I would treat each of them the same and would hold each person accountable.

I earned the trust of people that I thought it would take a long time to earn. Nurses came to me with issues that they fully expected me to do something about. There were many regulatory issues that I had no clue about and had to quickly research them. I felt it was odd for people to ask me for permission to do certain things, especially since I am one of the youngest people on the unit. I still go out on the floor to help clean and move patients. I answer phones, and I am very visible on the floor. I think it is important to let the staff know that I am not out of touch with what they are going through, but at the same time they do not expect me to carry a full team. They have a certain respect for me that came overnight, one that still takes me by surprise at times.

Management is complicated. We must set boundaries, be professional, knowledgeable, and support the staff. We must hold people accountable and establish a way for people to take ownership of their practice. When I have a rough day, I remind myself why I am in this position: to help empower the staff through information sharing, support, and presence.

Marietta Carter, RN, AND, OCN
RN-BSN student at the University of Oklahoma College of Nursing
Nurse Manager, Oncology Clinic, Valley View Regional Hospital, Ada, Oklahoma

Nursing leadership is one of the most rewarding and challenging jobs available to RNs. I was previously an assistant manager of ICU and home health care units and have been nurse manager of a hospital-based outpatient oncology clinic for almost 17 years. The main drawback of a leadership position is that your work is never really finished. It is extremely important to learn to prioritize and let go of the things that can wait till tomorrow. The best part of leadership is the opportunity to mentor new nurses and take them from a point of being scared to death and questioning every little care decision to be made, into a professional nurse who is knowledgeable and confidant in the care he or she provides. Transformational leadership is the theory I mostly use, and I've always felt and seen, evidenced in practice, that the best leaders lead by example. Staff nurses develop respect for leaders who work right alongside them, and this method also allows the leader to impart skills and knowledge to the new nurse. A big challenge for nursing leaders today is leading through change, in a climate of almost daily changes in rules and regulations, policies, reimbursement, etc. The participative theory allows shared decision making to get staff involved in how changes will be managed. Shared governance and allowing for autonomous practice will almost always help to get the staff to "buy-in" to new methods and policies.

References

American Association of Colleges of Nursing. (2007). *White paper on the education and role of the clinical nurse leader.* Washington, DC: Author.

American Nurses Association. (2007a). *Health system reform.* Retrieved December 3, 2007, from http://www.nursingworld.org/MainMenuCategories/HealthcareandPolicyIssues/HSR.aspx

American Nurses Association. (2007b). *About nursing.* Retrieved December 3, 2007, from http://www.nursingworld.org/MainMenuCategories/CertificationandAccreditation/AboutNursing.aspx

Cover the Uninsured. (2007). Retrieved December 3, 2007, from http://covertheuninsured.org/

Curtin, L. (2001). Healing healthcare's organizational culture. *Seminars for Nurse Managers, 9,* 218–227.

Dewan, S., & Sack, K. (2008, January 8). A safety-net hospital falls into financial crisis. *The New York Times,* pp. A1, A18–A19.

Ferguson, S., & Brindle, M. (2000). Nursing leadership: Vision and the reality. *Nursing Spectrum, 10*(21DC), 5.

Hess, R. (1995). Shared governance: Nursing's 20th-century tower of Babel. *Journal of Nursing Administration, 25*(5), 14–17.

Jones, K., & Redman, R. (2000). Organizational culture and work redesign: Experiences in three organizations. *Journal of Nursing Administration, 30,* 604–610.

Porter-O'Grady, T. (1999). Quantum leadership: New roles for a new age. *Journal of Nursing Administration, 29*(10), 37–42.

Reuters Health Information. (2007). *47 million Americans lack health insurance.* Retrieved October 2, 2008, from http://www.reuters.com/article/healthNews/idUSN313728120071101

Ritter-Teitel, J. (2002). The impact of restructuring on professional nursing practice. *Journal of Nursing Administration, 32*(1), 31–41.

Section III

Core Healthcare Professional Competencies

Section III focuses on the core healthcare professional competencies. These competencies were first identified by the Institute of Medicine (IOM) in its 2003 report, *Health Professions Education*. The competencies are based on the need to improve the safety and quality of health care and the recognition that healthcare professional education was not including these five critical competencies. The IOM does not recommend that these are the only competencies required, but rather that these competencies form the core competencies for all healthcare professional education: nurses, physicians, pharmacists, allied health professionals, and healthcare administrators. Each chapter in this section discusses one of the core competencies in relation to nursing. The core competencies are:

- **Provide patient-centered care:** Identify, respect, and care about patients' differences, values, preferences, and expressed needs; relieve pain and suffering; coordinate continuous care; listen to, clearly inform, communicate with, and educate patients; share decision making and management; and continuously advocate disease prevention, wellness, and promotion of healthy lifestyles, including a focus on population health.

- **Work in interdisciplinary teams:** Cooperate, collaborate, communicate, and integrate care in teams to ensure that care is continuous and reliable.
- **Employ evidence-based practice:** Integrate best research with clinical expertise and patient values for optimum care and participate in learning and research activities to the extent feasible.
- **Apply quality improvement:** Identify errors and hazards in care; understand and implement basic safety design principles, such as standardization and simplification; continually understand and measure quality of care in terms of structure, process, and outcomes in relation to patient and community needs; and design and test interventions to change processes and systems of care, with the objective of improving quality.
- **Utilize informatics:** Communicate, manage knowledge, mitigate error, and support decision making using information technology.

All these competencies are interrelated, and all should be applied to most clinical interactions. However, not every competency applies to every clinical situation. This competency-based approach to healthcare education should lead to improved quality because educators should be able to gather data about outcomes that could then be associated with better patient care. This is the desired goal.

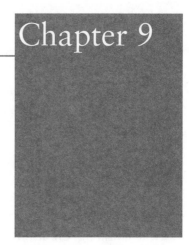

Chapter 9

Provide Patient-Centered Care

KEY TERMS

❏ Bias
❏ Care coordination
❏ Care map
❏ Clinical judgment
❏ Clinical reasoning
❏ Consumer/customer
❏ Critical thinking
❏ Culture
❏ Disparity
❏ Diversity
❏ Ethnicity
❏ Ethnocentrism
❏ Health literacy

❏ Macro consumer
❏ Micro consumer
❏ Nursing process
❏ Patient advocacy
❏ Patient-centered care
❏ Prejudice
❏ Race
❏ Self-management of care
❏ Stereotype
❏ Therapeutic use of self
❏ Unlicensed assistive personnel

Introduction

This chapter begins the discussion of the core competencies identified by the Institute of Medicine (IOM) for nurses and all healthcare professionals. The first core competency focuses on patient-centered care. The U.S. healthcare system is patient centered, but it is not at the level it could be. This content describes patient-centered care, relevant nursing theories, consumerism as a critical factor in healthcare delivery, cultural diversity and disparities, patient advocacy, care coordination to meet patient-centered care needs, self-management of care, and therapeutic use of self in the nurse–patient relationship. As students enter their nursing education, it is assumed that they are in a nursing program because of their concern about patients; however, providing patient-centered care does not come naturally. It takes knowledge, time, critical thinking, clinical reasoning, and judgment to ensure that care is coordinated and that the implementation process focuses on patient-centered care.

Our overall goal is to help physicians and other health professionals identify and utilize strategies to reduce disparities in health outcomes through integrating disease prevention and health promotion into routine medical care. The need for this approach is driven by changes in the health status of the population and provision of healthcare in our nation. (Peters & Elster, 2002, p. 9)

These changes include the following:

- The U.S. population is becoming older and more diverse.
- Preventive care and chronic care are increasingly joining curative and acute primary care.
- Chronic disease management is becoming more prominent in many medical practices.
- More patients want active involvement in their health care.

- Financial mechanisms that support health care are changing.
- Emphasis is increasingly being placed on concerns about access, cost, quality, and outcomes.

The IOM Competency: Provide Patient-Centered Care

As discussed in the introduction to Section III, the IOM has identified five key core competencies for all healthcare professionals, and this chapter focuses on the first core competency: provide **patient-centered care**. The IOM definition follows:

Identify, respect, and care about patients' differences, values, preferences, and expressed needs; relieve pain and suffering; coordinate continuous care; listen to, clearly inform, communicate with, and educate patients; share decision making and management; and continuously advocate disease prevention, wellness, and promotion of healthy lifestyles, including a focus on population health. (IOM, 2003a, p. 4)

On the surface, this definition may seem simple, but it is not; patient-centered care includes multiple factors and activities—all aimed at making the patient the center of care. The content in this chapter will focus on the key elements of the core competency as illustrated in Figure 9–1.

Support of Patient-Centered Care

Why is patient-centered care included in the core competencies? What is the basis for emphasizing patient-centered care? Figure 9–2 describes the relationship of the core competencies. Note that "provide patient-centered care" is the center. Evidence-based practice, quality improvement, and utilizing informatics all impact patient-centered care, and interdisciplinary teams encircle all and bring care to the patient.

Figure 9–1 Providing patient-centered care: Key elements.

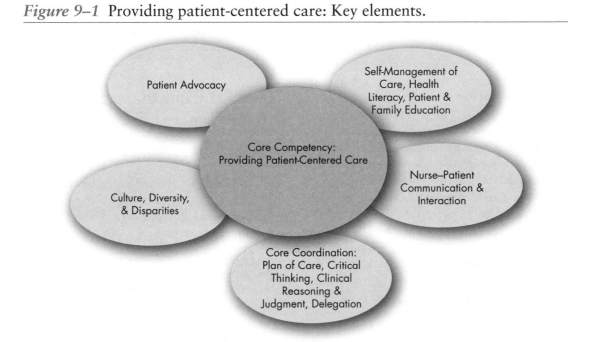

Crossing the Quality Chasm: A New Health System for the 21st Century (IOM, 2001) describes 10 rules for redesigning patient care, as shown in Exhibit 9–1.

How do these rules relate to the competency of providing patient-centered care? The first four rules specifically apply to patient-centered care, supporting the need to include patient-centered care in the core competencies. These four rules are:

1. Care is based on continuous health relationships.
2. Care is customized according to patient needs and values.
3. The patient is the source of control.
4. Knowledge is shared and information flows freely.

The other six rules are not directly related to patient-centered care. The rules are a major part

of the framework to improve the quality of care. Improving health care requires improved competencies in all healthcare professionals, beginning with providing patient-centered care.

The IOM has named patient-centered care as one of six domains of quality. The IOM has summarized issues related to specific skills that are needed to ensure patient-centered care. A description of these skills provides additional information about what is meant by patient-centered care (IOM, 2003a, pp. 52–53):

- Share power and responsibility with patients and caregivers (family, significant others). (e.g., involve the patient in care, make the patient the center of care and decision making; work to increase patient understanding, acceptance, and cooperation; help caregivers as they provide care to

Figure 9–2 IOM relationship core competencies.

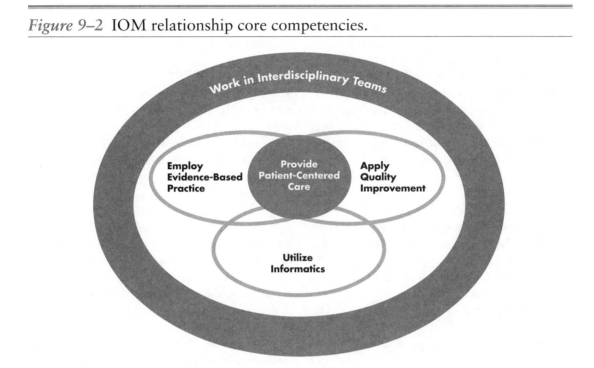

Source: Reprinted with permission from the National Academies Press, Copyright 2003, National Academy of Sciences.

EXHIBIT 9–1 SIMPLE RULES FOR THE 21ST-CENTURY HEALTHCARE SYSTEM

Current Approach (Old Rule)	New Rule
Care is based primarily on visits.	Care is based on continuous healing relationships.
Professional autonomy drives variability.	Care is customized according to patient needs and values.
Professionals control care.	The patient is the source of control.
Information is a record.	Knowledge is shared and information flows freely.
Decision-making is an individual responsibility.	Decision-making is evidence-based.
Do no harm is an individual responsibility.	Safety is a system property.
Secrecy is necessary.	Transparency is necessary.
The system reacts to needs.	Needs are anticipated.
Cost reduction is sought.	Waste is continuously decreased.
Preference is given to professional roles over the system.	Cooperation among clinicians is a priority.

Source: From *Crossing the Quality Chasm: A New Health System for the 21st Century* (p. 67), by Institute of Medicine, 2001, Washington, DC: National Academies Press. Copyright 2001 by the Institute of Medicine. Reprinted with permission.

family member [education for patient and family]; support self-management; provide comfort and emotional support; manage pain and suffering; relieve anxiety; provide expert care to manage symptoms)

- Communicate with patients in a shared and fully open manner. (e.g., patients have access to information, communication with healthcare providers (including nurses), use of technology to communicate)
- Take into account patients' individuality, emotional needs, values, and life issues. (e.g., culture, whole person)
- Implement strategies for reaching those who do not present care on their own, including care strategies that support the broader community. (e.g., underserved members of the community)
- Enhance prevention and health promotion. (e.g., population focus, consider risk factors, health promotion, and prevention strategies)

Patient-centered or person-centered care is the key focus for all nurses. This care

alleviates vulnerability in all of its forms. That care should and must then be delivered at the right time, at the right level, in the right place, and so on. If care were on a compass, it would be true north and all other functions would stand in line to provide added value and service to that fact. (Hagenow, 2003, p. 204)

The IOM has stimulated much discussion and many publications in nursing about patient-centered care. The Quality and Safety Education for Nurses initiative focuses on the five core competencies and nursing education. This initiative describes providing patient-centered care as "recogniz[ing] the patient or designee as the source of control and full partner in providing compassionate and coordinated care base on respect for patient's preferences, needs, values, and needs"

(Cronewett et al., 2007, p. 123). This definition does not conflict with the IOM's description of patient-centered care.

Levels of Patient-Centered Care

There are three levels of concern when discussing patient-centered care. The first relates directly to the identification of patient-centered care as the core healthcare professional competency, focusing on the care provided by an individual healthcare professional. What must each healthcare professional, such as a nurse, know and apply in order to provide patient-centered care? This level will be discussed later in the chapter. The second level focuses on the organizational level. How do healthcare organizations situate themselves to be patient-centered organizations? The third level is the macro focus; how does the healthcare system, as viewed from the local, state, and national perspectives, ensure that the healthcare system is patient centered? Strategies to ensure the third level are primarily healthcare policy concerns, as discussed in Chapter 5.

How can patient-centered care be described at the healthcare systems level? There is consensus about the key attributes of patient-centered care. In a systematic review of nine models and frameworks used to define patient-centered care, the following six core elements were identified most frequently (Shaller, 2007):

1. Education and shared knowledge
2. Involvement of family and friends
3. Collaboration and team management
4. Sensitivity to nonmedical and spiritual dimensions of care
5. Respect for patient needs and preferences
6. Free flow and accessibility of information

What are the factors that contribute to reaching these six core elements? What factors have an impact on patient-centered care at the organizational level (Shaller, 2007)?

- **Leadership,** at the level of the Chief Executive Officer and board of directors, sufficiently committed and engaged to unify and sustain the organization in a common mission.
- **A strategic vision clearly and constantly communicated** to every member of the organization.
- **Involvement of patients and families** at multiple levels, not only in the care process, but as full participants in key committees throughout the organization.
- **Care for the caregivers through a supportive work environment** that engages employees in all aspects of process design and treats them with the same dignity and respect that they are expected to show patients and families.
- **Systematic measurement and feedback** to continuously monitor the impact of specific interventions and change strategies.
- **Quality of the physical environment** that provides a supportive and nurturing physical space and design for patients, families, and employees alike.
- **Supportive technology** that engages patients and families directly in the process of care by facilitating information access and communication with their caregivers.

An example of an approach to improve patient-centered care within healthcare organizations is the Planetree Institute initiative, "Putting Patients First." The Planetree Institute was discussed in Chapter 8. It is a nonprofit membership organization that partners with hospitals and health centers to develop and implement patient-centered care in healing environments.

The Planetree Model is patient-centered rather than provider-focused and is committed to improving medical care from the patient's perspective. It empowers patients and families through information and education, and encourages "healing partnerships" with care givers. Planetree's approach is holistic and encourages healing in all dimensions—mental, emotional, spiritual and social, as well as physical. It seeks to maximize healthcare outcomes by integrating optimal medical therapies. Access to arts and nature are also incorporated into the healing environment. (Planetree Institute, 2007)

In addition to focusing on services and relationships, the "Planetree Model recognizes the importance of architectural and interior design in the healing process. A growing body of scientific data points to improved patient outcomes and satisfaction as a result of design factors which are home-like, barrier free, support patient dignity and encourage family participation in care" (Planetree Institute, 2007). This description of an environment to support patient-centered care is also an integral part of nursing. Nursing has long emphasized the importance of the environment, or milieu in which a patient recovers, and its relationship to physical, emotional, and spiritual well-being. When nursing care is planned and implemented, these factors are considered.

Does a Patient-Centered Healthcare System Exist in the United States?

Throughout its *Quality Chasm* reports, the IOM emphasizes the need for patient-centered care.

Research shows that orienting healthcare around the preferences and needs of patients has the potential to improve patients' satisfaction with care as well as their clinical outcomes. Yet, one of five American adults reports that they have trouble communicating with their doctors and one of 10 says that they were treated with disrespect during a healthcare visit. Patients often report that test results or medical records were not available at the time of a scheduled appointment or that they received conflicting information from their providers. (Commonwealth Fund, 2008)

Patients want to be partners in their care, but why? This approach offers patients improved:

- Provider–patient communication
- Educational materials about their health concerns
- Self-management tools to help them manage their illness or condition and make informed decisions
- Access to care (timely appointments, off-hours services, and so on), use of information technology (one of the IOM core competencies discussed in more detail in Chapter 13—for example, automated patient reminders and patient access to electronic medical records)
- Continuity of care
- Posthospital follow-up and support
- Effective management of drug regimens and chronic conditions
- Access to reliable information about the quality of physicians and healthcare organizations, with the opportunity to give feedback

"Ensuring that all patients have a medical home would be an important first step toward creating a patient-centered care system" (Commonwealth Fund, 2008). People need a regular place to receive care and the opportunity to develop a relationship with healthcare providers.

A serious difficulty in developing and maintaining a patient-centered healthcare system is that much of what is described as patient-centered care is not reimbursable. For example, care coordination is not covered by insurers; it is just considered a natural part of care delivery. However, this really does not account for the time that staff must spend on coordinating care, communicating with team members, and so on.

In addition, alternative methods are not typically covered, such as communication with patients over the Internet or telephone. To really change the system, this critical issue of reimbursement must be addressed. Just as providers are told by insurers that they need to be more productive and that they have less time to spend with patients, providers are also told that they have to be more patient centered. The latter requires more time, not less time, with patients. The nursing shortage (covered in more detail in Chapter 14) also comes at a time when nurses are expected to provide patient-centered care, and yet the shortage impacts the nurses' ability to provide this care—less time, more stress, more acutely ill patients requiring more time, not enough staff, and so on.

The growing number of diverse patients also demands more patient-centered care. Diversity, discussed later in this chapter, is a driver toward change in healthcare delivery. Along with the changes in diversity is the grave concern about disparities in health care, with some ethnic and culture populations receiving different care than others; as noted by the IOM (2003a), treatment is unequal.

The concept of patient-centered healthcare is beginning to take hold. Increasingly, patients expect physicians to be responsive to their needs and preferences, to provide them with access to their medical information, and to treat them as partners in care decisions. But despite being named one of the key components of quality healthcare by the Institute of Medicine, "patient-centeredness" has yet to become the norm in primary care. (Davis, Schoenbaum, & Audet, 2005, pp. 953–954)

How can this goal of patient-centered care be reached, improving insurance coverage, access to care, and quality of care in the United States? But also, as the IOM recommends, all healthcare professionals need to be competent in providing patient-centered care, or change will not occur across the continuum of care in all healthcare settings. The following attributes of patient-centered care indicate what needs to be done to reach this goal (Davis et al., 2005, p. 954), with examples as to how they might be described.

1. *Superb access to care* (e.g., patients can easily make appointments; waiting times are short; off-hours service is available)
2. *Patient engagement in care* (e.g., patients have the option of being informed and engaged partners in their care; patients are given information on treatment plans; assistance with self-care and counseling are provided)
3. *Clinical information systems that support high-quality care, practice-based learning, and quality improvement* (e.g., healthcare organizations maintain patient registries and monitor adherence to treatment; patients receive decision support and information on recommended treatments)
4. *Care coordination* (e.g., care is coordinated across the continuum and settings; systems are in place to prevent errors that occur when multiple healthcare providers are involved; post-hospital follow-up and support are provided)
5. *Integrated and comprehensive team care* (e.g., there is a free flow of communication among physicians, nurses, and other health professionals)
6. *Routine patient feedback to doctor/healthcare providers* (e.g., low-cost, Internet-based patient surveys are used to learn from patients and inform treatment plans)
7. *Publicly available information* (e.g., patients have accurate, standardized information on healthcare providers (physicians, hospitals) to help them choose where they will get their care)

Other experts and researchers have recommended the following strategies to improve patient-centered care (Gerteis, Edgman-Levitan, Daley, & Delbanco, 1993; Halpern, Lee, Boulter, & Phillips, 2001; IOM, 2001; Lewin, Skea, Entwistle, Zwarenstein, & Dick, 2001; Pew Health Professions Commission, 1995; Stewart, 2001, as cited in IOM, 2003a, pp. 52–53): "(1) Share power and responsibility with patients and caregivers, and (2) engage in an ongoing discussion with patients to increase understanding, acceptance, cooperation, and identification of common goals and related care plans."

Reaching the goal of improved patient-centered care within a healthcare organization will require redesigning care processes to improve its delivery. It requires partnerships among practitioners, patients, and patients' families as appropriate, and even greater partnerships between schools of nursing and clinical organizations to enable students to gain more experience (Finkelman & Kenner, 2007). Care decisions need to respect patient (1) values, (2) needs, (3) preferences, and (4) cultural issues, incorporating active use of the patient input and making the patient a partner in all aspects of care delivery. The IOM reports on quality indicate that it is more common for the patient to have to adapt to the healthcare delivery system, rather than the system adapting to the patient's needs and preferences. This approach needs to change. Patients who are involved in their own care tend to have better outcomes. There is greater and greater access to information among healthcare providers, and this means that patients also have more access to information. Information provides more power and control, not just for healthcare providers but also for patients. This all leads to a growing need for greater patient empowerment; this topic is discussed further in this chapter in the sections on consumerism and self-management. There is a great need to develop patient-centered models that focus on particular populations, such as those with chronic illness, populations in rural areas, urban populations, minority groups, women, children, the elderly, people with special needs, and patients at the end of life. Nurses are playing major roles in these new models and will continue to be active as new models are developed. Taking the priority areas of care, the IOM has considered how these areas of concern apply across the life span, through all age periods from birth to death, each with its unique health issues. Within this continuum are many opportunities for new patient-centered models. Some that are already in use are palliative care and end-of-life care.

Greater Emphasis on Chronic Illness

Another factor that supports including patient-centered care as a core competency is the growing number of patients with chronic illnesses and conditions. The IOM identified the priority areas of care, along with the need to move away from a disease- and clinician-focused approach to one that includes the patient, moving the patient to the center. What are the priority areas of care? Exhibit 9–2 identifies these areas.

The IOM recognizes that the priority areas may change over time as care improves in some areas and needs increase in new ones. Chronic illnesses dominate the list. The number of persons with chronic illnesses has increased, as has the

---

EXHIBIT 9–2 INSTITUTE OF MEDICINE PRIORITY AREAS FOR NATIONAL ACTION

- Care coordination
- Self-management/health literacy
- Asthma—appropriate treatment for persons with mild/moderate persistent asthma
- Cancer screening—evidence-based, with a focus on colorectal and cervical cancer
- Children with special needs—who are at increased risk for chronic physical, developmental, and behavioral conditions
- Diabetes—focus on appropriate management of early disease
- End-of-life with advanced organ system failure—focus on congestive heart failure and chronic obstructive pulmonary disease
- Frailty associated with old age—preventing falls and pressure ulcers, maximizing function, and developing advanced care plans
- Hypertension—focus on appropriate treatment of early disease

- Immunization—children and adults
- Ischemic heart disease—prevention, reduction of recurring events, and optimization of functional capacity
- Major depression—screening and treatment
- Medical management—preventing medication errors and overuse of antibiotics
- Nosocomial infections—prevention and surveillance
- Pain control in advanced cancer
- Pregnancy and childbirth—appropriate prenatal and intrapartum care
- Severe and persistent mental illness—focus on treatment in the public sector
- Stroke—early treatment in the public sector
- Tobacco dependence treatment in adults
- Obesity

Source: From *Priority Areas for National Action: Transforming Healthcare Quality* (p. 3), by Institute of Medicine, 2003, Washington, DC: National Academies Press. Copyright 2003, the Institute of Medicine. Reprinted with permission.

number of people with more than one chronic illness. Data related to this problem include (Anderson, 2002, as cited in IOM, 2003b, p. 49; Partnership for Solutions, 2001):

- 124 million Americans have some type of chronic condition, representing nearly half of the U.S. population.
- 1.7 million Americans die annually from a chronic illness, representing 7 out of 10 deaths.
- 60 million have more than one chronic condition.
- Chronic illnesses cause major limitations in daily living for more than 1 out of 10 Americans (25 million).
- More than 3 million (2.5 million women and 750,000 men) live with five conditions.
- Inappropriate or avoidable hospitalizations have increased from 7 per 1,000 for those with one chronic condition to 95 per 1,000 for those with five chronic conditions. (Appropriate ambulatory care might have prevented these hospitalizations.)
- Chronic illness accounts for 70% of the $1 trillion spent on healthcare annually in the United States.

Why does the United States have these problems with chronic illness? One reason is that there is better treatment today, so people with chronic illnesses live longer; consequently, there are more people with chronic illness. The second reason is that the United States needs to improve care provided for chronic illness. Figure 9–3 describes the Chronic Care Model, which is highlighted by the IOM (2003a).

This is a multidimensional solution for planned, clinically integrated care to meet the complex care needs of people with chronic illness. The focus is on primary care teams (interdisciplinary) that provide care focused on chronic illness. As seen in Figure 9–3, there are two major delivery focus areas. (1) The community needs to have resources and health policies that support care for chronic illnesses. (2) The health system needs to have healthcare organizations that support self-management and that recognize that the patient is the source of control (patient-centered); a delivery system design that identifies clear roles for staff in relation to chronic illness care; decision support, with integration of evidence-based guidelines into daily practice; and clinical information systems to ensure rapid exchange of information, and reminder and feedback systems. If this is all in place and effective, the results should be productive interactions with an informed, active patient and a prepared, proactive care team. The ultimate result should then be improved outcomes. This model reinforces the strong need to have a healthcare team that is patient centered.

Methods for delivering care for chronic illness have improved, though much more needs to be done. Greater use of disease management, which is a systematic approach to managing a chronic illness, is one method that has had an impact. Typically, interventions used in disease management have been tested with large groups and thus can be more effective. Disease management emphasizes interdisciplinary teams with expertise in the specific disease; use of evidence-based clinical guidelines (discussed in more detail in Chapter 11); clear descriptions of interventions and procedures, and recommended timelines; patient support and education; and measurement of outcomes. Nurses play important roles in disease management; they may be on the team or lead the team. Disease management programs are sponsored by insurers, hospitals, and other healthcare providers. The major goals are to assist the patient in maintaining the best lifestyle possible and to prevent complications that can lead to deterioration and increased costs of care.

Figure 9–3 Chronic Care Model.

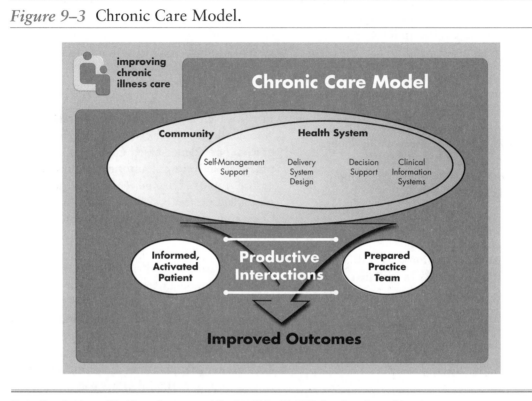

Source: From Institute of Healthcare Improvement. Retrieved May 26, 2008, from http://www.ihi.org/ IHI/Topics/ChronicConditions/AllConditions/Changes/. Reprinted with permission.

Disease management programs also empha-size prevention, although it is important to emphasize prevention throughout the healthcare system. Examples of prevention services include tobacco cessation counseling, screening (breast cancer, colorectal cancer, prostate cancer, dia-betes, hypertension, hearing, vision, cholesterol, and so on), and immunizations. Prevention is not always successful. Some of the barriers to success are (Peters & Elster, 2002):

1. Lack of reimbursement for these services
2. Lack of time for services
3. Inaccessible to populations who need these services

4. Inadequate consumer education to support need
5. Uncertainty as to effectiveness (from con-sumer and from provider perspectives)

Health promotion is also important in patient-centered care. This includes strategies that are directed at maintaining and improving health. Some of these strategies involve educa-tion about healthy lifestyles, such as diet, exer-cise, and stress reduction, and improvement in environmental status, such as control of pollu-tion or water purity. Chapter 7 includes content on *Healthy People 2010*. This initiative focuses on health promotion and prevention and is relevant to patient-centered care. The tendency is to focus on sickness when patient-centered care is discussed, but patient-centered care means that all aspects of the patient's health status are important, including promoting health and preventing disease and illness.

Related Nursing Theories

Nursing theories were discussed in Chapter 2. Some of these theories are particularly relevant to the issue of patient-centered care. These theories are Watson's theory on caring, Orem's self-care theory, Peplau's interpersonal theory, Leininger's cultural theory, and some theories related to learning. Why are these theories relevant to this content?

- Watson's theory on caring: This theory focuses on caring. Patient-centered care has a major emphasis on caring—how the patient receives care, how the patient perceives care, and how nurses and other healthcare providers perceive their roles and implement care.
- Orem's self-care theory: This theory focuses on providing support and guidance to patients so that they can be actively involved in their own care. Self-management of care is part of patient-centered care and one of the overall priority areas of care identified by the IOM.
- Leininger's cultural diversity theory: This theory focuses on cultural issues and their importance in health and healthcare delivery. The IOM's definition of patient-centered care includes cultural aspects of care, and IOM reports also discuss disparity in health care due to cultural issues, which are discussed later in this chapter.
- Peplau's interpersonal relations theory: This theory emphasizes the importance of the nurse–patient relationship and com-

munication. It is difficult to discuss or provide patient-centered care without considering the patient–provider relationship and communication.

- Learning theories: Knowles's adult learning and the health belief model (HBM): These two theories particularly relate to a patient-centered approach to patient education. Patient and family education about health and illness is a critical part of patient-centered care. This education emphasizes the active role of the patient in the care delivery process and the patient as a decision maker—the center of care. If the patient does not have adequate information and, in some cases, necessary skill to care for self, patient-centered care is diminished. The first theory, adult learning (Knowles, 1972), emphasizes that adult learners are different from younger learners and that this must be considered in any educational endeavor with adults. Patient education certainly does include children; however, there are more adult patients, and often their patient education is approached in a paternalistic manner in which they are not treated as adult learners. This is considered in more detail later in the chapter, in the section on patient education. The second theory, the HBM, also referred to as the Theory of Reasoned Action, focuses on health promotion (Hochbaum, 1958). The model was developed to predict if a person would follow medical recommendations and to gain a better understanding of patient motivation. According to this model, a person is more likely to respond to a health threat if any of the following factors are present (Masters, 2005, p. 173):
  - The person's perception of the severity of the illness

- The person's perception of susceptibility to illness and its consequences
- The value of the treatment benefits (e.g., Does the cost and side effect of treatment outweigh the consequences of the disease?)
- Barriers to treatment (e.g., expense, complexity of treatment, access to care)
- Costs of treatment in physical and emotional terms
- Cues that stimulate taking action toward treatment of illness (e.g., mass media campaigns, pamphlets, advice from family or friends, and postcard reminders from healthcare providers)

Through assessing these factors, nurses can develop a more effective patient education plan.

Consumerism: How Does It Impact Health Care and Nursing?

Consumerism may appear to be a strange term to use in a nursing textbook. It is commonly used in business, particularly in advertising. However, consumerism in health care has become a very important concept, and it relates directly to patient-centered care. As far as nursing is concerned, nursing has long viewed the patient as an integral part of the nursing process, but what does this really mean, and has nursing grasped the concept of consumerism so that it is not only spoken about, but actually a critical part of the implementation of nursing care?

Many consumers directly access the services of licensed nurses for health-related education, support and consultation. Assistive personnel are often independently hired by consumers to assist them in a wide range of activities from daily living, to childbirth, to health maintenance or wellness promotion. When patients (consumers)

are significantly health impaired and unable or incompetent to make care decisions, the nurse is often the care manager and assistive personnel carry out direct nursing care activities through the delegation process. (National Council of State Boards of Nursing, 1998, p. 1)

Nursing speaks of **patient advocacy**, and yet how patient advocacy is actively included in nursing care can vary widely. Patients, on the other hand, expect more and more to be active in their care at all levels. They do not like it when they are ignored and left out of decision making. Families are also much more assertive. Patients and families are more concerned about quality and costs. The 1999 IOM report on safety did much to bring out the major problem of safety in health care. When this report was published, the media used the content and widely shared it via newspapers, radio and television, and the Internet. The statistics in the report about the high level of errors were frightening and consequently woke up the public (consumers) to the need to be more vigilant. This report is discussed in more detail in Chapter 12.

Who Are the Consumers or Customers?

There are two major types of **consumers/customers** in health care. The *macro consumers* are the major purchasers of care: the government and insurers. They pay for care and thus are consumers in that they have expectations of the product (the care delivered) and can influence that care. The *micro consumer* is the patient. Patient families and significant others, when they play a role in the patient's care and decision-making process, are also micro consumers. Patients are turning more to nurses and asking questions about their health care and the healthcare delivery process. In the past, nurses knew little about reimbursement and the delivery process, but today, nurses need to be prepared to answer patient questions or to direct patients to resources for answers.

Customer-centered health care means that the nurse must be more aware of customer/patient needs, but this is not a simple description. Typically, one thinks of the statement, "the customer is always right"; however, in health care, this may not always be the case. The patient may not have all the information to make an informed decision and may need the expertise of healthcare professionals to meet his or her needs. Nurses need to find a balance—meeting patient needs, including the patient, and respecting the patient's opinion. Customer service goals that are important in today's healthcare system and are related to nursing include (Leebov, 2008, pp. 21–23):

1. **Caring with compassion**: This is not a foreign concept for nurses. Nurses know that patients have multiple needs and often feel vulnerable in the healthcare setting and when they are sick.
2. **Making sure caring comes across**: It is easy to wonder why caring should even be discussed in relation to nursing because caring is so much a part of nursing and its image; however, a key question needs to be asked: Does the caring come across to patients? Do nurses say and do things that really do not support caring? Yes, they do.
3. **Paying quality attention**: With the nursing shortage today, it is very easy, and in some cases critical, to focus on quantity; we do not have enough staff. However, in doing this, quality becomes less visible. The skill of presence or mindfulness involves controlling attention. This allows the persons (patient, family, others) that are on the receiving end to feel like the center at that moment. The nurse is not distracted, and the patient connects; caring occurs.
4. **Reducing patient anxiety**: This is where there is a clear deviation from what one typically thinks about when considering customers. Sales staff in a retail store want to make customers happy, but nurses and other healthcare staff want to reduce patient anxiety and support them. Making patients feel happy is not a bad result, but it may not reduce anxiety or provide support.
5. **Your personal calling**: Are you committed to improvement and caring, and how do you demonstrate this in your practice?

Critical in understanding patients is having knowledge about what they want and what they think their care outcomes should be. With increasing out-of-pocket patient expenses, as discussed in Chapter 8, there is greater need for patients to know about their needs and care, and to influence care decisions. If one compares this to shopping for a product, the buyer typically wants the best quality for the best price. Consumers are expressing concerns about the limits in their healthcare choices (e.g., employers offering fewer choices of health plans; plans with restricted or limited services; restrictions on provider use). Though healthcare consumers have changed over the years, quality of care and access to services continue to be important consumer issues. Managed care actually was a stimulus for consumers; they became more active in their complaints about the changes made by managed care in healthcare reimbursement.

Patient Rights

The Patient Self-Determination Act of 1990 is a law that has significantly impacted patient information and process. It applies to all healthcare organizations that receive Medicare or Medicaid reimbursement, and because few healthcare organizations do not receive this form of reimbursement, this law applies to most healthcare organizations. It requires that all these organizations or providers give their patients certain information that relates to confidentiality; consent; the right to make medical decisions, to be informed about diagnosis and treatment, and to refuse treatment; and use of advance directives. There is, however, no federal legislation that specifically addresses patients' rights, though there have been attempts to pass this type of legislation. "One of the most valuable aspects of the American healthcare system is its long-standing orientation to serving the needs of individual patients. . . . Much of the excellence of America's style of healthcare can be traced to the importance of the one-on-one relationship of the caregiver to the patient" (O'Neil & the Pew Health Professions Commission, 1998, pp. 34–35). It is with the patient–healthcare provider (nurse) relationship that patient-centered care can be best actualized.

Information Resources and Consumers

Today, technology provides easy access to information not only for healthcare providers but also for consumers. Chapter 13 discusses this in more detail, but it relates to patient-centered care. Through the use of new technologies, there are multiple ways to communicate with current customers/consumers/patients, such as e-mail, the Internet, and cell phones, and extensive methods to collect, manage, and use healthcare information. Patients use information to self-manage their health and care, expanding their knowledge of self-care and wellness. They seek medical advice, learn about their treatment options, and obtain information about reimbursement. The patient can increasingly obtain information to help him or her evaluate providers (physicians, hospitals, and so on), such as "report cards" about practice and outcomes, which are now more available to the public.

Customer or patient satisfaction is a critical topic in most healthcare organizations. Hospitals expend energy and monies to assess how patients feel about their services. External companies, such as Press Ganey (listed in the Internet links for this chapter), assist in data collection and analysis. Customer/patient satisfaction data can be helpful, but this information must be viewed carefully. The following are some issues and related comments about satisfaction data that can be important (Zimmerman, 2001, pp. 255–256):

1. Patient satisfaction is objective and straightforward. *This is not true. Surveys are difficult to develop, and they are often poorly designed.*
2. Patient satisfaction is easily measured. *Satisfaction is complex and not easily measured. Patient expectations play a major role in the process, and there are many factors that can affect patient responses that are not always easy to identify.*
3. Patient satisfaction is accurately and precisely measured. *This is not possible at this time. Attitudes are being measured.*
4. It is obvious who the customer is. *A healthcare organization actually has many different types of customers—more than just patients, for example, families, physicians, insurers, and internal customers (staff within the organization become customers to other staff, e.g., laboratory provides services to the units and thus nursing staff on the units are the laboratory's customers). A complete customer satisfaction analysis should include multiple types of customers in the healthcare organization.*

Exhibit 9–3 lists some consumer tips.

When it comes to quality of care, there is no clear universal definition of quality of care. A patient often sees quality of care and services differently than a nurse or physician would. An

---

---

insurer may look at quality mostly from a cost perspective. This makes it difficult to analyze satisfaction data objectively. In a study about views on quality, data from patients, nurses, and physicians were collected and compared (Shannon, Mitchell, & Cain, 2002). The sample included 489 patients, 518 nurses, and 515 physicians from 25 intensive care units in 14 hospitals. Standardized instruments were used to collect the data. What were the results? Physicians rated the quality of care higher than did either the patients or the nurses, and they were more likely to overestimate patient satisfaction. Patients and nurses were more similar in how they assessed quality of care. The overall results concluded that there was considerable variation within the three groups (patients, nurses, physicians) and among the 25 intensive care units, with patients, nurses, and physicians viewing patient satisfaction and quality of care differently. It is important to be careful not to assume that when a healthcare provider has a positive view of the quality of care and patient satisfaction, the patient agrees. When patients in ambulatory care express different views of quality from hospitalized patients, this is a concern. Root cause analysis needs to be done. In examining the issue, the ambulatory care patients were found to be more concerned with access issues, wait time for appointments, how much time the provider spends with him or her, response from office or clinic staff, follow-up, and access to information. These patients were not as interested in care out-

comes. The hospitalized patient data focused more on physical care, emotional support, response from staff when they were called for assistance, involvement of family and how this is accepted, sharing of information and communication, respect for patient's values and preferences, and education provided to assist the patient in understanding treatment and aftercare.

A government survey about patient satisfaction conducted in 2006–2007 (U.S. Department of Health and Human Services, 2008a) indicated that patients are dissatisfied with hospitals. Although 65% said that they would recommend the hospital to others, some of the results indicated serious problems. Patients indicated that they were not treated with courtesy and respect by doctors and nurses, that they had not received adequate pain medication after surgery, and that they did not understand instructions that they were given for discharge. A total of 25% felt that nurses did not always communicate well with them.

Culture, Diversity, and Disparities in Health Care

Healthy People 2010 identified two major goals for the health of U.S. citizens. The second goal is to "eliminate health **disparities**, which focuses on a variety of factors that have an impact on health disparities such as gender, **race** and **ethnicity**, income and education, disability, geographic location, sexual orientation to achieve equity" (U.S. Department of Health and Human Services, 1998). This goal also indicates that providers throughout the healthcare system, including nurses, need to know more about **culture**, as indicated in the definition of patient-centered care.

Culture

Culture is "generally defined as a shared system of values, beliefs, traditions, behavior, verbal and nonverbal patterns of communication that hold a group of people together and distinguish them from other groups" (Salimbene, 1999, p. 25). Nurses view patients through their personal experiences with culture and their personal histories. This may lead to problems, such as misinterpretation of communication and behavior, that result in limitations in planning and implementing patient-centered care that meets the patient's needs. Culture and language may influence the following (U.S. Department of Health and Human Services, 2008b):

- Health, healing, and wellness belief systems
- Patient/consumer perception of causes of illness and disease
- Patients/consumer behaviors and their attitudes toward healthcare providers
- Provider perceptions and values

In the United States, there is increasing population growth of different racial and ethnic communities and linguistic groups. Each population, with its own cultural traits and health profiles, presents a challenge to the healthcare delivery system and providers. The provider and the patient bring their individual learned patterns of language and culture to the healthcare experience. This has an impact on the care process and may influence the increase in healthcare disparities. The demographics indicate that more nurses are caring for patients from different cultural, racial, and ethnic backgrounds. In some areas, there are clusters of different cultural populations, such as African Americans, Hispanics, Native Americans, and Asians. It is predicted that by 2010, the U.S. population will be 32% minority ethnic (Institute for the Future, 2000). Areas of the United States that have the highest **diversity** in order of size are the South, the West, the Northeast, and the Midwest. This all requires greater emphasis on providing care that is respectful of, and responsive to, the health beliefs, practices, and cultural and linguistic needs of diverse patient populations (U.S. Department of Health and Human Services, 2008a).

Cultural Competence

Cultural and linguistic competence is a set of congruent behaviors, attitudes, and policies that come together in a system, agency, or among professionals that enables effective work in cross-cultural situations. "Culture" refers to integrated patterns of human behavior that include the language, thoughts, communications, actions, customs, beliefs, values, and institutions of racial, ethnic, religious, or social groups. "Competence" implies having the capacity to function effectively as an individual and an organization within the context of the cultural beliefs, behaviors, and needs presented by consumers and their communities. (IOM, 2003a, adapted from Cross, Bazron, Dennis, & Isaacs, 1989)

Schools of nursing and healthcare organizations are working to improve cultural competence in students, faculty, and practicing nurses (Finkelman & Kenner, 2007). This has been driven by the IOM reports that indicate healthcare disparities. Competence "implies having the capacity to function effectively as an individual and as an organization within the context of the cultural beliefs, behaviors, and needs presented by consumers and their communities" (Anderson, Scrimshaw, Fullilove, Fielding, & Normand, 2003, pp. 68–69). What are some of the components of cultural competencies (Salimbene, 1999)?

- Recognition that patient-centered care includes the patient's culture and background
- An awareness of, sensitivity to, and tolerance of differences in culture and language
- An ability to avoid the use of inappropriate stereotyping, **prejudice**, and **bias**
- Understanding the role that culture plays in health care (health/illness and practices)
- Recognizing one's own culture and background and its impact on attitudes and beliefs, and the ability to make adaptations to meet the needs of the patient
- Knowledge of cultures relevant to the patient populations served and incorporation of this knowledge into planning and implementation of care
- Providing patient education that considers culture and language issues (**health literacy**)
- Ability to be flexible to ensure effective patient-centered care

Disparities in Health Care

Disparities in health care are defined as "racial or ethnic differences in the quality of healthcare that are not due to access-related factors or clinical needs, preferences, and appropriateness of intervention" (IOM, 2002a, pp. 3–4). The IOM looked at two issues when determining the existence of disparities in health care. The first is how the healthcare system functions, and legal and regulatory issues that may make it difficult for patients to get equal care. The second is discrimination at the patient provider level. Discrimination is defined as "differences in care that result from bias, prejudices, stereotyping and

uncertainty in clinical communication and decision-making" (IOM, 2002a, p. 4). What do some of these terms mean?

- *Bias*: Predisposed to a point of view
- *Ethnicity*: Shared feeling of belonging to a group—peoplehood.
- ***Ethnocentrism:*** Belief that one's group or culture is superior to others.
- *Prejudice*: Making assumptions or judgments about the beliefs, behaviors, needs, and expectations of patients or other healthcare staff of a different cultural background than oneself because of emotional beliefs about the population; involves negative attitudes toward the "different" group.
- *Race*: A biological designation of a group; belonging to the group based on biological factor(s).
- *Stereotyping*: This is a "process by which people use social groups (such as sex and race) to gather, process, and recall information about other people . . . these are labels" (IOM, 2002a, p. 475). It is natural for people to organize information, and organizing information about people is part of this. However, this process can be negative if it involves unfairly classifying people or using incorrect information about an individual who may or may not meet the characteristics.

After the IOM report on disparities in health care indicated that there were problems in the United States, it was recognized that more effective monitoring of diversity in health care was necessary. In 2001, the National Healthcare Disparities Report was created. This annual report, accessible via the Internet, focuses on five critical areas (IOM, 2002b, p. 2):

1. Measurement of socioeconomic status in disparities research

2. Measurement of disparities in healthcare services and quality

3. Measurement of disparities in healthcare access

4. Measurement of geographic units in disparities research

4. Sub-national datasets

Critical issues of socioeconomic status, service and quality, and access, as well as geographic issues, are covered in this annual report. Healthcare disparities occur consistently across a variety of illnesses and delivery services and are associated not with specific types of illnesses but with a broad spectrum.

The U.S. Department of Health and Human Services (DHHS) (2008c) has published information on its Web site about culture and health care. The DHHS describes health disparities as the persistent gaps between the health status of minorities and nonminorities in the United States. How has it happened that there is inequity in healthcare services and health? As defined by the IOM, equity in health services involves "providing care that does not vary in quality because of personal characteristics such as gender, ethnicity, geographic location and socioeconomic status" (2001, p. 6). Despite continued advances in health care and technology, racial and ethnic minorities continue to have more disease, disability, and premature death than nonminorities. African Americans, Hispanics/Latinos, American Indians and Alaska Natives, Asian Americans, Native Hawaiians, and Pacific Islanders have higher rates of infant mortality, cardiovascular disease, diabetes, human immunodeficiency virus infection/ acquired immune deficiency syndrome, and cancer, and lower rates of immunizations and cancer screening. Two major factors impact these results:

1. *Inadequate access to care*: Barriers to care can result from economic, geographic, linguistic, cultural, and healthcare financing issues. Even when minorities have similar levels of access to care, health insurance, and education, the quality and intensity of health care they receive are often poor.

2. *Substandard quality of care*: Lower quality care has many causes, including patient–provider miscommunication, provider discrimination, stereotyping, and prejudice. Quality of care is usually rated on four measures: effectiveness, patient safety, timeliness, and patient-centeredness.

DISPARITIES: EXAMPLES AND IMPORTANCE

Disparities in health status and health outcomes can be categorized by individual factors and healthcare system factors (Peters & Elster, 2002):

1. *Individual factors*: Sociodemographic characteristics (e.g., age, race/ethnicity, gender), socioeconomic status (e.g., income, occupation, and education), or other personal characteristics such as disabilities, rural or urban residency, and sexual orientation. Although biological and genetic factors account for some of these group differences, other contributing factors include cultural norms and values, literacy levels, familial influences, environmental and occupational exposures, and patient preferences for care and treatment. Uneven distribution of societal resources, including social and political advantages such as knowledge and social connections, has a negative impact on health. Individual health behaviors also vary by race/ethnicity, income, and education and may explain group differences in mortality and morbidity, but this does not account for all of the disparities found in mortality and morbidity rates. Promoting healthy lifestyles and reducing health risk behaviors are interventions that nurses and other healthcare providers can use to intervene in reducing healthcare disparities.

2. *Healthcare system factors*: The rates of access to, and utilization of, health care vary among population groups. Explanations for these differences include insurance status and affordability, transportation and geographic barriers to needed services, health beliefs, attitudes, level of self-confidence in complying with treatment, racial concordance of patient and physician, cultural preferences for less invasive procedures, and provider bias, racism, and discrimination.

STRATEGIES TO OVERCOME DISPARITIES

It is most likely not possible to totally eliminate disparities in health care; however, much can be done to improve care for all persons and improving equity in health care. Ensuring access is critical. Can patients get the care they need from experts in a timely manner? Access involves multiple factors, such as appointments, transportation to appointments, availability of qualified staff, wait times, service hours, and so on. Disparity issues require that all healthcare professionals actively consider patient values and preferences (a critical component of patient-centered care). These values and preferences can vary between groups and within groups. It is easy to **stereotype** and assume that everyone in a specific ethnic group is the same, but this is not the case. Monitoring data on disparities is important to assist in identifying current status and to develop and improve effective interventions to reach desired outcomes. This monitoring is now being done annually in the National Disparities Report, but individual healthcare provider organizations such as hospitals can also monitor their own data and outcomes.

Diversity in the Healthcare Workforce

The Sullivan Commission report (Sullivan, 2004), which is separate from the IOM reports,

examined disparities in health care from a different perspective. This commission concluded that a key contributor to the growing healthcare disparity problem is the disparities in the nation's health professional workforce. This limits minorities' access to health care and to healthcare providers who understand their needs. The commission suggested that there should be an increase in the number of minority health professionals. This comes at a time when there is a shortage of nurses and other healthcare providers. There must be greater efforts to increase minority admissions to nursing programs and to retain students. The federal government is providing grants to encourage schools of nursing to increase minority enrollment, develop support services, and increase minority enrollment in graduate school to increase the number of minority nursing faculty. It will take time to improve the level of minority participation in nursing. The American Organization of Nurse Executives (AONE) issued a position statement on diversity in 2005, stating that the AONE, as the voice for nursing leadership, is "committed to advocate for and achieve diversity within the community of nurse leaders and in the workplace environment" (p. 10). The statement also recognizes that "perceptions regarding health and illness, patterns of communication, approaches to work, decision-making, leadership styles, and team-building are inherently influenced by an individual's culture" (p. 11). This demonstrates the complexity of the issue of culture; it impacts all aspects of work within the healthcare environment.

Patient Advocacy

Advocacy has always been a major aspect of the nursing role with the consumer and requires leadership skills. Nursing standards developed by the American Nurses Association, nursing specialty organizations, and healthcare institutions, as well as those developed by accrediting organizations and other healthcare professional organizations, support advocacy and consumerism. Throughout the care delivery process, nurses participate in, and support actions that emphasize, patient advocacy. They support patient and family education, patient satisfaction and the complaint process, and efforts to improve care, and they support and ask for patient participation in healthcare decision making. As each nurse provides care, he or she has numerous opportunities to be the patient's advocate. The nurse coordinates the care and in doing so represents the patient, but the nurse needs to recognize the patient's values and preferences in this process, thus supporting patient-centered care. This means that the nurse must know about the patient's values and preferences—for example, cultural issues and how they might impact the patient. This should lead to an improved collaborative relationship with the patient. Collaboration is "the process of joint decision-making among interdependent parties, involving joint ownership of decisions and collective responsibility for outcomes" (Disch, 2001, p. 275). When the nurse acts as the patient advocate, he or she remembers that the patient must be involved. Advocacy does not mean that the nurse makes the patient dependent on him or her. The nurse must also be persuasive with other healthcare team members to ensure better care for the patient that meets the patient's needs (outcomes). Advocacy means that the nurse is active in respecting the patient and patient rights, ensuring that the patient has the education to understand treatment and care needs. Support is given to the patient and family; if the patient makes a treatment decision based on information given to him or her, the nurse does not judge the patient's decision even though he or she may disagree with it.

Care Coordination: A Plan of Care

Care coordination is the first of the priority areas of care identified by the IOM. What is the purpose of care coordination? "To establish and support a continuous healing relationship, enabled by an integrated clinical environment and characterized by a proactive delivery of evidence-based care and follow-up" (IOM, 2003a, p. 49). To accomplish this, healthcare providers, including nurses, need to provide patient-centered care. The IOM also discusses the need for clinical integration and care coordination. What does this mean? It focuses on how care is coordinated across people, functions, activities, and sites (including the community and home) so that the patient receives effective care.

Critical Thinking, Clinical Reasoning, and Clinical Judgment

For a long time, nurse educators have included **critical thinking** in curricula; however, the content itself and how it is taught need to be revised. There are 15 patterns of change in thinking and learning that are relevant in today's healthcare delivery system and important to include in nursing education (Rubenfeld & Scheffer, 2006, p. 236). The following patterns are an important part of effective critical thinking that can improve nursing competency. There is a need to change:

- **From** passivity **to** engagement/presence
- **From** answers **to** questions
- **From** separate thinking and doing **to** thinking and doing together
- **From** destinations **to** journeys
- **From** reactive learning **to** proactive learning
- **From** mechanistic models **to** living systems models

- **From** dichotomous thinking **to** relativistic thinking
- **From** thinking of pieces **to** thinking of wholes
- **From** thinking alone **to** systems thinking
- **From** reduction **to** complexity
- **From** matching existing patterns **to** new patterns
- **From** linear **to** maps/knots/shapes
- **From** constant success **to** failure possibilities
- **From** valuing only objectivity **to** being open to intuition
- **From** reviewing **to** reflecting

Critical thinking and **clinical reasoning** and judgment should be used throughout the nursing process. They are important to effective nursing practice, but it takes time and experience to develop all three and to use them effectively.

Critical thinking requires nurses to generate and examine questions and problems, use intuition, examine feelings, and clarify and evaluate evidence. It means being aware of change and willing to take some risks. Critical thinking allows the nurse to avoid using dichotomous thinking—seeing things either as good or bad, or black or white. This limits possibilities and clinical choices for patients (Finkelman, 2001). An expert panel of 55 nurses defined critical thinking

as an essential component of professional account-ability and quality nursing care. Critical thinkers in nursing exhibit these habits of the mind: confidence, contextual perspective, creativity, flexibility, inquisitiveness, intellectual integrity, intuition, open-mindedness, perseverance, and reflection. Critical thinkers in nursing practice use the cognitive skills of analyzing, applying standards, discriminating, information seeking, logical reasoning, predicting, and transforming knowledge. (Scheffer & Rubenfeld, 2000, p. 357)

Clinical reasoning is the "practitioner's ability to assess patient problems or needs and analyze data to accurately identify and frame problems within the context of the individual patient's environment" (Murphy, 2004, p. 227).

The key components of critical thinking are information seeking (in-depth searching and asking questions), reflecting (reviewing experiences broadly, evaluating, examining cognitive processes), assigning meaning (identifying relevant data and interpreting), problem-solving, predicting, planning (knowing what to do next and making decisions), and applying novel contexts (Twibell, Ryan, & Hermiz, 2005).

Clinical judgment requires more than recall and understanding of content or selection of the correct answer; it also requires the ability to apply, analyze, and synthesize knowledge (Del Bueno, 2005). Nursing clinical judgment is the process, or the "ways in which nurses come to understand the problems, issues or concerns of clients/patients, to attend to salient information, and to respond in concerned and involved ways" (Benner, Tanner, & Chesla, 1996, p. 2). This process includes both deliberate, conscious decision making and intuition. "In the real world, patients do not present the nurse with a written description of their clinical symptoms and a choice of written potential solutions" (Del Bueno, 2005, p. 282). Beginning nursing students, however, are looking for the clear picture of the patient that matches what he or she has read about in the textbook. This patient really does not exist, and so critical thinking and clinical reasoning and judgment become more important as the student learns to compare and contrast what might be expected with what is reality.

Nursing Process

The **nursing process** is a systematic method for thinking about, and communicating how, nurses provide patient care. It is a step-by-step tool that guides nurses as they plan and provide care in a variety of clinical settings. The process requires that nurses use critical thinking, clinical reasoning, and clinical judgment. Students are asked to use the process often by developing extensive care plans for patients. As students become registered nurses and move into practice, this process is adapted for daily use with multiple patients.

What is included in the nursing process? The process is similar to the problem-solving process in that there is a concern that requires more information to determine the best approach to solving it. In the nursing process, there are five steps, as described in Figure 9–4.

1. Assessment: Information, or data about the patient, is required to describe the patient's health status and needs. The information is collected during assessment by multiple methods, such as a description of the patient's health history, interviews, observation, physical exam, and review of medical records. The nursing process is not linear; it is ongoing, and one step leads to the next step and then begins again. Assessment does begin the process; however, assessment is ongoing because a patient's health status and needs change, which may require a change in diagnosis, plan, and how a plan is implemented. This also impacts outcomes and evaluation. During assessment, the nurse must evaluate the quality of the information to determine if further information is needed, and the best method to obtain the information. It is during this step that the nurse begins to establish the nurse–patient relationship, which is discussed in a later section of this chapter. Patient-centered care means that the patient's values, preferences, needs, culture, and history play a critical role in the planned care. The nurse needs to document the assessment in a manner that is clear and that informs other staff. As will be discussed in Chapter 10, effective care is delivered by an interdisciplinary team. This means that the nursing plan of care should not be separate from other aspects of the patient's care needs. The team needs to consider all aspects of care and collaborate. There needs to be greater movement toward a patient plan of care rather than a focus on a specific profession's plan of care, such as the nursing care plan or medical care plan.

Patients often complain that many staff from different healthcare disciplines ask them the same questions. Some healthcare organizations are trying to address this problem by eliminating repetition in assessment forms—for example, making sure that the assessment forms that physicians use and the nursing assessment forms are not repetitive without sufficient rationale. Some have been more successful than

Figure 9–4 Nursing care process.

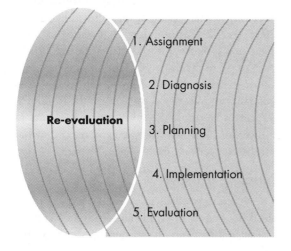

1. Assignment
2. Diagnosis
3. Planning
4. Implementation
5. Evaluation

Re-evaluation

others in this endeavor. Nurses do hear these complaints from patients, and it is inefficient.

The assessment is a critical time to communicate to the patient that he or she is the center of concern. This requires attention on the part of the nurse. Patient rights are also important—for example, maintaining privacy during the assessment, ensuring confidentiality of information obtained, and explaining to the patient the process and his or her rights. As part of the assessment, nurses (Alfaro-LeFevre, 2006, p. 91):

- Collect data
- Identify cues and make inferences from the data
- Validate the data
- Organize (cluster) the data
- Identify patterns in the data
- Report and record the data/documentation

2. Diagnosis: Diagnosis occurs as the nurse analyzes and interprets the information/data to determine the patient's nursing problems and needs, actual and potential. Nursing diagnoses have been identified and categorized through a system referred to as the North American Nursing Diagnosis Association (NANDA) (Carpenito-Moyet, 2007). As part of the diagnosis step, nurses (Alfaro-LeFevre, 2006, p. 91):

- Create a list of suspected problems/diagnoses
- Rule out similar problems/diagnoses
- Identify actual and potential problems/diagnoses and clarify possible causes (etiology) or contributors
- Determine risk factors that need to be managed
- Identify resources, strengths, limitations, and areas for health promotion

3. Planning: The care plan directs the care that will be given, promotes communication and sharing of information, and provides a record of the plan. The plan identifies the interventions or actions that the nurse may take to manage or resolve problems; to monitor the patient; to decrease risks of injury or illness; to promote health or prevent injury or illness; to support patient self-management; and to provide patient-centered care. Interventions may be direct or indirect care. Direct care interventions are "actions performed through direct interaction with the patient" (Alfaro-LeFevre, 2006, p. 170)—for example, administering medication, helping the patient get out of bed, changing a dressing, teaching the patient, and assessing or monitoring patient status. Indirect care interventions are "actions performed away from the patient, but on behalf of the patient" (Alfaro-LeFevre, p. 170)—for example, documenting in the medical record, preparing medications, giving a report on a patient's status, talking to the physician about the patient, reviewing medical orders, and delegating care to **unlicensed assistive personnel**, such as explaining what needs to be done for the patient during daily care. Nursing care and interventions can also be classified as (1) dependent care, meaning that the nurse cannot legally prescribe medications or act without a physician order (after the physician orders the medical intervention, the nurse may follow the orders); (2) independent care, meaning that the nurse may make decisions about interventions to prevent, reduce, or alleviate the problem; and (3) interdependent care, including care in which both the nurse and physician collaborate. State nurse practice acts identify

the types of care that are independent, dependent, and interdependent within each state.

Planning takes time and must be connected to the assessment data and the diagnoses/problems identified for the patient. The patient needs to be part of the planning, the identification of care needs, and the explanation of the plan. This supports patient-centered care. The key activities in the planning step are (Alfaro-LeFevre, 2006, p. 154):

- Focus on urgent problems
- Clarify expected outcomes (results)
- Decide which problems need to be recorded
- Determine individualized nursing interventions
- Ensure that the plan is adequately recorded

The plan identifies interventions; responsibility for implementing interventions; timeline; and expected outcomes. Outcomes are particularly important in evaluation. Some schools of nursing and some hospitals use lists of typical nursing interventions and outcomes. The lists are the Nursing Intervention Classification (Bulechek, Butcher, & Docterman, 2007) and Nursing Outcomes Classification (Johnson, Meridean, & Moorehead, 2007).

4. Implementation: The plan is developed so that the patient can receive the care required, and this requires implementation of the plan. Change may be required at any time during the process. It is possible that as the plan is implemented, the patient's status changes, or maybe an intervention is not effective. Many factors impact implementation, such as the nurse's competency, how delegation is handled, staffing levels, acuity levels of all the patients whom the nurse is caring for at the time, availability of supplies and resources, the number of interruptions, the needs of the patient's family, patient cooperation and acceptance of the plan, time management and priorities, and much more. As part of the implementation, nurses (Alfaro-LeFevre, 2006, p. 197):

- Prepare for report and get report
- Set daily priorities
- Assess appropriateness of (and readiness for) interventions
- Perform interventions and reassess to determine responses
- Make immediate changes as needed
- Document to monitor progress and communicate care
- Give report

Throughout the implementation step, it is critical that the nurse coordinate, collaborate, and communicate with the interdisciplinary team and other nursing staff. Delegation is part of implementation, which is described later in this chapter.

5. Evaluation: This step focuses on each of the nursing care process steps. Was the assessment adequate? (assessment); Are there changes in the patient's status that require attention? (assessment); Are there new diagnoses/problems? (diagnosis); What are the outcomes for the identified nursing diagnoses/problems? (diagnosis); Were the interventions completed, and what were the outcomes? (planning, implementation); Are new interventions required? (planning, implementation). Reevaluation should take place throughout the process as the patient's health status changes. This may require that the nurse return to a previous step in the nursing process. The key activities in the evaluation step are (Alfaro-LeFevre, 2006, p. 229):

- Determine outcomes achievement.
- Identify variables (factors) that affect outcome achievement.
- Decide whether to discharge the patient or continue or change the plan. (Nurses do not typically discharge the patient, but they should participate in the decision process with the treatment team.)

Getting patients involved in their care can be challenging. Most patients want to be involved, but nurses must use strategies to support patient-centered care. Box 9–1 provides some examples of strategies to help encourage patient participation in the thinking process, which is an important part of care planning.

Care/Concept Mapping

The traditional format for the nursing care plan, which focuses on the five steps just outlined, has been used for a long time; however, it has been the subject of some criticism. Its length is one issue, but it might also limit critical thinking, clinical reasoning, and clinical judgment because of its rigid format. "The concept map care plan is an innovative approach to planning and organizing nursing care. In essence, a concept map care plan is a diagram of patient problems and interventions. Your ideas (concepts) about patient problems and treatments are the 'concept' that will be diagrammed" (Schuster, 2002, p. 2). Using concept mapping for care plans develops critical thinking and clinical reasoning.

How are concept map plans developed? The steps include the following.

1. *Develop the basic skeleton diagram.* The nurse begins with the patient's reason for care (often the medical diagnosis), putting this in the center of the page or diagram. Around this central point, general problems (nursing problems) are identified. This is the first concept map.
2. *Analyze and categorize data.* In this step, the focus is on the information (assessment data) that is known; categorization provides evidence for the medical and nursing diagnoses. The information is obtained

---

BOX 9–1 STRATEGIES TO HELP HEALTHCARE PROVIDERS ENCOURAGE PATIENT PARTICIPATION IN THE THINKING PROCESS

- Stay in the room. Don't talk to patients from the doorway.
- Pay attention to your body language and to theirs.
- Sit down so that you are at eye level with the patient.
- Use open questions and comments, such as "Tell me about . . .," instead of closed questions that imply that you expect a short answer.
- Touch patients, but be respectful of their space and cultural norms.
- Use collaborative thinking language, such as "We should think this through," "Let's look at some possible conclusions," and "Can we analyze this together?"
- Use phrases that let the patient know that his or her situation is not so unusual that he or she cannot discuss it. For example, "Some people feel anxious when . . ."
- Address patients respectfully. Find out if they prefer Mr. or Mrs., Professor, Reverend, and so on.
- Do not look at your watch no matter how busy you are.
- Be direct and honest. For example, tell patients when the schedule is backed up and why.
- If you feel like avoiding a patient, reflect on why you feel that way.

Source: From *Critical Thinking Tactics for Nurses*, by M.G. Rubenfeld and B. Scheffer, 2006, Sudbury, MA: Jones and Bartlett Publishers.

from history, assessment, medical records, and interviews with the patient. This information is added to the **care map**—problems/diagnoses with related data.

3. *Analyzing nursing diagnoses relationships.* Taking the data map that also includes the problems with related data identified per problem, the nurse begins to make connections by analyzing relationships among the diagnoses, drawing lines to identify the relationships and numbering each problem/diagnosis. The goal is a holistic view of the patient.

4. *Identifying goals, outcomes, and interventions.* On a separate page, the nurse identifies the patient's goals and outcomes. He or she then identifies interventions to meet these goals and outcomes for each of the problems/diagnoses numbered on the care map. This step is similar to the planning process in the nursing care process.

5. *Evaluate the patient's responses.* On the page with the goals, outcomes, and interventions for each of the problems, the nurse adds the patient's responses (outcomes) to each of the interventions after they have been implemented and evaluated. This information is then used in documentation.

The concept map approach is more visual; the nurse creates the diagram and can add to it. It is similar to traditional nursing care because all the components are included. However, it allows for more creative thinking because the nurse creates a visual of the patient's status, care needs, and the plan for care.

Self-Management of Care

Regardless of whether healthcare providers accept it, patients (consumers) are very active in managing their own care. Even if they choose not

to receive health care, they have made a decision about the importance of their health and what they want to do about it. In some cases, the consumer is pushed into greater responsibility for his or her own care; he or she may have inadequate reimbursement or no reimbursement at all, or he or she may not have support from family and others. It is recognized that critical strategies in preventing health problems and reducing healthcare costs is self-management, health promotion, and disease and illness prevention. When patients use self-management effectively and are supported by healthcare providers to use self-management, the outcomes are (1) greater collaboration with healthcare providers, (2) greater understanding of treatment choices and patient and healthcare provider responsibilities, and (3) improved follow-up to treatment. Patients who are involved in their healthcare decisions are more satisfied with their health care and health status. The IOM defines self-management support as "the systematic provision of education and supportive interventions to increase patients' skills and confidence in managing their health problems, including regular assessment of progress and problems, goal setting, and problem-solving approach" (2003b, p. 52). Health literacy plays an important role in self-management. Based on this definition of self-management, it is critical to consider two important factors in nursing care: health literacy and its impact, and patient education.

Health Literacy: A Barrier

Nearly 90 million Americans (almost half of all adults) have difficulty understanding and using health information. This serious problem has increased the rate of hospitalizations and the use of emergency services, and it increases healthcare costs. How does this happen? If a patient cannot understand directions given to him or her and does not follow the directions, the patient may need more intensive care, including hospitalization. A patient who does not understand the diabetic diet or how to use insulin correctly will have health problems; he or she may then seek out help in the emergency room and consequently need to be hospitalized. Healthcare literacy includes reading, writing, and arithmetic skills; listening and speaking abilities; and conceptual knowledge. Health literacy is defined as "the degree to which individuals have the capacity to obtain, process, and understand basic information and services needed to make appropriate decisions regarding their health" (IOM, 2004, p. 2). Even well-educated people can find themselves in a health literacy position and not understand medical information. The Joint Commission has highlighted that communication problems are the most common root cause of healthcare errors (The Joint Commission, 2008). Safety and errors are discussed in more detail in Chapter 12, but it is important for this discussion about patient-centered care to recognize the connection between healthcare literacy and self-management.

With the increase in the number of patients from diverse backgrounds, healthcare organizations are seeking more and more language interpreters, particularly Spanish but also other languages. Families are not the best source for interpretation because they are not trained in medical terminology, and they may influence the process because of their personal connection to the patient. An interpreter interprets only the language or words and is not involved in how the patient should respond. Some healthcare organizations have bilingual staff, who can be a useful source of interpreting services if they are easily accessible and still able to complete their usual work. In 2006, the U.S. Department of Health and Human Services Office of Minority Health issued a new guide to help healthcare organizations implement effective language access services and improve care for patients with limited English skills. The report, *A Patient-Centered Guide to Implementing Language Access Services in Healthcare Organizations,* is a practical and basic step-by-step approach to implementing language services. Activities such as this one have been influenced by the IOM reports and their recommendations.

> *A growing number of healthcare organizations and providers are working to improve patients' access to and understanding of basic health information. They note that low health literacy represents a major barrier to high-quality care, particularly among low-income, underserved and minority patients. Dennis O'Leary, president of The Joint Commission, calls low health literacy "a silent epidemic that threatens the quality of healthcare." He says the issue remains largely unaddressed by providers in many settings. While cultural and linguistic issues can hinder health literacy, health experts note that low health literacy is most prevalent among patients who are elderly, low income or chronically ill. To raise awareness among providers and patients of health literacy's importance, The Joint Commission in early February, 2007, issued 35 recommendations on the subject. The guidelines call on providers to adopt more effective provider-patient communication techniques, simplify consent forms, use less medical jargon and post patient-friendly navigation signs in health facilities. (Boodman, 2007)*

Nurses are in direct contact with patients daily and encounter many patients who are experiencing health literacy problems. This has an impact on how effective nurses can be in providing care, in assisting patients with self-management of their care, and in teaching patients what they need to know to understand their health, illness, and care needs.

Patient/Family Education: Inclusion in Plan of Care

Patient and family teaching is best defined by Travelbee: "The core of health teaching in nursing is (if necessary) to assist ill individuals to find meaning in illness, as well as the very measures they must take to conserve health and control symptoms of illness" (1971, p. 11). This presents patient teaching from two perspectives: (1) helping the patient to understand the illness experience and cope with it effectively, and (2) provide information and direction for **self-management of care**. One of the major nursing activities is patient education. It is not an activity that the nurse can delegate unless the learning need is best addressed by another healthcare professional. The RN cannot delegate patient education to non-RNs because this is a nursing responsibility. It is not easy to provide effective patient education. The barriers to meeting patient education needs may include:

- Inadequate assessment of the patient's education needs; inadequate patient education plan
- Lack of time to provide the education required
- Interruptions that limit concentration
- Medical status of the patient (Patient is unable to participate.)
- Unclear assessment of the role of the family/significant others (Does the family want or need to participate in the education?)
- Patient education in settings such as ambulatory care typically not reimbursed; less emphasis placed on education as a result
- Confusion regarding who is responsible for patient education
- Lack of effective learning strategies and tools to meet individual patient education needs
- Lack of nursing staff (Nurses must see to other aspects of nursing that are more critical.)

- Lack of follow-up and evaluation of patient outcomes related to the education provided

Given the realities of the healthcare workplace today, it is difficult to plan and implement education for patients and their families. This can be very frustrating for the nurse and the patient. Patients are discharged early, but they are often still sick. While in the hospital, they may not be able to concentrate on what they need to learn, and then they are sent home and feel at a loss. Home care is one resolution, but most home care is not 24-7, and patients still need to know about their illness or injury, and treatment. Home health nurses provide a lot of the education, but patient education needs to be provided in the hospital as well. Patients who do not have home health services are particularly vulnerable.

When nurses are rushed, the typical scenario is to hand the patient and/or family some written information. The nurse may ask if there are questions. This is not effective patient education. What is effective education?

1. *The nurse assesses the patient's education status and needs.* What does the patient need to know? How much does he or she know?
2. *The nurse identifies (diagnoses) learning needs; for example, the patient needs to know how to administer insulin and how to plan a diet.*
3. *The nurse develops a learning plan with specific interventions.* These interventions are based on expected outcomes. The nurse identifies who is responsible for providing the learning intervention and creates the time line. Here the nurse must consider the patient's values and preferences, age, family support, cultural background and issues, and health literacy. For example, the nurse will teach the diabetic patient about equipment and where to get it; how to draw up insulin, including checking dosage and so on; how to prepare the skin; and how to administer the medication. He or she will talk

about complications and aftercare needs. The nurse discusses how the patient will keep track of the insulin administered and address storage issues. The nurse plans several sessions with the patient and uses a variety of teaching-learning strategies, such as discussion, visuals, equipment, demonstration, and return demonstration. The family is included as appropriate. The patient needs time to ask questions and express concerns.

4. *The nurse implements the plan.* Typically, this is not delegated unless assigned to another RN. Many of the barriers mentioned earlier come into play when implementing the plan. It takes planned effort to make sure the patient gets the education that he or she needs at the proper time.

5. *The nurse evaluates the plan/interventions.* Were the expected outcomes met? This is commonly a weak part of the process, often because the patient goes on to another setting or home. It is important, whenever possible, to assess outcomes, such as through questions, return demonstrations, and so on, and to ask the patient how he or she feels about the process and outcomes. Often the patient is discharged, preventing complete evaluation of patient education.

For nursing care to be patient centered and each patient to develop effective self-management of health and care needs, the patient will need information and skills to meet his or her individual needs.

Therapeutic Use of Self in the Nurse–Patient Relationship

When a nursing student begins to care for patients, eventually he or she realizes that the relationship is different from other relationships that the student has experienced. It is not a parent–child relationship, a teacher–student relationship, or a personal or friend relationship. As the student progresses in the nursing program and then becomes an RN, this difference becomes even more evident. In the beginning, students often try to make the nurse–patient relationship into something it is not (e.g., in many cases, the nurse tries to be friends with the patient). The key difference between the nurse–patient relationship and a friendship is that in a friendship, there is an expectation, on both sides, that friends will help one another, listen to one another, and be there for each other. This is not the case in a nurse–patient relationship. There should not be any expectation that the patient will listen to the nurse's concerns, feelings, or problems, nor is the patient there to support the nurse. The nurse is expected to listen to the patient, work with the patient (even if the nurse does not really like the patient), and meet his or her care needs. This is difficult to learn, but it does come with experience.

The nurse–patient relationship has been described as therapeutic. What does *therapeutic* mean?

Therapeutic means treatment. Using this term to describe this special relationship emphasizes that this relationship is part of the care process. **Therapeutic use of self** requires the nurse

to use his/her personality consciously and in full awareness in an attempt to establish relatedness and to structure nursing intervention. . . . This requires self-insight, self-understanding, an understanding of the dynamics of human behavior, ability to interpret one's own behavior, as well as the behavior of others, and the ability to intervene effectively in nursing situations. (Travelbee, 1971, p. 19)

This relationship should not be minimized.

Professional successes, especially at the bedside, are most often measured objectively through such sources as patient outcome data, length of stay, response to treatment, patient satisfaction, and the like. But other measurements, which are often therapeutic but less tangible, cannot be discounted as measures of success. These patient outcomes may take the form of relief in a troubled countenance, tears of joy, or a peaceful, pain-free sleep. (Parker, 2006, p. 28)

In this relationship, the patient expects the nurse to be competent and to have expertise in nursing care. There is no such expectation of the patient. The nurse plans and initiates care for the patient, but patient-centered care must include the patient in the process. The center of the nurse–patient relationship is the patient. Even when a patient asks a nurse about his or her life or personal reactions, the patient is still more focused on self. Through the nurse–patient relationship, the patient is given support and guidance in coping with the illness experience. Patients with acute illness recover, but they still need help with coping during their illness, and they may need time to reflect on the illness after recovery. As has been discussed, more and more people have chronic illnesses that do not resolve. These patients need support and to learn coping skills to help them during the ups and downs of their illness process.

Communication is a critical component of the nurse–patient relationship. Chapter 10 discusses communication in more detail. The nurse needs to be clear and consistent with the patient and provide explanations about the care. Verbal and nonverbal communications are integrated throughout the communication process. The nurse needs to be aware of his or her own communication patterns and nonverbal messages, as well as those of the patient and people around the patient (family, friends, and other members of the healthcare team). Exhibit 9–4 identifies some examples of therapeutic and nontherapeutic communication responses.

Box 9–2 identifies examples of validation remarks to promote patient participation in decisions. These communication examples illustrate how communication, the nurse–patient relationship, and patient-centered care are interrelated.

The National Council of State Boards of Nursing (NCSBN; 1996) has identified key information about boundaries in the nurse–patient relationship. A professional boundary is an invisible line that provides limits to a nurse's behavior. This allows for professional nurse–patient behavior that has the patient in the center. The patient expects that the nurse will act for the patient and respect his or her values and preferences. There should be no personal gain for the nurse. Figure 9–5 lists critical descriptors of professional boundaries.

The NCSBN highlights guiding principles (1996):

- The nurse's responsibility is to delineate and maintain boundaries [*e.g., it is not the patient's responsibility to know the boundaries or enforce them*].
- The nurse should work within the zone of helpfulness [*The zone of helpfulness falls between being underinvolved with the patient and being overinvolved with the patient. The most common boundary issue involves being overinvolved and thus forgetting one's professional boundary*]. Figure 9–6 describes a continuum of professional behavior.
- The nurse should examine any boundary crossing, be aware of its potential implications, and avoid repeated crossings [*e.g., if a patient offers the nurse a gift and the nurse does not take the gift, the nurse should analyze the situation and may consider discussing this with a supervisor, mentor, or colleague to get feedback*].
- Variables such as the care setting, community influences, patient needs and the

---

Exhibit 9–4 Therapeutic and Nontherapeutic Communication Responses

Therapeutic	Nontherapeutic
Using silence	Giving false reassurance
Accepting	Giving approval or disapproval
Giving recognition	Rejecting
Offering self	Agreeing or disagreeing
Giving broad openings	Giving advice
Offering general leads	Probing
Placing an event in time or sequence	Defending
Making observations	Demanding explanation
Encouraging description or perceptions	Indicating the existence of an external source or
Encouraging comparison	power
Restating	Belittling feelings
Reflecting	Making stereotyped, biased, or prejudicial state-
Focusing	ments
Exploring more fully	Using denial
Seeking clarification	Interpreting without validation
Presenting reality	Confronting
Voicing doubt	
Verbalizing the implied, then asking for validation	
Attempting to translate words into feelings	
Formulating a verbal contract	
Assessing, evaluating with client	

Source: From *Role Development in Professional Nursing Practice*, by K. Masters, 2005, Sudbury, MA: Jones and Bartlett Publishers.

Box 9-2 Validation Remarks to Promote Patient Participation in Decisions

- Here's what I think; do you agree?
- What would you say is going on here?
- How is all of this affecting you?
- Does it seem that way to you? It does to me.
- Let's think about this together for a minute.
- Only you know your daily living situation.
- Can we find a way through this together?
- Let me explain my thinking to you.

- What do you think?
- Does this feel OK?
- Do you agree with this?
- This is what I'm thinking; what do you think?
- I'm interested in your take on all of this.
- If you could change this, what would be different?
- If you had a magic wand, what would you have it do?

Source: From *Critical Thinking Tactics for Nurses*, by M.G. Rubenfeld and B. Scheffer, 2006, Sudbury, MA: Jones and Bartlett Publishers.

---

nature of therapy affect the delineation of boundaries [*e.g., patients in mental health settings are particularly vulnerable to boundary issues, and nurses have to be clear about the boundaries*].

- Actions that overstep established boundaries to meet the needs of the nurse are boundary violations [*e.g., the nurse does not describe his or her personal problems to patients, does not accept money or individual gifts from*

Figure 9–5 Professional Boundaries: Definitions.

Professional boundaries are the spaces between the nurse's power and the client's vulnerability. The power of the nurse comes from the professional position and the access to private knowledge about the client. Establishing boundaries allows the nurse to control this power differential and allow a safe connection to meet the client's needs.	*Boundary violations can result when there is confusion between the needs of the nurse and those of the client.* Such violations are characterized by excessive personal disclosure by the nurse, secrecy or even a reversal of roles. Boundary violations can cause distress for the client, which may not be recognized or felt by the client until harmful consequences occur.
Boundary crossings are brief excursions across boundaries that may be inadvertent, thoughtless or even purposeful if done to meet a special therapeutic need. Boundary crossings can result in a return to established boundaries but should be evaluated by the nurse for potential client consequences and implications. Repeated boundary crossings should be avoided.	*Professional sexual misconduct is an extreme form of boundary violation and includes any behavior that is seductive, sexually demeaning, harassing or reasonably interpreted as sexual by the client.* Professional sexual misconduct is an extremely serious violation of the nurse's professional responsibility to the client. It is a breach of trust.

Source: From *Professional boundaries: A nurse's guide to the importance of appropriate professional boundaries*, by National Council of State Boards of Nursing (NCSBN), 1996, Chicago: Author. Retrieved September 24, 2008, from https://www.ncsbn.org/Professional_Boundaries_2007_Web.pdf Reprinted with permission.

Figure 9–6 A continuum of professional behavior.

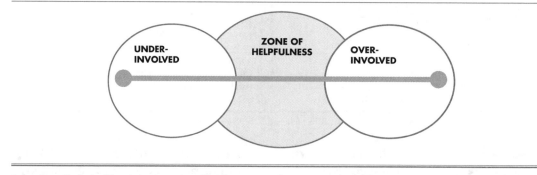

Source: From *Professional boundaries: A nurse's guide to the importance of appropriate professional boundaries*, by National Council of State Boards of Nursing (NCSBN), 1996, Chicago: Author. Retrieved September 24, 2008, from https://www.ncsbn.org/Professional_Boundaries_2007_Web.pdf Reprinted with permission.

patients, and does not give money or gifts to patients].

- The nurse should avoid situations where the nurse has a personal or business relationship, as well as a professional one [*e.g., the nurse should not date a patient, develop a friendship outside the nurse–patient relationship, or have a business transaction with a patient*].
- Post-termination relationships are complex because the client/patient may need additional services and it may be difficult to determine when the nurse–patient relationship is truly terminated [*e.g., postcare personal relationships with patients are not recommended*].

How does a nurse know that there may be a boundary violation with a patient? There are some red flags to watch for (Ohio Nursing Law, 2007):

- Self-disclosure of your own personal information to a patient
- Secretive behavior between you and a patient
- "Super nurse" behavior (You think you are the only one who can care for the patient.)
- Special treatment by the nurse
- Selective communication (not open communication)
- "You and me against the world" thinking
- Failure to protect the patient

All nurses need to watch for these red flags and use them to alter communication and behavior if boundary violation problems may be occurring.

Conclusion

This chapter has discussed the first of the five IOM core competencies for healthcare providers: provide patient-centered care. Nurses work with patients with many different health problems and in many different settings. Through the nursing process, nurses need to consider how they can better provide patient-centered care. This is care that puts the patient first and considers the patient's values, preferences, needs, culture, and background. The nurse–patient relationship can be an important element in supporting and recognizing the patient as the center of care. Nurses provide patient and family education to allow patients to more actively participate in their care and care decisions, and to encourage effective self-management of health and illness.

CHAPTER HIGHLIGHTS

1. The IOM Competency: Provide Patient-Centered Care refers to considering the patient's needs, cultural values, preferences, and unique situation instead of centering on the provider's prospective.
2. Four rules underpin patient-centered care: (1) care is based on continuous health relationships; (2) care customization is based on patient needs and preferences; (3) patients are the source of control; and (4) there is shared knowledge and free flow of information.
3. Patients who are involved in their care have better outcomes.
4. Four nursing theories related to patient-centered care are: Watson's theory on caring, Oren's self-care theory, Leininger's cultural diversity theory, and Peplau's interpersonal relations theory.
5. Macro consumers of health care are government and insurers.
6. Micro consumers of health care are the patient and family.
7. Patient satisfaction is a key factor that many healthcare institutions measure as a part of their delivery of care.

8. The health disparities problem comprises access to care, level of care, and whether care is equal across races and ethnic groups.

9. Strategies to overcome disparities include addressing access-to-care issues, such as wait times, appointment availability, and hours of service, to meet the needs of the population served. Another strategy is to include patient values and preferences in the delivery of care.

10. Patient advocacy means the nurse is active in respecting patient rights, ensuring that the patient has the education to understand treatment and care needs.

11. Care coordination is a priority of the IOM, but it is an aspect of care that is not generally reimbursable.

12. Clinical reasoning is different from critical thinking. It focuses on putting the care needs within the context that the patient presents—environment, values, and preferences—as gathered in the assessment.

13. The nursing process is a systematic method for thinking about and communicating how nurses provide patient care.

14. A concept map care plan is a diagram of patient problems and interventions that offers a more interactive plan than the traditional care plan.

15. Healthcare literacy includes reading, writing, and arithmetic skills; listening and speaking ability; and conceptual knowledge. Lack of healthcare literacy can present a barrier to care because patients may not understand aspects of their care.

16. A professional boundary is an invisible line that provides limits to a nurse's behavior.

Linking to the Internet

- National Council State Boards of Nursing
  https://www.ncsbn.org/index.htm
- Planetree Institute
  http://www.planetree.org
- The Commonwealth Fund: Health Care Disparities
  http://www.cmwf.org/programs/programs_list.htm?attrib_id=9133
- Unequal Treatment: Two-Part PowerPoint Slide Presentation
  Part 1: http://www.iom.edu/CMS/3740/4475/13172.aspx
  Part 2: http://www.iom.edu/CMS/3740/4475/13174.aspx
- Press Ganey: Partners in Improvement
  http://www.pressganey.com/
- Remaking American Medicine (Patient-Centered Care)
  http://www.pbs.org/remakingamericanmedicine/care.html
- The Center for Nursing Classification
  http://www.ncvhs.hhs.gov/970416w6.htm
- NANDA International
  http://www.nanda.org/
- Department of Health and Human Services: Minority Health
  http://www.omhrc.gov/templates/browse.aspx?lvl=1&lvlID=6
- Patients First (Massachusetts Hospitals)
  http://www.patientsfirstma.org/psa.cfm

DISCUSSION QUESTIONS

1. What does patient-centered care mean, and why is it relevant to nursing?
2. Describe a nursing theory that relates to patient-centered care.
3. How is diversity related to patient-centered care?
4. Explain consumerism in health care and its relevance to nursing.
5. Describe healthcare disparity and its importance.
6. What is health literacy?
7. Why is patient advocacy important?
8. Compare and contrast the nursing process, nursing care plan, and concept mapping.
9. What is the relationship between care coordination and delegation?
10. What is self-management of care?
11. Discuss the importance of patient education.

CRITICAL THINKING ACTIVITIES

1. The *Guidance for the National Healthcare Disparities Report* (Institute of Medicine, 2002b) outlines the annual National Healthcare Disparity Report (http://www.ahrq.gov/qual/nhdr03/nhdrsum03.htm). This report tracks four measurements: (1) socioeconomic status, (2) access to the healthcare system, (3) healthcare services and quality, and (4) geographic disparities in health care. Go to the site. What can you learn about disparity in health care? Summarize a key point related to each of the four measurements.

2. *The Provider's Guide to Quality and Culture* is an extensive compendium of information about diversity. Review one of sections on this site that interests you (http://erc.msh.org/mainpage.cfm?file=1.0.htm&module=provider&language=English). (When you get to the end of the screen, please note whether there is a "next" page noted; if so, click to continue the assigned section.) What is relevant, in the content that you reviewed, to your view of nursing?

3. Watch an episode of a favorite TV show, including the commercials. This does not have to be a health-related TV show. As you watch the show, keep notes describing ethnic, racial, and culture issues that arise. Note who is playing what types of the roles. Also note communication, clothing, attitudes, values, and any other factors related to diversity. Do the same for the commercials. Share your findings in an online course discussion forum.

4. Respond to the following questions with brief, clear responses.
   a. How would you describe yourself ethnically/racially/culturally? Has your view of ethnicity/race/culture changed over time? If so, how?
   b. If you are a member of an ethnic or racial group, describe the group.

(continues)

CRITICAL THINKING ACTIVITIES (continued)

    c. Do you think people are treated differently because of race or ethnicity? If so, describe an example.

    d. If you are a member of an ethnic or racial group, have you been treated differently yourself because of your own ethnicity or race? If so, how?

    e. When did you first become aware that people were different ethnically or racially?

5. If you were a member of a minority group, would you want to have a healthcare professional who is a member of that minority group care for you? Why?

6. Review *Healthy People 2010*, Chapter 11: Health Communication (http://www.healthy people.gov/document/html/volume1/11healthcom.htm). What is important about health communication? How does this content relate to patient-centered care?

7. Review the following material on Health Literacy: http://nnlm.gov/outreach/consumer/hlthlit.html

With your team, discuss the identified vulnerable populations and their relevance to health literacy.

8. Learn more about critical thinking by visiting these two sites: http://www.criticalthinking.org/aboutCT/definingCT.cfm and http://www.critical thinking.org/aboutCT/ourConceptCT.cfm

Describe how you might apply some of this information to your own critical thinking.

9. Visit the Joint Commission Web site and learn what this important healthcare organization is emphasizing about diversity in healthcare (http://www.jointcommission .org/PatientSafety/HLC/). What can you learn that might help you be more culturally competent? How does information like this improve health care?

10. Divide into teams. Have each team member review one of the following.

    a. *What Health Care Consumers Need to Know About Racial and Ethnic Disparities in Health-care*. Find commentary at http://www.iom.edu/CMS/3740/4475/4176.aspx

    b. *What Health Care System Administrators Need to Know About Racial and Ethnic Disparities in Healthcare*. Find commentary at http://www.iom.edu/CMS/3740/4475/14973.aspx

    c. *Unequal Treatment: What Healthcare Providers Need to Know about Racial and Ethnic Disparities in Health-Care*. Find commentary at http://www.iom.edu/Object.File/Master/4/175/Disparitieshcproviders8pgFINAL.pdf

Discuss your findings together, noting similarities and differences.

11. The Sullivan report is a government report on diversity issues in the healthcare workforce. Read what the American Association of Colleges of Nursing (AACN) had to say about this important landmark report (http://www.aacn.nche.edu/Media/NewsReleases/2004/SullivanCom04.htm).

What is your opinion about what you have learned from the AACN statement?

CASE STUDY

A 45-year-old woman has fallen during an ice storm. She goes to the emergency department (ED) because she thinks she may have broken her rib. When the X-ray results came back, the physician told her and her husband that they found a carcinoid tumor in one lung. The patient had never smoked and was healthy. There was no history of lung cancer in her family. The couple left devastated, with a list of specialists for follow-up. They spent 3 weeks in testing. Both the patient and husband assumed from the term *carcinoid* that she had malignant lung cancer. The patient and her husband had college degrees and held management positions. The physician in the ED did not discuss what *carcinoid* meant. Their anxiety rose with each passing day. It was at a later appointment that it became evident that the couple were not clear on what *carcinoid* meant and that the couple's interpretation had more life-threatening implications.

What does *carcinoid* mean? The National Cancer Institute in the National Institutes of Health defines it as a slow-growing type of tumor usually found in the gastrointestinal system (most often in the appendix) and sometimes in the lungs or other sites. Carcinoid tumors may spread to the liver or other sites in the body, and they may secrete substances such as serotonin or prostaglandins, causing carcinoid syndrome. This patient's tumor was localized, and it was removed.

Case Questions

1. What do you see in this case that could have been done differently?
2. What role might a nurse have played, and what specifically might the nurse have done?
3. Is this an example of health literacy? If so, in what way?
4. How might patient-centered care be applied to this case? (Please be specific.)

WORDS OF WISDOM

Josepha Campinha-Bacote, PhD, MAR, APRN, BC, CNS, CTN, FAAN
President, Transcultural C.A.R.E. Associates

The literature clearly reveals a strong relationship between patient-centered care and culturally competent care, for both concepts center on the core essential of respecting and incorporating the patient's worldview into the delivery of care. The concept of culture and its relationship to health is critical to comprehend, for cultural values give an individual a sense of direction and meaning to life. One of the most influential factors for understanding an individual's health behaviors and practices is to understand their worldview. There is compelling research and documentation supporting that the lack of cultural competence among healthcare professionals can result in poor health outcomes. Therefore, to positively impact on health outcomes, nursing must engage in the process of becoming culturally competent. Culturally competent nursing care can be viewed as the ongoing process in which the nurse continuously strives to achieve the ability and availability to work effectively within the cultural context of the patient (individual, family, community). Cultural competence, like patient-centered care, will render quality patient care that is individualized and equitable.

References

Alfaro-LeFevre, R. (2006). *Applying nursing process.* Philadelphia: Lippincott Williams & Wilkins.

American Organization of Nurse Executives. (2005, September). *AONE position statement on diversity.* Retrieved October 7, 2008, from http://www.aone.org/aone/advocacy/statement_on_diversity.html

Anderson, G. (2002). Testimony by Dr. Gerard Anderson, director of Partnership for Solutions at Johns Hopkins, before the House Ways and Means Health Subcommittee, April 16, 2002. Congressional Record.

Anderson, L., Scrimshaw, S., Fullilove, M., Fielding, J., & Normand, J. (2003). Culturally competent healthcare systems: A systematic review. *American Journal of Preventive Medicine, 24*(3S), 68–79.

Benner, P., Tanner, C., & Chesla, C. (1996). *Expertise in nursing practice: Caring, clinical judgment and ethics.* New York: Springer.

Boodman, S. G. (2007, February 20). A silent epidemic. *Washington Post.* Retrieved January 8, 2007, from http://www.washingtonpost.com/wp-dyn/content/article/2007/02/16/AR2007021602260.html

Bulechek, G., Butcher, H., & Docterman, J. (2007) *Nursing interventions classification (NIC)* (5th ed.). St. Louis, MO: Mosby.

Carpenito-Moyet, L. (2007). *Handbook of nursing diagnosis* (12th ed.). Philadelphia: Lippincott, Williams & Wilkins.

Commonwealth Fund. (2008). *Patient-centered care: An overview.* Retrieved January 8, 2008, from http://www.commonwealthfund.org/General/General_show.htm?doc_id=319061

Cronewett, L., Sherwood, G., Barnsteiner, J., Disch, J., Johnson, J., Mitchell, P., et al. (2007). Quality and safety education for nurses. *Nursing Outlook, 55,* 122–131.

Cross, T., Bazron, B., Dennis, K., & Isaacs, M. (1989). *Towards a culturally competent system of care: A monograph on effective services for minority children who are severely emotionally disturbed.* Washington, DC: CASSP Technical Assistance Center, Georgetown University.

Davis, K., Schoenbaum, S., & Audet, A. (2005). A 2020 vision of patient-centered primary care. *Journal of General Internal Medicine, 15,* 953–957.

Del Bueno, D. (2005). A crisis in critical thinking. *Nursing Education Perspectives, 26,* 278–282.

Disch, J. (2001). Strengthening nursing and interdisciplinary collaboration. *Journal of Professional Nursing, 17*(6), 275.

Finkelman, A. (2001, December). Problem-solving, decision-making, and critical thinking: How do they mix and why bother? *Home Care Provider,* 194–199.

Finkelman, A., & Kenner, C. (2007). *Teaching IOM: Implications of the Institute of Medicine reports for nursing education.* Silver Spring, MD: American Nurses Association.

Gerteis, M., Edgman-Levitan, S., Daley, J., & Delbanco, T. (Eds.). 1993. *Through the patient's eyes.* San Francisco: Jossey-Bass.

Hagenow, N. (2003). Why not person-centered care? The challenges of implementation. *Nursing Administration Quarterly, 27,* 203–207.

Halpern, R., Lee, M., Boulter, P., & Phillips, R. (2001). A synthesis of nine major reports on physicians competencies for the emerging practice environment. *Academic Medicine, 76,* 606–615.

Hochbaum, G. (1958). *Public participation in medical screening programs: A sociological study* (Public Health Service Publication No. 572). Washington, DC: U.S. Government Printing Office.

Institute for the Future. (2000). *Health and healthcare 2010: The forecast, the challenge.* San Francisco: Jossey-Bass.

Institute of Medicine. (1999). *To err is human.* Washington, DC: National Academies Press.

Institute of Medicine. (2001). *Crossing the quality chasm: A new health system for the 21st century.* Washington, DC: National Academies Press.

Institute of Medicine. (2002a). *Unequal treatment: Confronting racial and ethnic disparities in healthcare.* Washington, DC: National Academies Press.

Institute of Medicine. (2002b). *Guidance for the national healthcare disparities report.* Washington, DC: National Academies Press.

Institute of Medicine. (2003a). *Health professions education.* Washington, DC: National Academies Press.

Institute of Medicine. (2003b). *Priority areas for national action: Transforming healthcare quality.* Washington, DC: National Academies Press.

Institute of Medicine. (2004). *Health literacy: A prescription to end confusion.* Washington, DC: National Academies Press.

Johnson, M., Meridean, M., & Moorehead, S. (Eds.). (2007). *Nursing outcomes classification (NOC).* St. Louis, MO: Mosby.

Joint Commission on Accreditation of Healthcare Organizations. (2008). *Facts and figures.* Retrieved March 14, 2008, from http://www.jointcommission.org/NewsRoom/PressKits/Health_Literacy/facts_figures.htm

Knowles, M. (1972). *The modern practice of adult education.* New York: Associated Press.

Leebov, W. (2008). Beyond customer service. *American Nurse Today, 3*(1), 21–23.

Lewin, S., Skea, Z, Entwistle, V., Zwarenstein, M., & Dick, J. (2001). Interventions for providers to promote a patient-centered approach to clinical consultations. *Cochrane Database System Review, 4,* CD003267.

Masters, K. (2005). *Role development in professional nursing practice.* Sudbury, MA: Jones and Bartlett.

Murphy, J. (2004). Using focused reflection and articulation to promote clinical reasoning. *Nursing Education Perspectives, 24,* 226–231.

National Council of State Boards of Nursing. (1996). *Professional boundaries: A nurse's guide to the importance of appropriate professional boundaries.* Chicago: Author.

National Council of State Boards of Nursing (NCSBN). (1998). *The continuum of care: A regulatory perspective.* Retrieved October 7, 2008, from https://www.ncsbn.org/contcarepaper.pdf

O'Neil, E., & the Pew Health Professions Commission. (1998). *Recreating health professional practice for a new century.* San Francisco: Pew Health Professions Commission.

Ohio Nursing Law. (2007, December 2). *2006 Ohio nursing law program-boundaries* (Vol. 4).

Parker, D. (2006). Establishing a passion for nursing: The role of the nurse leader. *Nurse Leader, 4*(5), 28–32.

Partnership for Solutions, Johns Hopkins University. (2001). *Partnership for solutions: A national program of the Robert Wood Johnson Foundation.* Retrieved December 12, 2002, from http://www.partnershipforsolutions.org/

Peters, K., & Elster, A. (2002). *Roadmaps for clinical practice: A primer on population-based medicine.* Chicago: American Medical Association.

Pew Health Professions Commission. (1995). *Critical challenges: Revitalizing the health professions for the twenty-first century.* San Francisco: UCSF Center for the Health Professions.

Planetree Institute. (2007). Retrieved January 8, 2007, from http://www.planetree.org

Rubenfeld, M., & Scheffer, B. (2006). *Critical thinking TACTICS for nurses.* Sudbury, MA: Jones and Bartlett.

Salimbene, S. (1999). Cultural competence: A priority for performance improvement action. *Journal of Nursing Care Quality, 13*(3), 23–25.

Scheffer, B., & Rubenfeld, M. (2000). A consensus statement on critical thinking in nursing. *Journal of Nursing Education, 39,* 352–359.

Schuster, P. (2002). *Concept mapping: A critical thinking approach to care planning.* Philadelphia: F. A. Davis.

Shaller, D. (2007). *Patient-centered care: What does it take?* New York: Commonwealth Fund. Retrieved April 5, 2008, from http://www.commonwealthfund.org/publications/publications_show.htm?doc_id=559715

Shannon, S., Mitchell, P., & Cain, K. (2002). Patients, nurses, and physicians have differing views of quality of critical care. *Journal of Nursing Scholarship,* 173–179.

Stewart, M. (2001). Towards a global definition of patient-centered care. *British Medical Journal, 322*(7284), 444–445.

Sullivan, L. (2004). *Missing persons: Minorities in the health professions: A report of the Sullivan Commission on diversity in the healthcare workforces.* Washington, DC: Sullivan Commission on Diversity in the Healthcare Workforce.

Travelbee, J. (1971). *Interpersonal aspects of nursing.* Philadelphia: F. A. Davis.

Twibell, R., Ryan, M., & Hermiz, M. (2005). Faculty perceptions of critical thinking in student clinical experiences. *Journal of Nursing Education, 44,* 71–79.

U.S. Department of Health and Human Services. (1998). *Healthy People 2010.* Washington, DC: U.S. Government Printing Office.

U.S. Department of Health and Human Services. (2008a). *Hospital compare.* Retrieved April 17, 2008, from the Agency for Healthcare Research and Quality Web site: http://www.hospitalcompare.hhs.gov

U.S. Department of Health and Human Services. (2008b). *The Office of Minority Health.* Retrieved February 6, 2008, from http://www.omhrc.gov/templates/browse.aspx?lvl=1&lvlID=3

U.S. Department of Health and Human Services. (2008c). *National Partnership for Action to End Healthcare Disparities.* Retrieved February 6, 2008, from http://www.omhrc.gov/npa/templates/browse.aspx?lvl=1&lvlid=13

Zimmerman, P. (2001). The problems with healthcare customer satisfaction surveys. In J. Dochterman & H. Grace (Eds.), *Current issues in nursing* (6th ed., pp. 255–260). St. Louis, MO: Mosby.

Chapter 10

Work in Interdisciplinary Teams

CHAPTER OBJECTIVES

At the conclusion of this chapter, the learner will be able to:

- Discuss the Institute of Medicine competency: Work in interdisciplinary teams.
- Define teamwork and types of teams.
- Describe effective team functioning.
- Discuss communication and its relationship to patient care and teams.
- Discuss collaboration and its relationship to patient care and teams.
- Discuss coordination and its relationship to patient care and teams.
- Describe the change process and implications for health care and teams.
- Describe delegation.
- Explain conflict and conflict resolution.

CHAPTER OUTLINE

KEY TERMS

- ❏ Collaboration
- ❏ Communication
- ❏ Conflict
- ❏ Conflict resolution
- ❏ Coordination
- ❏ Delegatee
- ❏ Delegation
- ❏ Delegator

- ❏ Empowerment
- ❏ Followers
- ❏ Power
- ❏ Team
- ❏ Team leader
- ❏ Teamwork
- ❏ Types of power

Introduction

This chapter focuses on working in teams, a critical competency for every nurse. The content includes an explanation of the Institute of Medicine (IOM) core competency, teams and teamwork, and critical components of effective teams: communication, collaboration, and coordination. In addition, delegation is a part of the daily work for every nurse and is part of planning care and teamwork. Teams must cope with change and learn to make effective change decisions. The last topic in the chapter is conflict and conflict resolution—improving teamwork. Teams need to recognize the importance of patient-centered care and how the patient participates in the healthcare team. Through its assessment of the healthcare system, the IOM has determined that the system "is in need of fundamental change. Many patients, doctors, nurses and healthcare leaders are concerned that the care delivered is not, essentially, the care we should receive. The frustration levels of both patients and clinicians have probably never been higher. Yet the problems remain. Healthcare today *harms too frequently and routinely fails to deliver its potential benefits*" (2001, p. 1). Technology and new drugs, among many other care advances, can improve health and health care, but something is wrong with the care delivery models. This is

what the IOM is most concerned about, and this has resulted in the focus on core competencies. This chapter looks at the core competency that most directly addresses the need for changes in the care delivery models. Figure 10–1 highlights the key elements for this competency.

The IOM Competency: Work in Interdisciplinary Teams

Chapter 9 discussed the first of the IOM healthcare professions core competency: provide patient-centered care. This chapter covers the second core competency: work in interdisciplinary teams. This is described as "cooperate, collaborate, communicate, and integrate care in teams to ensure that care is continuous and reliable" (IOM, 2003a, p. 4). As a reminder, these core competencies were developed for all healthcare professions, not just nursing; however, this

Figure 10–1 Working in interdisciplinary teams: Key elements.

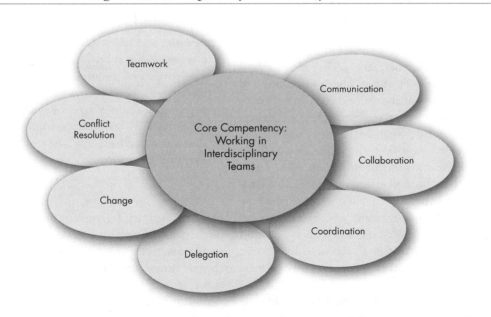

chapter focuses on nurses and interdisciplinary teams, and also teams of nursing staff. The Quality and Safety Education for Nurses describes this competency as having essential features: "Essential features of this competency include sections related to self, team, team communication and conflict resolution, effect of team on safety and quality, and the impact of systems on team functioning" (Cronewett et al., 2007, p. 123). The IOM further supports the need for effective interdisciplinary needs by identifying care coordination as one of the 20 priority areas of care (2003b).

One has to ask why there is such emphasis on this core competency, because it makes sense that teams are important. The critical issue is whether healthcare professionals are prepared to participate effectively in teams, particularly interdisciplinary teams. The IOM has concluded that they are not. Healthcare profession education takes place in isolation; each healthcare profession provides its own education, with limited regard to other healthcare professionals. The result is that nursing, medical, pharmacy, and allied health students (e.g., physical therapists, occupational therapists, and so on) have limited, if any, contact with each other in their programs (Finkelman & Kenner, 2007). They have limited knowledge of roles of the other professions and how they must collaborate and coordinate care to provide patient-centered care. This is a serious problem because when healthcare professionals graduate and meet licensure requirements, they are expected to work together. The IOM states that there is limited effective interdisciplinary teamwork. In addition, nurses need to know how to work with nursing teams whose focus is nursing care. In most cases, this too leads to isolation and limited recognition of the need for greater reaching out to other healthcare disciplines. Nurses tend to focus on the nursing care plan to the detriment of the total plan of care for the

patient—a nursing care plan, as opposed to a care plan that is patient centered. Nursing education reinforces this by emphasizing just the nursing care plan. This is not to say that the same scenario does not exist in other healthcare professions, because it does. Nursing students need a broader view of health care along with the nursing perspective (Barnsteiner, Disch, Hall, Mayer, & Moore, 2007). The product is patient-centered care—care that

> *alleviates vulnerability in all of its forms. That care should and must then be delivered at the right time, at the right level, in the right place, and so on. If care were on a compass it would be true north and all other functions would stand in line to provide added value and service to that focus. (Hagenow, 2003, p. 204)*

Interdisciplinary teams are best suited to achieving this patient-centered care. One individual healthcare profession cannot do it.

Teamwork and Types of Teams

The IOM stated that

> *an interdisciplinary team is composed of members from different professions and occupations with varied and specialized knowledge, skills, and methods. The team members integrate their observations, bodies of expertise, and spheres of decision making to coordinate, collaborate, and communicate with one another in order to optimize care for a patient or group for patients. (2003a, p. 54)*

With the increasing complexity of care and concerns about the fragmented healthcare system, interdisciplinary teams are even more important. In addition to the complex needs of patients with chronic illness, critical acute care, geriatric care, and care at the end of life all require effective planning to ensure improved outcomes. These patients have multiple, complex needs. The types of settings, complexity of settings, and great need to share information and planning across settings require more **teamwork**. As noted by the IOM (2003a), use of interdisciplinary teams tends to result in improved quality and decrease health-care costs. Throughout this content, when the term **team** is used, it applies to both interdisciplinary teams and nursing staff teams; nurses are members of interdisciplinary teams and also members of nursing teams (nursing teams include nursing staff such as RNs, licensed practical/vocational nurses [LPN/LVNs], and unlicensed assistive personnel [UAP]). Why are teams important in health care?

Clarification of Terms

The IOM uses the term *interdisciplinary*; however, in the literature and in practice, nurses encounter other terms that seem similar, such as *multidisciplinary* and *interprofessional*. Are these different? Interdisciplinary "refers to people with distinct disciplinary training working together for a common purpose, as they make different, complementary contributions to patient-focused-care" (Leathard, 1994, as cited in McCallin, 2001, p. 419). Multidisciplinary refers to "a team or collaborative process where members of different disciplines assess or treat patients independently and then share information with each other" (Sorrels-Jones, 1997, as cited in McCallin, p. 420). The key difference between these two descriptions of teams is that multidisciplinary focuses on how individual team members do their work but encourages sharing of information with others who are providing care. Nurses share information about the nursing care plan with physicians and the social workers, and vice versa. This is typically what has been done in health care, but this is not what the IOM is recommending in the core competency. Interdisciplinary is much more involved and emphasizes

collective action and in-depth collaboration. Less emphasis is placed on what individual team members do, and more emphasis is placed on what individual members can do to contribute to the joint team plan and initiatives. Interprofessional is more closely related to interdisciplinary, though interdisciplinary is the term that the IOM chose to use. Table 10–1 compares multidisciplinary, interdisciplinary, and interprofessional teams.

Following are advantages of using interdisciplinary teams:

- Decreased fragmentation in a complex care system
- Effective use of multiple expertise (e.g., medicine, nursing, pharmacy, allied health, social work, and so on)
- Decreased utilization of repetitive or duplicate services
- Increased creative or innovative solutions to complex problems
- Increased learning for team members about different roles and responsibilities, communication and coordination, and how to better plan care
- Provides motivation and increased self-esteem in team and individual performance
- Greater sharing of responsibility
- Empowers members to speak up

Team Leadership

Teams typically have designated leaders. The leader may be a nurse, and for a nursing team, the leader is an RN. Interdisciplinary teams may have different leaders, and in some cases, the leader may be a nurse. Regardless of who is the leader, all team members are critical to the success of a team. What makes an effective **team leader**? A team leader must first recognize that it is the work of the team that is critical; he or she should not focus on personal success as a leader or on the

Table 10–1 COMPARISON OF MULTIDISCIPLINARY, INTERDISCIPLINARY, AND INTERPROFESSIONAL TEAMS

	Multidisciplinary Teams (adapted from Siegler, 1998)	Interdisciplinary Teams (adapted from Siegler, 1998)	Interprofessional Teams (adapted from Simpson et al., 2001)
Membership	Professionals from a variety of disciplines	All necessary disciplines	A partnership among professionals, individuals, families, and communities
Sources of information	Members contribute information from their own area of expertise within the roles of their specific discipline	Patients and/or significant others provide information along with members of the disciplines	Patients and/or significant others, members of the disciplines related to the patient's care provide information
Leadership	Leadership and membership are fixed	Leadership and membership vary depending on the situation	Leadership is based on expertise that matches the situation
Decision making	One person makes the final treatment decisions	All members work together to come up with both alternative solutions and final decisions	A shared responsibility for decision making and problem solving
Focus of Care	Task orientation	Collaboration to see the bigger picture	A shared biopsychosocial paradigm

Source: From *Critical Thinking Tactics for Nurses*, by M.G. Rubenfeld and B. Scheffer, 2006, Sudbury, MA: Jones and Bartlett Publishers.

success of any one team member. This is not always easy to do, but truly effective team leaders shine through the effectiveness of the team. Leaders need to know when to guide, when to let the team function, and when to be directive. If the team is on task as planned, direction is not as critical, but if the team is floundering and not able to get work done, the leader needs to be more active and direct the team. Leaders need to encourage and accept members' ideas and actively seek information and ideas from team members. Some of the responsibilities of team leaders are:

- Lead the team—meetings and the team's work.
- Determine or clarify the team's purpose and operating rules or guidelines. Some of this may be predetermined by the organization.
- Select team members. In many cases, this is done by someone other than the team leader or by simple structure; for example, the team members may be assigned to a unit or a particular patient.
- Orient team members to the team, including coaching and training new members.

- Determine the plan of action with team members' participation. After the team reviews information, discusses issues, and arrives at team decisions, the team leader ensures that there is an effective plan of action. If it is a clinical team, keep the focus on the patient(s).
- Determine how to make the team more effective given time constraints.
- Provide resources and information for the team as needed.
- Update the team as necessary.
- Ensure that the team's plan of action is implemented as designed.
- Recognize the team's work as well as individuals.
- Resolve conflict when it occurs.
- Evaluate the team's outcomes, and include input from all team members; strive for improvement.
- Encourage team learning to improve effectiveness.
- Ensure that required information about team functioning, decisions, and actions implemented is recorded as documentation.
- Accept feedback from team members and others who may be involved.
- Provide feedback to team members and the team as a whole.
- Ensure that the team effectively uses collaboration, coordination, and delegation.

An important role for team leaders is to lead the team's activities, and much of this is done through team discussion. Leading discussion can be informal or formal. When the team leader seeks out individual team members to discuss team issues and the team's work, this is informal discussion. In this situation, the leader is seeking an open discussion of issues and sharing of ideas. It can help the leader to better understand team members and to identify the issues. Informal discussion can be used for the team members to get to know the leader on a different level.

FORMAL TEAM MEETINGS

Formal meetings are an important part of teamwork, and these are usually led by the team leader or someone designated by the leader. Formal meetings can be held in a variety of settings. The most common is a conference room in the healthcare setting. The setting should be private and conducive to fostering communication. Space should be provided for team members to sit and to take notes. In clinical settings, telephone access is important, although members should be encouraged to keep interruptions to a minimum. Another method for conducting meetings today is virtual conferencing: conference calls, video conferencing, and even Internet conferencing. These methods also require planning and equipment. Members must be informed about access requirements, and technological support may be needed to assist with possible connection problems. The following is a guide for leading formal meetings.

1. Planning the Meeting: Planning before the meeting is important. Avoid scheduling meetings just to have a meeting. Time is too limited. Staff will be reluctant to attend, and may not be productive in, meetings that they do not feel are worthwhile. Prior to completing the final agenda, the leader can survey members via e-mail for additional agenda items.
2. Steps Prior to the Meeting: Arrange for meeting space. Send out the agenda, any necessary handouts, and minutes from the last meeting. Allow time for this material to be reviewed. Typically, these are now sent electronically. If there is no designated

minute-taker or secretary, the leader may ask a member to take this role.

3. Meeting Time: Meetings should begin and end on time. All members should make an effort to be on time, come prepared, and follow the agenda. The leader should guide the meeting so that the agenda is followed. Minutes should be reviewed and approved because they are the team's documentation. The leader is responsible for making sure all members have the opportunity to participate. If the discussion digresses from the agenda or becomes volatile, the leader needs to guide the discussion back to the topic and away from personal reactions. Decisions made should be clearly identified. The minutes should reflect action items, person responsible, and timeline for completion. Planning and conducting a meeting in an orderly fashion indicate that a team member's time is valued and that accountability for actions is an expectation.

4. Postmeeting: Minutes are finalized. Actions that require follow-up are taken by the leader and members as designated by the decision plan. A report of these actions would be addressed at the next meeting.

5. Evaluation of meetings should consider these questions: (1) Was there a clearly defined purpose (agenda) for the meeting? (2) Were there measurable outcomes (do the minutes provide data)? (3) What was the attendance level? (4) Did members participate in the meeting(s), or was it primarily the leader?

Another type of meeting that is common for clinical teams is the patient-planning meeting. These meetings may take place daily, each shift, or several times a week. The purpose of these meetings is to assess patient care and determine the patient plan of care. This type of meeting is typically less structured than the formal meeting (e.g., no structured agenda or minutes). However, the team leader does need to plan the topics for discussion, which might be patients. The team may develop a common order in which patient issues will be discussed. Notes do need to be kept, though they may not be formal minutes. The team may add changes to the patient's plan of care or other standard clinical document. The responsibilities noted earlier for team leaders remain the same for the clinical planning team as for other types of teams. In many hospitals, patient rounds are used for planning. Staff go to the patient's bedside to talk with the patient and assess needs. The patient should be an active participant in the rounds, though this is not always the case. Rounds can be interdisciplinary (the ideal method) or can be focused on a specific profession (such as nursing rounds or physician rounds).

Healthcare Team Members: What Knowledge and Skills Do They Need?

Team members can be viewed as **followers**. This is not a negative term. If there were no members or followers, there would be no need for a leader. There may be times when a follower, leader of a subgroup, and so on, must take over the leadership role, such as in the absence of the team leader; however, in most cases, team members are followers. This should not be a passive role, but a very active one. Each member needs to feel a responsibility to participate actively in the work of the team and to feel the right to help the team determine its rules, structure, and activities. "The organization is essentially a community of many leaders and many followers, frequently changing places depending on the particular activity that is occurring" (Sullivan, 1998, p. 477).

Effective teams require members (healthcare professionals) who (IOM, 2003a):

- Learn about other team members' expertise, background, knowledge, and values.

- Learn individual roles and processes required to work collaboratively.
- Demonstrate basic group skills, including communication, negotiation, delegation, time management, and assessment of group (team) dynamics.
- Ensure that accurate and timely information reaches those who need it at the appropriate time.
- Customize care and manage smooth transitions across settings and over time, even when the team members are in entirely different physical locations.
- Coordinate and integrate care processes to ensure excellence, continuity, and reliability of the care provided.
- Resolve conflicts with other members of the team.
- Communicate with other members of the team in a shared language, even when the members are in entirely different physical locations.

Development of Effective Teams

A team implies a group of people, but how do they develop into a team? To just say "today this group of staff is a team" does not mean that it is functioning as a team. It takes time to develop a team. Within a team, members have roles, and some members may play multiple roles at different times as the team interacts. What are some of these roles? They are (Heller, 1999, p. 42):

- *Coordinator*: Pulls together the work of the team
- *Critic*: Keeps an eye on the team's effectiveness
- *Ideas Person*: Encourages the team to be innovative
- *Implementer*: Ensures that the team's functioning is effective
- *External Contact*: Looks after the team's external contacts and relationships

- *Inspector*: Ensures that standards are met
- *Team Builder*: Develops the team spirit

The IOM (Fried, Topping, & Rundall, 2000, as cited in IOM, 2001, p. 132) noted four areas of particular concern that need to be considered when evaluating team effectiveness:

1. Team make-up, such as having the appropriate team size and composition of members, and the ability to reduce status differences (for example, between nurses and physicians).
2. Team processes, such as communication structure, conflict management, leadership that emphasizes excellence, and clear goals and expectations.
3. Nature of team tasks, such as matching roles with knowledge and experience, and promoting cohesiveness when work is highly interdependent.
4. Environment context, such as obtaining needed resources and establishing appropriate rewards.

"Effective teams have a culture that fosters openness, collaboration, teamwork, and learning from mistakes" (IOM, 2001, p. 132). Health care has a problem with development of effective teams because it overemphasizes personal accountability of healthcare professionals such as nurses and physicians. Teams often resort to uncoordinated or sequential action rather than collaborative work, which is required for effective teams (IOM, 2001).

Teams and Decision Making

Teams make decisions about the work that they need to do. Any decision is affected by the amount and quality of information that is required and the number of possible solutions for a problem. The time schedule is very important; for example, is an immediate decision required, or can time be taken to consider options carefully?

Many clinical teams must act quickly in response to clinical problems. These teams need to develop quick-thinking and analysis skills (depending on the expertise of team members), trust one another, weigh benefits and risks, and move to a decision. At other times, teams may have more time to fully analyze an issue or problem, brainstorm possible solutions, and develop a consensus regarding the best decision. Teams must recognize that there may not be a perfect solution (there rarely is) and that there is risk, but decisions need to be made. Not making a decision is really making a decision—to do nothing. Several decision-making styles may be used (Milgram, Spector, & Treger, 1999). *Decisive decision making* depends on minimal data to arrive at a single solution or decision. The *integrative style* uses as much data as possible to arrive at several reasonable solutions or decisions. The *hierarchic style* uses a large amount of data and organizes them to arrive at one optimal decision. The *flexible style* relies on minimal data but generates several different options or will shift focus as the data are interpreted. A team leader and the team typically use more than one style, depending on the issue or problem.

Key questions that are asked during decision making are: (1) What is the issue, problem, or task to be done and the desired outcome? (2) What kind of data are needed? How complicated and substantial is the issue, problem, or task? (3) How many possible solutions or approaches are there, and what are they? (4) Can the desired outcome(s) be met with acceptable cost-benefit standards? (Note that cost is more than financial; it could refer to the patient's health status, for example.) Figure 10–2 describes team thinking. Box 10–1 provides a team thinking inventory that teams can use to assess their thinking.

Communication

All nurses communicate—with other nurses, other staff, patients, families, and others who impact patient care. The assumption is that people know how to communicate effectively, and this is not true. It takes practice and awareness of communication. What is important is the effectiveness of this communication. Teams must communicate, too; the effectiveness of this communication can also vary, but it is clear that communication makes a difference in results and decreases errors. Individuals have communication styles, and understanding one's style is important. Some people are more passive, others use a lot of nonverbal communication, others prefer to see important information in writing, and so on.

Assertiveness

Assertiveness is a communication style that is often confused with aggression and thus can be viewed as negative. Assertiveness, however, is important, though many have to learn how to use this style. Using assertiveness, a person stands up for what he or she believes in but does not push or control others. The assertive nurse uses "I" statements when communicating thoughts and feelings, and "you" statements when persuading others (Fabre, 2005). Other suggestions for improving assertiveness are (Fabre, 2005, p. 78):

- Intervene in situations calmly and confidently.
- Respond to problems in a timely way to avoid accumulation of negative feelings. Those who are passive for a long time run the risk of overreaction to small incidents.
- Clearly articulate the importance of using nursing perspectives.
- Use language that others understand (the audience; for example, the team, management, etc.).

Communication is the sharing of a message between one person or group and another. It is important to know if the message was received

Figure 10–2 Interdisciplinary team thinking.

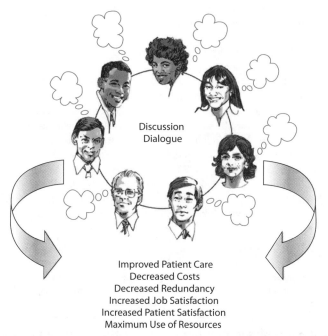

Discussion
Dialogue

Improved Patient Care
Decreased Costs
Decreased Redundancy
Increased Job Satisfaction
Increased Patient Satisfaction
Maximum Use of Resources

Source: From *Critical Thinking Tactics for Nurses*, by M.G. Rubenfeld and B. Scheffer, 2006, Sudbury, MA: Jones and Bartlett Publishers.

as sent. Interpretation plays a major role, and sometimes interpretation confuses or changes the original message. Nonverbal communication has an impact on the message sent. If a team member says that he or she is committed to an action but his or her facial expression shows a lack of interest (such as no eye contact or a hurried manner), the message of commitment may be viewed as noncommitment. As team members get to know one another, they learn each other's communication styles, including nonverbal methods. This knowledge has an advantage in that it can improve and speed up communication, but in some cases, team members may jump to conclusions, and communication may not be clear. Nurses need to break the code of silence (Fabre, 2005). What does this mean? Nurses are often silent, keeping their opinions to themselves

rather than being open with the treatment team. This most likely has occurred because of low self-esteem of the profession as a whole, which has a very negative impact—loss of valuable nursing input. Speaking up takes risk, but the results can be worthwhile. It may take time for team members to value each other's opinions and expertise. But if done in a professional manner with the goal of collaboration and coordination, over time, most team members begin to respect and trust one another and see value in the team's diversity of multiple healthcare professionals and variety in experience.

Listening

Listening is an important skill to develop. It is important when delivering care—listening to the patient and family—and when listening in

---

BOX 10–1 TEAM THINKING INVENTORY

1. What strategies are used to help team members think about the big picture as well as the parts?
2. What strategies are used to help team members see the situation from different perspectives?
3. What strategies are used to help team members see their biases and assumptions?
4. What strategies help team members think about patterns and interrelationships of issues and parts of problems?
5. What strategies are used to help team members think beyond cause and effect consequences?
6. Does the thinking that occurs in the team resemble simple sharing of information or discussion/dialogue? Why? How can you move in the direction of discussion/dialogue?
7. What is done to encourage team members to share their thinking or feel comfortable enough to talk about it?
8. How is conflict managed in the team to promote thinking instead of discouraging it?
9. What other sources of gratification, besides interdisciplinary teamwork, are available for team members to socialize, obtain recognition, and interact?
10. How were the interdisciplinary team members prepared for their thinking roles?
11. How does the team deal with ambiguity? How long can team members tolerate not having a solution?
12. How does the team examine its own thinking processes (e.g., how it works, not what it is doing), and who is doing it?

Source: From *Critical Thinking Tactics for Nurses,* by M.G. Rubenfeld and B. Scheffer, 2006, Sudbury, MA: Jones and Bartlett Publishers. Data adapted from *The fifth discipline: The art and practice of the learning organization,* by Senge, P., 1998, New York: Doubleday; *Redesigning collegiate leadership: Teams and teamwork in higher education,* by Bensimon, E. & Neumann, A., 1993, Baltimore: The Johns Hopkins University Press; and *Discussion as a way of teaching: Tools and techniques for Democratic classrooms,* by Brookfield, S. & Peskill, S., 1999, San Francisco: Jossey-Bass.

---

work teams and to colleagues. Most people probably would say that they listen, but listening takes practice. There are also a lot of barriers to effective listening, such as

- Anxiety and stress
- Interruptions
- Too many tasks to do
- Fatigue and hunger
- Lack of self-esteem
- Anger
- Reaction from the past
- Confusing message

In addition, the team member may not think that his or her opinion would be valued, so he or she tunes out or exhibits a lack of concern or respect for the communicator. When a nurse finds that he or she is not listening, he or she should think about what is interfering with listening. What is the barrier(s) at the moment? From this process, the listener can learn more about the listening process and improve his or her listening, and thus communication. Why is listening important, other than to say that it generally improves communication (Fabre, 2005; McConnell, 2001)?

- Listening helps us identify problems.
- Listening exposes feelings—those invaluable but sometimes inconvenient traits that make us truly human. We need to manage our feelings and give them a positive focus instead of denying them.
- Listening jump-starts the solution process because answers pop up during candid conversations.
- Listening relieves stress. Bottling up thoughts and feelings only depletes our energy.
- Active listening is more than hearing; it requires communicating to the other person that you are listening.

- Saying "yes" and "no" is not active listening.
- Paraphrasing communicates that you have listened; you share back what you have heard to make sure the message is clear.

Nurse–physician communication has long been an important topic, probably more so in nursing than in medicine. Studies have looked at this issue and how collaboration impacts care (Baggs et al., 1999; Fairchild, Hogan, Smith, Portnow, & Bates, 2002; Higgins, 1999; Thomas, Sexton, & Helmreich, 2003). These studies indicate that there are communication problems, and these problems can impact collaboration and, consequently, patient outcomes. Two nurses and one physician conducted a study using focus groups of nurses and physicians, and they identified methods to improve nurse–physician communication (Burke, Boal, & Mitchell, 2004). The researchers noted that some communication problems require major organizational changes—system changes. The suggested methods that are not so system focused include:

1. Develop a personal connection, which helps to increase colleagueship.
2. Use humor.
3. Make the assumption that you are on the same team.
4. Recognize that team members are equal in the expertise that can be important to patient care.
5. If you speak frequently to a physician over the phone, arrange to meet in person.
6. Report good news about patients— improvements, not just problems.
7. Recognize that conflict will occur, but this does not mean that communication and collaboration cannot be maintained.
8. Discuss preferred methods of communication (telephone, e-mail, pager, in person, voice message) and under what circumstances they should be used.

9. Ask for parameters regarding when the physician wants to be called.
10. Plan ahead for meetings or times of contact so that you are prepared with information and know what you want to communicate. Provide clinically pertinent information.
11. Work with the physician to determine the best methods for communicating with the family, and determine who should contact whom and for what purposes.

Collaboration

Collaboration is an integral part of patient-centered care and safe, quality care. When staff or team members work in an environment where there is collaboration, it is a more satisfying experience, and there is less conflict. Collaboration means that all the people involved are listened to and that decisions are developed together. Views are respected; however, at some point, decisions must be made, and not all views or opinions can be chosen as the decision. The goal is to arrive at the best possible decision. Working with others increases the possibility of having the best decision because there is greater availability of ideas and dialogue about ideas and solutions. This diversity improves decision making. A definition of collaboration is "a joint communication and decision-making process with the goal of satisfying the healthcare needs of a target population. Quality of care is best achieved through this process and members contribute based on their knowledge and expertise" (Arcangelo, Fitzgerald, Carroll, & Plumb, 1996, p. 106).

The American Nurses Association (ANA) stated that "collaboration among healthcare professionals involves recognition of the expertise of others within and outside the profession, and referral to those other providers when appropriate. Collaboration involves some shared functions and a common focus on the same over-all mission" (2003, p. 8). The common focus on the same overall mission should be patient-centered care. The ANA professional performance standards address collaboration by identifying the need for nurses to collaborate with the patient, family, and others as care is provided (ANA, 2004). This requires nurses to communicate, collaborate when a plan of care is developed, partner with others for change, and document referrals that enhance continuity of care.

Collaboration requires that there be open communication and that team members feel comfortable expressing their opinions. Team members of different healthcare professions must work across professional boundaries to gain a team culture of working together. The goal is not to make an individual's profession "look good," but rather to focus on the team. Even when the team is composed of members from the same healthcare profession, such as a nursing team, the focus is on the team, not individuals. This does not mean that conflicts will not occur, but some can be prevented; when conflict does occur, there are effective methods for coping in order to reach a common goal.

Nurses work closely with physicians, and this relationship has a long history of conflict. Often it is stereotyped as "we versus them," which is an unhealthy approach. With the greater emphasis on teamwork, nurses and physicians are slowly being forced into improving their work relationship. As has been discussed, this really needs to begin at the student level. Organizations need to stand behind improving team collaboration, coordination, and communication. One area that has received notice is abuse—usually verbal—from physician to nurse. Many organizations now have zero-tolerance policies related to this type of abuse as well as code-of-conduct policies. However, just having a written policy does not mean that attitudes and behaviors improve. Staff

need to know policy content and consequences, and consequences must be employed when needed. It is very easy to say that this is all the physicians' fault when it is not. Many nurses enter the profession with a negative attitude toward physicians and feel that they do not want to be controlled by physicians. The better approach is for new nurses to enter the profession with a positive attitude toward nursing as a profession, knowledgeable about what nursing is, competent, and with a reasonable level of self-esteem. What is needed is someone who wants to work with others, not against others, and someone who approaches issues and problems with an open mind and who is not tied to an "I know better" mindset. If all healthcare professionals could approach practice in this manner, then collaboration, coordination, and communication would improve. There would be limited incidents of verbal abuse, and the work environment would be positive and healthy for all team members. Another method for dealing with verbal abuse is to try and remove the emotion from the situation—step back for a breather, and then discuss the issue or problem on a factual basis. This may require a third party to act as neutral party in the discussion. This is not easy to do when parties are emotional and often tired and stressed, but it does make a difference. This provides time to gain more a objective perspective. Why is there interest in this topic of verbal abuse and disruptive behavior among team members? There is concern about their impact on patient care. Examples of disruptive behavior are verbal abuse, negative behavior, and physical abuse (e.g., profanity, innuendo, demeaning comments), reprimanding or insulting another in public and inappropriately, threatening, telling racial or ethnic jokes, undermining team cohesion, scapegoating, silence (not speaking to team member), assaulting another, throwing objects, and outbursts of rage (Lower, 2007).

A study was conducted that explored the impact of work relationships on clinical outcomes (Rosenstein & O'Daniel, 2005). This study was published in a nursing journal and conducted by a physician and a healthcare administrator. It was a follow-up study that looked at the impact of disruptive behavior on job satisfaction and retention (Rosenstein, 2002). In the 2005 study, 1,500 surveys from nurses and physicians were evaluated. What were the results of this study? First, nurses were reported to exhibit disruptive behavior as frequently as physicians did. Both groups felt that disruptive behavior (which includes verbal abuse) negatively impacted relationships and created stress, leading to frustration, lack of concentration, poor communication, and the inability to effectively collaborate and provide effective information transfer in the workplace. Given that this chapter discusses the need for greater use of effective interdisciplinary teams to provide quality, safe patient-centered care, it is easy to see how these results can be disturbing. The participants also felt that disruptive behavior was adversely affecting patient safety, patient mortality, the quality of care, and patient satisfaction. This further emphasizes the need to improve teamwork and professional relationships. The researchers recommended that the following be done in organizations to improve workplace relationships.

- The organization should conduct a self-assessment to determine the prevalence of disruptive behavior and better understand its nature.
- The organization should then share results with staff to increase awareness of the problem.
- The organization should open up lines of communication between nurses and physicians (and any other staff who are experienc-

ing disruptive behavior) in a nonantagonistic environment to discuss issues.
- The organization should provide education about mutual respect among coworkers and the benefits of team collaboration; communication; team building; and conflict management. (This is a good way to emphasize the IOM core competency.)
- The organization should develop and implement policies and procedures that reinforce acceptable codes of behavior.

All these strategies should promote better patient care and clinical outcomes.

Coordination

Nurses coordinate patient care through planning and implementing care. Effective **coordination** needs to be interdisciplinary. Coordination and collaboration should be interconnected. Dessler described coordination as "the process of achieving unity of action among interdependent activities" (2002, pp. 143–144). Why is this so important? Care is complex, and patients require healthcare providers with different expertise to meet these needs. With this type of situation, the different providers need to collaborate to reach a plan and an implementation of care that makes sense—meeting the timeline required, with minimal conflict and confusion. Coordination—working to see that the pieces and activities fit together and flow as they should—can help to meet desired patient outcomes. Patients often complain about the number of care providers. They may not know who is responsible for what aspects of their care, and they receive confusing and often conflicting communication and information. The patient needs to have an anchor—a healthcare provider whom the patient can turn to for support and knowledge of the plan. Basically, patients are saying that they are not the center of care and that their care appears fragmented. This leads to an increased risk of errors and decreases the quality of care. The ANA (2004) standards of practice include coordination of care. Care is coordinated through the implementation of the care plan and in documentation of care.

Barriers and Competencies Related to Coordination

Coordination is not easy to achieve even when team members want to achieve it. Some of the barriers to effective coordination are listed next.

- Team members who do not understand the roles and responsibilities of other team members, particularly members from different healthcare professions.
- Lack of a clear interdisciplinary plan of care.
- Limited leadership.
- Overwork and excessive burden of responsibilities for team members.
- Ineffective communication, both oral and written.
- Lack of inclusion of the patient and family/significant others in the care process.
- Competition among team members to control decisions.

Despite these barriers, coordination can be achieved. First, the team must recognize that coordination is critical and work to achieve it. The team needs to understand its purpose and goals and implement them. This means that the team evaluates its work and is willing to identify weaknesses and figure out methods to improve coordination. Team members need to communicate openly and in a timely manner. Teams that can effectively solve problems together will improve their coordination. Delegation, to be discussed in the next section, is an important part of coordination. Not everything can be done by one person (and that one person may not even

be the best person for the task or activity). Coordination requires team members to understand different roles and the expertise of the members, to determine the best member to make or deliver care and in what timeline, and to evaluate the outcomes.

Tools to Improve Coordination

Health care has developed tools and methods to increase coordination. From a chronic illness perspective, disease management is a tool to improve coordination and collaboration. Disease management has been discussed in earlier chapters. Two other methods are practice guidelines, which will be discussed in Chapter 11 in relation to evidence-based practice, and clinical protocols or pathways. What is a clinical protocol or pathway?

A clinical protocol or pathway is a written guide to provide direction for specific clinical problems. It considers interventions, timeline, and resources needed; it identifies expected outcomes; and it provides a sequencing of interventions to reach the outcomes. Typically, a pathway is laid out in a chart, as illustrated in Figure 10–3, which provides examples of information categories that might be found in a clinical pathway.

Pathways are developed in a number of ways. Healthcare organizations may develop them by identifying focus areas based on needs—for example, pathways that focus on the care of a diabetic patient who has been hospitalized, a patient who needs a hip replacement, or a patient who is severely depressed and suicidal. A team of interdisciplinary experts then develop the pathway. The team should use current literature and evidence from research, and team members may even seek out examples from other hospitals or examples found in professional literature. In other situations, the healthcare organization may decide to use a published clinical pathway. After the clinical pathway is developed or selected, staff need training about the pathway and its

Figure 10–3 Categories of information found in clinical pathways.

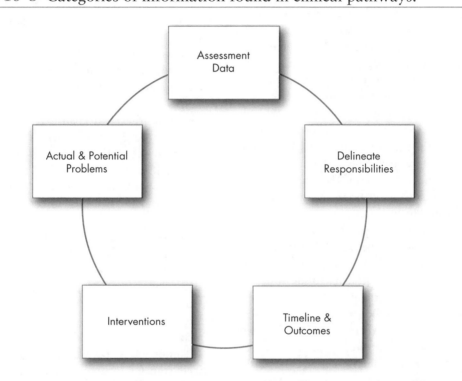

Note: Within these five categories of information in the clinical pathway is specific information such as tests and procedures; predetermined length of stay based on the usual length of stay; medications; patient activity; diet/nutrition; and patient/family education. When appropriate, trigger points are identified to indicate when certain actions would typically be done—for example, when a lab test or procedure should be done (e.g., Day 1), or a time schedule for medication.

use. Pathways can be used to evaluate care and outcomes by collecting data about their use and the patients' outcomes. Does the pathway, or specific interventions within a pathway, make a difference?

There are a number of advantages to using clinical protocols or pathways. First, this type of tool improves coordination and ensures that outcomes are met. Because they are written and based on evidence, there is a standard for care and greater consistency. However, whenever a pathway is used, it must be reviewed to ensure that

it meets the individual needs of the patient and adapted accordingly. Other advantages include more effective use of expertise and resources, better management of healthcare costs, improved collaboration and communication, a decrease in errors, improvement in quality of care, improved patient satisfaction (because patients feel that their care is organized and they are more informed), improved care documentation (because it follows a consistent plan), improved identification of responsibilities, and a clear statement of interventions.

Delegation

Delegation is part of the daily work of nurses. Care is planned and coordinated to meet patient needs, but at some point, the registered nurse (RN) may need to delegate work to others. This action involves giving another staff member the responsibility and authority to complete a task or activity. Before an RN can delegate, he or she needs to have responsibility and authority, or the power over the activity or task. An RN cannot delegate something that he or she cannot do. An extreme example is that an RN cannot delegate prescriptive authority (prescribing of medications) because he or she typically cannot do this activity. An advanced practice nurse can have prescriptive authority because he or she has met special requirements, but even this nurse cannot delegate prescriptive authority to someone who has not met the requirements.

When an RN delegates to another staff member, such as UAP or an LPN/LVN, the RN is not avoiding work and is still held accountable for the outcomes, but the care is provided in a more efficient manner. Accountability is "being responsible and answerable for actions or inactions of self or others in the context of delegation" (National Council of State Boards of Nursing [NCSBN], 1995). The UAP is "any unlicensed individual who is trained to function in an assistive role to the licensed nurse in the provision of patient activities as delegated by the nurse. The term includes, but is not limited to nurse aides, orderlies, assistants, attendants, or technicians" (ANA, 1997, p. 3). There is no national standard that is accepted and enforced in every state as to employment requirements, training, or position descriptions for UAP (Zimmerman, 2002). The RN (the **delegator**) is still responsible for supervising the work (activity, task) that the other staff member (the **delegatee**) is to do.

Key Terms

Supervision, assignment, and *delegation* are key terms that are easy to confuse (Zimmerman, 2002). They are related to one another. When a nurse is monitoring care and the work, this is supervision. The nurse may be in a formal management position, such as a nurse manager, a team leader, or an RN who has delegated work to another and ensures that it is done effectively. Assignment moves an activity from one person to another, including the responsibility and accountability. For example, the nurse manager assigns an RN to lead a team or to administer medications to the patients. An assignment can be given only to staff who have the required qualifications to complete the tasks and who can carry the responsibility and accountability; however, the accountability is shared. The person doing the activity has the accountability for the actual action or activity, whereas the person who made the assignment is responsible for the assignment decision. An RN cannot *assign* to a UAP; "delegation is the partial transfer of authority and responsibility regarding care activities, while accountability for completion and outcome remains with the delegator" (Yoder-Wise, 1999, as cited in Zimmerman, 2002).

Importance of Delegation

Why is delegation important, and why is it part of care coordination? One RN cannot always do everything that is required for a patient. There must be effective use of resources—expertise and time. Through delegation, work can be allocated to those who can most effectively accomplish it. Delegation is a critical part of providing cost-effective care. It is more cost-effective if care can safely be provided by an UAP or an LPN whose salary is lower than that of an RN, with the RN providing overall supervision. The NCSBN, through the state boards of nursing, identifies the standards and describes the delegation process. The NCSBN (1995) defines delegation as "transferring to a competent individual authority to perform a selected nursing task in a selected situation. The nurse retains the accountability for the delegation." What does this definition really say?

1. Transferring means that the RN can do something that will be passed on to someone else to do. The RN has the right to do this. The RN cannot delegate something that he or she has no right to do. (*For example, a patient needs a bed bath. The RN can do the bed bath, but it is more efficient to have the UAP complete the bed bath while the RN assesses the patient's overall status at the beginning of a shift.*)
2. The RN transfers this activity to a competent person—someone who can complete the task because that person has the skills and experience to do so. (*For example, the UAP has been trained to give bed baths and report to the nurse any problems encountered.*)
3. In the delegation process, the delegator or RN is giving the delegatee the authority or power to do the act or task. (*For example, RNs have overall responsibility and authority for all nursing care—from basic care, such as bed bath, to complex care needs. The RN determines who is the best staff member to complete a task. In some cases, the RN may decide that because of the critical status of the patient and the need for intensive interaction and assessment, he or she should complete the bed bath. Or, the RN may decide that the UAP is best suited.*)
4. The delegatee must then do something—that something is specific and is attached to a specific situation. (*For example, the UAP completes the bed bath, documents the care, and informs the RN that there was nothing unusual to report.*)

Five Rights

It is natural to wonder who is responsible for the care. The delegatee is responsible for the care that he or she provides or the performance. What is the role of the delegator? The delegator is responsible for the delegation process. This process is not a simple one and requires experience. The RN must consider the five rights of delegation (NCSBN, 1995).

1. **Right Task:** The task must be delegatable for a specific patient or situation. What is the task? If the RN or delegator is not clear about the task, the RN will not be able to clearly identify what needs to be done and by whom.
2. **Right Circumstances:** Appropriate setting, available resources, and other relevant factors need to be considered. Where should the task be done? What is needed to complete the task? It may be that the RN will need to tell the delegatee where to complete the task and to identify what supplies, equipment, and other resources are needed to complete the task effectively.
3. **Right Person:** The right person delegates the right task to the right person, to be performed by the right person. The RN must consider the best staff member to complete the task (type of staff, his or her experience and skills, if he or she has time to complete task without negatively impacting other work, and so on).
4. **Right Direction/Communication:** Providing a clear, concise description of the task, including its objective, limits, and expectations, is part of effective delegation. The delegator must explain to the delegatee what is to be done, how to do it (if not clear), the timeframe, outcomes, and so on. The delegatee needs to feel comfortable asking questions for clarification or expressing concern about his or her

inability to complete the task. The delegator must be an effective communicator and sensitive to concerns and issues in order to establish a communication environment that allows for open discussion. This is critical to ensure patient-centered care that is focused on safety and quality. If the delegatee is afraid of speaking up and saying, "I do not know how to do something," or "Would you explain more about what you want done?" then this is an ineffective delegation process that can harm the patient. The delegatee may need help in organizing work and setting priorities, or he or she may need to be told what to report to the RN and when. The delegator needs to ask directly if there are questions or concerns and be open to the response. All of this is part of providing clear directions.

5. **Right Supervision:** Appropriate monitoring, evaluation, intervention (as needed), and feedback are part of delegation. The RN as a delegator does not just delegate a task and then forget about it. The RN needs to supervise as required. Monitoring methods include observation, verbal feedback, written feedback, and review of records in which the delegatee documented what he or she did. In some situations, supervision is minimal, and in other situations, there may be a greater need for monitoring. Factors such as the expertise of the delegatee, the patient's status, the complexity of the task, and timing may all impact the monitoring process. Another factor that cannot be ignored is how comfortable the delegator feels in delegating, and how well the delegator knows the delegate. New RNs can be very nervous about delegating; trusting another to complete a task can be risky. Some new RNs may be overly concerned because they feel that

they could perform the task better. In both situations, the result could be excessive "hovering," or overmonitoring; the delegatee may interpret the delegator's behavior or attitude as indicating a lack of confidence in the delegatee. This message can have a negative impact on staff team relationships. Finding the balance takes experience. New RNs need time to learn how to delegate effectively, and they need to seek guidance from their own supervisors or mentors to assess their delegation competencies. Figure 10–4 highlights the five delegation rights.

Delegation Principles

The ANA and the NCSBN collaborated to identify the key delegation principles that should be applied by every RN (ANA & NCSBN, 2006, pp. 2–3):

- The RN takes responsibility and accountability for the provision of nursing practice.
- The RN directs care and determines the appropriate utilization of any assistant involved in providing direct patient care.
- The RN may delegate components of care but does not delegate the nursing process itself. Nursing judgment cannot be delegated.
- The decision of whether or not to delegate or assign is based upon the RN's judgment concerning the condition of the patient, the competence of all members of the nursing team, and the degree of supervision that will be required of the RN if a task is delegated.
- The RN delegates only those tasks for which he or she believes the other healthcare worker has the knowledge and skill to perform, taking into consideration training, cultural competence, experience, and facility/agency policies and procedures.

Figure 10–4 Five rights for effective delegation.

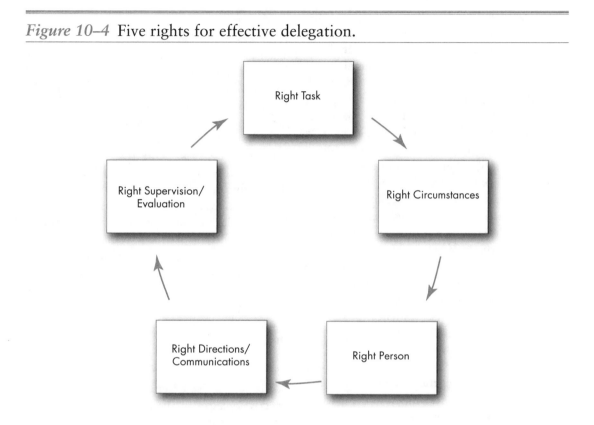

- The RN individualizes communication regarding the delegation to the nursing assistive personnel and client situation, and the communication should be clear, concise, correct and complete. The RN verifies comprehension with the nursing assistive personnel and that the assistant accepts the delegation and the responsibility that accompanies it.
- Communication must be a two-way process. Nursing assistive personnel should have the opportunity to ask questions and/or for clarification of expectations.
- The RN uses critical thinking and professional judgment when following the five rights of delegation.

- Chief Nursing Officers are accountable for establishing systems to assess, monitor, verify and communicate ongoing competence requirements in areas related to delegation.
- There is both individual accountability and organizational accountability for delegation. Organizational accountability for delegation relates to providing sufficient resources.

It is important that the RN, as the delegator, thank the delegatee and recognize the work that he or she has done. Compliment work when it is done well, and provide constructive feedback. *Constructive* means that the RN does not criticize work negatively, but discusses the work and outcomes and makes recommendations for improvement. It is easy to take things for granted and not recognize the work of team members. It really takes little time to give positive feedback and a thank you, and yet this can go a long way toward building teams. Will there be times when the RN as delegator must "take back" a task that has been delegated? If so, why would this occur? In the monitoring process, the delegatee could ask for help. The RN needs to listen to this and intervene. There may be times when the patient's condition changes, and someone else, including the RN, may be better suited to complete the task. The RN may recognize that the delegatee is not as qualified to complete the task as originally thought. The RN must be aware of the need to avoid being negative, hurting the delegatee's self-confidence, or embarrassing the delegatee in front of others. How the RN communicates and intervenes can make the situation a positive learning experience for the delegatee. In addition, the RN must recognize the impact on the patient—how the patient views the change of assignment and if he or she wonders what is going on. Supervision plays a critical role in delegation. The ANA and NCSBN have similar definitions of supervision (ANA & NCSBN, 2006). The ANA defines supervision as the "active process of directing, guiding, and influencing the outcome of an individual's performance of a task," whereas the NCSBN defines it as "the provision of guidance or direction, oversight, evaluation and follow-up by the licensed nurse for the accomplishment of a delegated nursing task by assistive personnel" (ANA & NCSBN, 2006). It is important to note that supervision does not necessarily mean that the RN is in a management position. RNs who are not in management positions must also supervise when they delegate. Figure 10–5 describes the decision tree for delegation.

Evaluation

How does the RN evaluate his or her delegation? The first focus is the role of the delegator. Were the right tasks delegated, and why? The second concern is the directions. Were they clear? The RN should consider to whom the task was delegated, and the delegatee's strengths and limitations. Did the delegatee have the resources to complete the task? Did the delegatee have the time to complete the task? What impact did performing the specific task have on other responsibilities that the delegatee may have had? Did the delegatee have the authority to complete the task? Was the delegator available to the delegatee if questions arose or problems occurred? This availability is more than just physical; it concerns not just whether the delegatee is able to reach the delegator, but also whether the delegator is able to listen and hear the delegatee and then respond effectively.

EFFECTIVE DELEGATION

What is effective delegation? RNs want to be effective delegators, and new RNs struggle with how to delegate. The following are some characteristics of effective delegation (Milgram et al., 1999, p. 245):

- Do not give employees just menial tasks; include tasks that offer opportunities for learning and growth.
- Distribute tasks with an understanding of each employee's job status, abilities, and total workload.
- Delegate when there is someone skilled available or when the task can be completed by a subordinate whose time is less expensive.
- Use benchmarks to monitor progress along the way; having only a final deadline can be overwhelming. (This applies to activities or tasks that take a longer time to complete.)

Figure 10–5 Decision tree for delegation to nursing assistive personnel.

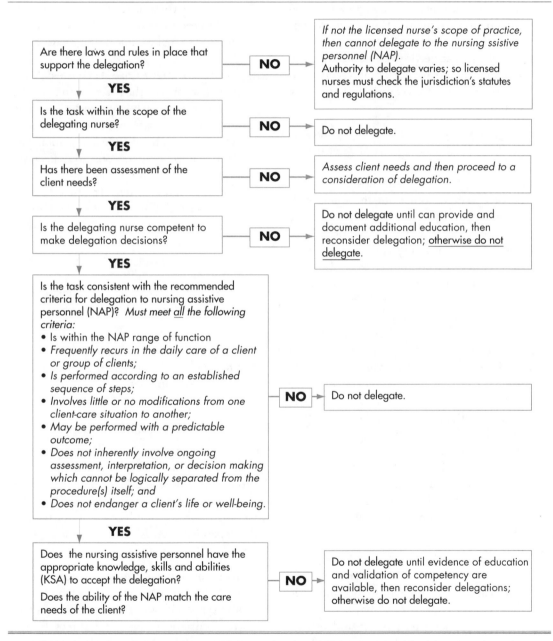

Source: From *Delegation decision-making tree*, by National Council of State Boards of Nursing, 1997, Chicago: Author. Retrieved September 24, 2008; from https://www.nesbn.org/delegation_Decisions__Making_Tree_NEW Reprinted with permission.

- Do not micromanage subordinates. Experienced employees usually have the skills necessary for managing complex tasks on their own (particularly if the tasks are typically done by them).
- Establish what needs to be done, and then provide support for the employee as he or she decides how to accomplish the activity or task.

Exhibit 10–1 provides a delegation self-assessment tool that can be used to determine if a nurse feels ready to delegate.

The focus of this discussion thus far has been on RNs delegating to other nursing staff—staff who are not RNs. However, it is important to recognize that RNs may assign work or tasks to RNs, but this is not delegation. A team may include several RNs, and one may be the team leader. The nurse manager or nurse coordinator of a unit assigns work to RN staff routinely.

Effective delegation takes practice. It does not just happen. There are barriers to delegation. Staff may be uncomfortable with delegating and with criticism, depending on whether they are the delegator or delegatee. This can interfere with effective delegation and positive outcomes. The RNs typically delegate to UAPs. RNs need to know what an UAP can do. What are the UAP role and job responsibilities? UAPs cannot do the following or be delegated these activities: health counseling; teaching; and activities that require independent, specialized nursing knowledge, skills, or judgment. The ANA (1997) has identified the UAP direct and indirect patient care activities.

1. **Direct Patient Care Activities:** Activities that assist the patient in meeting basic human needs (settings may be hospitals, home, long-term care, and other). Activities include assisting with feeding, drinking, ambulation, grooming, toilet-

ing, dressing, and socializing. Collection, reporting, and documentation of data related to these activities is important. UAPs need to report data to RNs that then are used to make clinical judgments about patient care.

2. **Indirect Patient Care Activities:** Activities that support the patient and his or her environment, such as providing a clean, efficient, and safe patient care milieu. Activities might include companion care; simple meal preparation; housekeeping; providing transportation; and clerical, stocking, and maintenance tasks. Many of these activities would take place in the patient's home, where UAPs may be working one-on-one with a patient through a home health agency or some type of community agency.

Generally, tasks that can be delegated are those that (NCSBN, 1998):

- Frequently occur
- Are considered technical by nature
- Are considered standard and unchanging
- Have predictable results
- Have minimal potential for risks

Levels of Patient Health Status

Another aspect to consider is the continuum of care as it relates to the patient's needs and the roles of the RN and UAP. There are three levels of patient health status and needs that the nurse must consider: independent status, partially dependent status, and dependent status (NCSBN, 1998, pp. 2–3).

1. **Independent Status**—A patient with or without a health impairment who has the ability for self-care. The patient at this level may initiate, accept, and direct health-related interventions. Interventions may be provided by licensed nurses or assistive

---

Exhibit 10–1 Delegation Self-Assessment

Answer the following with Strongly Agree (SA), Agree (A), Unsure (U), Disagree (D), or Strongly Disagree (SD).

_____ 1. I hate risk: I don't think risk of any kind should be present in healthcare delivery.

_____ 2. It's very difficult for me to trust the people I work with. How can I be sure they'll do what I want them to?

_____ 3. Letting go of the tasks I like to do is impossible for me. I get all my positive feedback from doing my clinical tasks exceptionally well.

_____ 4. There's so little I can control about my daily work that I find it very difficult to lose the control I gain by doing it all myself. How can I control others enough to be certain everything is done my way?

_____ 5. I'm finding that overcoming my old habits of doing it all myself is more difficult than giving up (choose one) cigarettes, or chocolate, or fine wine. Giving up things that are comfortable for me and are a part of my daily life is not my cup of tea.

_____ 6. I feel very little achievement when someone else does the nuts and bolts of the care. I want to do that myself so I can feel the satisfaction of crossing tasks off my list.

_____ 7. If everyone else does the tasks on the care plan, I'm confused about what's left for me to do.

_____ 8. When people tell me they have time to help me, it's difficult for me to tell them what they could do to help. I could use some help with organizing my work.

_____ 9. I do all the work in my area better than most people. I am an expert clinician, and I would hate for the clients to receive an "inferior" product if I am not the person actually performing that care.

_____ 10. I really hate to make people mad when I assign them work. I'd rather do it myself than give out a bad assignment.

_____ 11. There are a few people who work as hard as I do. I often find myself with the most challenging assignments. I rarely ask for help. Often, I'm behind doing my charting after the shift is over while the "slackers" go out for pizza.

_____ 12. I am uncertain about what can be delegated to the personnel in our department. The roles are unclear, and I'm not comfortable with the state regulations and rules.

_____ 13. I hate to even think about delegating care to anyone else!

_____ 14. If I don't do the tasks I'm used to doing, I wonder if I will still be a real nurse? I've worked too hard to become a clinical "has-been."

_____ 15. I've never seen or worked with anyone who is a good delegator. I wouldn't know what it's like.

Source: From *Clinical Delegation Skills: A Handbook for Professional Practice*, by R. Hansten and M. Jackson, 2009, Sudbury, MA: Jones and Bartlett Publishers.

---

personnel to the extent that the actions of assistive personnel do not constitute the practice of nursing. For the patient without an identified health impairment, interventions may include general education and support to promote wellness, health maintenance and disease prevention. For the patient with identified health impairment, the nurse may also provide consultation, initiated by the patient or nurse, to support and maintain the patient's independent status.

2. **Partially Dependent Status**—A patient with self-care deficits who needs assistance in activities of daily living and/or health maintenance activities. The nurse's primary responsibilities for partially dependent patients may be described as care coordination. Such responsibilities may include consultation, needs assessment, providing education, support, and other direct care activities; ongoing evaluation of the care provided by self and others; and teaching and validating the competencies of assistive personnel who perform care activities. Whether the patient or the nurse directs the care will depend upon the degree of self-care deficit and the level of monitoring and interventions required by health professionals. Assistive personnel may be directed by the patient or authorized to perform care through the nursing delegation process.

3. **Fully Dependent Status**—A patient whose responsibility for care has been transferred to licensed health professionals within a healthcare system. This patient may or may not be competent or capable of participating in self-care. The nurse is accountable for the overall management of nursing care. When assistive personnel are utilized, they are authorized to perform care through the delegation process.

What are the desired outcomes of delegation (NCSBN, 1997)?

1. Allows protection of public/patient safety.
2. Achievement of desirable patient outcomes.
3. Achievement of potential benefits for the RN and UAP (or staff delegated to).
4. Reduction of healthcare costs (better use of resources).
5. Facilitation of access to appropriate level of care (better use of resources may allow for increased access to providers who can bet-

ter provide care; allowing others to be used for other needs).
6. Delineation of the spectrum of accountability for nursing care (supports each team member's role in providing care).
7. Decrease nurse liability (promotes more effective use of provider skills that may decrease risk of liability).

In summary, Figure 10–6 illustrates the key to delegation and highlights the key aspects of delegation.

Change

Change was discussed in Chapter 8 in relation to changes in the healthcare delivery system.

Figure 10–6 The key to delegation.

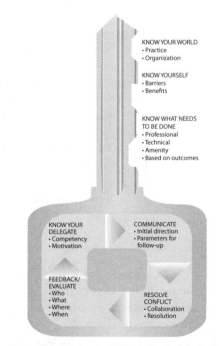

Source: From *Clinical Delegation Skills: A Handbook for Professional Practice*, by R. Hansten and M. Jackson, 2009, Sudbury, MA: Jones and Bartlett Publishers.

Change is also a part of collaboration and coordination, which are difficult to accomplish without some change; change may be required from an individual team member, the entire team, a unit, or the organization. Patients are asked to change all the time. Why do team members often not like change? They may be fearful of the results, particularly of the unknown; they may fear losing something of value, such as control, job responsibility, and so on; or they may have a belief that change will not make things better. The other view of change is its potential, an opportunity for improvement. Sometimes change does not lead to positive outcomes. This has to be dealt with, but not changing means stagnation and lack of improvement.

What methods can be used to decrease these barriers to change and increase team involvement in change? Explanation and education about the issue or problem and the need for change is the first step. Including team members in the discussion about the need for change and possible solutions allows members to buy into the change process. They will participate more and be more invested in the results. Change is stressful; this stress needs to be recognized and, when possible, interventions to reduce stress should be used. Experiencing too many changes at one time or too quickly can make effective change difficult. Sometimes there are situations in which change is dictated. When this occurs, team members still need an explanation, and all attempts to include them in some aspects of the change process should be encouraged. Asking for feedback and listening are important. Changing is risky. Sometimes it will fail. Teams need to learn from errors and ineffective decisions, and then move on. Effective collaborative teams do not place blame on individuals; rather, they look at results in an objective manner and realize that the team works together and sometimes can make mistakes.

Conflict and Conflict Resolution

Conflict is inevitable; however, what is important is how it is handled. In many cases, it can be prevented. It is natural for misunderstandings to occur among people who work together, such as in teams. Often, causes of conflict relate to whether resources are shared equitably; to insufficient explanation of expectations, leading to performance being questioned; to unexplained changes that disturb routines and process and that team members are not prepared for; and to stress resulting from changes that team members do not understand and may see as threatening. Each of these causes can be prevented from developing into conflict, or at least conflict can be lessened. The method for doing this is engaging in clear, timely communication and including team members in the process. There is another cause of conflict that is more difficult to manage: an individual's personal responses, behavior, or issues that increase conflict in the team. Examples are the team member who does not do his or her work, the team member who is late to meetings, the team member who does not listen to others, the team member who complains, the team member who is overly critical of others, the team member who does not know how to communicate effectively, and the team member who wants to be the "star" and take all the credit. Figure 10–7 shows a conflict flowchart.

Conflict resolution takes leadership and participation from team members. When difficult issues or problems arise, it is best to deal with them rather than postpone decisions (which usually means that the problem has time to get worse). Using threats and negativity with little positive feedback can lead to conflict, so these approaches need to be avoided. Listening can go a long way in preventing conflict, and, if conflict does occur, in resolving it. When team members treat each other with respect and communicate clearly, conflict can be decreased. Respect means

Figure 10–7 Conflict flowchart.

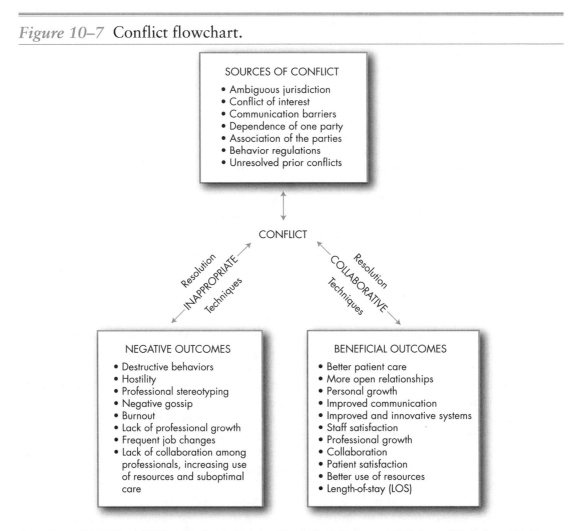

Source: From *Clinical Delegation Skills: A Handbook for Professional Practice*, by R. Hansten and M. Jackson, 2009, Sudbury, MA: Jones and Bartlett Publishers; Dennis Burnside.

to recognize another's right to have opinions and to listen and discuss these opinions. Nonverbal communication can give important clues as to when conflict is increasing. When teams or individual members experience stress, the risk of conflict increases. Open communication is key to resolution of conflict, and it is key to preventing conflict when possible. When conflict occurs, it is important to provide opportunities to identify the facts, determine the purpose of the actions or activities at the time, and review team member perspectives. When members are emotional, this can interfere with effective resolution, so sometimes the best first approach is to "step back" and allow some time for everyone involved to lower his or her emotional reactions. However, the issue needs to be resolved, so this time period needs to be monitored; it should not go on too long. Sometimes one or two members need to be persuaded to reexamine the issue. This may or may not be successful. Teams need to learn that individual team members will not always get their viewpoint accepted by all. Compromise is required; however, when this occurs, it must be done in a manner that respects divergent opinions and that does not use negativity or reduce self-esteem. All this requires leadership—on the part of the designated team leader and members who commit to the team and its effectiveness. Figure 10–8 describes a collaborative resolution method.

Power and Empowerment

Empowerment was discussed in earlier chapters, but it is also important to consider here how power and empowerment relate to teams. As people work together, the issue of **power** arises. Simply put, power can be described as when healthcare provider A wants something that healthcare provider B has and does not need or want as much; healthcare provider B then has more power in the relationship. Herzberg's theory on job satisfaction relates to power and teams (Herzberg, Mausner, & Snyderman, 1959). Typically, there is not a balance of power in a team, particularly when it is first formed. This is most

Figure 10–8 Hansten & Washburn's Collaborative Resolution Method.

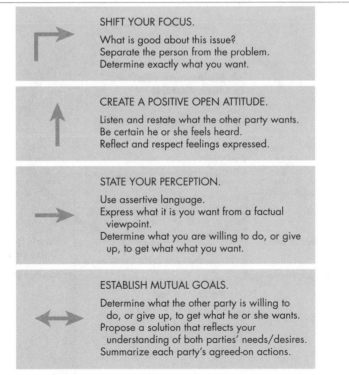

SHIFT YOUR FOCUS.
What is good about this issue?
Separate the person from the problem.
Determine exactly what you want.

CREATE A POSITIVE OPEN ATTITUDE.
Listen and restate what the other party wants.
Be certain he or she feels heard.
Reflect and respect feelings expressed.

STATE YOUR PERCEPTION.
Use assertive language.
Express what it is you want from a factual
viewpoint.
Determine what you are willing to do, or give
up, to get what what you want.

ESTABLISH MUTUAL GOALS.
Determine what the other party is willing to
do, or give up, to get what he or she wants.
Propose a solution that reflects your
understanding of both parties' needs/desires.
Summarize each party's agreed-on actions.

Source: From *Clinical Delegation Skills: A Handbook for Professional Practice*, by R. Hansten and M. Jackson, 2009, Sudbury, MA: Jones and Bartlett Publishers.

commonly seen with nurses and physicians; physicians have more power because of their profession, experience, and history. This, however, can change and should change as the team develops, with members recognizing one another's value and experience. But an imbalance can be difficult to overcome and makes the work situation stressful.

How a person feels about his or her work and job has an impact on how that person functions on a team. Herzberg's theory, as described in Figure 10–9, identifies job maintenance factors or extrinsic factors that influence job satisfaction; however, there is more to job satisfaction than these hygiene factors, as Herz-

berg calls them. The motivator factors (intrinsic factors) must also be considered. Herzberg suggested that because of these factors, organizations that increase accountability, create teams, remove controls, provide feedback, introduce new tasks, allocate special assignments, and grant additional authority would increase staff motivation (Norman & Crowley, 1999, as cited in Michalopoulos & Michalopoulos, 2006). Staff will feel increased personal achievement and more empowered. The same authors noted that the factors to increase staff motivation are part of the need for nurses to "increase responsibility, control over their work, and the opportunity to use their own initiative, all of

Figure 10–9 Herzberg's theory on job satisfaction.

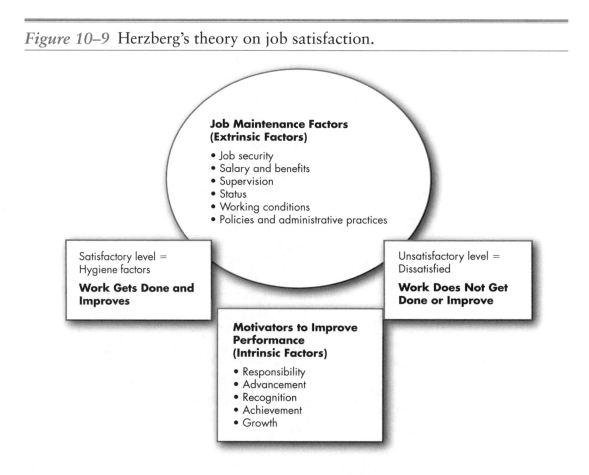

Job Maintenance Factors (Extrinsic Factors)

- Job security
- Salary and benefits
- Supervision
- Status
- Working conditions
- Policies and administrative practices

Satisfactory level = Hygiene factors

Work Gets Done and Improves

Unsatisfactory level = Dissatisfied

Work Does Not Get Done or Improve

Motivators to Improve Performance (Intrinsic Factors)

- Responsibility
- Advancement
- Recognition
- Achievement
- Growth

Table 10–2 Types of Power

Type of Power	Description
Legitimate/Formal Power	Power that originates from serving in a formal position (for example, a team leader, nurse manager, or chief nursing officer).
Referent/Informal Power	Power that originates from others recognizing that an individual has leadership qualities and choosing to follow that person.
Informational Power	Power that originates from information a person has and others need.
Expert Power	Power that originates from a person's expertise, which can be useful to others and enable the person to provide guidance (for example, a nurse clinical specialist).
Reward Power	Power that originates from a person's ability to reward others (for example, the ability to grant a salary increase, promotion, or assign an interesting project) if they agree to do something.
Coercive Power	Power that originates from a person's ability to punish others (for example, the ability to assign an unpleasant task or project, or deny a promotion) if they do not do what is asked.Expectations

which are offered in team nursing and the nursing process" (Michalopoulos & Michalopoulos, 2006, pp. 54–55). Table 10–2 describes the **types of powers**.

Empowering teams means that the leader of the team needs to be less assertive over time and allow the team to lead. The team needs to find the best solutions by using the expertise of all the members. The team then takes on the leadership, and this actually strengthens the team leader's leadership—with the result of better team outcomes.

Conclusion

This chapter has discussed the important healthcare profession core competency: work in interdisciplinary teams. The content explored the meaning of this competency, its relationship to nursing, and what is involved in teams and teamwork. Collaboration, coordination, communication, delegation, and conflict and conflict resolution are major team activities.

CHAPTER HIGHLIGHTS

1. The essential features of the interdisciplinary team include examination of self as it relates to the team effort, interdisciplinary communication and conflict resolution, and the impact of the team's efforts on quality, safety, patient-focused or patient-centered care, and overall delivery of care.

2. Care coordination is a key factor in healthcare delivery and requires an interprofessional or interdisciplinary team effort.

3. Healthcare profession education takes place in isolation, with each healthcare

profession providing its own education with limited regard to other healthcare professionals.

4. Multidisciplinary teams are not the same as interdisciplinary ones. In the former, members of each profession report aspects of care from their vantage point, whereas members of the interdisciplinary team solve problems and plan care together.

5. A team leader must first recognize that it is the work of the team that is critical and avoid focusing on personal success as a leader.

6. Formal meetings are an important part of teamwork.

7. Planning before any team meeting is very important to the overall success of the meeting itself.

8. Effective teams value openness and collaboration.

9. Communication is the sharing of a message between one person or group and another. It is important to know if the message was received as sent. Interpretation plays a major role, and sometimes interpretation confuses or changes the original message sent.

10. Listening is critical to good communication.

11. Collaboration means that all people involved are listened to and that decisions are developed together.

12. Coordination—working to see that the pieces/activities fit together and flow as they should—can help to meet desired patient outcomes.

13. A clinical protocol or pathway is a written guide that provides direction for specific clinical problems; considers the inter-

ventions, timeline, and resources needed; and identifies expected outcomes.

14. Delegation refers to transferring responsibility for a task to another person. First, the person delegating must have the authority to transfer this task, and second, it must be handed off to someone whose scope of responsibilities includes this work.

15. There are five rights of delegation: right task, right circumstances, right person, right direction, and right supervision.

16. Change is also a part of collaboration and coordination, which are difficult to accomplish without some change—change may be required from an individual team member, the entire team, a unit, or the organization.

17. Often, causes of conflicts relate to whether resources are shared equitably; to insufficient explanation of expectations, leading to performance being questioned; to unexplained changes that disturb routines and process and that team members are not prepared for; and to stress resulting from changes that team members do not understand and may see as threatening.

18. Resolving conflict takes leadership and participation from team members.

19. Empowering teams means that the leader of the team must be less assertive over time and allow the team to lead.

Linking to the Internet

- National Council of State Boards of Nursing
  https://www.ncsbn.org/index.htm

DISCUSSION QUESTIONS

1. Explain the healthcare core competency; work in interdisciplinary teams. Why is this important to address in healthcare education, and what is its impact on practice?
2. What is a team, and how does it function?
3. How does collaboration impact team effectiveness?
4. Why is coordination a key activity of a clinical interdisciplinary team? Of a nursing team?
5. Explain the communication process.
6. Discuss the five delegation rights.
7. What is conflict resolution? How can conflict be prevented?

CRITICAL THINKING ACTIVITIES

1. For a week, keep a log of your critical communications. Note who was involved in the communication; the context or situation in which it occurred; the time of day and day of the week; what the message was; effectiveness of the communication; and what could have been done to improve it. Compare four communication examples from your log.
2. Describe a group experience that you have had. Consider the structure, process, and communication of the group. For example, you might use a committee that you have been on, a group that you were in for a course project, a community service group, and so on. Consider how your experience relates to content in this chapter. Be sure and include your role(s) in the group.
3. If you were to make a list of what you would like to improve in your communication, what would you put on that list, and why is it important to you?
4. Why do you think delegation might be easy or difficult for you as an individual?
5. Have you been a member of a group or in a work situation in which there was conflict? Describe the situation, what occurred, your role in the situation, and the resolution. How did you feel about the experience? Could something have been done to prevent the conflict? Were you satisfied with the resolution? If not, what could have improved it?
6. If you can observe a team, use the following to guide your assessment of the team (not all the questions may apply) (District of Columbia Area Health Education Center [AHEC], 2008):
   • What is the team's mission? How is it interdisciplinary? How does it relate to its larger organization?
   • Who is the team's leader at any given time? Is leadership the same or does it change? How is leadership determined? How is it shared?

(continues)

CRITICAL THINKING ACTIVITIES (continued)

- What are the roles and qualifications of team members? How does each profession contribute to the team's task?
- What is the climate for the team's functioning? Is it constructive and open?
- How are specific objectives generated and agreed upon for each task?
- What are the team's communication patterns?
- How does the team make decisions?
- How does the team review and evaluate its progress and decisions?

7. Visit the AHEC Web site (http://dcahec.gwumc.edu/education/session3/index.html) and review the information on interdisciplinary healthcare teams. What can you learn about the models suggested and the various team members?

CASE STUDY

A 96-year-old man in very good health experiences a syncopal episode after standing unsupported for 20 minutes. His pulse was 46 and color ashen with circumoral cyanosis. Paramedics were called, and he was taken to the nearest emergency department. After extensive tests and 3 weeks of home monitoring, it was determined that he needed a pacemaker. Following the pacemaker insertion, it was determined that his cholesterol was elevated, and he was started on medication. He stated that he had been put on statins once before by his primary care physician and not able to tolerate them. So this time, the medication was to be closely monitored. One month following his pacemaker insertion and the start of this medication, he saw his primary care physician. The physician went over his labs, which were drawn prior to the visit. When the patient asked about his cholesterol, he was told that no lipid levels had been drawn. When the patient further asked about the report on his pacemaker surgery, the physician replied that he had no report. This case presents a lack of care coordination, a lack of effective communication among team members, and potential for error, resulting in patient safety and quality-of-care issues.

Case Questions

1. What could have been done to prevent the confusion that this patient experienced?
2. Where and when might errors have occurred?
3. How does this case reflect the need for interdisciplinary teamwork?
4. Have you or a family member experienced similar situations when receiving health care? What happened? Now that you know more about teamwork, safety, and quality, what is your perspective of the experience?

WORDS OF WISDOM

Gayla D. Freeman, RN, MS, Acting Associate Chief Nurse Specialty Services, Department of Veterans Affairs Medical Center, Oklahoma City, Oklahoma

I am the operating room nurse manager for the past 5 years, I was the nurse manager for the surgical intensive care unit from 1988 to 1999, and nurse manager of the surgical clinics from 1999 to 2003.

Teamwork is the one of the most important tasks of our time. Teamwork is like the invasive Kudzu vine that covers everything in its path and is found growing everywhere in the southern part of the United States. Teamwork allows the healthcare team to bond together in a manner that promotes timely completion of patient care and support of each other's life struggles. Without teamwork, we are ineffective in our efforts; we struggle to pull all of the factors together; and we are obligated to duplicate the efforts of others. Without teamwork, healthcare is like a single stalk growing in the desert without anyone to nurture us. With teamwork we are the Kudzu vine, grasping, connecting, and supporting one another. I learned a long time ago that I was nothing without my staff, my patients, my doctors, and ancillary staff. In fact, I couldn't exist without all of the team members.

References

American Nurses Association. (1997). *Position statement: Registered nurse utilization of unlicensed assistive personnel.* Washington, DC: Author.

American Nurses Association. (2003). *Nursing's social policy statement* (2nd ed.). Silver Spring, MD: Author.

American Nurses Association. (2004). *Scope and standards of practice.* Silver Spring, MD: Author.

American Nurses Association & National Council of State Boards of Nursing. (2006). *Joint statement on delegation.* Retrieved October 7, 2008, from https://www.ncsbn.org/Joint_statement.pdf

Arcangelo, V., Fitzgerald, M., Carroll, D., & Plumb, J. (1996). Collaborative care between nurse practitioners and primary care physicians. *Primary Care, 23*(1), 103–113.

Baggs, J. G., Schmitt, M. H., Mushlin, A. I., Mitchell, P. H., Eldredge, D., Oakes, D., et al. (1999). Association between nurse-physician collaboration and patient outcomes in three intensive care units. *Critical Care Medicine, 27*, 1991–1998.

Barnsteiner, J., Disch, J., Hall, L., Mayer, D., & Moore, S. (2007). Promoting interprofessional education. *Nursing Outlook, 55*, 144–150.

Burke, M., Boal, J., & Mitchell, R. (2004). Communicating for better care: Improving nurse-physician communication. *American Journal of Nursing, 104*(12), 40–47.

Cronewett, L., Sherwood, G., Barnsteiner, J., & Disch, J., Johnson, J, Mitchell, P., et al. (2007). Quality and safety education for nurses. *Nursing Outlook, 55*, 122–131.

Dessler, G. (2002). *Management: Leading people and organizations in the 21st century.* Upper Saddle River, NJ: Prentice Hall.

District of Columbia Area Health Education Center. (2008). *Interdisciplinary healthcare teams.* Retrieved February 11, 2008, from http://dcahec.gwumc.edu/index.htm

Fabre, J. (2005). *Smart nursing.* New York: Springer.

Fairchild, D., Hogan, J., Smith, R., Portnow, M., & Bates, D. W. (2002). Survey of primary care physicians and home care clinicians. *Journal of General Internal Medicine, 17*, 243–261.

Finkelman, A., & Kenner, C. (2007). *Teaching IOM: Implications of the Institute of Medicine reports for nursing education.* Silver Spring, MD: American Nurses Association Publishing.

Fried, B., Topping, S., & Rundall, T. (2000). Groups and teams in health services organizations. In S. Shortell & A. Kaluzny (Eds.), *Healthcare management: Organization and design behavior* (4th ed., pp. 233–250). Albany, NY: Delmar.

Hagenow, N. (2003). Why not person-centered care? The challenges of implementation. *Nursing Administration Quarterly, 27*(3), 203–207.

Heller, R. (1999). *Learning to lead.* New York: DK Publishing.

Herzberg, F., Mausner, B., & Snyderman, B. (1959). *The motivation to work.* New York: Wiley.

Higgins, L. (1999). Nurses' perceptions of collaborative nurse-physician transfer decision making as a predictor or patient outcomes in a medical intensive care unit. *Journal of Advanced Nursing, 29*, 1434–1443.

Institute of Medicine. (2001). *Crossing the quality chasm.* Washington, DC: National Academies Press.

Institute of Medicine. (2003a). *Health professions education: A bridge to quality.* Washington, DC: National Academies Press.

Institute of Medicine (2003b). *Priority areas for national action: Transforming healthcare quality*. Washington, DC: National Academies Press.

Lower, J. (2007, September). Creating a culture of civility in the workplace. *American Nurse Today*, pp. 49–51.

McCallin, A. (2001). Interdisciplinary practice—a matter of teamwork: An integrated review. *Journal of Clinical Nursing, 10*, 419–428.

McConnell, E. (2001, April). *About communicating clearly*. Retrieved June 21, 2002, from http://www.findarticles.com/cf_0/m3231/4_31/74091631/pring.jhtml

Michalopoulos, A., & Michalopoulos, H. (2006). Management's possible benefits from teamwork and the nursing process. *Nurse Leader, 4*(3), 52–55.

Milgram, L., Spector, A., & Treger, M. (1999). *Managing smart*. Houston, TX: Gulf Publishing.

National Council of State Boards of Nursing. (1995). *Delegation: Understanding the concepts and decision-making process*. Retrieved October 1, 2008, from https://www.ncsbn.org/323.htm

National Council of State Boards of Nursing. (1997). *Role development: Critical components of delegation curriculum outline*. Retrieved October 1, 2008, from https://www.ncsbn.org/roledevelopment.pdf

National Council State Boards of Nursing. (1998). *The continuum of care: A regulatory perspective. A resource paper for regulatory agencies*. Chicago: Author.

Rosenstein, A. (2002). Original research: Nurse-physician relationships; Impact on nurse satisfaction and retention. *American Journal of Nursing, 102*(6), 26–34.

Rosenstein, A., & O'Daniel, M. (2005). Disruptive and clinical behavior outcomes. *American Journal of Nursing, 105*(1), 54–63.

Siegler, E. (1998). *Geriatric interdisciplinary team training*. New York: Springer.

Simpson, G., Rabin, D., Schmitt, M., Taylor, P., Urban, S., & Ball, J. (2001). Interprofessional healthcare practice: Recommendations of the National Academics of Practice expert panel on healthcare in the 21st century. *Issues in Interdisciplinary Care, 3*(1), 5–19.

Sullivan, T. (1998). Transformational leadership. In T. Sullivan (Ed.), *Collaboration: A healthcare imperative* (pp. 469–497). New York: McGraw-Hill.

Thomas, E., Sexton, J. B., & Helmreich, R. L.(2003). Discrepant attitudes about teamwork among critical care nurses and physicians. *Critical Care Medicine, 31*, 956–959.

Zimmerman, P. (2002). Delegating to unlicensed assistive personnel. *Nursing Spectrum Online*. Retrieved November 5, 2002, from http://nsweb.nursingspectrum.com/ce/ce124.htm

Chapter 11

Employ Evidence-Based Practice

CHAPTER OBJECTIVES

At the conclusion of this chapter, the learner will be able to:

- Discuss the core competency: Employ evidence-based practice (EBP).
- Define research.
- Describe the research steps.
- Discuss the relevance of nursing research.
- Define EBP.
- Explain examples of EBP models.
- Describe the EBP process.
- Identify two key EBP tools.
- Discuss the barriers to implementing EBP in nursing practice.
- Compare and contrast EBP with research and quality improvement.

CHAPTER OUTLINE

KEY TERMS

- ❏ Applied research
- ❏ Basic research
- ❏ Evidence-based practice
- ❏ Experimental design
- ❏ Hypothesis
- ❏ Integrative review
- ❏ Nonexperimental design
- ❏ Meta-analysis
- ❏ Metasynthesis
- ❏ Outcomes research
- ❏ Patient, Intervention, Comparison, Outcome (PICO)
- ❏ Procedures
- ❏ Quality improvement (QI)

- ❏ Quasi-experimental design
- ❏ Qualitative study
- ❏ Quantitative study
- ❏ Randomized controlled trial (RCT)
- ❏ Research
- ❏ Research analysis
- ❏ Research design
- ❏ Research problem statement
- ❏ Research proposal
- ❏ Research purpose
- ❏ Research question
- ❏ Research utilization (RU)
- ❏ Systematic review

Introduction

This chapter focuses on the third Institute of Medicine (IOM) core competency that emphasizes the need to use **evidence-based practice (EBP)** by all healthcare professionals, including nurses. The content explores this core competency. Because research is an important component in understanding and using EBP, an introduction to nursing research is discussed. EBP and its impact on nursing care and the nursing profession are described.

The IOM Competency: Employ Evidence-Based Practice

The third healthcare profession core competency is to employ EBP. The IOM (2003a) definition of EBP is to "integrate best research with clinical expertise and patient values for optimum care, and participate in learning and research activities to the extent feasible" (p. 4). EBP as a core competency is connected to providing patient-centered care and to interdisciplinary teams. Teams need to use EBP to provide the most effective patient-centered care. Why is there emphasis on EBP today in health care? "The lag between the discovery of more effective forms of treatment and their incorporation into routine patient care is, on average, 17 years" (Balas, 2001, as cited in Institute of Medicine, 2003a, p. 33). Clearly, there is a great need to get research results to the patient sooner. Increasing use of evidence can improve the quality of care and avoid underuse, misuse, and overuse of care (Chassin, 1998). What does this really mean in practice? To the nurse, it means the ability to get to the evidence, know what the evidence is, and apply the evidence as appropriate at the point of care. Using evidence might impact interventions such as prevention, diagnostic tests, or therapy; affect the ability to compare alternatives; and, in some cases, lead to the decision that no intervention is the best choice. Figure 11–1 illustrates the key elements related to this core competency.

Nursing Research

The first step to understanding EBP is to describe **research**. Research is a systematic investigation that includes research development, testing, and evaluation. It is designed to develop or contribute to generalizable knowledge. Knowledge about research and the research process is important to EBP. One of the major sources of best evidence for practice comes from research results. As discussed at the beginning of this book, nursing is a science discipline in that much of the knowledge base for nursing practice includes theoretical and evidence-based knowledge (American Nurses Association [ANA], 2003).

There are two major types of research approaches: basic and applied. **Basic research** is

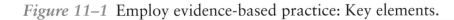

Figure 11–1 Employ evidence-based practice: Key elements.

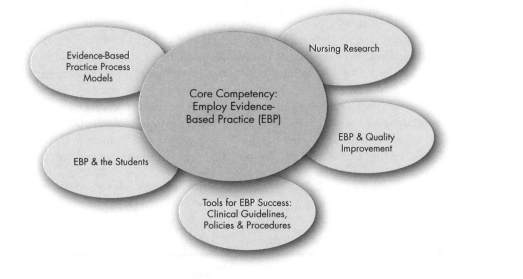

designed to broaden the base of knowledge rather than solve an immediate problem. Results from basic research may be used to develop applied research. **Applied research** is designed to find a solution to a practical problem. Nurses typically are involved in more applied research, though some do basic research. Outcomes research is a newer approach. This type of research focuses on determining the effectiveness of healthcare services and patient outcomes. Research is closely related to theory and practice.

Historical Background

How has the nursing profession developed nursing research (ANA, 2004)? Florence Nightingale was interested in clinical nursing research, which she emphasized in the data that she used to measure patient outcomes and improve care; however, the nursing community really did not pay much attention to research until the early 1990s. Nurses began to earn advanced degrees, which resulted in some studies about nurses and nursing education, but research was not an important part of nursing. Studies that focused more on nursing care were carried out in the 1920s and 1930s; some of these studies were published in the *American Journal of Nursing*, making them the first studies to be published in a nursing journal. It took time for more studies to be done; in the 1950s, there was greater interest in nursing research, and the journal *Nursing Research* was first published. In the 1970s and 1980s, more nurses conducted studies and more nurses obtained graduate degrees (including doctoral degrees), so nursing researchers were more qualified. Nursing theorists were very active in the 1960s and 1970s, adding to the scholarly work.

The American Association of Colleges of Nursing (AACN) position statement on nursing research states, "Nursing research worldwide is committed to rigorous scientific inquiry that provides a significant body of knowledge to advance nursing practice, shape health policy, and impact the health of people in all countries. The vision for nursing research is driven by the profession's mandate to society to optimize the health and well-being of populations" (International Council of Nurses, 1999; as cited in American Association of Colleges of Nursing, 2006, p. 1). The statement continues, "Nursing researchers bring a holistic perspective to studying individuals, families, and communities; their research takes a biobehavioral, interdisciplinary, and translational approach to science. The priorities for nursing research reflect nursing's commitment to the promotion of health and healthy lifestyles, the advancement of quality and excellence in health care, and the critical importance of basing professional nursing practice on research" (American Association of Colleges of Nursing, 2006, p. 1). The position statement identifies major research focus areas. Clinical research includes interventions that might be used, from acute to chronic care experiences across the entire life span; health promotion and preventive care to end-of-life care; and care for individuals, families, and communities in diverse settings. The second area is health systems and **outcomes research**, which focuses on identifying ways that the organization and delivery of health care influence quality, cost, and the experience of patients and their families. The third focus is on nursing education: research that explores more effective and efficient educational processes and new ways to incorporate technology in the learning process; intergenerational learning differences and their impact on education; and the development of methods to improve lifelong learning and commitment to leadership.

THE NATIONAL INSTITUTE OF NURSING RESEARCH

The National Institute of Nursing Research (NINR), established in 1985, is part of the

National Institutes of Health (NIH). It is important that nursing have a presence in the most prestigious national research system in the United States. The NINR conducts research that has an impact within the discipline of nursing, but interdisciplinary research is encouraged and funded as well.

The NINR is physically located at the NIH in Rockville, Maryland. When funded research is conducted at the NINR campus, it is referred to as an intramural or internal study. Grants are also awarded for outside, or extramural, studies that are conducted at the researcher's home institution. Areas of NINR research current priorities are:

- Promoting health and preventing disease.
- Improving quality of life; this includes self-management, one of the IOM priority areas of care, symptom management, and caregiving.

- Eliminating health disparities.
- Setting directions for end-of-life research.

The Research Process

The research process is similar to the nursing process. It is a problem-solving method. Exhibit 11–1 describes the steps of the process.

First, the researcher develops a plan or proposal. This written document describes recent relevant literature on the problem area, describes the research topic or problem, and defines the processes or steps that will be followed to answer the **research question** or questions. The proposal is used to plan the research and also may be used to apply for research funding. The proposal is written in the future tense because the research has not yet been done.

There must be an assessment to identify and describe the problem, formulating the **research problem statement**. The researcher does this

---

EXHIBIT 11–1 STEPS IN THE QUANTITATIVE RESEARCH PROCESS

I. Describe Problem Statement, Including Background and Significance

II. Identify Research Question(s) and Hypothesis

III. Identify the Purpose(s) of the Study
Explain what use will be made of findings.

IV. Review of Literature
Provide a summary of critical literature (theoretical and research literature) that applies to the study.

V. Theoretical Framework
Use theories and conceptual models to organize research findings into a broader conceptual context. Include conceptual and operational definitions of the variables (independent and dependent) in the framework. Identify assumptions.

VI. Ethical Considerations

VII. Research Design and Methods
A. Research Design
   1. Name the research design. Is the study a quantitative study or qualitative? What specific design (such as experimental, quasi-experiemental, descriptive, etc.) is being used?

continues

Exhibit 11–1 (continued)

2. Provide an adequate rationale for choosing the research design.
3. Identify independent and dependent variables (if experimental).

Or

1. Explain why variables were not designated as independent or dependent (if not an experimental study).

B. **Sample and Sample Selection**
   1. Name the sample population.
   2. Provide sample criteria (inclusion and exclusion criteria).
   3. Describe sample size using power analysis.
   4. Describe how those subjects who met the criteria were selected as study subjects (how were eligible subjects located?)
   5. If applicable, describe how groups or treatments were assigned.
   6. Name and justify the sampling method.

C. **Setting**
   Briefly describe the setting for the study.

D. **Measurement and Instrumentation**
   1. Discuss origin and type of measurement instruments.
   2. Describe why the instrument or instruments are clearly appropriate to study the problem (i.e., why the instrument can produce data that can answer the study question).
   3. Ensure that the instrument is compatible with the conceptual/theoretical framework.
   4. If an instrument was developed, describe how it was developed, how it was tested for reliability/validity, and its pilot use.
   5. Describe the reliability and validity of the instrument. Evaluate and report relevant reliability and validity data from previous research.

E. **Data Collection**
   1. Describe how access to facilities was obtained.
   2. Describe the data collection process and procedures chronologically and clearly enough to allow for replication (describe so that a stranger could use this procedure and collect the data as intended).
   3. Note who collected the data and the training required. Provide data collection forms as required.
   4. Discuss control features of study procedures.

F. **Data Analysis**
   1. Answer each hypothesis or study question according to a specific plan for each.
   2. Identify appropriate statistical tests and the rationale for their use in analyzing each study question or hypothesis and participant demographic data. Include level of measurement of each variable, and selected level of significance.
   3. Specify and justify level of significance (.05, .01) for statistical results and findings.

G. **Limitations**
   Ensure that limitations are clearly identified and appropriate.

VIII. **Results and Conclusions**

assessment using his or her individual expertise and by reviewing the literature. The review of literature is included in the research proposal and in the subsequent research report of results. The researcher (or researchers) primarily examines previous studies by reading their published reports of results.

The researcher then identifies the study question(s) and hypothesis(ses). The research question is concise; it is stated before the research is conducted, and it should be in the research proposal. Questions may focus on

1. Describing a variable or variables. (A variable is an attribute or characteristic that varies, such as anxiety level, pain, blood pressure, a lab value, and so on.)
2. Determining the differences between two or more variables.
3. Examining relationships among variables; how do they relate to each other?
4. Using an independent variable to predict a dependent variable. (An independent variable is the variable that the researcher thinks causes or influences the dependent variable. The independent variable is the intervention that the researcher manipulates if the study is experimental. The dependent variable is the variable that the researcher thinks depends on, or is caused by, the independent variable; for example, turning a patient every hour [independent variable] decreases skin damage [dependent variable]).

The **hypothesis** is the formal statement of the expected relationship or relationships between two or more variables in a specified population, which is the sample. The hypothesis is stated before the research is conducted, and it is included in the proposal. Some studies typically do not have hypotheses, such as qualitative studies in which the emphasis is on describing a situation or perception rather than on measuring the variable of interest. The question and hypothesis flow from the description of the research problem statement. The researcher also needs to consider the **research purpose**—what potential uses the results would have.

In nursing research, the researcher typically identifies a theory or a conceptual model to organize the findings, although this is not done for all studies. The theory or model is described and related to the research question. For example, if a study was developed to investigate patient education about diabetes, Orem's theory on self-care might be used as the framework for the study. Not all nursing research that uses a conceptual framework relies on nursing theory. It is important that the framework represent the phenomenon of interest and guide the question and how the variable is to be measured. For example, if the nurse is studying blood pressure in a premature infant, the study would most likely use a scientific, physiologically based framework to support factors that influence blood pressure.

This all sets the stage for the actual research; the assessment and problem identification should be clear. Comparing this to the nursing process, these steps are the assessment and nursing diagnosis phases. The specific plan for conducting the study is the research design and methods. In the proposal, the researcher would describe what *will* be done, and in the research report or published article, poster, or presentation after the study, the researcher describes what *was* done.

The **research design** is complex. It includes the details related to type of study (research approach and design); the sample and how the sample is selected; the setting for the study; measurement and instrumentation to collect data; data collection (what exactly will be done to collect the data?) and data analysis (how will the data be analyzed?); and a description of potential limitations. The plan should be clear and detailed. The **research proposal** can be compared to the nursing care plan and another step in the nursing process. This information, or the plan, is called a proposal until the research is conducted. The study is conducted after funding is received. At this point, this step could be compared to implementing a care plan.

The last part of the research process is the **research analysis** and description of the results and conclusions. The proposal describes how the data will be analyzed, but the actual analysis of data cannot occur until the study has been conducted and data collected. What did the analysis of data demonstrate, and what are the implications of the data? The researcher has to consider the proposal—what was planned, how the study was implemented, and how the data were to be analyzed—so that the outcomes are identified, just as in the nursing process. This can be compared to the evaluation that determines if patient outcomes were met based on the nursing process or care plan.

Types of Research Design

The research design describes the plan for the study in detail. It can be compared to a nursing care plan because the design describes information about the study and how to conduct the study, as well as planned assessment or analysis of the results. Research study designs are categorized as either quantitative or qualitative. In **quantitative studies**, the research question focuses on "how many" or "how much", and in **qualitative studies**, the research question focuses on "feel" or "experience." Not all quantitative research is experimental, but to be experimental, a study must meet three criteria:

1. *Manipulation*: The researcher administers an intervention to the participants (sample). This intervention represents the independent variable or variables. The researcher wants to see the effect of the independent variable on the dependent variable or if the independent variable causes the dependent variable.

2. *Control*: The researcher controls some of the experimental situation and uses a control group. Total control is not usually possible, but efforts must be made to have as much control of the situation as possible. This is more difficult in applied or clinical research as compared with a laboratory setting.

3. *Randomization*: The researcher assigns participants in the sample to the experimental or control groups using systematic methods. The control group does not experience the intervention identified as the independent variable.

Data collection in a quantitative study is highly structured. Examples of data collection methods are structured interviews; collection of physical data, such as blood pressure, blood and urine, and other physiological parameters; questionnaires; rating scales; structured observation; and many other methods. Analysis of data involves the use of statistics.

Data collection in qualitative studies is less structured than in a quantitative study. A qualitative study might use focus groups, diaries, logs, observation, and open-ended interviews; analysis of data does not rely on statistics or mathematical equations. The researcher is less detached and may interact actively with the participants to obtain the best data possible. In fact, the researcher is often considered the instrument of the qualitative research. Data are analyzed as the study progresses and may lead the researcher in a different direction or to collect additional data. However, data that are not covered in the informed consent cannot be collected without an Institutional Review Board (IRB) approval for the change. The goal is to understand the issue deeply, not to intervene, and to see results or compare groups.

There are two other major classifications of quantitative studies other than experimental. In a study that uses **quasi-experimental design**, there is some manipulation of the independent variable, but there is no randomization or control, which is why it is not a true **experimental design**. The **nonexperimental design** uses no manipulation of the independent variable.

There are also research design subtypes for qualitative studies. Some examples are:

- *Phenomenology*: Focuses on the meaning of people's experiences of some phenomenon—looks at the person's perceptions. An example is understanding the caregiver's role with a family member who has terminal cancer.
- *Ethnography*: Focuses on trying to understand the participants' (sample) world view—cultural behavior is important; often includes long periods of observation.
- *Case Study*: Uses an in-depth case; may focus on an individual or group; examines the case to understand issues.

Research Funding

Funding is a critical part of any research because it provides the resources to conduct the research. Funding sources are varied: universities, private donations, foundations and organizations, local and state governments, and the federal government. The federal government is the largest source of grant monies. There are three approaches that a researcher can take.

1. Identify a problem and develop a proposal. This proposal is sent to funding sources that would have an interest in the particular problem.
2. Develop a research proposal that specifically addresses a problem area that a funding source has identified as a critical need area. This is called a request for proposals or request for applications.
3. Sometimes funding sources require that the researcher conduct a pilot study or have data that indicate greater need for research about a particular problem.

Once the required written proposal is completed and submitted, there are very specific requirements for proposals. These requirements can vary from one funding source to another, and deadlines differ. The proposal then goes through the grant review process, which can take months. Typically, grants are reviewed by peer groups identified by the funding source. It is extremely difficult to get funding. The federal government grants are highly competitive, and the major source is the NIH. The NIH budget is designated by the Congress. Nursing research is funded by similar sources, as is other healthcare research. There are also funds for training programs—for example, to develop a new graduate program for nurse practitioners or for doctorate of nursing practice; to develop a nurse residency program; and to develop programs to increase student retention. Funding for these types of projects typically comes from Health Resources and Services Administration, which is part of the U.S. Department of Health and Human Services.

Ethics and Legal Issues

When ethics and legal issues are considered in relation to research, the first concern is to protect the rights of human subjects (participants). A second area that the researcher considers is how best to balance benefits and risks in the studies. There are many studies in which participants may be harmed. Research ethics emphasizes the need to be clear about risks whenever possible. The third ethical and legal issue is informed consent, which is also important in healthcare service delivery. The last concern is review of the proposal to ensure that participant rights are protected and that the study is planned in an effective manner that meets standards. This is called institutional review.

Several major historical research projects have been influential in increasing attention to the ethical conduct of research, particularly studies that involve human subjects. The most familiar is the Nazi medical experiments conducted during World War II. These "research" studies violated many aspects of basic human rights and provided little gain in scientific knowledge. In 1947, 27 Nazi physicians were tried at Nuremberg, Germany, for research atrocities that they performed. The U.S. Holocaust Memorial Museum maintains a Web site where the official trial record can be accessed. The transcripts of testimony by persons who were forced to serve as subjects in these experiments reveal incredible violations of human rights. An important outcome of this experience and the trial was the publication of the first internationally recognized code of research ethics, *The Nuremberg Code*, which has served as a prototype for the development of many later codes of research ethics. The core of any of the research code comprises the following rights that must be protected.

- Right to self-determination
- Right to privacy
- Right to anonymity and confidentiality
- Right to fair treatment
- Right to protection from discomfort and harm

Other important examples of human rights violations have occurred in the United States. The two best known are the Tuskegee syphilis study (1932–1972) and the Willowbrook study (mid-1950s–1970s). The Tuskegee study used African Americans in the sample to examine the natural course of syphilis. Many of the participants did not receive informed consent, and some did not even know that they were participants in a study. Even though it was clear within a few years that participants with syphilis had severe complications and high death rates, nothing was done to institute treatment. The Willowbrook study looked at hepatitis at an institution for the mentally retarded. The children were deliberately infected with hepatitis. It is clear that all three of these examples abused vulnerable subjects and that there were few, if any, controls. Today, because of standards and ethics, there is greater control to prevent these types of experiences from happening again. An example is the extensive informed consent process and documentation. Table 11–1 highlights guidelines for protecting human subjects.

After these experiences of abuse in research, efforts were instituted to prevent further problems. One of the strategies was the creation of the IRB. This is a committee that reviews research before it is conducted to ensure that the study is conducted ethically. Researchers conducting any study that involves human subjects have to obtain approval from their institution's IRB. IRBs are mandated to review all research that involves human subjects in institutions that receive federal funds. The purpose is to protect subjects from unnecessary risk or from risks that outweigh potential benefits. Particularly vulnerable populations are:

- Neonates (newborns)
- Children
- Pregnant women and fetuses
- Persons with mental illness
- Persons with cognitive impairment
- Terminally ill persons
- Persons confined to institutions (e.g., prisons, long-term care hospitals)

Examples of questions that might be considered by an IRB include:

Table 11–1 ANA GUIDELINES FOR PROTECTING THE RIGHTS
OF HUMAN SUBJECTS

Rights/Guidelines	Obligations
Right to Self-Determination	• Employers must inform nurses in writing if participating as a subject in research is a condition of employment • Risks must be clarified to potential subjects
Right to Freedom from Risk or Harm	• Nurses must ensure freedom from harm • Researchers must monitor vulnerable or captive subjects to reduce potential risk of injury
Scope of Application	• All nurses must ensure that all human subjects enjoy protection of their rights
Responsibilities to Support Knowledge Development	• All nurses must support the development of scientific knowledge
Informed Consent	• Nurses must ensure that informed consent from potential subjects (or legal guardians) protects right to self-determination
Participation on IRB	• Nurses should support inclusion of nurses on IRB • Nurses have an obligation to serve on IRB

Source: From *Evidence-Based Practice for Nurses: Appraisal and Applications of Research*, by N.A. Schmidt and J.M. Brown, 2009, Sudbury, MA: Jones and Bartlett Publishers. Data adapted from *Guidelines for nurse in clinical and other research*, by American Nurses Association, 1985, Kansas City, MO: Author.

1. Is the subject being deceived, and if so, is it necessary to the integrity of the research?
2. Does the subject understand the purpose of the project and completely understand his or her role in the project?
3. Are there obvious costs or hidden costs to people if they participate? Can they withdraw at any time?
4. What are the benefits, if any, to the subject?
5. What are the risks, immediate and long term (if known), to the subject?
6. How will the researcher protect the subject's right to confidentiality?
7. Whom should the subjects contact with questions?
8. What will be done with the results of the study?

Barriers and Facilitators to Research

Research is not easy to accomplish. Barriers need to be turned into facilitators for research to be successful.

1. *Lack of funding*: Researchers need to obtain adequate funding.
2. *Lack of sufficient time*: Good research takes planning and time to accomplish. The researcher needs blocks of time to work on a study. Some do research full time.
3. *Lack of research competencies*: Research expertise is developed over a period of years.

Finding a mentor or mentors is important; working with researchers who have been successful can assist a novice researcher.

4. *Lack of participants for the sample*: If the study requires participants, it is not always easy to find them in the number required. This takes time and creativity, and ethical principles must be considered.

5. *Inability to find the right setting*: Finding and securing a setting that agrees to participate in the study can be problematic because it requires contacts and communication.

6. *Lack of statistics expertise*: Find an expert to consult; researchers work in teams.

Evidence-Based Practice

What is the purpose of EBP? The use of EBP in nursing leads to more effective decision making to guide the use of limited resources, control costs, and improve quality (Jennings & Loan, 2001). An EBP review is not nursing research; an EBP review involves looking for evidence: (1) evidence of research results, (2) evidence from a patient's assessment and other sources, (3) evidence from clinical expertise, and (4) evidence

from information about patient preferences and values.

Now, how do you get from EBP to research? You may not. At the conclusion of an EBP review, one could find that there is sufficient evidence to support the clinical question. If this is the case, is more research needed? No. So an EBP review does not mean that research is conducted or that it must be conducted. But if an EBP review indicates that evidence is already available, there is no need for additional research. In most cases in nursing, however, there is insufficient nursing research to support most nursing questions. This means that research may be needed to fill the gap in the knowledge base. Exhibit 11–2 shows a five-step approach for EBP.

Definitions

Evidence-based practice is the conscientious use of current best evidence in making decisions about patient care. It is a problem-solving approach to clinical practice that integrates: a systematic search for and critical appraisal of the most relevant evidence to answer a burning clinical question; one's own clinical expertise; and patient preferences and values. (Sackett,

---

Exhibit 11–2 Five-Step Approach for Evidence-Based Nursing Practice

Ask	Identify the research question. Determine if the question is well constructed to elicit a response or solution.
Acquire	Search the literature for preappraised evidence or research. Secure the best evidence that is available.
Appraise	Conduct a critical appraisal of the literature and studies. Evaluate for validity and determine the applicability in practice.
Apply	Institute recommendations and findings and apply them to nursing practice.
Assess	Evaluate the application of the findings, outcomes, and relevance to nursing practice.

Source: From *Evidence-Based Practice for Nurses: Appraisal and Applications of Research*, by N.A. Schmidt and J.M. Brown, 2009, Sudbury, MA: Jones and Bartlett Publishers. Adapted from *Introduction to teaching evidence-based health care*, by S. Straus, 2005, University of Toronto Knowledge Translation Program (Powerpoint Presentation). Retrieved October 10, 2008, from http://www.cebm.net/?o=1021

Straus, Richardson, Rosenberg, & Haynes, 2000 as cited in Melnyk & Fineout-Overholt, 2005, p. 6)

This definition does not mean that all patient care decisions are based on research evidence or only research evidence. There are multiple sources of knowledge:

- *Best research evidence:* This evidence is ranked and described in another section of this chapter.
- *Clinical expertise*: The knowledge and experience of the clinician (nurse, physician, and others on the healthcare team).
- *Patient values and preferences/circumstances*: These are the individual patient's own concerns, preferences, expectations, and social and financial resources that impact health and health care. All these factors can change over time and with each unique healthcare need and encounter.
- *Clinical data (assessment) and history*: A patient's assessment includes important evidence that should be considered in treatment decisions.

As nursing students soon discover when they search for nursing EBP literature, there is a problem. Nursing and allied health are not as far along in EBP as medicine is. Why is this so? First, the amount of nursing research must increase—not just in quantity but also in quality and in relevance to nursing practice. Second, nursing health interventions are not captured effectively in medical records, and this impacts whether nursing data are included in research studies (IOM, 2003a). Examples of data are patient pain, dehydration, skin breakdown, lifestyle change, patient knowledge deficiencies, and noncompliance with treatment. A third issue is that nursing interventions often are evaluated in descriptive or qualitative studies rather than quantitative studies. Quantitative studies are ranked higher than qualitative studies when evaluating or ranking evidence from research studies. How is this different from **research utilization (RU)** (Levin, 2006)?

- EBP and RU are not the same but can easily be confused. RU includes only research results as a source of evidence. How does RU compare with EBP?
- EBP critically summarizes multiple relevant studies and uses a designated hierarchy to rate the studies as to their quality. RU also critically appraises research, but usually only one or two studies, and it does not attempt to evaluate the state of current research about a certain topic or focus on a clinical question (PICO, or Patient, Intervention, Comparison, Outcome) as does EBP. RU does not use a hierarchy rating scale to evaluate the studies.
- EBP includes clinical expertise, patient preferences and values, and patient assessment and history as part of the evidence for best practice. RU is concerned only with research and does not include these other elements.

The **PICO** question should be part of every search for evidence to improve practice. What is the PICO? The goal is to ask a searchable and answerable question. The acronym stands for the following (Melnyk & Fineout-Overholt, 2005, p. 30):

1. The "P" (patient) needs to be specific—describing the population such as age, gender, diagnosis, ethnicity, other.
2. The "I" (intervention) can be related to prognostic factors, risk behaviors, exposure to disease, or clinical intervention or treatment.
3. The "C" (comparison) can be with another treatment or no treatment.

4. The "O" is the outcome; what will it be, such as risk of disease, complication, or side effect, or adverse outcome.

There are five steps in the PICO process (Melnyk & Fineout-Overholt, 2005, p. 9):

1. Identify a burning clinical issue or question.
2. Collect the best evidence relevant to the question.
3. Critically appraise that evidence before it is used.
4. Integrate the evidence with the other parts of EBP: patient preferences and values, your clinical expertise, assessment information about the patient and patient's history.
5. Evaluate the practice decision or change.

Exhibit 11–3 describes the templates that can be used to develop PICO questions.

EBP Models

A number of models are used to describe EBP in nursing. Why is a model important? A model provides a description of a process and includes the impact of EBP on practice. Two of the major examples are:

- *The Iowa Model of Evidence Based Practice to Promote Quality of Care*: This model was created by the University of Iowa Medical Center nursing administration as a method to support EBP to improve quality of care (Titler et al., 2001; Vratny & Shriver, 2007). The critical elements of this model are examining clinical excellence and improving quality of care by addressing barriers to its implementation. The model includes these questions: (1) What are the "triggers" for EBP? (2) What will make an organization include patient-focused care? (3) How does the workforce get educated on EBP to implement it? Critical thinking, staff empowerment, and professional development are key components, along with the use of EBP ambassadors for each unit (Vratny & Shriver, 2007).
- *ACE Star Model of the Cycle of Knowledge Transformation*: This model is also referred

---

Exhibit 11–3 Templates for PICO Questions

PICO Question Templates:

- **Therapy:** In _____ , what is the effect of _____ on _____ compared with _____ ?

- **Etiology:** Are _____ who have _____ at _____ risk for/of _____ compared with _____ with/without _____ ?

- **Diagnosis or Diagnostic Test:** Are (is) _____ more accurate in diagnosing _____ compared with _____ ?

- **Prevention:** For _____ does the use of _____ reduce the future risk of _____ compare with _____ ?

- **Prognosis:** Does _____ influence _____ in patients who have _____ ?

- **Meaning:** How do _____ diagnosed with _____ perceive _____ ?

Source: From *Evidence-based practice in nursing and healthcare* (p. 31), by B. Melnyk & E. Fineout-Overholt, 2005, Philadelphia: Lippincott Williams & Wilkins. Reprinted with permission.

to as the Star Model of Knowledge Transformation (Stevens, 2004). It uses the five points of a star to indicate the steps that are important to follow when examining whether the research findings exist and their relationship to practice. These steps are discovery, summary, translation, integration, and evaluation (Stevens, 2004). The underlying theme is that in order to complete the five steps, there must be education as well as a shift in knowledge (Stevens, 2004).

Figure 11–2 and Exhibit 11–4 describe these two models.

Types of EBP Literature

EBP literature is different from typical clinical literature and even research literature (i.e., published articles about studies). The key component of EBP literature is a **systematic review**. A systematic review is a "summary of evidence typically conducted by an expert or a panel of experts on a particular topic, that uses a rigorous process (to minimize bias) for identifying, appraising, and synthesizing studies to answer a specific clinical question and draw conclusions about the data gathered" (Melnyk & Fineout-Overholt, 2005, p. 594). Another definition of systematic review is that it is "the consolidation of research evidence that incorporates a critical assessment and evaluation of the research (not simply a summary) and addresses a focused clinical question using methods designed to reduce the likelihood of bias" (DiCenso, Guyatt, & Ciliska, 2005, p. 570). There are several types of systematic reviews, but all the types (1) have prescribed criteria for conducting the review process, (2) review not only research reports but also some data from large databases and may include published articles that are opinion or essay, and (3) try to find as much available evidence as possible (Brown, 2009). During the assessment process, when evidence is reviewed, a standard hierarchy or rating system is used (described in Figure 11–3).

Three types of systematic reviews are important in EBP literature.

1. *Integrative research review*: Panels or groups of experts conduct **integrative reviews** and begin by identifying the topic or question. The result is a "narrative summary of past research in which the reviewer(s) extract findings from original studies and use analytical reasoning to produce conclusions about the findings of a body of research" (Brown, 2009, p. 195).

2. *Meta-analysis*: This is a research technique in which entire studies on a particular topic or question (PICO) are appraised to determine the state of knowledge on that topic. **Meta-analysis** is the "process of using quantitative methods to summarize the results of multiple studies, obtained and critically reviewed using rigorous process to minimize bias for identifying, appraising, synthesizing studies to answer a specific question and draw conclusions about the data. The purpose is to gain a summary statistic (e.g., measure of a single effect) that represents the effect of the intervention across multiple studies" (Melnyk & Fineout-Overholt, 2005, p. 590). Another definition of meta-analysis is: "a statistical technique for quantitatively combining the results of multiple studies that measure the same outcome, into a single pooled or summary estimate" (DiCenso et al., 2005, p. 560).

   An example of a topic/question for a meta-analysis is, To what extent does *patient education on hypertension in adults impact patient outcomes?* The reviewer or

Figure 11–2 The Iowa Model of evidence-based practice to promote quality care.

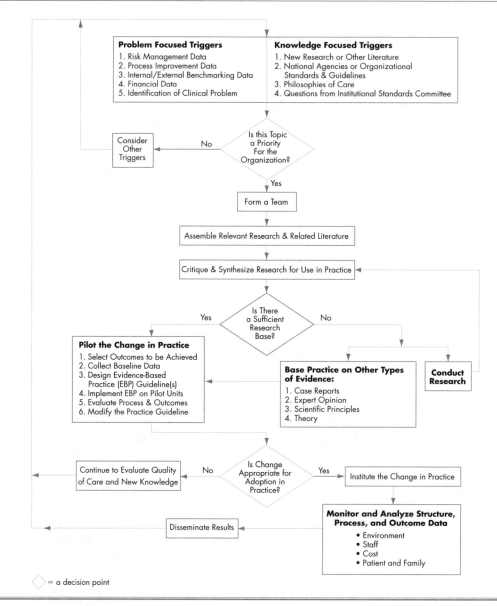

Source: From The Iowa Model of Evidence-Based Practice to Promote Quality Care, by M. G. Titler, C. Kleiber, V. Steelman, B. Rakel, G. Budreau, K. C. Buckwalter, et al., 2001, *Critical Care Nursing Clinics of North America, 13*(4), 497–509. Reproduced with permission.

EXHIBIT 11–4 ACE STAR MODEL OF THE CYCLE OF KNOWLEDGE TRANSFORMATION

ACE Star Model of Knowledge Transformation©
Academic Center for Evidence-Based Practice
The University of Texas Health Science Center at San Antonio

BACKGROUND

The health care we provide does not reflect current knowledge due to a number of hurdles. In order to achieve science-based care, two principal hurdles must be addressed: the complexity of knowledge, including volume, and the form of available knowledge.

HURDLES AND SOLUTIONS

HURDLE: COMPLEXITY OF LITERATURE

One obstacle in moving research rapidly into patient care is the growing complexity of science and technology. "No unaided human being can read, recall, and act effectively on the volume of clinically relevant scientific literature"
(IOM, 2001, 25).

EBP SOLUTION

Evidence summaries, including systematic reviews and other forms, reduce the *complexity and volume* of evidence by integrating all research on a given topic into a single, meaningful whole.

HURDLE: FORM OF KNOWLEDGE

Not only is the volume of literature a hurdle, but the *form* of the knowledge is a hurdle as well. Literature contains a variety of knowledge forms, many of which are NOT suitable for direct practice application.

EBP SOLUTION

From the point of discovery, knowledge can be transformed through a series of stages to increase meaning to the clinician and utility in clinical decision making.

The stages of converting knowledge are explained by the ACE Star Model of Knowledge Transformation.

The Star Model of Knowledge Transformation© is a model for understanding the cycles, nature, and characteristics of *knowledge* that are utilized in various aspects of evidence-based practice (EBP). The Star Model organizes both old and new concepts of improving care into a whole and provides a framework with which to organize EBP processes and approaches. Known as the **ACE Star Model**, it is a simple, parsimonious depiction of the relationships between various stages of knowledge transformation, as newly discovered knowledge is moved into practice. It is inclusive of familiar processes and also emphasizes the unique aspects of EBP. The ACE Star Model places nursing's previous scientific work within the context of EBP, serves as an organizer for examining and applying EBP, and mainstreams nursing into the formal network of EBP.

ACE Star Model of Knowledge Transformation

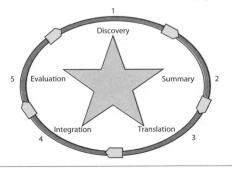

continues

EXHIBIT 11–4 (continued)

The Star Model depicts various *forms* of knowledge in a relative sequence, as research evidence is moved through several cycles, combined with other knowledge and integrated into practice. The ACE Star Model provides a framework for systematically putting evidence-based practice processes into operation.

Configured as a simple 5-point star, the model illustrates five major stages of knowledge transformation: 1) knowledge discovery, 2) evidence summary, 3) translation into practice recommendations, 4) integration into practice, and 5) evaluation. Evidence-based processes and methods vary from one point on the Star Model to the next.

Definition of Knowledge Transformation—the conversion of research findings from primary research results, through a series of stages and forms, to impact on health outcomes by way of EB care.

UNDERLYING PREMISES OF KNOWLEDGE TRANSFORMATION

1. Knowledge transformation is necessary before research results are useable in clinical decision making.
2. Knowledge derives from a variety of sources. In healthcare, sources of knowledge include research evidence, experience, authority, trial and error, and theoretical principles.
3. The most stable and generalizable knowledge is discovered through systematic processes that control bias, namely, the research process.
4. Evidence can be classified into a hierarchy of strength of evidence. Relative strength of evidence is largely dependent on the rigor of the scientific design that produced the evidence. The value of rigor is that it strengthens cause-and-effect relationships.
5. Knowledge exists in a variety of forms. As research evidence is converted through systematic steps, knowledge from other sources (expertise, patient preference) is added, creating yet another form of knowledge.
6. The form ('package') in which knowledge exists can be referenced to its use; in the case of EBP, the ultimate use is application in healthcare.
7. The form of knowledge determines its usability in clinical decision making. For example, research results from a primary investigation are less useful to decision making than an evidence-based clinical practice guideline.
8. Knowledge is transformed through the following processes:
   o summarization into a single statement about the state of the science
   o translation of the state of the science into clinical recommendations, with addition of clinical expertise, application of theoretical principles, and client preferences
   o integration of recommendations through organizational and individual actions
   o evaluation of impact of actions on targeted outcomes

EXPLANATION OF EACH STAGE

STAR POINT 1. Discovery

This is a knowledge generating stage. In this stage, new knowledge is discovered through the traditional research methodologies and scientific inquiry. Research results are generated through the conduct of a single study. This may be called a *primary research study* and research designs range from descriptive to correlational to causal; and from randomized control trials to qualitative. This stage builds the corpus of research about clinical actions.

STAR POINT 2. Evidence Summary

Evidence summary is the first unique step in EBP—the task is to synthesize the corpus of research knowledge into a single, meaningful statement of the state of the science. The most advanced EBP methods to date are those used to develop evidence summaries (i.e., evidence synthesis, systematic reviews, e.g., the systematic review methods outlined in the Cochrane Handbook) from randomized control trials. Some evidence summaries employ more rigorous methods than others, yielding more credible and reproducible results.

This stage is also considered a knowledge generating stage, which occurs simultaneously with the summarization. Evidence summaries produce new knowledge by combining findings from all studies to identify bias and limit chance effects in the conclusions. The systematic methodology also increases reliability and reproducibility of results. The following terms are used to refer to various forms of evidence summaries: *evidence synthesis* (Agency for

Healthcare Research and Quality), *systematic review* (Cochrane Collaboration), *meta analysis* (a statistical procedure), *integrative review, review of literature*, and *state of the science review* (*less rigorous and therefore less reliable summary process*). This field of science is referred to as the 'science of research synthesis.'

The rigorous evidence summary step distinguishes EBP from the old paradigm of research utilization. Largely due to the work of the Cochrane Collaboration, rigorous methods for systematic reviews have been greatly advanced, using meta analytic techniques and developing other statistical summary strategies, such as Number Needed to Treat (NNT).

Advantages of an Evidence Summary

An evidence summary has the following advantages:

- Reduces large quantities of information into a manageable form
- Establishes generalizability across participants, settings, treatment variations and study designs
- Assesses consistency and explains inconsistencies of findings across studies
- Increases power in suggesting the cause and effect relationship
- Reduces bias from random and systematic error, improving true reflection of reality
- Integrates existing information for decisions about clinical care, economic decisions, future research design, and policy formation
- Increases efficiency in time between research and clinical implementation
- Provides a basis for continuous updates with new evidence (Mulrow, 1994)

STAR POINT 3. Translation

The transformation of evidence summaries into actual practice requires two stages: *translation* of evidence into practice recommendations and *integration* into practice.

The aim of translation is to provide a useful and relevant package of summarized evidence to clinicians and clients in a form that suits the time, cost, and care standard. Recommendations are generically termed *clinical practice guidelines* (*CPGs*) and may be represented or embedded in care standards, clinical pathways, protocols, and algorithms.

CPGs are tools to support informed clinical decisions for clinician, organization, and client. Well-developed CPGs state benefits, harms, and costs of various decision options. The strongest CPGs are developed systematically using a process that is explicit and reproducible. Summarized research evidence is interpreted and combined with other sources of knowledge (such as clinical expertise and theoretical guides) and then contextualized to the specific client population and setting. Evidence-based CPGs explicitly articulate the link between the clinical recommendation and the strength of supporting evidence and/or strength of recommendation.

STAR POINT 4. Integration

Integration is perhaps the most familiar stage in healthcare because of society's long-standing expectation that healthcare be based on most current knowledge, thus, requiring implementation of innovations. This step involves changing both individual and organizational practices through formal and informal channels. Major aspects addressed in this stage are factors that affect individual and organizational rate of adoption of innovation and factors that affect integration of the change into sustainable systems.

STAR POINT 5. Evaluation

The final stage in knowledge transformation is evaluation. In EBP, a broad array of endpoints and outcomes are evaluated. These include evaluation of the impact of EBP on patient health outcomes, provider and patient satisfaction, efficacy, efficiency, economic analysis, and health status impact.

As new knowledge is transformed through the five stages, the final outcome is evidence-based quality improvement of health care.

Source: From *ACE Star Model of EBP: Knowledge Transformation*, by K. R. Stevens, 2004, San Antonio: Academic Center for Evidence-based Practice, University of Texas Health Science Center at San Antonio, http://www.acestar.uthscsa.edu. Reproduced with permission.

Figure 11–3 Rating evidence-based practice.

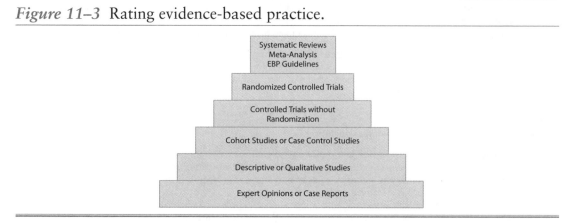

Source: From *Evidence-Based Practice for Nurses: Appraisal and Applications of Research,* by N.A. Schmidt and J.M. Brown, 2009, Sudbury, MA: Jones and Bartlett Publishers. Adapted from Melnyk and Fineout-Overholt, 2005, p. 10, Philadelphia: Lippincott Williams & Wilkins.

reviewers must first identify the criteria to select the reports and studies on the topic or question. Typical criteria are the design, the number of groups, the type of control groups, and the outcome variables used. To limit bias by reviewers, only published evidence should be used. Each study is evaluated for the presence, absence, or degree of the different variables and rated using a recognized rating scale. Meta-analysis is really a statistical specialty and requires extensive training.

3. *Metasynthesis*: **Metasynthesis** is "a systematic review in which findings from several or many qualitative studies examining an issue are merged to produce generalizations and theories" (Brown, 2009, p. 370). This review does not use statistical methods to combine the findings.

Exhibit 11–5 describes questions that are asked when evaluating studies.

Who uses systematic reviews?

- Clinicians (nurses, physicians, pharmacists, allied health professionals)

- Healthcare administrators in developing effective services
- Healthcare policy makers
- Healthcare insurers

What are the advantages of using systematic reviews within the healthcare delivery system (Academic Center for Evidence-Based Nursing, 2008)?

- Reduces large quantities of information into a manageable form
- Establishes generalizability across participants, settings, treatment variations, and study designs
- Assesses consistency and explains inconsistencies of findings across studies
- Increases power in suggesting the cause-and-effect relationship
- Reduces bias from random and systematic error, improving true reflection of reality
- Integrates existing information for decisions about clinical care, economic decisions, future research design, and policy formation

---

EXHIBIT 11–5 QUESTIONS TO EVALUATE STUDIES

General Questions:

Is the research question clearly stated and significant to nursing?

Is an unbiased synthesis of the recent literature provided?

What are the theoretical foundations for the study?

Was the selection of subjects explicit and appropriate?

Were the methods of data collection and analysis explicit and appropriate?

Was the type of analysis appropriate for the question posed?

Were the conclusions drawn within the scope of the study?

Were limitations of the study discussed?

Were ethical considerations discussed?

Questions Related to Systematic Reviews and Meta-Analyses:

Does it describe a comprehensive and detailed search for relevant studies?

Were the individual studies assessed for validity?

Questions Related to Quantitative Studies:

Was the assignment to treatment randomized?

Was the randomization concealed?

Were groups similar at the start of the study?

Was data collection sufficiently long and complete?

Were patients, clinicians, and study personnel kept blind to the study treatment?

Were groups equally treated apart from the experimental therapy?

Questions Related to Qualitative Studies:

Were strategies used to ensure trustworthiness?

Was there prolonged engagement to assure saturation?

Source: From *Evidence-Based Practice for Nurses: Appraisal and Applications of Research*, by N.A. Schmidt and J.M. Brown, 2009, Sudbury, MA: Jones and Bartlett Publishers.

- Increases efficiency in time between research and clinical implementation
- Provides a basis for continuous updates with new evidence

SEARCHING FOR EBP LITERATURE: EVIDENCE

The first step in finding evidence is to look for a systematic review that addresses the PICO. If these reviews cannot be found, a **randomized controlled trial (RCT)**/study should be sought. RCT is often referred to as the "gold standard" in research design. This is the true experiment; there is control over variables, randomization of the sample with a control group and an experimental group, and an intervention or interven-

tions (independent variable). It provides the strongest support for a cause-and-effect relationship. Not all studies meet these criteria.

Where should the search begin? Two important EBP databases are the Cochrane database and the Joanna Briggs Institute Evidence-Based Practice database. A third source is the Agency for Healthcare Research and Quality (AHRQ) and its collection of evidence-based clinical guidelines.

1. *The Cochrane Collaboration*: This center develops, maintains, and updates systematic reviews of healthcare interventions to allow practitioners to make informed decisions.

2. *Joanna Briggs Institute*: This represents an international collaboration among nursing and allied health centers. The main purpose is to train professionals to conduct systematic reviews. Some of the centers, like the Joanna Briggs Institute of Oklahoma (housed at the University of Oklahoma College of Nursing), focus on educational awareness of EBP in practice and education. (http://www.joannabriggs.edu.au/about/home.php)

3. *National Clinical Guidelines*: This source is government based, though the guidelines come from many different sources. Guidelines are discussed further in the chapter. (http://www.guideline.gov/).

Exhibit 11–6 identifies other, less specific databases that can be used to find EBP literature.

Sigma Theta Tau International is also active in the area of EBP through its online publication, *Online Journal of Knowledge Synthesis for Nursing*. This journal provides full-text systematic reviews to guide nursing practice. This is a subscription journal; university libraries may have access via a university subscription, so students can access the journal through the library.

THE ROLES OF STAFF NURSES AS RELATED TO SYSTEMATIC REVIEWS

Nurses may be involved in developing systematic reviews by reviewing studies based on spe-

---

EXHIBIT 11–6 SUBJECT-SPECIFIC DATABASE

CINAHL	http://www.cinahl.com	CINAHL is the premier database covering the areas of nursing and allied health. Online coverage is usually comprehensive back to 1982 with monthly updates. After beginning with the indexing of five journals in the 1940s, there are currently over 2,800 journals indexed, resulting in over 1 million records.
MEDLINE via PubMed	http://www.ncbi.nlm.nih.gov/sites/entrez?db=pubmed	Providing coverage of MEDLINE and other medical sciences and biomedical literature back to the 1950s, PubMed is a service of the U.S. National Library of Medicine, providing free access on the Internet to over 17 million citations. While this link is to the free version available on the Internet, your library might provide access to other vendor-created versions that might provide a familiar search environment and then also link directly to library resources (and it will be called MEDLINE, not PubMed).
PubMed Clinical Queries	http://www.nchi.nlm.nih.gov.entrez/query/static/clinical.shtml	The Clinical Queries search supports specialized PubMed queries for clinicians in areas of clinical studies, systematic reviews, and medical genetics.

Source: From *Evidence-Based Practice for Nurses: Appraisal and Applications of Research*, by N.A. Schmidt and J.M. Brown, 2009, Sudbury, MA: Jones and Bartlett Publishers.

Evidence-Based Nursing/ EBN Online	http://ebn.bmjjournals.com	EBN Online seeks to help practicing nurses keep up with the evidence-based literature in a manageable manner. Each study presented at the Web site begins with a brief but detailed abstract followed by expert commentary on the potential for clinical application of the study.
Joanna Briggs Institute	http://www.joannabriggs.edu.au/ about/home.php	Based in the Royal Adelaide Hospital and the University of Adelaide (Australia), the institute was established in 1996 to offer collaboration in EBP with healthcare professionals and researchers across the professional continuum in over 40 countries.
The Cochrane Collaboration and Library	http://www.cochrane.org/index.htm	An international not-for-profit organization, The Cochrane Collaboration seeks to provide timely, up-to-date research evidence. Not a physical entity, The Cochrane Library is a database collection, providing access to systematic reviews, controlled trials, methodology registry, technology assessment, and more. DARE (Database of Abstracts of Reviews of Effects) is also part of the library.
Centre for Evidence-Based Medicine	http://www.cebm.net/?o=1013	Established in Oxford, England, the Centre's mission is to provide free and open access to support and resources in the field of evidence-based health care to anyone who wants to make use of them.
TRIP Database	http://www.tripdatabase.com/ AboutUs/Index.html	In support of EBP, the TRIP database aims simply to provide healthcare professionals with easy access to high-quality material on the Web. Its contents are evaluated by the Centre for Evidence-Based Medicine. After four years of being a subscription only service, it resumed as an open access service in September 2006.
Virginia Henderson International Nursing Library	http://www.nursinglibrary.org/Portal/ main.aspx?PageID=4001	With a primary goal of becoming a comprehensive nursing resource, the library and its Registry of Nursing Research database offers nurses access to reliable, easy-to-use information.
Agency for Healthcare Research and Quality (AHRQ): Evidence-based Practice	http://www.ahrq.gov/clinic/epcix.htm	This site provides open Internet access to categorized EBP resources, reports, and related issues. There are links to other parts

continues

Exhibit 11–6 (continued)

		of the AHRQ site as well, in clinical practice guidelines, outcomes and effectiveness, technology assessments, and preventive services.
National Guideline Clearinghouse	http://www.guideline.gov/	An initiative of the AHRQ, the clearinghouse serves as an open access, public resource for evidence-based clinical practice guidelines.
National Quality Measures Clearinghouse	http://www.qualitymeasures.ahrq.gov/	Another resource sponsored by AHRQ, this site serves as a public repository for evidence-based quality measures and measure sets.
National Institute of Nursing Research	http://www.nih.gov/ninr	NINR is a foundational resource in supporting and improving health across the spectrum. Among other initiatives, the institute supports and conducts its own clinical research and provides training on health and illness issues.
BMJ Clinical Evidence	http://www.clinicalevidence.com/ceweb/index.jsp	Owned by the British Medical Journal Publishing Group Ltd., this Internet site adds the fluidity of Web-based updates to an already respected, authoritative peer reviewed journal that provides access to systematic reviews of clinical conditions.
EMBASE	http://info.embase.com/embase_com/about/index.shtml	With more than 18 million records, EMBASE provides comprehensive online access to recent literature in pharmacological and bio-medical literature. It includes MEDLINE records in topic areas from 1966-forward.
ClinicalTrials.gov	http://clinicaltrials.gov/ct/gui	A collaboration between the National Library of Medicine and the Food and Drug Administration, ClinicalTrials.gov offers access to more than 36,000 clinical studies sponsored by various federal agencies and private industry. The Web site offers up-to-date information on the various federal and private clinical trials. All 50 states and over 130 countries have trials listed within the collection.
American FactFinder	http://factfinder.census.gov/home/saff/main.html?_lang=eng	The definitive source for population, housing, economic, and geographic data as provided by the U.S. Census Bureau.

PsycINFO	http://www.apa.org/psycinfo/	Dating back to 1987 in its electronic coverage, PsycINFO is the definitive source of psychology literature, claiming that over 97 percent of its content is peer reviewed.
ERIC	http://www.eric.ed.gov	The Educational Resources Information Center (ERIC) is the definitive source of education literature. While this link is to the free version available on the Internet, your library might provide access to other vendor-created versions that might provide a familiar search environment and also link directly to library resources.
Sociological Abstracts	http://www.csa.com/factsheets/ socioabs-set-c.php	Sociological Abstracts provides access to international literature in sociology and in the related social sciences and behavioral disciplines.
Social Services Abstracts	http://www.csa.com/factsheets/ ssa-set-c.php	Social Services Abstracts provides access to current research in social work, human services, social welfare, social policy, and community development.
ABI/Inform	http://proquest.com/products_pq/ descriptions/abi_inform.shtml	Serving as an example of an excellent business literature source, ABI/Inform is the comprehensive business database, covering all areas of business conditions and related topics. While some business-related materials are within CINAHL, searching the business literature for issues of human resources, staffing, customer service, and so on, can be helpful.
UMI Dissertation Publishing	http://proquest.com/products_pq/ products_umi/dissertations	Coverage includes dissertations and theses from the United States, Canada, Britain, and European countries. Searching dissertation topics is a great way to learn what is new in the disciplines as well as gain access to comprehensive reference lists.
Google Scholar	http://scholar.google.com/	Google Scholar allows you to use the familiarity of Google to search the Internet in an interdisciplinary way. Citation results are scholarly in nature and will direct you to full content if it is available on the Internet. Google Scholar also partners with libraries to set up linking with their full content resources. Your librarian can tell you if this is possible in your system.

cific criteria, but this is not common (Jennings & Loan, 2001). As with meta-analysis, this requires specialized statistical knowledge. Over time, more nurses will get more involved. The Joanna Briggs Institute provides an opportunity to increase nursing involvement. The staff nurse's most important role is that of a consumer of the systematic reviews. Nurses search for the systematic reviews through databases (Cochrane and Joanna Briggs) and then use the evidence in practice. Most nurses are, and will be over time, involved at this level. After evidence is found, the nurse looks at the validity of the evidence, its relevance, and its applicability to the nurse's focus question.

Importance of EBP to the Nursing Profession

As noted by the IOM, EBP can improve care. Nursing care should be supported by evidence, but it is not uncommon for nursing care to be provided in a manner that is best described as "we have always done it this way." This type of approach may not always lead to quality care that best meets patient outcomes, and it may not be the most cost-effective approach. "Evidence-based practice is a problem-solving approach to making clinical, educational, and administrative decisions that combines the best available scientific evidence with the best practical evidence" (Newhouse, 2006, p. 337). In this process, EBP increases nurses' clinical knowledge; this leads to greater freedom to act, increasing nurses' autonomy (Kramer & Schmalenberg, 2005). EBP can empower nurses. Following are the critical questions for each nurse to ask:

1. Will the evidence help me provide care?
2. Were all clinically relevant outcomes considered?
3. Are the benefits worth the potential harm and costs?

Changing how care is delivered is a major undertaking because there are barriers. It takes an organized approach to implement EBP into a healthcare delivery system. The reimbursement for services—medical and nursing—are increasingly based on whether the guidelines for care are evidence based. As this financial incentive grows, so will integration of EBP. For example, the Case Management Practice at the University of Oklahoma College of Nursing provides elder care to Medicare and Medicaid patients. No reimbursement is possible if the care is not grounded in evidence. Exhibit 11–7 describes nursing role criteria for the staff nurse, nurse manager, advanced practice nurse, and nurse executive in relation to EBP.

Barriers to EBP Implementation

It has not been easy to incorporate EBP into practice. Some healthcare organizations have been more successful than others. Over time, this will occur, but some barriers need to be overcome by most organizations:

- *Lack of knowledge about EBP and its value*—EBP has only been added to nursing curricula in the last 5 years, so most practicing nurses have limited knowledge. This requires healthcare organizations to play catchup to improve staff knowledge of EBP.
- *Limited time in practice settings*—Staff are rushed and just able to keep up with required care.
- *Nursing shortage*—There are not sufficient staff to allow nurses time to consider EBP effectively.
- *Greater need to emphasize both knowledge and practical approaches*—This applies to both nursing education and practice settings.
- *Concern that EBP represents a cookbook approach to care*—EBP is a cookbook approach if it is used without assessment and clinical rea-

---

Exhibit 11–7 Sample EBP Performance Criteria for Nursing Roles

Staff Nurse (RN)
- Questions current practices
- Participates in implementing changes in practice based on evidence
- Participates as a member of an EBP project team
- Reads evidence related to one's practice
- Participates in QI initiatives
- Suggests resolutions for clinical issues based on evidence

Nurse Manager (NM)
- Creates a microsystem that fosters critical thinking
- Challenges staff to seek out evidence to resolve clinical issues and improve care
- Role models EBP
- Uses evidence to guide operations and management decisions
- Uses performance criteria about EBP in evaluation of staff

Advanced Practice Nurse (APN)
- Serves as coach and mentor in EBP
- Facilitates locating evidence
- Synthesizes evidence for practice
- Uses evidence to write/modify practice standards
- Role models use of evidence in practice
- Facilitates system changes to support use of EBPs

Nurse Executive
- Ensures the governance reflects EBP if initiated in councils and committees
- Assigns accountability for EBP
- Ensures explicit articulation of organizational and department commitment to EBP
- Modifies mission and vision to include EBP language
- Provides resources to support EBPs by direct care providers
- Articulates value of EBP to CEO and governing board
- Role models EBP in administrative decision making
- Hires and retains NMs and APNs with knowledge and skills in EBP
- Provides learning environment for EBP
- Uses evidence in leadership decisions

Source: From *Evidence-Based Practice for Nurses: Appraisal and Applications of Research*, by N.A. Schmidt and J.M. Brown, 2009, Sudbury, MA: Jones and Bartlett Publishers. Adapted from Titler, 2006, p. 472, *Critical Care Nursing Clinics of North America, 13*, 497–509.

---

soning and judgment. Every patient must be viewed as an individual (patient-centered care).
- *Lack of knowledge about EBP resources*—To make evidence available and usable, more information is needed regarding searching for resources, accessing resources, and analyzing resources.
- *Lack of resources to find information*—For example, easily accessible Internet access, access to appropriate databases, and library support are lacking.

- *Limited recognition by employers regarding the value of EBP*—Nurses are not given time to find EBP evidence and then apply it.

IMPROVING EBP IMPLEMENTATION

The IOM recommends that for EBP to be used effectively, healthcare professionals should be able to (Institute of Medicine, 2003a, pp. 57–58):

- Know where and how to find the best possible sources of evidence.
- Formulate clear clinical questions.
- Search for the relevant answers to the questions from the best possible sources of evidence, including those that evaluate or appraise the evidence for its validity and usefulness with respect to a particular patient or population.
- Determine when and how to integrate these new findings into practice.

Nursing services within a healthcare organization (or any type of healthcare organization) need to plan carefully how they will prepare staff for EBP, implement EBP, and evaluate the outcomes. The first step is staff preparation. Most staff are not ready. Given that most did not graduate from nursing education programs within the last few years (the average age of nurses is older than 45 years), and few had any EBP content in their nursing programs, this is a major hurdle. In a study published in 2005 (Pravikoff, Tanner, & Pierce, 2005), 760 registered nurses responded to a 93-item questionnaire about readiness of nurses for EBP. The results indicated that

> *although these nurses acknowledge that they frequently need information for practice, they feel much more confident asking colleagues or peers and searching the Internet and World Wide Web than they do using bibliographic databases such as PubMed or CINAHL to find specific*

information. They don't understand or value research and have received little or no training in the use of tools that would help them find evidence on which to base their practice. (Pravikoff et al., 2005, p. 40)

Table 11–2 describes strategies to use to overcome barriers to EBP.

Tools to Ensure a Higher Level of EBP

EBP evidence can be incorporated into standards of care that guide nursing practice and education. This can reduce practice variation and provide greater consistency based on evidence to improve quality and safety (Newhouse, 2006). In practice, two common major tools can be used to ensure a higher level of EBP: (1) policies and procedures used by healthcare organizations, which should be based on evidence, and (2) clinical guidelines.

POLICIES AND PROCEDURES BASED ON EBP

"The stark reality [is] that we invest billions in research to find appropriate treatments, we spend more than $2 trillion on healthcare annually, we have extraordinary capacity to deliver the best care in the world, but we repeatedly fail to translate that knowledge and capacity into clinical practice" (IOM, 2003b, p. 2). Much of the care in healthcare organizations is defined by policies and **procedures**. Policies and procedures are important guides for care within healthcare settings (they are described in more depth in Chapter 12). The organizations develop these guides to inform staff about expectations related to specific policies and procedures. They are written documents. Policies and procedures are not new to health care, and many have been developed by reviewing resources such as research results. However, in many cases, they have been developed without an EBP approach.

Table 11–2 Strategies to Overcome Barriers to Adopting EBP

Barrier	Strategy
Time	→ Devote 15 minutes a day to reading evidence related to a clinical problem → Sign up for e-mails that offer summaries of research studies in your area of interest → Use a team approach when considering policy changes to distribute the workload among members → Bookmark Web sites having clinical guidelines to promote faster retrieval of information → Evaluate available technologies (i.e., PDA) to create time-saving systems that allow quick and convenient retrieval of information at the bedside → Negotiate release time from patient care duties to collect, read, and share information about relevant clinical problems → Search for already established clinical guidelines because they provide synthesis of existing research
Research in practice not valued	→ Make a list of reasons why healthcare providers should value research, and use this list as a springboard for discussions with colleagues → Invite nurse researchers to share why they are passionate about their work → When disagreements arise about a policy or protocol, find an article that supports your position and share it with others → When selecting a work environment, ask about the organizational commitment to EBP → Link measurement of quality indicators to EBP → Participate in EBP activities to demonstrate professionalism that can be rewarded through promotions or merit raises → Provide recognition during National Nurses Week for individuals involved in EBP projects
Lack of knowledge about EBP and research	→ Take a course or attend a continuing education offering on EBP → Invite a faculty member to a unit meeting to discuss EBP → Consult with advance practice nurses → Attend conferences where clinical research is presented and talk with presenters about their studies → Volunteer to serve on committees that set policies and protocols

continues

Table 11–2 (continued)

Barrier	Strategy
Lack of knowledge about EBP and research	→ Create a mentoring program to bring novice and experienced nurses together
Lack of technological skills to find evidence	→ Consult with a librarian about how to access databases and retrieve articles → Learn to bookmark important Web sites that are sources of clinical guidelines → Commit to acquiring computer skills
Lack of resources to access evidence	→ Write a proposal for funds to support access to online databases and journals → Collaborate with a nursing program for access to resources → Investigate funding possibilities from others (i.e., pharmaceutical companies, grants)
Lack of ability to read research	→ Organize a journal club where nurses meet regularly to discuss the evidence about a specific clinical problem → Write down questions about an article and ask an advance practice nurse to read the article and assist in answering the questions → Clarify unfamiliar terms by looking them up in a dictionary or research textbook → Use one familiar critique format when reading research
Communication gap between researchers and nursing staff	→ Identify clinical problems and share them with nurse researchers → Participate in ongoing unit-based studies → Subscribe to journals that provide uncomplicated explanations of research studies
Resistance to change	→ Listen to people's concerns about change → When considering an EBP project, select one that interests the staff, has a high priority, is likely to be successful, and has baseline data → Mobilize talented individuals to act as change agents → Create a means to reward individuals who provide leadership during change
Organization does not embrace EBP	→ Link organizational priorities with EBP to reduce cost and increase efficiency → Recruit administrators who value EBP → Form coalitions with other healthcare providers to increase the base of support for EBP → Use EBP to meet accreditation standards or gain recognition (i.e., Magnet Recognition)

Source: From *Evidence-Based Practice for Nurses: Appraisal and Applications of Research*, by N.A. Schmidt and J.M. Brown, 2009, Sudbury, MA: Jones and Bartlett Publishers.

What is the evidence to support a policy or procedure? The difficulty in nursing is that there may not yet be evidence, but policies and procedures should state what the evidence is (if it exists) to support the content. Many healthcare organizations are now trying to improve their policies and procedures by reviewing them from an EBP perspective. This is a time-consuming process.

CLINICAL GUIDELINES BASED ON EBP

Clinical practice guidelines are developed by expert panels or professional organizations and are EBP based. An important source for guidelines is the National Guideline Clearinghouse, which is sponsored by the AHRQ primarily, but also the American Medical Association and the American Health Insurance Plans. This is a searchable database of guidelines that are used to improve patient outcomes.

> *Variation in practice patterns and a continued gap between evidence and practice has resulted in recognition for the need to assess the value of interventions and to use evidence-based decision-making. Practice guidelines and other forms of standardized protocols such as clinical pathways (see Chapter 10) have been defined as both the engines and the vehicles for improving an organization. (Kaegi, 1996, as cited in Goode, Tanaka, Krugman, & O'Connor, 2000, p. 202)*

An EBP guideline is one of the strongest sources for EBP, along with systematic reviews (Melnyk & Fineout-Overholt, 2005). Clinical guidelines are described as "systematically developed statements to assist clinicians and patients in making decisions about care; ideally the guidelines consist of a systematic review of the literature, in conjunction with consensus of a group of expert decision-makers, including administrators, policy-makers, clinicians, and consumers who consider the evidence and make recommendations" (Melnyk & Fineout-Overholt, 2005, p. 585).

Confusion: Difference in Research, EBP, and Quality Improvement

Research, EBP, and **quality improvement (QI)** are not the same. QI will be discussed in detail in Chapter 12; however, it is important to clarify the differences in these three terms and processes in this chapter. Research is systematic investigation of a problem, question, issue, or topic that uses a specific process to gain new knowledge. As has been discussed, results from studies can be used as evidence to support clinical decisions, though not all research is about clinical decisions. An example of research is a nurse questioning the best method for preventing patient falls in a long-term care facility and wanting to consider new interventions. This nurse develops a study to gather data to examine how two different groups of patients respond to a new intervention to prevent falls. The nurse follows the research process described earlier in the chapter.

As has been described, EBP focuses on a systematic review and appraisal of evidence, including research results but also the patient's assessment and history data, the clinician's expertise, and the patient's preferences and values. In this case, the same nurse who wondered about factors related to falls might take a different approach, the EBP approach. The nurse would pose a PICO question, such as, What factors influence patient falls in a long-term care facility? The nurse would look for systematic reviews on this question to guide practice.

QI is "a process by which individuals work together to improve systems and processes with the intention to improve outcomes" (Committee on Assessing the System for Protecting Human Research Participants, 2002, as cited in Newhouse, 2007, p. 433). Healthcare organizations are involved in QI on a daily basis as the healthcare organization staff try to understand outcomes and improve them. In the same example noted with falls, a QI project might include a monthly collecting of data related to the number of falls, and specific information about those falls (i.e., factors related to the falls). The facility would be looking to see how serious the problem is. The facility then might institute a change, such as requiring that patients at risk for falls be identified in medical records and on labels in the patient areas. The facility would then track data to see if there was a change in the number of falls for at-risk patients.

Applying EBP as a Student

Nursing curricula are including more content on EBP for both undergraduate and graduate students. The location of this content in the curriculum can vary from school to school, and typically it is associated with nursing research content and then emphasized throughout the curriculum. This content is not something that should be presented in isolation from other nursing content and from clinical experiences. Students need to actively pursue evidence—in the literature and in published studies. Relying only on textbooks that are out of date by the time they are published is not the best preparation. When students are assigned or select patients for clinical experiences, part of the preparation for clinical experience or practicum should be to search for current evidence and incorporate this evidence into the care plan and practice. Students typically do include the other types of EBP evidence: patient values and preferences, patient history, and assessment data. Students less often include research evidence and do not know how to consider their own clinical expertise level. The more a student does with EBP, the more it will become an integral part of his or her practice, and practice after graduation. Merely completing a few assign-

ments on EBP or taking an exam on EBP will not develop the IOM core competency to use EBP practice. Each student needs to make a commitment to practice at the best possible level; to get there takes practice, and that practice should include EBP.

Conclusion

This chapter examined the important core competency of using EBP. Research was discussed as a major source of evidence. The research process and some elements used to describe studies were provided as necessary information for understanding how research is reviewed and used in EBP. Every nurse needs to be using EBP, and this requires understanding the topic and implications for nursing practice and the profession.

CHAPTER HIGHLIGHTS

1. EBP as a core competency is connected to providing patient-centered care and interdisciplinary teams.
2. EBP's use has grown because of the translation gap between bench, or scientific, research and the impact, or use in practice. Translation is taking about 17 years.
3. Research is a systematic investigation of a specific problem.
4. The relationship between research and EBP is that the best evidence comes from research findings.
5. Basic research is designed to broaden the base of knowledge rather than solve an immediate problem.
6. Applied research is designed to find a solution to a practical problem.
7. Nursing research is inextricably linked to the profession's mandate to protect the

public and promote the best possible patient outcomes.

8. The NINR was established by Dr. Ada Sue Hinshaw in 1985.

9. The research process, like the nursing process, is based on problem solving.

10. Research can be either quantitative or qualitative. In quantitative studies, the research question or questions focus on "how many" or "how much", and in the qualitative design, the research question or questions focus on "feel" or "experience."

11. IRBs focus on participant rights. The IRB is charged with the responsibility of ensuring that a research subject's rights are protected and that the study is planned in an effective manner that meets scientific standards, particularly theory and informed consent.

12. *The Nuremberg Code* aims to protect research subjects by addressing five rights:
    a. Right to self-determination
    b. Right to privacy
    c. Right to anonymity and confidentiality
    d. Right to fair treatment
    e. Right to protection from discomfort and harm.

13. EBP uses evidence from research results, patient assessment and other sources, clinical expertise, and information about patient preferences and values.

14. EBP and RU are not the same but can easily be confused. RU includes only re-search results as a source of evidence. The EBP clinical question is often referred to as a PICO question.

15. EBP models include the Iowa Model and the ACE Star Model.

16. The key component of EBP literature is systematic reviews.

17. EBP reviews include integrative reviews, meta-analysis, and metasynthesis.

18. The involvement of staff nurses in the EBP process is critical to its eventual integration into the organization's culture of care delivery.

19. Research, EBP, and QI are not the same. Research focuses on the scientific method to deduce answers to questions. EBP focuses on the use of supporting data to ground interventions. QI is focused on a system or process to measure and systematically examine quality of care at a macro (or system) level, or a micro (or patient) level.

20. Nursing education has begun to shift from pure research content with additive information on EBP, to a focus on EBP while teaching how research underlies much of EBP.

Linking to the Internet

- National Institute of Nursing Research
  http://www.ninr.nih.gov/
- National Institutes of Health
  http://www.nih.gov/
- Health Resources and Services Administration
  http://www.hrsa.gov/
- Academic Center for Evidence-Based Practice, University of Texas, San Antonio (ACE Star Model)
  http://www.acestar.uthscsa.edu/
- The Joanna Briggs Institute
  http://www.joannabriggs.edu.au/
- Arizona State University College of Nursing Center for Advancement of Evidence-Based Practice
  http://nursing.asu.edu/caep/index.htm
- Agency for Healthcare Research and Quality Click "Evidence-based Practice" for a list of evidence reports and technical reviews.

http://www.ahrq.gov/ and http://www
.ahrq.gov/clinic/epcix.htm

- National Guideline Clearinghouse Review EBP guidelines on many topics. http://www.guideline.gov/

DISCUSSION QUESTIONS

1. What does the core competency "employ evidence-based practice" mean?
2. What is the research process?
3. How does research relate to EBP?
4. What is a systematic review, and what are the types of systematic reviews? How do they relate to EBP? What is their value to practice?
5. Why is EBP important to nursing practice?
6. What are the barriers to implementing EBP, and how might some of them be overcome?
7. What factors would you consider when implementing EBP in a nursing unit?

CRITICAL THINKING ACTIVITIES

1. Visit the Web site for the Academic Center for Evidence-Based Practice, University of Texas School of Nursing, San Antonio, to learn more about the school's EBP center (http://www.acestar.uthscsa.edu/). What is the ACE Star Model? What do you think about this model? Can you connect this model to what you know about nursing practice?
2. Where do you begin with an EBP review? By describing the clinical problem or scenario. See http://healthlinks.washington.edu/ebp/pico.html—you will find examples of clinical problems and scenarios. The PICO method is used to clearly define a specific clinical problem. This site shows you how to move from the clinical problem/scenario to a clinical question using PICO.
3. Write a PICO question using one of the templates described in this chapter. After you have written your PICO, compare it with others (this can be done in a small group). Ask members of the group to identify the P, I, C, and O in your question, and do the same with other questions. Select one PICO and see if the group can find a systematic review on the question. If you cannot, discuss what this means. Identify PICOs for your clinical patients.
4. Visit the National Institute of Nursing Research Web site and review the strategic plan (http://www.ninr.nih.gov/AboutNINR/NINRMissionandStrategicPlan/). What examples are given on the site to demonstrate how nursing research is making a difference?

Do any of these surprise you (nursing involvement, type of study, results)? What is your own school doing in the area of nursing research?

5. Visit http://bioethics.od.nih.gov/ and select "Bioethics Resources." Review one of the posted topics. Why did you select this topic? Summarize what you have learned from this site.

6. If you are interested in learning more about the Tuskegee study, visit http://www.tuskegee.edu/Global/Story.asp?s=1207598. What happened in this study? What were the ethical issues that should have been considered? Does your school have an IRB office? If so, visit its Web site and review the informed consent forms and Health Insurance Portability and Accountability Act forms.

CASE STUDY

Health professionals noticed that ventilator-dependent adults often developed pneumonia. They started questioning what might be going on. They reviewed the literature and found that there was little "evidence" to support this phenomenon, but there was some. Over the past few years, more and more institutions examined ventilator-associated pneumonia (VAP). Based on these reviews, guidelines or best practices were developed to decrease the incidence of VAP in adults. Now, research and EBP studies examine VAP as a measure of quality of care; consider costs associated with VAP versus preventative costs; and use VAP as a benchmark-ing tool for quality care and patient safety (Ruffell & Adamcova, 2008; Uckay, Ahmed, Sax, & Pittet, 2008).

Case Questions

1. Can you find a systematic review on VAP and care? If so, what evidence does it provide?
2. Can you find a clinical guideline on VAP? What evidence is provided?
3. What care approach is used in a clinical setting in which you have practicum? How does it relate to what you have learned from the systematic review and/or clinical guideline?

WORDS OF WISDOM

Lisa English Long, MSN, RN, CNS, Evidence-Based Practice Mentor, Director, Evidence-Based Practice, Cincinnati Children's Hospital Medical Center, Cincinnati, Ohio

EBP is an approach that promotes scholarly inquiry, a sense of autonomy, and control over practice. The growth that nurses have experi-enced through the use of EBP has been instru-mental in leading practice changes that improve patient, family, and staff outcomes. My experi-ences in working with staff whose goal is to establish a practice based on evidence is exciting and one that instills a sense of pride. I have found point-of-care staff eager to learn, work collabo-ratively, and support each other in establishing and sustaining that "questioning attitude." Engaging in the EBP process motivates staff to learn about change theory, use of EBP models in guiding work, and the barriers to implementation of EBP. The challenges that permeate through the evidence work relate, many times, to system issues of which they have less control. The barriers have not limited staff in their efforts to change practice from "the way we have always done it" to "the way that is the best based on critically appraised research, clinical expertise, and patient/family preferences." My experiences with those involved in evidence work have allowed me to witness change in policy, policy and procedure development, dissemination of findings, and presentations at regional, local, national, and international forums. Truly the growth in colleagues both personally and professionally is impressive, as they not only grow but also improve outcomes in patients, families, and colleagues through engagement in evidence-based practice.

References

Academic Center for Evidence-Based Nursing. (2008). *Star Model*. Retrieved April 5, 2008, from http://www.acestar.uthscsa.edu/

American Association of Colleges of Nursing. (2006). *AACN position statement on nursing research*. Washington, DC: Author.

American Nurses Association. (2003). *Nursing's social policy statement* (2nd ed.). Silver Spring, MD: Author.

American Nurses Association. (2004). *Scope and standards of practice*. Silver Spring, MD: Author.

Balas, E. (2001). Information systems can prevent errors and improve quality. *Journal of the American Medical Informatics Association, 8*, 398–399.

Brown, S. (2009). *Evidence-based nursing*. Sudbury, MA: Jones and Bartlett.

Chassin, M. (1998). Is healthcare ready for Six Sigma quality? *Milbank Quarterly, 76*, 565–591.

Committee on Assessing the System for Protecting Human Research Participants. (2002). *Responsible research: A systems approach to protecting research participants*. Washington, DC: National Academies Press.

DiCenso, A., Guyatt, G., & Ciliska, D. (2005). *Evidence-based nursing. A guide to clinical practice*. St. Louis, MO: Elsevier Mosby.

Goode, C., Tanaka, D., Krugman, M., & O'Connor, P. (2000). Outcomes from use of an evidence-based practice guideline. *Nursing Economics, 18*, 202–207.

Institute of Medicine. (2003a). *Health professions education: A bridge to quality*. Washington, DC: National Academies Press.

Institute of Medicine. (2003b). *Priority areas for national action: Transforming healthcare quality*. Washington, DC: National Academies Press.

International Council of Nurses. (1999). *Position statement on nursing research*. Geneva, Switzerland: Author.

Jennings, B., & Loan, L. (2001). Misconceptions among nurses about EBP. *Journal of Nursing Scholarship, 33*, 121–127.

Kramer, M., & Schmalenberg, C. (2005). Best quality patient care: A historical perspective on magnet hospitals. *Nursing Administration Quarterly, 29*, 275–287.

Levin, R. (2006). Evidence-based practice in nursing: What is it? In R. Levin & H. Feldman (Eds.), *Teaching evidence-based practice in nursing* (pp. 5–13). New York: Springer.

Melnyk, B., & Fineout-Overholt, E. (2005). *Evidence-based practice in nursing and healthcare*. Philadelphia: Lippincott Williams & Wilkins.

Newhouse, R. P. (2006). Examining the support for evidence-based nursing practice. *Journal of Nursing Administration, 36*, 337–340.

Newhouse, R. P. (2007). Diffusing confusion among evidence-based practice, quality improvement, and research. *Journal of Nursing Administration, 37*(10), 432–435.

Pravikoff, D., Tanner, A., & Pierce, S. (2005). Readiness for U.S. nurses for evidence-based practice. *American Journal of Nursing, 105*(9), 40–50.

Ruffell, A., & Adamcova, L. (2008). Ventilator-associated pneumonia: Prevention is better than care. *Nursing Critical Care, 13*(1), 44–53.

Sackett, D., Straus, S., Richardson, W., Rosenberg, W., & Hayes, R. (2000). *Evidence-based medicine: How to practice and teach EBM*. London: Churchill Livingstone.

Stevens, K. R. (2004). *ACE Star Model of EBP: Knowledge transformation*. San Antonio: Academic Center for Evidence-Based Practice, University of Texas Health Science Center at San Antonio.

Titler, M. G., Kleiber, C., Steelman, V. J., Rakel, B. A., Budrequ, G., Everett, L. Q., et al. (2001). The Iowa model of evidence-based practice to promote quality care. *Critical Care Nursing Clinics of North America, 13*, 497–509.

Uckay, I., Ahmed, Q., Sax, H., & Pittet, D. (2008). Ventilator-associated pneumonia as a quality indicator for patient safety? *Clinical Infectious Disease, 46*(4), 557–563.

Vratny, A., & Shriver, D. (2007). A conceptual model for growing evidence-based practice. *Nursing Administration Quarterly, 31*, 162–170.

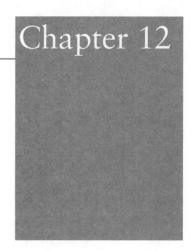

Chapter 12

Apply Quality Improvement

CHAPTER OUTLINE

KEY TERMS

- ❏ Accreditation
- ❏ Adverse event
- ❏ Benchmarking
- ❏ Blame-free environment
- ❏ Clinical pathways
- ❏ Effective care
- ❏ Efficient care
- ❏ Equitable care
- ❏ Error
- ❏ Failure to rescue
- ❏ Healthcare report card
- ❏ The Joint Commission
- ❏ Misuse
- ❏ Near miss
- ❏ Outcomes
- ❏ Overuse

- ❏ Patient-centered care
- ❏ Process
- ❏ Protocols
- ❏ Quality
- ❏ Quality improvement (QI)
- ❏ Risk management (RM)
- ❏ Root cause analysis
- ❏ Safety
- ❏ Sentinel event
- ❏ Structure
- ❏ Surveillance
- ❏ System
- ❏ Timely care
- ❏ Underuse
- ❏ Utilization review/management (UR/UM)

Introduction

This chapter's content discusses the fourth IOM healthcare core competency: apply quality improvement. The content includes information about the key IOM quality and safety reports and their recommendations. Through further exploration of safety issues and quality care, the role of accreditation of healthcare organizations (HCOs) is related to the need to improve care.

Nurses and nursing as a profession play major roles in ensuring that care is safe and that outcomes are reached.

The IOM Competency: Apply Quality Improvement

The fourth healthcare profession core competency is to apply **quality improvement (QI)** . The IOM (2003) description of this core competency is: "identify errors and hazards in care; understand and implement basic safety design principles, such as standardization and simplification; continually understand and measure quality of care in terms of **structure**, **process**, and **outcomes** in relation to patient and community needs; and design and test interventions to change processes and systems of care, with the objective of improving quality" (p. 4). As will be described in this chapter, current data indicate that there are serious problems with health care in the United States—its safety, its quality, and waste and inefficiency. The healthcare **system** is the focus of

quality improvement. The system is fragmented and in need of improvement. A system

can be defined by the coming together of parts, interconnections, and purpose. While systems can be broken down into parts which are interesting in and of themselves the real power lies in the way the parts come together and are interconnected to fulfill some purpose. The healthcare system in the United States consists of various parts (e.g., clinics, hospitals, pharmacies, laboratories) that are interconnected (via flows of patients and information) to fulfill a purpose (e.g., maintaining and improving health). (Plsek, 2001, p. 309)

This does not mean that individual patient needs and improvement of individual patient care are not important. Each patient's care is part of this overall emphasis on healthcare improvement. Ultimately, the goal is that each patient's outcomes will be met. Figure 12–1 illustrates the key elements related to this core competency as discussed in this chapter.

Figure 12–1 Apply quality improvements: Key elements.

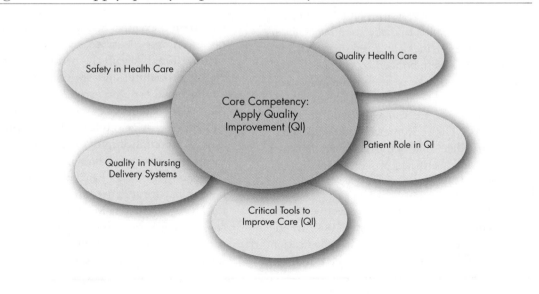

Safety in Health Care

There is no question that healthcare providers, including nurses, have long been concerned about providing safe care for their patients. If one interviewed healthcare providers, there is no doubt that they would say that they want to keep their patients safe and that care is safe. This belief was somewhat shattered when the IOM was directed by Congress to begin an exploration of healthcare safety and quality and to make recommendations based on its findings. The following section in this chapter explores the topic of safety in health care: what it is and what can be done to better ensure safe care for all.

To Err Is Human: *Impact on Safety*

The first IOM report in the Quality Series was *To Err Is Human: Building a Safer Health System* (1999). This report explored the status of safety within the healthcare delivery system. The results were dramatic, with data indicating serious safety problems in hospitals. This investigation did not include other types of healthcare settings, such as ambulatory care, home care, long-term care, and many other types of sites. We do not know the status of safety in these settings at this time, and more data are needed to make statements about safety in these settings. This report and its recommendations were noticed by the media, and soon there were stories on the evening news and in newspapers; special in-depth news reports asked, "How safe are you when you go in for health care?" The consumer began to ask questions. What were some of the data that disturbed the public and healthcare providers (Institute of Medicine, 1999, pp. 1–2)?

- When data from one study were extrapolated, the result was at least 44,000 Americans die each year as a result of a medication error. Another study indicated the number could be as high as 98,000 (American Hospital Association, 1999).
- More people die in a given year as a result of medical errors than from motor vehicle accidents (43,458), breast cancer (42,297), or acquired immune deficiency syndrome (AIDS) (16,516) (Centers for Disease Control and Prevention, 1998).
- Healthcare costs represent over one-half of total national costs, which includes lost income, lost household production, disability, and healthcare costs (Thomas et al., 1999).

Later in this chapter, accreditation is discussed in detail; however, it is important to note here that accreditation, focusing on the quality of care, has been active for a long time in health care. It is clear from *To Err Is Human* (1999) that this has not been enough to improve care at the level that is needed. What happens when there are errors? Why is it so important?

- *Complications may occur and increase costs.* In the fall of 2007, the Centers for Medicare and Medicaid Services (CMS) introduced a major change: CMS will not pay for complications that occur in the hospital that could have been prevented. Specific types of complications were identified, such as falls, hospital-acquired decubiti, performing the wrong procedure, and administering the wrong blood type. In early 2008, some of the major insurers came out in support of this approach—zero tolerance for hospital-acquired complications. This policy has major implications; who will pay for this? Ultimately, the HCO may hold the bill and have to pay for it. There are limits to what the HCO can charge a Medicare patient. It is complex and serious, but the major message is that when errors are made, there are costs involved. For many reasons, HCOs have problems with maintaining a stable budget, as discussed in Chapter 8. This change will have a major impact on the financial status of hospitals, and it is uncertain how hospitals will respond to this change.

- *Opportunity costs increase.* What does this mean? Opportunity costs relate to situations in which diagnostic tests must be repeated or in which a change in the plan of care is needed because of adverse reactions to treatment. This may put the patient at greater risk for harm depending on the test and may increase costs of care.
- *Decrease in patient trust.* As mentioned, the report *To Err Is Human* had a major impact on consumers and was shared via the media across the country. The result is that patients and families are now questioning their care more. Some patients do not want to be in the hospital without having a family member or friend with them at all times. When a patient experiences an error, his or her trust level drops, and this has an impact on how he or she approaches future care. There is a positive side to this situation: More patients are demanding that they be informed about their care and thus are more involved in the care process.

Recognizing that there are major safety concerns in the U.S. healthcare system, what can be done? The first important issue is that there is not a specific answer to this problem; the IOM report (1999) makes this clear. Changing the status of safety will require multiple planned strategies in practice and an increase in safety education in professional healthcare programs and staff training.

CRITICAL SAFETY TERMS

The IOM has expanded knowledge about safety and errors, and part of this is identification of key terms. This identification of common language is important for shared communication and also has an impact on data collection and analysis. To do this effectively nationally, there must be a shared language. The following terms are part of this effort, and they have relevance to nurses who need to be directly involved in initiatives to improve care, including decreasing errors and improving safety. The definitions are identified by the IOM (1999; Chassin & Galvin, 1998).

- *Safety*: Freedom from accidental injury. Example: The patient leaves the hospital after surgery and a 3-day stay with no complications and expected outcomes reached.
- *Error*: The failure of a planned action to be completed as intended or the use of the wrong plan to achieve an aim; errors are directly related to outcomes. There are two types of errors: *error of planning* and *error of execution*. Errors harm the patient, and some that injure the patient may have been *preventable adverse events*. Example: The patient is given the wrong medication.
- *Adverse Event*: An injury resulting from a medical intervention; in other words, it is not due to the underlying patient condition. Not all adverse events are due to errors, and not all are preventable. It requires greater investigation and analysis to determine the relationship between an error and an adverse event. When an adverse event is the result of an error, it is considered a *preventable adverse event*. Example: A patient is given the wrong medication and experiences a seizure. If the patient does not have a seizure disorder, this is most likely an adverse event, but much more needs to be known about the causes. How did the error that led to the adverse event happen?
- *Misuse*: Avoidable complications that prevent patients from receiving full potential

benefit of a service. Example: The patient receives a medication that is not prescribed and that conflicts with his or her allergies; the patient experiences anaphylaxis.

- *Overuse*: The potential for harm from the provision of a service that exceeds the possible benefit. Example: An elderly patient is on multiple medications, and his or her multiple healthcare providers do not know the medications that have been prescribed by different specialists.

- *Underuse*: Failure to provide a service that would have produced a favorable outcome for the patient. Example: The patient is not able to get a specialty service needed for cancer because of his or her distance from resources, or the patient's insurer will not cover a medication for arthritis that could make the patient more mobile.

- *Near Miss*: Recognition that an event occurred that might have led to an adverse event. This does not mean that the error happened, but that it *almost* happened. It is important to understand these errors because they provide valuable information for preventing future actual errors. Example: The surgical team is preparing for surgery to repair a knee. The right knee is prepped, but soon after, the team checks the records and goes through safety check to ensure that the correct knee is exposed— only to find out that it is the left knee that requires surgery. The team stops and replans the surgery.

- *Sentinel Event*: An event that had a negative patient outcome (unexpected death, serious physical or psychological injury, or serious risk). A root cause analysis or a systematic review of the event is conducted to assess the process, not the individual staff who were involved; blame is not the goal, but rather prevention of further events. Example: A patient commits suicide while

in the hospital for treatment of diabetes or for treatment of depression.

- *Root Cause Analysis*: An in-depth analysis of an error to assess the event and identify causes and possible solutions. The Joint Commission root cause analysis matrix includes the following dimensions that need to be assessed (The Joint Commission, 2004): Behavioral assessment process (includes assessment of patient risk to self and to others as appropriate); physical assessment process (includes search for contraband); patient identification process; patient observation procedures; care planning process; continuum of care; staffing levels; orientation and training of staff; competency assessment/credentialing; supervision of staff (includes supervision of physicians-in-training); communication with patient/family; communication among staff members; availability of information; adequacy of technological support; equipment maintenance/management; physical environment (includes furnishings and hardware, such as bars, rooks, rods, lighting, distractions, security systems and processes); and medication management (includes selection and procurement, storage, ordering and transcribing, preparing and dispensing, administration, and monitoring). Not all of these dimensions apply to every event, but each needs to be considered and then eliminated if not applicable.

If the IOM had stopped its investigation into healthcare quality with the *To Err Is Human* report, the major impact of the report and its recommendations would most likely have been diluted. This, however, did not happen. In 2004, the IOM published a follow-up report, which has been the approach of the IOM—describe a problem area, identify recommendations to respond to the problem, and then identify monitoring methods. *Patient Safety: Achieving a New Standard for Care* (IOM, 2004b) focuses on the need to establish a national information infrastructure and the need for data standards. This is needed to better monitor outcomes. Is the safety problem decreasing? As mentioned earlier in this chapter, having a common language about safety and errors is critical in meeting the goal of having a national information infrastructure. The fifth IOM healthcare professions core competency focuses on informatics and is discussed in Chapter 13. This is just another example that illustrates how the IOM reports, data, recommendations, and methods to monitor change are all interconnected; they are clearly connected to the need to develop core competencies so that healthcare providers can meet the need to improve care. Table 12–1 illustrates the simple rules related to quality that were identified by the IOM for the healthcare system.

A CULTURE OF SAFETY AND A BLAME-FREE WORK ENVIRONMENT

The typical approach to errors in health care has been to identify the staff member who made the error or to ask staff to report their errors by completing an incident report that describes the error. This type of approach has been punitive in nature and has not been effective. Why has it not been effective? Most errors are not made by an individual, but are complex and have been described as system errors. When an error occurs, the question should not be "Who is at fault?" but rather "Why did our defenses fail?" (Reason, 2000). Communication, collaboration, and coordination (interdisciplinary teamwork); lack of staff; patient acuity level; equipment; delivery processes; the role of the patient in care; and many other factors affect any action taken or not taken in health care. The IOM (1999) reported that the healthcare system was focusing on the

Table 12–1 SIMPLE RULES FOR THE 21ST CENTURY

Current Approach (Old Rule)	New Rule
Care is based primarily on visits.	Care is based on continuous healing relationships.
Professional autonomy drives variability.	Care is customized according to patient needs and values.
Professionals control care.	The patient is the source of control.
Information is a record.	Knowledge is shared and information flows freely.
Decision-making is an individual responsibility.	Decision-making is evidence-based.
Do no harm is an individual responsibility.	Safety is a system property.
Secrecy is necessary.	Transparency is necessary.
The system reacts to needs.	Needs are anticipated.
Cost reduction is sought.	Waste is continuously decreased.
Preference is given to professional roles over the system.	Cooperation among clinicians is a priority.

Source: From *Crossing the Quality Chasm: A New Health System for the 21st Century* (p. 67), by Institute of Medicine, 2001, Washington, DC: The National Academies Press. Reprinted with permission.

"blame game" and not really finding out more about all the factors related to an error. Staff members need to feel comfortable, not fearful, in reporting errors. The goal should be a **blame-free environment** in which staff can practice and openly discuss potential errors or near misses as well as actual errors. If they are worried about implications, they may not report an error, and this can have serious consequences for patients and prevent the system from improving. This type of fear may also prevent staff from communicating near misses, from which much can be learned about potential errors. In the past, if a nurse made a medication error, he or she might have been required to take a medication review course with an exam. Does this intervention really get to an understanding of the error? Does it consider factors such as: Was the correct medication sent by pharmacy? Did the error involve placing patient medication in the incorrect box? Was the prescription transcribed correctly? Was there a computer error? What were the distractions and interruptions when the medication was prepared and administered? Did the nurse check the patient's identification correctly? Was an error made in what the physician intended to order or what the team agreed would be the best approach? These are just a few examples of questions that could be asked in this situation.

There is a strong recommendation to move to a culture of safety within a blame-free enviroment. To accomplish this, there must be (1) greater understanding of its essential elements, (2) a decrease in barriers to creating the culture, (3) development and implementation of strategies to create the safety culture, and (4) evaluation of outcomes (IOM, 2004a). Trust is important in this type of culture. Moving away from blame means that staff must trust that they will not be individually blamed or punished for errors that are out of their individual control. Another aspect of this issue is related to individual staff expectations: Nurses feel that they should not make mistakes, that their care should be perfect. This is not a reality-based perspective. Errors will be made that are due to many factors. Improvement is, of course, critical, but to think that errors will never be made is an extreme scenario. There is no doubt that errors need to decrease, with the level being so high. There is no doubt that what has been done to address errors has not been effective. Hospitals and other HCOs are moving toward cultures of safety, but it will take time and effort to change attitudes and behaviors. Particularly important is how the HCO leadership guides and supports the development of a culture of safety (Anderson, 2006). A topic that comes up often from all types of healthcare professionals is concern about revealing errors and near misses. This is based on past experiences. To be truly effective, disclosure has to be present with maximum transparency. Ensuring transparency and involving patients are the hardest aspects of ensuring a culture of safety (Anderson, 2006). "A fundamental principle of the systems approach to error reduction is the recognition that all humans make mistakes and that errors are to be expected, even in the best organizations" (Reason, 2000, p. 768).

Staff Safety

To Err Is Human (1999) focused on patient safety not staff safety, but the report did state the committee believes that "creating a safe environment for patients will go a long way in addressing issues of worker safety as well" (IOM, 1999, p. 20). This does not mean that staff safety is not important; it is very important. The IOM report *Keeping Patients Safe: Transforming the Work Environment for Nurses* (2004a) does include content related to staff safety, particularly nurses. Nursing staff are not immune to injury at work. The Occupational Safety and Health Administration

(OSHA) is the federal agency that is responsible for monitoring safe workplaces.

The American Nurses Association (ANA) is a strong advocate for safety for nurses in all types of healthcare settings. Its position statements on staff safety provide guidelines for work environments for staff. Examples of some of the position statements that are available at the ANA Web site (http://www.nursingworld.org) are Personnel Policies and HIV in the Workplace, HIV Infection and Nursing Students, and HIV Testing. Some of the key safety issues for nursing staff other than those mentioned are:

- *Needlesticks*: Healthcare workers (HCWs) suffer between 600,000 and one million injuries from conventional needles and sharps annually. These exposures can lead to hepatitis B, hepatitis C, and human immunodeficiency virus (HIV), the virus that causes AIDS. At least 1,000 HCWs are estimated to contract serious infections annually from needlestick and sharps injuries. Registered nurses (RNs) working at the bedside experience the majority of these exposures. Over 80% of needlestick injuries could be prevented with the use of safer needle devices. More disturbing is that less than 15% of U.S. hospitals use safer needle devices and systems.
- *Infections*: As noted, HCWs are often exposed to communicable diseases via needlesticks. These include HIV and hepatitis B and C. Other examples are tuberculosis, which is rising in this country, staphylococcus, cytomegalovirus, influenza, and bacteria. Influenza has been linked to suboptimal vaccination levels of HCWs (Polygreen et al., 2008). Bacterial infections have sometimes been linked to glove contamination (Diaz et al., 2008).
- *Ergonomic Safety*: There are a significant number of work-related back injuries and

other musculoskeletal disorders among nurses. ANA's Handle with Care campaign addresses work-related musculoskeletal disorders (Castro, 2004). Because of these injuries, nurses transfer to other units or other healthcare settings, and they may leave nursing. Typical injuries are to the neck, shoulder, and back. Nursing includes a lot of patient handling, and factors such as the patient's weight, height, body shape, age, dependency, and medical status are important. There has been an increase in weight in the adult population in general, and this has made the risk of injury higher. The physical setting also is a factor in increasing risk. Is there enough room to move around when moving the patient? What are the types of equipment available to assist with moving patients? Handle with Care (ANA, 2003) is a national campaign that was established in September 2003 by the ANA. Its goal is to develop and implement a proactive, multifaceted plan to promote the issue of safe patient handling and the prevention of musculoskeletal disorders among nurses in the United States. Through a variety of activities, the campaign seeks to educate and to advocate and facilitate change from traditional practices of manual patient handling to emerging technology-oriented methods. Nursing education needs to include content and experiences to teach the most effective handling methods. In addition, more emphasis is placed on assistive patient handling equipment and devices. Students need to learn how to use this equipment, too.
- *Violence*: Violence may not be a typical staff safety concern that a student would first think of when asked about safety in the healthcare workplace, but it is a concern. There is greater risk for violence in emer-

gency departments, psychiatric/substance abuse departments, and long-term care facilities; however, it could occur anywhere. Patients and families may not be able to control their anger appropriately. The nurse may be in a situation in which violence occurs that is not directly related to the nurse or health care, such as providing home care in a community in which there is violence. The four types of violence are (1) violence committed during a robbery or similar crime (this accounts for 85% of all workplace homicides); (2) violence that involves customers who become violent during the course of a transaction; (3) violence related to worker-on-worker assault; and (4) violence as a spillover of domestic violence (Gates & Kroeger, 2007).

Staff need training so that they can prevent violence when possible—particularly identification of signs of escalation and how to deescalate a situation when possible—and they need to know how to protect themselves when violence cannot be prevented. In areas such as psychiatry, this training is more common. Signs of escalation include a sudden change in behavior, clenched jaws or fists, threats, pacing, increased movement, shouting, use of profanity, increased respirations, and staring or pointing. These signs do not mean that the person will become violent, but rather that the nurse should be more aware of the person's behavior and communication to determine if the person is escalating. Protecting oneself is very important; the nurse may leave the room, stay near the door or keep the door open, ask other staff to be present, or call for security assistance.

OSHA has developed guidelines for preventing workplace injuries due to exposure to chemicals, (OSHA, 2004).

An online survey of workplace exposures and disease conditions among 1,500 nurses was conducted by the Environmental Working Group (EWG) and Healthcare Without Harm (HCWH), in collaboration with the American Nurses Association and the Environmental Health Education Center of the University of Maryland's School of Nursing, and supported by numerous state and specialty nursing organizations. This comprehensive survey indicates that participating nurses who were exposed frequently to sterilizing chemicals, housekeeping cleaners, residues from drug preparation, radiation, and other hazardous substances report increased rates of asthma, miscarriage, and certain cancers, as well as increases in cancers and birth defects, in particular musculoskeletal defects, in their children. There are workplace safety standards for only six of the hundreds of hazardous substances to which nurses are exposed on the job. (EWG, HCWH, ANA, & Environmental Health Education Center of the University of Maryland's School of Nursing, 2007).

Specific risks identified include anesthetic gases, hand and skin disinfection, housekeeping chemicals, latex, medications such as antiretroviral medications and chemotherapeutic agents, mercury-containing devices, personal care products, radiation, and sterilization and disinfectant agents such as ethylene oxide and glutaraldehyde.

Examples of Safety Initiatives

A number of important safety initiatives have been stimulated by the IOM work on safety. The Institute for Healthcare Improvement (IHI) was established in 1991, and it describes itself as "a reliable source of energy, knowledge, and support for a never-ending campaign to improve healthcare worldwide. The Institute helps accelerate change in healthcare by cultivating promising concepts for improving patient care and turning those ideas into action" (IHI, 2008). It focuses on safety, effectiveness, patient-centeredness, timeliness, efficiency, and equity, all of which are emphasized in the IOM quality series. The 5 Million Lives Campaign is one example; it is a voluntary initiative to protect patients from five million incidents of medical harm over 2 years (December 2006–December 2008).

Another initiative, a collaborative effort between IHI and the Robert Wood Johnson Foundation (RWJF), is Transforming Care at the Bedside (TCAB). TCAB is a "unique innovation initiative that aims to create, test, and implement changes that will dramatically improve care on medical/surgical units, and improve staff satisfaction as well" (IHI, 2008). TCAB is discussed in more detail in Chapter 15.

Another example of a safety initiative is The Joint Commission's annual safety goals, which began in 2003. Each year, The Joint Commission identifies safety goals that should be the focus of every Joint Commission-accredited HCO. These goals are based on the critical, current safety concerns. Surveyors also emphasize the goals during accreditation visits. HCOs typically provide staff education related to the goals and monitor related progress. The current goals are available on The Joint Commission Web site (http://www.jointcommission.org).

Quality Health Care

There is no universal definition of healthcare **quality**, and this has made it difficult to assess. For this discussion, the IOM definition of *quality care* will be used; this is the definition used throughout the IOM quality series of reports. The IOM defines quality as the "degree to which health services for individuals and populations increase the likelihood of desired health outcomes

and are consistent with current professional knowledge" (1990, p. 4). Quality is a very complex concept, and who is defining it can make a difference; for example, a nurse, a physician, and a patient may have different definitions of quality. There are three elements to quality that are included in the IOM definition and that are usually included in a discussion about quality care and monitoring care (Donabedian, 1980):

- *Structure*: The environment in which services are provided; inputs into the system, such as patients, staff, and environments
- *Process*: The manner in which services are provided; the interactions between clinicians and patients
- *Outcome*: The result of services; evidence about changes in patients' health status in relation to patient and community needs.

Crossing the Quality Chasm: *Impact on Quality Care*

Crossing the Quality Chasm (IOM, 2001a) is the report that followed *To Err Is Human* (IOM, 1999) as part of the quality series. The report's major message is that the healthcare system is in need of fundamental improvement. Although it is a system that has undergone many changes—such as in the area of new drugs, medical technology, and informatics—that have improved care and care options, more needs to be done. This report provides valuable information to help nurses better understand quality issues in the healthcare system; however, if this information is not applied to improve care, it serves little purpose.

The report identifies six aims or goals for improvement. These aims state that care should be (IOM, 2001a, pp. 5–6):

1. *Safe*: Avoiding injuries to patients from the care that is intended to help them.
2. *Effective*: Providing services based on scientific knowledge (evidence-based practice—

EBP) to all who could benefit and refraining from providing services to those not likely to benefit (avoiding underuse and overuse).

3. *Patient-centered*: Providing care that is respectful of and responsive to individual patient preferences, needs, and values and ensuring that patient values guide all clinical decisions.

4. *Timely*: Reducing waits and sometimes harmful delays for both those who receive and those who give care.

5. *Efficient*: Avoiding waste, including waste of equipment, supplies, ideas, and energy.

6. *Equitable*: Providing care that does not vary in quality because of personal characteristics such as gender, ethnicity, geographic location, and socioeconomic status. (disparity concern)

All the healthcare professions' core competencies relate to these aims. The IOM quality series is unique in that each report does not stand alone, but rather expands on previous reports in the series. This interconnectedness makes it important that readers understand the general information in each report, how the reports relate to one another, and the recommendations and joint implications for nursing and health care.

To ensure an improved healthcare system that will meet the six aims, the IOM developed new rules for the 21st century to guide care delivery. These rules are directly related to the six aims and to the healthcare professions' core competencies. The rules are described, along with examples of how they relate to nursing and healthcare delivery (IOM, 2001a):

1. **Care based on continuous healing relationships.** Patients should receive care whenever they need it—access is critical. *Consider these related examples: nurse–patient relationship, continuum of care, HCO services and systems, diversity, interdisciplinary teams.*

2. **Customization based on patient needs and values.** This rule relates directly to patient-centered care. Patient needs and values also constitute one of the sources of evidence for EBP. *Consider these related examples: nursing care and planning, interdisciplinary teams, patient-centered care, diversity, and patient education.*

3. **The patient as the source of control.** Patients need information to make decisions about their own care—patient-centered care. Healthcare systems and professionals need to share information with patients and bring patients into the decision-making process. *Consider these related examples: plan of care, interdisciplinary care, nursing care, informed consent, patient education, informatics.*

4. **Shared knowledge and the free flow of information.** Patients need access to their medical information, and clinicians also need access. This rule relates to all the core competencies, and particularly to the fifth competency—applying informatics—discussed in Chapter 13. *Consider these related examples: informatics, interdisciplinary teams, nursing care, patient-centered care, patient education, computerized documentation.*

5. **Evidence-based decision making.** Patients need care that is based on the best possible evidence available. Care should not vary illogically from clinician to clinician or from place to place. *Consider these related examples: patient-centered care, nursing research and other areas of research, plan of care.*

6. **Safety is a system property.** Patients need to be safe from harm that may occur within the healthcare system. There needs to be more attention placed on system errors rather than individual errors. *Consider these related examples: patient-centered*

care, nursing care, plan of care, patient safety and errors, staff safety, reimbursement (government, insurers).

7. **The need for transparency.** The healthcare system should make information available to patients and their families that allows them to make informed decisions when selecting a health plan, hospital, or clinical practice, or when choosing among alternative treatments. This should include information that describes the system's performance on safety, EBP, and patient satisfaction. *Consider these related examples: interdisciplinary teams, informatics, informed consent, research, patient education, report cards, and national reports on quality and disparity.*

8. **Anticipation of needs.** Healthcare providers and the health system should not just react to events that may occur with patients but should anticipate patient needs and provide care needed. *Consider these related examples: assessment, interdisciplinary teams, nursing care, plan of care, HCO services, patient satisfaction, diversity, outcomes.*

9. **Continuous decrease in waste.** Resources should not be wasted—including patient time. *Consider these related examples: care delivery, costs of care, access to care and services, and issues of misuse, overuse, and underuse.*

10. **Cooperation among clinicians.** Collaboration and communication are critical among healthcare professionals and systems (interdisciplinary teamwork). *Consider these related examples: interdisciplinary team, plan of care.*

Envisioning the National Healthcare Quality Report

Envisioning the National Healthcare Quality Report (IOM, 2001b) is the follow-up report to the *Quality Chasm* (IOM, 2001a) report. It describes a framework to be used in collecting annual data about healthcare quality and focuses on how the healthcare delivery system performs in providing personal health care. The Agency for Health Resources and Quality (AHRQ), part of the U.S. Department of Health and Human Services (DHHS), is mandated to collect the data using this framework and to publish the annual report, which is available on the Internet. This report should "serve as a yardstick or the barometer by which to gauge progress in improving the performance of the healthcare delivery system in consistently providing high-quality care" (IOM, 2001b, p. 2). Later in this chapter, healthcare report cards are discussed. This annual national report card does not replace the need for individual HCOs to monitor their own quality. The information from the national annual report can be used by HCOs in developing services, by insurers and health policy makers, and by nurse educators in planning curricula and teaching-learning strategies.

The framework for the annual report uses a matrix. "The matrix is a tool to visualize possible combinations of the two dimensions (consumer perspectives and components of healthcare quality) of the framework and better understand how various aspects of the framework relate to one another" (IOM, 2001b, p. 8). The matrix is shown in Table 12–2.

This annual national report is designed to do the following (IOM, 2001b, p. 31):

- Supply a common understanding of quality and how to measure it that reflects the best current approaches and practices
- Identify aspects of the healthcare system that improve or impede quality
- Generate data associated with major quality initiatives
- Educate the public, the media, and other audiences about the importance of healthcare quality and the current level of quality

Table 12–2 MATRIX FOR THE ANNUAL NATIONAL HEALTHCARE QUALITY REPORT

Consumer Perspectives on Health Care Needs	Components of Health Care Quality			
	Safety	Effectiveness	Patient Centeredness	Timeliness
Staying Healthy				
Getting Better				
Living with Illness or Disability				
Coping with the End-of-Life				

Source: From *Envisioning the National Health Care Quality Report* (p. 61), by Institute of Medicine, Ed. M. Hurtado, E. Swift, & J. Corrigan, 2001, Washington, DC: National Academies Press. Reprinted with permission.

- Identify for policy makers the problem areas in healthcare quality that most need their attention and action, with the understanding that these priorities may change over time and differ by geographic location
- Provide policy makers, purchasers, healthcare providers, and others with realistic benchmarks for quality of care in the form of national, regional, and population comparisons
- Make it easier to compare the quality of the U.S. healthcare system with that of other nations
- Stimulate the refinement of existing measures and the development of new ones
- Stimulate data collection efforts at the state and local levels (mirroring the national effort) to facilitate targeted quality improvements
- Incorporate improved measures as they become available and practicable
- Clarify the many aspects of healthcare quality and how they affect one another and quality as a whole
- Encourage data collection efforts needed to refine and develop quality measures and, ultimately, stimulate the development of a health information infrastructure to support quality measurement and reporting

Quality Improvement

Implementing IOM QI approaches "requires that health professionals be clear about what they are trying to accomplish, what changes they can make that will result in an improvement, and how they will know that the improvement occurred" (IOM, 2003, p. 59). Healthcare complexity is mentioned many times as a barrier to understanding safety and quality and to improving healthcare delivery.

Why is health care so complex? Its consumers are very diverse in their needs, diagnoses, ethnic and cultural backgrounds, and overall health status, including genetic background, socioeconomic factors, patient preferences for health care, community differences, and healthcare coverage/reimbursement. Health care cannot be viewed in the same manner as other businesses (such as the automobile industry) that might have one product or a series of highly related products. Healthcare products vary based on the medical problem, the setting, the expertise of clinical staff, desires of the patient, treatment options, patient prognosis, and health policy and legislation. In specialty areas such as obstetrics, psychiatry, emergency care, intensive care, home care, and long-term care there is great variation within services—in their interventions, roles of the patient and family, patient education needs, prognosis and outcomes, and so on. It is expensive to develop and maintain effective quality improvement programs, but The Joint Commission requires such programs for all its accredited organizations. QI programs can lead to improved safety and quality, making them critical regardless of any pressure from The Joint Commission.

Because of the complex nature of quality, developing a QI program that addresses monitoring and improving healthcare quality is in itself a complex process. Effective appraisal of the scientific facts suggests that health care can be improved by closing the wide gaps between prevailing practices and the best known approaches to care, and by inventing new forms of care. This takes planning and careful evaluation of results. One model for improvement focuses on three key questions (Berwick & Nolan, 1998):

1. What is the healthcare organization trying to accomplish?
2. How will the healthcare organization know whether a change is an improvement?
3. What change can the healthcare organization try that it believes will result in improvement?

For an HCO to have an effective QI program, nurses and other health professionals need to be knowledgeable and competent in the following areas (Institute of Medicine, 2003, p. 59).

- Continually understand and measure quality of care in terms of structure, or the inputs into the system, such as patients, staff, and environments; process, or the interactions between clinicians and patients; and outcomes, or evidence about changes in patients' health status in relation to patient and community needs.
- Assess current practices and compare them with relevant better practices elsewhere as a means of identifying opportunities for improvement.
- Design and test interventions to change the process of care, with the objective of improving quality.
- Identify errors and hazards in care; understand and implement basic safety design principles, such as standardization and simplification and human factors training.
- Both act as an effective member of an interdisciplinary team and improve the quality of one's own performance through self-assessment and personal change.

Figure 12–2 illustrates the importance of quality in the healthcare system.

The Joint Commission

Accreditation is the process by which organizations are evaluated on their quality, based on established minimum standards. The major organization that accredits HCOs is **The Joint Commission**, a nonprofit organization that accredits more than 17,000 HCOs, including hospitals, long-term care organizations, home care agencies, clinical laboratories, ambulatory care organizations, behavioral health organizations, and healthcare networks or managed care organizations. It has been accrediting HCOs since 1951, and over

that time, the accreditation requirements and process have changed. Participating in a Joint Commission survey is time consuming and costly, but it is necessary. For example, a hospital must have current Joint Commission accreditation to have nursing students use its facility for practicum. As The Joint Commission has changed, its emphasis on quality and safety has also changed. Continuous quality improvement is now the major focus of the accreditation process.

Nurses serve on The Joint Commission Nursing Advisory Council, which advises The Joint Commission about nursing concerns and care issues related to safety and quality. All nurses who work in HCOs eventually experience

Figure 12–2 Medallion of quality health care through critical thinking.

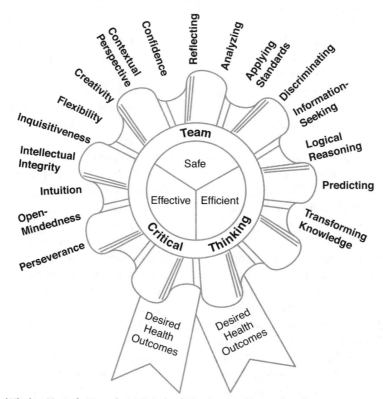

Source: From *Critical Thinking Tactics for Nurses*, by M.G. Rubenfeld and B. Scheffer, 2006, Sudbury, MA: Jones and Bartlett Publishers.

a Joint Commission survey. The Joint Commission makes a visit to the HCO every 3 years to complete its intensive survey and may even make unscheduled visits. For the scheduled visits, the HCO is given a date and has 9–12 months to prepare for the visit. Preparing for the visit involves gathering information and data for The Joint Commission, educating staff about the standards, conducting mock surveys to prepare staff, and so on. The HCO should meet standards at all times. In the past, great emphasis was placed on getting ready for The Joint Commission visit and surviving it; afterward, the HCO was less vigilant until the time to prepare for the next visit. This approach is less effective now because accredited HCOs must submit reports on certain data to The Joint Commission annually, with a plan of action for areas noted in the self-assessment requiring improvement (periodic performance review); in addition, now HCOs must be prepared for the chance of an unscheduled visit.

Nurses are very active in preparing for the survey and during the survey visit. The Joint Commission now involves more direct care staff in their visits by including them in meetings to discuss care in the HCO and asking individual staff questions during the survey. Students may even be asked questions. The goal is to find out if the patients are reaching expected outcomes, and if not, why. Examples of some outcomes that The Joint Commission assesses mortality rates, length-of-stay, adverse incidents, complications, readmission rates, patient/family satisfaction, referrals to specialists, patient adherence to discharge plans or treatment plans, and prevention adherence (e.g., mammogram, Pap smear, immunizations).

The Joint Commission standards have been developed, evaluated, and changed over the years to meet the changing needs of healthcare delivery. These standards form the framework for The Joint Commission accreditation. Standards cover three major areas:

1. *Patient-focused functions*: Ethics, rights, and responsibilities; provision of care, treatment, and services; medication management; and surveillance, prevention, and control of infection.
2. *Organization functions*: Improving organization performance; leadership; management of the environment of care; management of human resources; management of information.
3. *Structures and functions*: Medical staff; nursing.

Because The Joint Commission accredits a broad range of HCOs, there are differences in the minimal standards and in how different settings might monitor their safety and quality. One example is home care agencies; these agencies use national evaluation approaches that are not related to or led by The Joint Commission. The home care outcome-based approach to QI, the Outcome Assessment Information Set (OASIS), was developed in the 1990s by the DHHS to provide a "systematic process that would yield consistent data to improve care outcomes" (Mosocco, 2001, p. 205). The database focuses on a group of data elements that represent core items of a comprehensive assessment of home care patients. The key question is, Did the patient benefit from the home care services? In this type of system, home care agencies from all over the country input their QI data. OASIS is managed through the CMS.

Other organizations that focus on quality and safety in health care include those listed in Table 12–3.

Healthcare Report Cards

Healthcare report cards provide specific performance data on an organization at specific intervals, with a focus on quality and safety. The report can be used by the HCO to compare

Table 12–3 SELECTED QUALITY AND SAFETY ORGANIZATIONS AND SAMPLE OF INITIATIVES AFFECTING RNS IN HOSPITALS

Organization	Major National Initiatives Since 2000 Related to Nurses
Institute of Medicine	• Published high-profile reports on quality and safety of patient care: *To Err is Human: Building a Safer Health System* (2000) *Crossing the Quality Chasm: A New Health System for the 21st Century* (2001) *Keeping Patients Safe: Transforming the Work Environment of Nurses* (2004) • Advocated six aims to improve the quality of health-care systems (patient centered, safe, effective, equitable, timely, and efficient) (2001)
National Quality Forum	• Endorsed 15 national voluntary consensus standards for nursing-sensitive care in hospitals (2004)
Institute for Healthcare Improvement	• Implemented the national hospital 100,000 Lives Campaign (2005) • Implemented the national hospital 5 Million Lives Campaign (2006–2008)
The Joint Commission	• Established a national Nursing Advisory Committee (2003) • Endorsed the National Quality Forum's 15 national voluntary consensus standards for nursing-sensitive care in hospitals (2005) • Included nursing-sensitive measures in the hospital accreditation process (2005)
Robert Wood Johnson Foundation	• Developed the Transforming Care at the Bedside Initiative (2005) • Partnered with the Institute for Healthcare Improvement and American Organization of Nurse Executives (2007) • Developed Interdisciplinary Nursing Quality Research Initiative (2006)

Source: From *The Future of the Nursing Workforce in the United States: Data, Trends and Implications*, by P.I. Buerhaus, D.O. Staiger and D.I. Auerbach, 2009, Sudbury, MA: Jones and Bartlett Publishers.

its outcomes with report cards published by other HCOs or with a large state or national database. This information can be helpful in improving care in the HCO by identifying what the HCO is doing well and what needs improvement as compared with other similar HCOs. Some of these report cards are now accessible on the Internet and can be used by the consumer (patients, families). Nurses can use them when searching for new jobs to obtain evaluation data about a specific HCO. In some cases, insurers use them to assess an HCO and compare it with similar HCOs. The goal is to examine performance based on clearly defined criteria.

HOW DO REPORT CARDS RELATE TO NURSING?

In 1994, the ANA began an investigation of the impact of workforce restructuring and redesign on the safety and quality of patient care in acute care settings. This was around the time that the IOM was beginning to work on this issue, too. The ANA wanted to "explore the nature and strength of the linkages between nursing care and patient outcomes by identifying nursing quality indicators" (Pollard, Mitra, & Mendelson, 1996, p. 1). The result provided a framework for educating nurses, consumers, and policy makers about the contributions of nursing within the acute care setting by tracking the quality of nursing care provided in such settings. Databases and report cards that focus on measuring quality and that include nursing-specific quality indicators are needed. Patients come into the acute care setting primarily because they need 24-7 care, which is the focus of nursing care. This early study made it clear that data on nursing and outcomes were lacking. Old methods of collecting data were not nursing-specific.

This project identified 10 "nursing-sensitive indicators" that reflect characteristics of the nursing workforce, nursing processes, and patient outcomes. The ANA identified examples for each of these indicators (Montalvo & Dunton, 2007, p. 1):

- *Nursing Workforce*: Measures of the supply of nursing (e.g., total nursing hours per patient day); nursing skill (percent of nursing hours provided by RNs)
- *Nursing Processes*: Risk assessment; **protocol** implementation
- *Patient Outcomes*: Fall rates that are related to nursing hours; hospital-acquired pressure ulcer rates that are related to skill mix

After the 1994 survey, the ANA collaborated with seven state nurses associations on a pilot to test whether it was possible to collect data on the indicators from a large number of sites. As a result, in 1998, the ANA established the National Database of Nursing Quality Indicators (NDNQI). As of 2007, over 1,000 hospitals are participating. This initiative "provides each nurse the opportunity to review the evidence, evaluate their practice, and determine what improvements can be made" (Montalvo & Dunton, 2007, p. 3). The participating institutions submit their nursing-sensitive indicator data to the database. This allows for the collection of a large amount of data for evaluation and for research. What are the indicators (Montalvo & Dunton, 2007, p. 173)?

- Nursing Hours per Patient Day (RNs, licensed practical nurses (LPNs)/licensed vocational nurses (LVNs), unlicensed assistive personnel (UAPs)
- Patient Falls
- Patient Falls with Injury (injury level)
- Pediatric Pain Assessment, Intervention, Reassessment Cycle
- Pediatric Peripheral Intravenous Infiltration Rate
- Pressure Ulcer Prevalence (community acquired, hospital acquired, unit acquired)
- Psychiatric Physical/Sexual Assault Rate
- Restraint Prevalence
- RN Education/Certification
- RN Satisfaction Survey Options (Job satisfaction scales, practice environment scale)
- Skill Mix (Percent of total nursing hours supplied by RNs, LPNs/LVNs, UAPs; % of total nursing hours supplied by agency staff)

Indicators that will be added are voluntary nurse turnover, and nosocomial infections (urinary catheter-associated urinary tract infection, central line catheter-associated bloodstream infection, ventilator-associated pneumonia).

Data are collected quarterly for all indicators except for RN satisfaction, which is done annually. To assist with more effective comparison, reports are provided to hospitals with information about patient, unit type, and hospital bed size. This is the profession's quality report card. Participation in the process is voluntary.

The list of NDNQI indicators identifies some of the critical quality issues in health care that relate to nursing care. Other common issues in health care today are handwashing; medication errors; methycillin-resistant *Staphyloccus aureus* infection; wrong patient identification and consequences; wrong procedure; operating on the wrong area or limb; administering the wrong blood type; and using contaminated supplies, devices, and drugs. In nursing programs, students learn how to provide safe care through didactic content, simulation, laboratory experiences, and practicum. It is very important that as this learning occurs, students connect that care to the need to protect the patient and provide quality care.

Tools and Methods to Monitor and Improve Healthcare Delivery

HCOs use a variety of tools and methods to monitor safety and quality and to ensure improvement of quality. Nurses are involved in the use of all these tools and methods. Some examples follow.

Standards of Care

A standard is an authoritative statement that provides a minimum description of accepted actions that are expected from a healthcare organization or an individual healthcare provider, such as a nurse who has specific skill and knowledge levels. Standards are expectations about what should be done. Standards are developed by professional organizations and are derived from legal sources such as nurse practice acts and federal and state laws; they are also developed by regulatory agencies such as accreditation bodies and federal and state agencies as well as HCOs. These standards should be evidence based and supported by scientific literature. As discussed, there are standards of practice and standards for professional performance. Many are published by the ANA, and some specialty-area standards have been developed by specialty-focused nursing organizations. As discussed, The Joint Commission also uses standards in its accreditation process.

Policies and Procedures

Policies and procedures set standards within an HCO that guide decisions and how care is provided. Use of policies and procedures supports greater consistency in how care is delivered and can help to improve care. Policies and procedures should be evidence based, though there are care issues in nursing for which there is limited research evidence at this time. Policies and procedures for nurses and nursing care should not conflict with regulatory issues in the state (such as the state's nurse practice act), and they should be in agreement with nursing standards. A nurse uses policies and procedures daily in practice; for example, what is the accepted procedure in the hospital for administering blood products and medication administration, and for ensuring safety for patients at risk of falling? Policies and procedures need to be readily available to staff. Many HCOs have put their policies and procedures into their computer systems, reducing the need for hard copy policy and procedure manuals and making it easier for staff to access the information when needed. Nurses are expected to follow the HCO policies and procedures, which means that they need to know about them and how to seek out the information. Policies and procedures related to nursing care should be developed by nurses in the HCO and updated annually or as needed. As discussed in Chapter 11, many HCOs that are emphasizing EBP are reviewing and updating their policies and procedures based on EBP or evidence.

Licensure and Credentialing

Professional licensure verification is an important activity in all HCOs. This includes licensure for RNs, LPNs/LVNs, MDs, and others. Why is this done? A license means that the person has met expected minimal standards set by the state practice act. State laws require that certain healthcare providers have licenses. If an HCO allows someone to practice without a license, the HCO and the individual are breaking the law. Credentialing is different from checking licensure, though this is part of the process. Credentialing is a more in-depth review process that includes evaluation of licenses, certification if required in a specialty area, evidence of malpractice insurance as required, history of involvement in malpractice suits, and education. Credentialing is not done for all healthcare staff; it is primarily used for physicians who want to practice or admit to an HCO, for nurse-midwives, and for nurse practitioners. Credentialing would not be done for RNs who are not in an advanced practice position. Licensure and credentialing information is kept on file and may be reviewed by The Joint Commission during a survey.

UTILIZATION REVIEW/MANAGEMENT

Utilization review/management (UR/UM) is the process of evaluating the necessity, appropriateness, and efficiency of healthcare services for specific patients or in patient populations. Data from UR are used by the HCO in a number of ways—for example, to assess access and usage of services; to determine that a service is no longer needed; to determine that a new service is needed; and to review the relationship of data to patient outcomes. UR data are connected to financial concerns for the HCO and its budget (e.g., whether the HCO is serving enough patients to meet its budget, types of procedures and their reimbursement, and so on). UR is administered by the HCO administration, though nurses may participate as data collectors and in the analysis process. Data are primarily obtained from medical records to determine necessity, appropriateness, and timeliness of healthcare services.

RISK MANAGEMENT

The goal of **risk management (RM)** is "to maintain a safe and effective healthcare environment and prevent or reduce loss to the healthcare organization" (Pike, Janssen, & Brooks, 2002, p. 3). RM is concerned with decreasing financial loss to the HCO that is due to legal and malpractice issues. RM monitors errors and incidents and works with QI to decrease errors. If there is an error, RM would evaluate the risk for a lawsuit and take actions as required. HCO attorneys are very involved in RM, and in some HCOs, RNs with a legal background are hired to work in the RM department or to consult with the department. RNs have considerable knowledge about healthcare delivery and can be excellent resources.

BENCHMARKING

Many hospitals and other types of HCOs use benchmarking.

> *{Benchmarking is} the concept of discovering what is the best performance being achieved, whether in your company, by a competitor, or by an entirely different industry. Benchmarking is an improvement tool whereby a company measures its performance or process against other companies' best practices, determines how those companies achieved their performance levels, and uses the information to improve its own performance. Benchmarking is a continuous process whereby an enterprise measures and compares all its functions, systems and practices against strong competitors, identifying quality gaps in the organization, and striving to achieve competitive advantage locally and globally. (Six Sigma, 2008)*

One of the popular benchmarking approaches is Six Sigma.

> *This is a rigorous and a systematic methodology that utilizes information (management by facts) and statistical analysis to measure and improve a company's operational performance, practices and systems by identifying and preventing "defects" in manufacturing and service-related processes in order to anticipate and exceed expectations of all stakeholders to accomplish effectiveness. (Six Sigma, 2008)*

ASSESSMENT OF ACCESS TO HEALTHCARE SERVICES

Access to healthcare services is important to monitor and improve. Communities are concerned about whether their citizens have access to care. *Healthy People 2010* (U.S. DHHS, 2000) looks at access as a critical issue across the country and for all types of healthcare needs. When a patient does not have access, his or her health status is at risk, and further complications may occur. Access is not a simple concept; it can mean any of the following:

- Ability to get to a healthcare appointment (transportation, funds for transportation)
- Ability to get an appointment for needed care
- Ability to access specialty care when needed
- Ability to pay for care or having an outside source for payment, such as insurance
- Ability to understand when care is needed
- Ability to understand information and language
- Ability to get an appointment in the time frame needed (e.g., appointment time, day of week)
- Ability to access physical facility (does the facility have handicap provisions?)
- Ability to get diagnostic tests and reports in a timely manner
- Ability to choose providers

Vulnerable populations that often have limited access are low-income individuals, children and adolescents, minorities, homeless persons, the mentally ill, the uninsured, the disabled, elderly veterans, immigrants, and prisoners.

EVIDENCE-BASED PRACTICE

Evidence-based practice was discussed extensively in Chapter 11; however, it is relevant here because it is a method of improving the quality of care. Basing care decisions on evidence can better ensure that care needs are met in an effective manner. For example, clinical guidelines, as discussed in Chapter 11, are a source of evidence to improve care and implement EBP. The AHRQ is a government agency that develops guidelines and serves as a repository of guidelines (see http://www.guidelines.gov/). The AHRQ's goals are to (1) support improvements in health outcomes, (2) promote patient safety and reduce medication errors, (3) advance the use of information technology for coordinating patient care and conducting quality and outcomes research, and (4) establish an Office of Priority Populations (this office should ensure that low-income groups, minorities, women, children, the elderly, and individuals with special needs receive care). The IOM defines clinical guidelines as "systematically developed statements to assist practitioner and patient decisions about appropriate healthcare for specific clinical circumstances" (IOM, 1990, p. 38).

CLINICAL PATHWAYS/PROTOCOLS

Clinical pathways were discussed in Chapter 11; however, it is important here to recognize their use in the assessment of quality and cost of health care and how they increase consistency of care. Pathways describe how care is best provided for a specific patient population with specific problem(s); however, a pathway needs to be assessed for applicability to an individual patient's needs. The pathway helps the healthcare provider focus on outcomes and the assessment of achievement; in doing this, outcomes serve as a benchmarking method for individual patients. If outcomes are not met, the provider can consider the variances for the individual patient, and collecting and reviewing data from multiple patients can help to improve care for a certain patient population with certain problems.

INSTITUTIONAL REVIEW BOARD

Use of an Institutional Review Board (IRB), discussed in Chapter 11, is the key method for ensuring informed consent and protection of human participants in research. This method also ensures, through its process, that patients who are participants in studies are not harmed unnecessarily.

HEALTHCARE POLICY AND LEGISLATION

Healthcare policy and legislation may mandate how care should be delivered to ensure safe, quality care. A current example is legislation related to whether mandatory overtime can be used. This issue is important because there are questions about how many hours a nurse can work without increasing the risk for errors.

Patient Outcomes and Nursing Care: We Do Make a Difference

Keeping Patients Safe: Transforming the Work Environment of Nurses (IOM, 2004a) focuses on acute care or care that is provided in the hospital setting; however, it is relevant here because much of the content can be applied to nursing in other types of settings. As the report states, "When we are hospitalized, in a nursing home, or managing a chronic condition in our own homes—at some of our most vulnerable moments—nurses are the healthcare providers we are most likely to encounter, spend the greatest amount of time with, and be dependent upon for our recovery" (IOM, 2004a, p. ix). The report emphasizes designs for a work environment in which nurses can provide safer, higher quality patient care. The content discusses the nursing shortage, healthcare errors, patient safety risk factors, the central role of the nurse in patient safety, and work environment threats to patient safety. In discussing errors, the IOM emphasizes moving away from a punitive, blaming environment and states that errors need to be viewed more from a system perspective. Some of the factors that influence errors from a system perspective are highlighted in this report and include equipment failures, inadequate staff training, lack of clear supervision and direction, and inadequate staffing levels. The central message in the report is that we need a transformation of the work environment.

This critical report identifies six major concerns for direct care in nursing (IOM, 2004a):

1. *Monitoring patient status or surveillance*, which, according to the report, is different from assessment. **Surveillance** is defined as "purposeful and *ongoing* acquisition, interpretation, and synthesis of patient data for clinical decision-making" (McCloskey & Bulechek, 2000, p. 629). If surveillance is not successful, the result may be termed **failure to rescue**—missing an opportunity to prevent complications.
2. *Physiologic therapy*, the most common visible interventions that nurses perform.
3. *Helping patients compensate for loss of function*; many related activities are performed by UAPs under the direction of RNs, but RNs do this as well.
4. *Providing emotional support,* critical for patients and their families.
5. *Education for patients and families*, which has become more difficult for practicing nurses to provide because of work conditions, the staffing shortage, patient acuity, and shorter length of stay.
6. *Integration and coordination of care*; patients' needs are complex, and care is complex, often resulting in multiple forms of care provided by multiple providers. There is a high risk of failures in communication and inadequate collaboration, both of which increase the risk of errors. There is a critical need for interdisciplinary teams.

REPORT RECOMMENDATIONS AND IMPLICATIONS

The report recommends (1) adopting transformational leadership and evidence-based management, (2) maximizing the capability of the workforce, (3) understanding work processes so that they can be improved, and (4) creating and sustaining cultures of safety. Nursing leadership must be very active throughout the HCO; nurse leaders must represent staff, support the need for effective change, facilitate input from direct-care nursing staff, and expand communication and collaboration. The HCO needs to support ongoing learning—for example, through effective orientation for appropriate length of time; ongoing training; nursing residency programs; funding support for nurses to return to school; establishing partnerships with schools of nursing; providing opportunities for interdisciplinary educational experiences; and so on. All this requires resources that administrations must ensure are available. Adequate staffing is critical, and all HCOs are struggling with how to fill positions and retain staff. Staffing issues also include scheduling, nurse–patient ratios, and workloads (staffing is discussed in Chapter 14). The report comments on 12-hour shifts and the potential for greater risk of errors when staff are tired and stressed. Excessive paperwork can lead to less time for patients, which can impact safety and quality. There is a need for computerized documentation with decision-making support, as discussed in Chapter 13. Work design is discussed in depth in the report; physical space and design—for example, lighting, size of the unit, and the ability to get to equipment easily and quickly—and how these may impact safety are addressed.

The Joint Commission noted in 2004 that "inadequate orientation and training is a factor in 58% of serious medication errors. Staffing levels impacted 24% of 1,609 sentinel events over the past 5 years." As mentioned earlier in this chapter, the HCO needs to commit to developing and maintaining a culture of safety, and this must include staff safety issues. Throughout all of the recommendations is the need for EBP and the need to base decisions on evidence. "As nurses are the largest component of the healthcare workforce, and are also strongly involved in the commission, detection, and prevention of errors and adverse events, they and their work environment are critical elements of stronger patient safety defenses" (IOM, 2004a, p. 31). Table 12–4 provides examples of studies that examined quality and nursing care.

Conclusion

The IOM notes that with the need for change in the healthcare system, the following is critical:

> *The 21st century healthcare system envisioned by the committee—providing care that is evidence-based, patient centered, and systems-oriented—also implies new roles and responsibilities for patients and their families, who must become more aware, more participative, and more demanding in a care system that should be meeting their needs. And all involved must be united by the overarching purpose of reducing the burden of illness, injury, and disability in our nation. (IOM, 2001a, p. 20)*

CHAPTER HIGHLIGHTS

1. QI is aimed at processes that critically examine the level of care, any problems with care, and how to make patient outcomes better.
2. Safety goes hand in hand with quality care and improved patient outcomes.
3. In the fall of 2007, the CMS introduced a major change, stating that CMS will not

Table 12–4 REPRESENTATIVE STUDIES REPORTING AN ASSOCIATION BETWEEN HOSPITAL NURSE STAFFING AND PATIENT OUTCOMES

Patient Outcome	Study
Nosocomial infection	Flood & Diers (1988) Giraud et al. (1993) Archibald, Manning, & Bell (1997)
Sepsis/bloodstream infections	Pronovost et al. (1999) Amaravaid, Dimick, Pronovost, & Lipsett (2000) Dimick, Swoboda, Pronovost, & Lipsett (2001) Fridkin, Pear, Williamson, Galgiani, & Jarvis (1996) Cimiotti, Hass, Saiman, & Larson (2006)
Pneumonia	Needleman, Buerhaus, Mattke, Stewart, & Zelevinsky (2002) Kovner & Gergen (1998) Pronovost et al. (1999) Amaravaidi et al. (2000) Dimick et al. (2001) Network (2000) Unruh (2003)
Urinary tract infection	Needleman et al. (2002) Kovner & Gergen (1998) Network (2000) Blegen, Goode, & Reed (1998)
Falls	Blegen & Vaughn (1998) Wan & Shukla (1987) Sovie & Jawad (2001) Langemo, Anderson, & Volden (2002)
Upper gastrointestinal bleeding	Needleman et al. (2002)
Medication errors	Blegen et al. (1998) Blegen & Vaughn (1998)
Shock and cardiac arrest Pressure ulcers	Needleman et al. (2002) Network (2000) Unruh (2003) Blegen et al. (1998)
Longer than expected length of stay	Needleman et al. (2002) Schultz, van Servellen, Chang, McNeese-Smith, & Waxenberg (1998) Pronovost et al. (1999) Amaravaidi et al. (2000) Network (2000) Dimick et al. (2001) Flood & Diers (1988) Langemo et al. (2002)

Source: From *The Future of the Nursing Workforce in the United States: Data, Trends and Implications*, by P.I. Buerhaus, D.O. Staiger and D.I. Auerbach, 2009, Sudbury, MA: Jones and Bartlett Publishers.

pay for complications that occur in the hospital that could have been prevented.

4. Opportunity costs relate to situations in which diagnostic tests must be repeated or a change in the plan of care is necessary because of adverse reactions to treatment.

5. Because of a lack of trust of healthcare delivery, more patients are demanding that they be informed about their care and involved in the care process.

6. *Safety*: Freedom from accidental injury.

7. *Error*: The failure of a planned action to be completed as intended or the use of the wrong plan to achieve an aim; errors are directly related to outcomes.

8. *Adverse event*: An injury resulting from a medical intervention (in other words, the injury is not due to the patient's underlying condition).

9. *Misuse*: Avoidable complications that prevent patients from receiving the full potential benefit of a service.

10. *Overuse*: The potential for harm from the provision of a service exceeds the possible benefit.

11. *Underuse*: Failure to provide a service that would have produced a favorable outcome for the patient.

12. *Near miss*: Recognition that an event occurred that might have led to an adverse event.

13. *Sentinel event*: An event that had a negative patient outcome (unexpected death or serious physical or psychological injury or serious risk).

14. *Root cause analysis*: An in-depth analysis of an error to assess the event and identify causes and possible solutions.

15. Errors are generally systems errors, not individual problems.

16. There is a strong recommendation to move to a culture of safety. To accomplish

this, there must be (1) greater understanding of its essential elements, (2) a decrease in barriers to creating the culture, (3) development and implementation of strategies to create the safety culture, and (4) evaluation of outcomes (IOM, 2004a).

17. Some of the key safety issues for nursing staff are needlesticks, infections, ergonomic safety, violence, and chemical exposures.

18. Safety initiatives include the IHI 5 Million Lives Campaign; the IHI and RWJF's TCAB initiative; and The Joint Commission annual safety goals.

19. Quality of care is usually measured by structure, process, and outcomes.

20. The six aims, or goals for improvement, state that care should be safe, effective, patient-centered, timely, efficient, and equitable (IOM, 2001a).

21. The IOM developed new rules for the 21st century to guide care delivery. These rules, which are directly related to the six aims and to the healthcare professions core competencies, are (1) care based on continuous healing relationships, (2) customization based on patient needs and values, (3) the patient as control source, (4) shared knowledge and free flow of information, (5) evidence-based decision making, (6) safety as a system property, (7) the need for transparency, (8) anticipation of needs, (9) continuous decrease in waste, and (10) cooperation among clinicians

22. The IOM suggests collecting healthcare quality data annually. The data should focus on delivery of care within the context of personal health care. This is a published report to make health care transparent. It uses a matrix to visually depict consumer

perspectives and components of quality of care.

23. The Joint Commission standards for QI focus on patient-focused functions, organizational functions, and structural functions.

24. Healthcare report cards provide specific performance data about an organization at specific intervals, with a focus on quality and safety.

25. Nursing's report card resulted in the provision of a framework for educating nurses, consumers, and policy makers about nursing's contributions within the acute care setting by tracking the quality of nursing care provided in acute care settings. Data were collected in the areas of nursing-sensitive indicators that reflect the nursing workforce, nursing process, and patient outcomes.

26. Nursing-sensitive indicators include nursing hours per patient day, patient falls, pediatric pain assessment, pediatric peripheral intravenous infiltration rate, pressure ulcer prevalence (community acquired, hospital acquired, and unit acquired), psychiatric physical/sexual assault rate, restraint prevalence, RN education/certification, RN satisfaction, and skill mix.

27. Tools used to measure and monitor safety and quality include standards of care, policies and procedures, licensure and credentialing, UR/UM, risk management, benchmarking, access to care, EBP, clinical pathways, IRBs, and healthcare policy and legislation.

28. Nursing care contributes to health care because nurses are the interface between the patient and the system.

29. *Keeping Patients Safe* (IOM, 2004a) recommended the following: (1) adopting transformational leadership and evidence-based management, (2) maximizing the capability of the workforce, (3) understanding work processes so that they can be improved, and (4) creating and sustaining cultures of safety.

Linking to the Internet

- Institute for Healthcare Improvement
  http://www.ihi.org
- Centers for Medicare and Medicaid Services, OASIS Program
  http://www.cms.hhs.gov/OASIS/
- The Joint Commission
  http://www.jointcommission.org/
- American Nurses Association
  http://www.nursingworld.org
- U.S. Department of Labor, Occupational Safety & Health Administration
  http://www.osha.gov/
- Occupational Safety and Health Administration, Workplace Violence
  http://www.osha.gov/SLTC/workplaceviolence/

DISCUSSION QUESTIONS

1. How do the aims identified to improve quality relate to the rules for the 21st century and the healthcare core competencies?
2. Describe the culture of safety.
3. What is accreditation? Also describe the major source of accreditation for healthcare organizations.
4. Discuss the definition of quality.
5. If you had to explain the importance of the safety and quality reports to someone outside health care, how would you do this?
6. Describe four tools and methods used to improve care.

CRITICAL THINKING ACTIVITIES

1. Divide up into teams, with each team taking one of the rules for the 21st century. Develop a defense for this rule and share with other teams.
2. Visit the National Healthcare Quality Report site (http://nhqrnet.ahrq.gov/nhqr/jsp/nhqr.jsp). After reviewing data on the dimensions of quality, what have you learned? Select one of the clinical conditions and summarize key issues. Share this with others who have reviewed different clinical conditions.
3. Visit the OASIS site (http://www.cms.hhs.gov/OASIS/) and then visit http://www.cms.hhs.gov/HomeHealthQualityInits/10_HHQIQualityMeasures.asp#TopOfPage to review the specific quality measures in the database. Why would these be important in home care nursing?
4. Learn more about NDNQI by going to: http://www.nursingquality.org/FAQPage.aspx Review some of the frequently asked questions that interest you. Discuss in a small group.
5. Visit the OSHA Workplace Violence site (http://www.osha.gov/SLTC/workplaceviolence/) to learn about this important staff safety problem and possible solutions. Review the guidelines for healthcare workplace violence. What solutions are recommended, and what is your opinion of the solutions?
6. Select one of the common safety and quality care issues, such as handwashing, decubiti, and so on, and search for information about the topic and how care can be improved.

CASE STUDY

A 21-year-old-woman presents to the emergency department (ED) of an urban hospital with a history of systemic lupus. Her complaint is dehydration, dizziness, and feeling faint. The woman also has a recent history of being dehydrated, complicated by renal involvement from the lupus, and having to receive bolus fluids. She is currently on multiple medications, including steroids and methotrexate.

An IV is started and labs drawn. The ED physician returns to pronounce the lab values within normal limits, yet the young woman feels no better. She states that she still feels dehydrated, that her blood pressure is low, and that she normally receives more IV fluids and a steroid injection. The physician indicates that he feels no need, but when she insists on more fluids, he agrees to continue them for a while and to give her an injection of steroids. The patient states, "Do you want to give me antinausea medication first?" The physician states that there is no indication. Again, the patient tells him that she is always nauseated following steroids and some-times vomits if no antiemetic is administered first. The physician argues but finally grows tired and walks away. The steroid injection is given, and nausea ensues. The patient calls her rheumatologist and urologist (neither had been available when the illness occurred because of the late hour). They repeat her labs the next day, only to find that she is severely dehydrated, and many values, including renal panel, are outside normal limits. This case presents a lack of responsiveness to patient information and compromised patient safety and quality. It does not represent EBP nor patient-centered care.

References

American Hospital Association. (1999). *Hospital statistics*. Chicago: Author.

American Nurses Association. (2003). *Handle with care*. Retrieved February 28, 2008, from http://www.nursingworld.org/MainMenuCategories/Occupational andEnvironmental/occupationalhealth/handle withcare/Resources/FactSheet.aspx

Anderson, D. (2006). Creating a culture of safety: Leadership, teams, and tools. *Nurse Leader, 4*(5), 28–41.

Berwick, D., & Nolan, T. (1998). Physicians as leaders improving healthcare. *Annals of Internal Medicine, 128*, 289–292.

Castro, A. (2004). Handle with Care: The American Nurses Association's Campaign to address work-related musculoskeletal disorders. *Online Journal of Issues in Nursing, 9*(3). Retrieved May 15, 2008, from http://www.nursingworld.org/MainMenuCategories/ANAMarketplace/ANAPeriodicals/OJIN.aspx

Centers for Disease Control and Prevention, National Center for Health Statistics. (1998). Births and deaths: Preliminary data for 1998. *National Vital Statistics Report, 47*(25), 6.

Chassin, M., & Galvin, R. (1998). The urgent need to improve healthcare quality. *Journal of the American Medical Association, 280*, 1000–1005.

Diaz, M. H., Silkaitis, C., Malczynski, M., Noskin, G. A., Warren, J. R., & Zembower, T. (2008). Contamination of examination gloves in patient rooms and implications for transmission of antimicrobial-resistant microorganisms. *Infection Control and Hospital Epidemiology, 29*(1), 63–65.

Donabedian, A. (1980). *Explorations in quality assessment and monitoring, Vol. I: The definition of quality and approaches to its assessment*. Ann Arbor, MI: Health Administration Press.

Environmental Working Group, Healthcare Without Harm, American Nurses Association, & Environmental Health Education Center of the University of Maryland's School of Nursing. (2007). Retrieved February 28, 2008, from http://www.ewg.org/sites/nurse_survey/analysis/main.php

Gates, D., & Kroeger, D. (2007, December). Violence against nurses: The silent epidemic. *Ohio Nurse*, 8–10.

Institute of Healthcare Improvement. (2008). Retrieved February 26, 2008, from http://www.ihi.org/IHI/

Institute of Medicine. (IOM). (1990). *Clinical practice guidelines: Directions for a new program*. Washington, DC: National Academies Press.

Institute of Medicine. (1999). *To err is human*. Washington, DC: National Academies Press.

Institute of Medicine. (2001a). *Crossing the quality chasm*. Washington, DC: National Academies Press.

Institute of Medicine. (2001b). *Envisioning the national healthcare quality report*. Washington, DC: National Academies Press.

Institute of Medicine. (IOM). (2003). *Health professions education: A bridge to quality*. Washington, DC: National Academies Press.

Institute of Medicine. (2004a). *Keeping patients safe: Transforming the work environment for nurses*. Washington, DC: National Academies Press.

Institute of Medicine. (2004b). *Patient safety: Achieving a new standard for care.* Washington, DC: National Academies Press.

The Joint Commission. (2004). The Joint Commission press kit. Retrieved October 5, 2007, from http://www.jointcommission.org/NewsRoom/PressKits/

McCloskey, J., & Bulechek, G. (2000). *Nursing interventions classification (NIC).* St. Louis, MO: Mosby.

Montalvo, I., & Dunton, N. (2007). *Transforming nursing data into quality care: Profiles of quality improvement in U.S. healthcare facilities.* Silver Spring, MD: American Nurses Association.

Mosocco, D. (2001). Data management using outcomes-based quality improvement. *Home Care Provider, 12,* 205–211.

Occupational Safety and Health Administration. (2004). Retrieved February 28, 2008, from http://www.osha.gov/Publications/OSHA3148/osha3148.html

Pike, J., Jansen, R., & Brooks, P. (2002). Role and function of a hospital risk manager. *Journal of Legal Nurse Consultants, 13*(2), 3–13.

Plsek, P. (2001). Redesigning healthcare with insights from the science of complex adaptive systems. In Institute of Medicine, *Crossing the quality chasm* (pp. 309–322). Washington, DC: National Academies Press.

Pollard, P., Mitra, K., & Mendelson, D. (1996). *Nursing report card for acute care.* Washington, DC: American Nurses Publishing.

Polygreen, P. M., Chen, Y., Beekmann, S., Srinivasan, A., Neill, M. A., Gay, T., et al. (2008). Infectious Diseases Society of America's Emerging Infections Network. *Clinical Infectious Diseases, 46*(1), 14–19.

Reason, J. (2000). Human error: Models and management. *British Medical Journal, 320*(7237), 768–770.

Six Sigma. (2008). Retrieved February 27, 2008, from http://main.isixsigma.com/

Thomas, E., Studdert, J., Newhouse, J., Zbar, B., Howard, K., Williams, E., et al. (1999). Costs of medical injuries in Utah and Colorado. *Inquiry, 36,* 255–264.

U.S. Department of Health and Human Services. (2000). *Healthy People 2010.* Washington, DC: U.S. Government Printing Office.

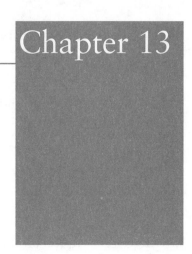

Chapter 13

Utilize Informatics

CHAPTER OUTLINE

INFORMATICS: TYPES AND METHODS
The Future of Informatics and Medical Technology
HIPAA: ENSURING CONFIDENTIALITY
TELEHEALTH
INTERNET
OTHER TECHNOLOGY: BIOMEDICAL AND PATIENT CARE EQUIPMENT
HIGH-TOUCH CARE VERSUS HIGH-TECH CARE
CONCLUSION
CHAPTER HIGHLIGHTS
LINKING TO THE INTERNET
DISCUSSION QUESTIONS
CRITICAL THINKING ACTIVITIES
CASE STUDY
WORDS OF WISDOM
REFERENCES

KEY TERMS

- ❏ Clinical data repository
- ❏ Clinical decision support systems
- ❏ Clinical information system (CIS)
- ❏ Coding system
- ❏ Computer literacy
- ❏ Data
- ❏ Data analysis software
- ❏ Databank
- ❏ Database
- ❏ Data mining
- ❏ Electronic medical record (EMR)
- ❏ E-mail list
- ❏ Encryption
- ❏ Health Insurance Portability and Accountability Act of 1996 (HIPAA)
- ❏ Informatics
- ❏ Information

- ❏ Information literacy
- ❏ Knowledge
- ❏ Minimum data set
- ❏ National Database of Nursing Quality Indicators
- ❏ Nomenclature
- ❏ Nursing informatics
- ❏ Personal digital assistants
- ❏ Personal health record (PHR)
- ❏ Professional order entry system (POES)
- ❏ Security protections
- ❏ Software
- ❏ Standardized language
- ❏ Telehealth
- ❏ Telenursing
- ❏ Wisdom

Introduction

This chapter concludes the section that focuses on the Institute of Medicine (IOM) healthcare profession core competencies with a discussion about

the fifth core competency: utilize informatics. Informatics/information technology (IT) is an important topic in all areas of life today, with the explosion of technology that provides many opportunities for communication and sharing of knowledge. The impact of informatics on nursing care is explored. Other issues that need to be addressed are documentation, confidentiality and privacy of information, and telehealth. This chapter also includes content about biomedical equipment; this is not necessarily directly related to informatics, but it is another example of the growth of technology in health care. Some of this equipment also uses IT. Nurses today cannot avoid technology, whether it is used for communication or for care provision. The chapter concludes with discussion of the concern about high-touch care versus high-tech care: How do they relate? This is an important issue for nurses to consider. Figure 13–1 identifies key elements in this chapter.

The IOM Competency: Utilize Informatics

The IOM description of the fifth healthcare profession core competency is: "communicate, man-age knowledge, mitigate error, and support decision making using information technology" (IOM, 2003, p. 4). **Informatics** is more than just understanding what IT is, but rather how that technology is used to prevent errors and improve care. From the initial use of computers to manage financial records to the current use of informatics, there has been a major move toward IT application in care. Some examples are greater use of informatics to find evidence to implement evidence-based practice (EBP); use of informatics in research; greater consumer access to information via the Internet; and more specific clinical applications, such as reminder and decision systems, telehealth, teleradiology, online prescribing, and use of e-mail for provider–provider communication and patient–provider communication. Additional details and examples are discussed later in this chapter. The IOM concludes that every healthcare professional should meet the following competencies (2003, p. 63):

Figure 13–1 Utilize informatics: Key elements.

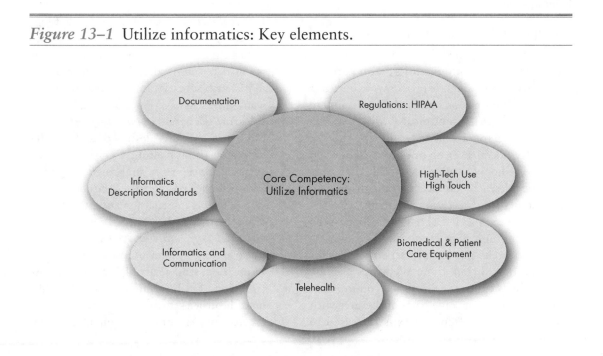

- Employ word processing, presentation, and data analysis software.
- Search, retrieve, manage, and make decisions using electronic data from internal information databases and external online databases and the Internet.
- Communicate using e-mail, instant messaging, e-mail lists, and file transfers.
- Understand security protections such as access control, data security, and data encryption, and directly address ethical and legal issues related to the use of IT in practice.
- Enhance education and access to reliable health information for patients.

Informatics

Informatics is complex, and the fact that it is changing daily makes it even harder to keep current. Healthcare delivery has been strongly influenced by the changes in informatics, but what is informatics?

Definitions and Description

Informatics has opened doors to many innovative methods of communication with patients and between providers. It often saves time, but can lead to information overload. Physicians are using e-mail to communicate with patients (e.g., sending appointment reminders, sharing lab results, and answering questions). The Web has provided opportunities to build communities of people with common chronic diseases to help them with disease management. Healthcare organizations (HCOs) have developed Web sites to share information about their organizations with the public (a marketing tool for services). In addition, these Web sites provide HCOs with a window for internal communication; staff can access some parts of the sites with special passwords. Informatics is also used to

evaluate the performance of the HCO and individual healthcare providers. IT has a major impact on quality improvement (QI); today, it is much easier to collect, store, and analyze large amounts of data that in the past were collected by hand. Insurers rely heavily on informatics to provide insurance coverage, manage data, and analyze performance, which has a direct impact on whether care is covered for reimbursement. Informatics has allowed governments at all levels—local, state, national, and international—to collect and use data for policy decision making and evaluation.

KEY TERMS RELATED TO INFORMATICS

Informatics has its own language and is a highly specialized area. Nurses do not have to be informatics experts, but they do need to understand the basics. Some terms have become so common that the majority of people know what they are (such as *Internet* and *e-mail*). Some terms that are useful to know are listed next.

- *Clinical data repository*: A physical or logical compendium of patient data pertaining to health; an "information warehouse" that stores data longitudinally and in multiple forms, such as text, voice, and images (American Nurses Association [ANA], 2008).
- *Clinical decision support systems*: Computer applications designed to facilitate human decision making. Decision support systems are typically rule based. They use a knowledge base and a set of rules to analyze data and information and provide recommendations (ANA, 2008).
- *Clinical information system*: A clinical information system (CIS) supports the acquisition, storage, manipulation, and distribution of clinical information throughout a healthcare organization, with a focus on electronic communication. This system

uses IT that is applied at the point of clinical care. Typical CIS components are electronic medical records (EMRs), clinical data repositories, decision support programs (such as application of clinical guidelines and drug interaction checking), handheld devices for collecting data and viewing reference material, imaging modalities, and communication tools such as electronic messaging systems.

- *Coding system*: A set of agreed-on symbols (frequently numeric or alphanumeric) that are attached to concept representation or terms to allow exchange of concept representations or terms with regard to their form or meaning. Examples are the Perioperative Nursing Data Set (PNDS) and the Clinical Care Classification (CCC) System (ANA, 2008).
- *Computer literacy*: The knowledge and skills required to use basic computer applications and computer technology.
- *Data*: Discrete entities that are described objectively without interpretation.
- *Data analysis software*: Computer software that can analyze data.
- *Data mining*: Locating and identifying unknown patterns and relationships within data.
- *Databank*: A large store of information; may include several databases.
- *Database*: A collection of interrelated data that are organized according to a scheme to serve one or more applications. The data are stored so that they can be used by several programs without concern for data structures or organization. An example is the **National Database of Nursing Quality Indicators** (ANA, 2008).
- *E-mail List*: A list of e-mail addresses that can be used to send one e-mail to many addresses at one time.

- *Encryption*: To change information into a code, usually for security reasons, to limit access.
- *Information literacy*: The ability to recognize when information is needed and to locate, evaluate, and effectively use that information (ANA, 2008).
- *Information*: Data that are interpreted, organized, or structured.
- *Knowledge*: Information that is synthesized so that relationships are identified and formalized (ANA, 2008).
- *Minimum data set*: The minimum categories of data with uniform definitions and categories; they concern a specific aspect or dimension of the healthcare system that meets the basic needs of multiple data users. An example is the Nursing Minimum Data Set (ANA, 2008).
- *Nomenclature*: A system of designations (terms) that is elaborated according to pre-established rules. Examples include Systematized Nomenclature of Medicine—Clinical Terms (SNOMED CT) International, and the International Classification for Nursing Practice (ANA, 2008).
- *Security protections* (access control, data security, and data encryption): Methods used to ensure that information is not read or taken by authorized persons.
- *Software*: Computer programs and applications.
- *Standardized language*: A collection of terms with definitions for use in informational systems databases. A standardized language enables comparisons to be made because the same term is used to denote the same condition. Standardized language is necessary for documentation in electronic health records (ANA, 2008).
- *Wisdom*: The appropriate use of knowledge to solve human problems; understanding

when and how to apply knowledge (ANA, 2008).

Nursing Standards: Scope and Standards of Nursing Informatics

Nursing informatics (NI) is a specialty that integrates nursing science, computer science, and information science to manage and communicate data, information, knowledge, and wisdom in nursing practice. NI supports consumers, patients, nurses, and other providers in their decision-making in all roles and settings. This support is accomplished through the use of information structures, information processes, and IT. The goal of NI is to improve the health of populations, communities, families, and individuals by optimizing information management and communication. (ANA, 2008, p. 1)

This specialty area has expanded, and all nurses need to understand basic IT concepts and their application to nursing practice. Undergraduate nursing programs often include IT in the curriculum, sometimes as a course on informatics, but not all programs include this content. This is now a problem because of the emphasis on informatics as a healthcare profession core competency. Some schools of nursing offer master's degrees in nursing informatics.

Three major concepts related to information are important to understand (Englebardt & Nelson, 2002):

- Data are discrete entities that are described objectively without interpretation.
- Information is defined as data that are interpreted, organized, or structured.
- Knowledge is information that is synthesized so that relationships are identified and formalized.

The flow from data to wisdom can be described as data naming, collecting, and organizing following this pattern: (1) information—organizing and interpreting; (2) knowledge—interpreting, integrating, and understanding; and (3) wisdom—understanding, applying, and applying with compassion. Figure 13–2 illustrates this flow.

"Wisdom is defined as the appropriate use of knowledge to manage and solve human problems. It is knowing when and how to apply knowledge to deal with complex problems or specific human needs" (Nelson & Joos, 1989, p. 6). "While knowledge focuses on what is known, wisdom focuses on the appropriate application of that knowledge. For example, a knowledge base may include several options for managing an anxious family, while wisdom would help decide which option is most appropriate for a specific family" (ANA, 2008, p. 5). Nurses first need to understand the importance of data collection and data analysis, and then how to apply data and knowledge—leading to wisdom. Data are important to the delivery of nursing care. In hospitals, data can be used to evaluate outcomes, identify problems for a specific group of patients, and assist in making plans for change to improve care. In the community, aggregated data are often collected to better understand the health issues in a population or community and to formulate a plan of action.

Figure 13–2 From data to wisdom.

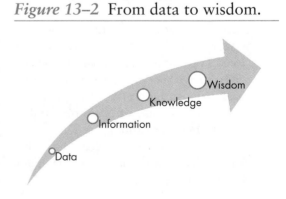

CERTIFICATION IN INFORMATICS NURSING

Nurses who practice in the area of informatics can be certified if they meet the eligibility criteria and complete the certification examination satisfactorily. Following are the eligibility criteria to apply for the informatics certification exam sponsored by the American Nurses Credentialing Center for 2008–2009 (ANA, 2007):

- Hold a current, active registered nurse license within a state or territory of the United States or the professional, legally recognized equivalent in another country
- Have practiced the equivalent of two years full time as an RN
- Hold a baccalaureate or higher degree in nursing or a baccalaureate degree in a relevant field
- Have completed 30 hours of continuing education in informatics within the last three years
- Meet one of the following practice hour requirements:
  a. Have practiced a minimum of 2,000 hours in NI within the last three years
  b. Have practiced a minimum of 1,000 hours in NI in the last three years and completed a minimum of 12 semester hours of academic credit in informatics courses that are a part of a graduate level NI program
  c. Have completed a graduate program in NI containing a minimum of 200 hours of faculty supervised practicum in informatics

These are not simple criteria, and they take time to meet. All criteria must be met before a nurse can apply to take the certification examination.

What does an informatics nurse do? The informatics nurse is involved in activities that focus on the methods and technologies of information handling in nursing. Informatics nursing practice includes the development, support, and evaluation of applications, tools, processes, and structures that help nurses to manage data in direct care of patients. The work of an informatics nurse can involve any and all aspects of information systems including theory formulation, design, development, marketing, selection, testing, implementation, training, maintenance, evaluation, and enhancement. "Informatics nurses are engaged in clinical practice, education, consultation, research, administration, and pure informatics" (ANA, 2007, p. 1). It is clear that a nurse who wants to function in this specialty area must have excellent computer skills, understand the practice needs for information, and know how best to apply IT to nursing practice. By speaking for the needs of the practicing nurse, the informatics nurse represents all nurses in practice when he or she practices in this area.

Informatics: Impact on Care

The IOM recommendations indicate that informatics can lead to safe, quality care, and it can. However, applying informatics is not perfect.

> *There is a perception that technology will lead to fewer errors than strategies that focus on staff performance; however, technology may in some circumstances lead to more errors. This is particularly true when the technology fails to take into account end users, increases in staff time, replicates an already bad process or is implemented with insufficient training. The best approach is not always clear, and most approaches have advantages and disadvantages. (Finkelman & Kenner, 2007, p. 55)*

Nurses need to take an active role in the development of IT for patient care and not wait to be asked to participate. When an HCO is choosing a system for an EMR, nurses need to be involved to ensure that the system meets nursing care documentation requirements and that relevant data can be collected to assist nurses in providing and improving care. Nurses may serve in key IT roles to guide development and implementation, and these nurses may have special training or education in informatics. Nurses may also serve as resources in identifying needs and testing systems to ensure that the systems are nurse-user-friendly. Many nurses who provide feedback about systems do not have special IT training; they review the system to determine if it is user-friendly for nurses who have limited informatics knowledge. All nurses must be skilled in managing and communicating information, and they are primarily concerned with the content of that information.

As discussed in Chapter 9 on patient-centered care, coordination of care is very important. One of the barriers to seamless coordination is the lack of interoperable computerized records (Bodenheimer, 2008). As of 2005, only 10–15% of physician offices and 20–25% of hospitals have implemented EMRs (Hillstead et al., 2005). This is far from what is needed to improve information sharing and coordination of care. Information can rarely be shared from one system to another, which is a deficit that needs to be resolved. Innovative methods to improve coordination that focus on informatics have been developed. One method is using electronic referral, or e-referral. This allows a healthcare provider to send an e-mail to another provider, such as a specialist, with information about the patient and to ask for consultation. In many situations, this eliminates the need to see the patient. The specialist reviews such information as lab reports, surgical reports, and so on, and can share his or her opinion with the healthcare provider. It is critical that this type of service be reimbursed, or it will not be used. Timely information flow from the hospital to posthospital care is also needed to improve coordination. This is a major drawback; even though the technology to improve it is available, it is not freely used.

Implications for Nursing Education and for Nursing Research

Informatics is important not only for practice but also for nursing education and nursing research. There is greater and greater use of IT in nursing education. The increased use of online courses throughout the nursing curriculum, both at the undergraduate and graduate levels, has revolutionized nursing education. It has required that faculty consider more interactive learning methods. Informatics has also impacted simulation, allowing faculty to create complex learning scenarios that use the computer and computerized equipment. This topic was discussed in Chapter 4. Students expect greater use of IT as they use it more in their personal lives. Such tools as iPods, **personal digital assistants (PDAs)**, Internet tools such as Facebook and MySpace, and mobile phones provide instant information and can be very interactive. These methods can be used to increase student–faculty communication and have the potential to provide different methods for student–faculty supervision in the clinical area. This is particularly true in areas like community health, when students visit multiple sites and faculty move from site to site to see students.

Nursing research uses informatics in data collection and analysis; it saves time and improves the quality of data collection and analysis. "The capacity for a mega-repository of clinical and research findings will allow for a richer science derived from multiple perspectives. Nurses have the responsibility to initiate practice-based inquiry, participate in clinical nursing research, and use nursing research to enhance patients' well-being and contribute to the body of nursing knowledge" (Appleton, 1998, as cited in Richards, 2001, p. 10).

Documentation

Over time, nursing documentation has increased in terms of its relevance to nurses and to other healthcare professionals, thus increasing its impact on patient care and patient outcomes. The format and content of nursing documentation have also changed. It is a professional responsibility to document planning, actual care provided, and outcomes. Care coordination and continuity are supported by documentation. With many staff caring for patients 24-7, it is critical that there be a clear communication mechanism, and this mechanism is documentation. Verbal communication is important, but a written document must be available. Staff can refer to documentation when other care providers are not available. Documentation serves as a record of the patient's care, it provides data for reimbursement and regarding quality improvement and staff performance, and it supports interdisciplinary teamwork. Through documentation, outcomes and evaluation of patient care are made clear. The medical record is a legal document, and as such, there are rules that must be followed. Once documentation has been created, changes to it must be accompanied by a note indicating who made the change(s) and when (date and time). Only certain staff can document; they must note the date and time on the documentation and include their name and credentials. If there are questions about care or a legal action, such as a malpractice suit, the medical record is the most important evidence. Medical records need to be saved. A nurse can say that he or she provided certain care, but if it was not documented, then it is as if it did not occur. Some critical concerns that should be addressed in documentation are (Iyer & Camp, 1999, p. 5):

- The medical record reflects the nursing process.
- The medical record describes the patient's ongoing status from shift to shift (inpatient care) or from patient visit to patient visit (ambulatory care).
- The plan of care and medical record complement each other.
- The documentation system is designed to facilitate retrieval of information for quality improvement activities and for research.
- The documentation system supports the staffing mix and acuity levels in the current healthcare environment.

What is effective documentation? The following provides a guide (Iyer & Camp, 1999):

- Documentation should not include opinion, but rather objective information. The nurse does not make subjective comments (e.g., comments about the patient being uncooperative, lazy, impolite, and so on). Nurses document only what they have done and objective data. A nurse would not document another nurse's action or another staff member's actions. Supervision of care can be documented.
- Write neatly and legibly (many HCOs now use computerized documentation, though not all HCOs have moved to an EMR system.) If a computerized system is used, typos may be a problem.
- Use correct spelling, grammar, and medical terminology.
- Use authorized abbreviations (using unapproved abbreviations can increase risk of errors).
- Use graphic records to record specified patient data, such as vital signs and medication administration.
- Record the patient's name on every page (hard copy medical records); this should be part of the EMR.

- Follow HCO rules about verbal and telephone orders.
- Transcribe orders carefully; double-check and ask questions if not clear. In computerized systems, orders do not need to be transcribed; however, this does not mean that there is no risk of an error in an order. All orders need careful review and may require follow-up if not clear.
- Document omitted care.
- Document medications and outcomes.
- Document patient noncompliance and reason(s).
- Document allergies and use this information to prevent errors and complications.
- Document sites of injections.
- Record all information about intravenous therapy and blood administration.
- Report abnormal laboratory results.
- Document as soon as possible after care is delivered. If documentation is done late, note this in the record. The nurse should not leave blank areas to come back to for later documentation.
- When quoting, use quotation marks and note who made the statement.
- When documentation is corrected because of a mistake, the nurse should follow the HCO policies regarding corrections. Medical records are never rewritten.
- Document patient status change.
- When contacting the physician, documentation of this contact should include time, date, name of physician, reason for the call, content, physician response, and steps taken after the call.

What content should be included in a medical record? The Joint Commission (2002, pp. 6–9) identifies the minimum information categories that are required for accreditation (accreditation was discussed in Chapter 12):

- The patient's name, address, date of birth, and the name of any legally authorized representative.
- The patient's legal status, as appropriate, such as if the patient has a court-appointed guardian or any legal judgment related to care.
- Emergency care provided to the patient before arrival.
- Record and findings of patient's assessment.
- A statement of conclusions or impressions drawn from the medical history and physical examination.
- The diagnosis or diagnostic impression—admitting diagnosis.
- The reason for admission or treatment.
- The treatment plan and goals of treatment.
- Evidence of known advance directives.
- Evidence of informed consent for procedures and treatments for which hospital policy requires informed consent.
- All diagnostic and therapeutic procedures performed, and the results.
- Test results relevant to managing the patient's condition.
- Records of all operative and other invasive procedures performed.
- Progress notes made by all healthcare providers as required.
- All reassessments and any revisions of the treatment plan.
- Clinical observations.
- The patient's response to care.
- Consultation reports.
- Every medication ordered or prescribed for inpatient care.
- Every medication dispensed to an ambulatory patient or an inpatient at discharge.
- Every dose of medication administered and any adverse reaction.
- All relevant diagnoses established during the course of care.

- Any referrals or communications made to external or internal care providers and to community agencies.
- Conclusions at the end of hospitalization.
- Discharge instructions to patients and family.
- Discharge summary; final progress note; transfer summary.

This list applies to hospital medical records. The content would be different for other types of settings, such as ambulatory care, long-term care, and home care, though some information would be the same. Nurses are not involved in documenting in all these categories because other staff members also have documentation responsibilities.

A Need: Standardized Terminology

Health care has expanded in multiple directions and includes the services of many different healthcare providers. Communication among the providers is not easy. Certainly, there are issues regarding willingness to communicate, lack of time to communicate, and so on, but a critical problem is the lack of a common professional language. For those entering health care, such as nursing students, this is probably a surprising comment. Each healthcare professional area has its own language; there are common medical terms, but each has a specific language that is often not known or understood by other healthcare professionals. "Creating a common language is no small task. Developing and adhering to distinct profession-specific terms may be a manifestation of professionals' desire to preserve identity, status or control" (IOM, 2003, p. 123). This problem affects all the core competencies and the ability to develop educational experiences that meet the competencies across healthcare professions, such as nursing, medicine, pharmacy, and allied health. It does not just

relate to informatics; however, because informatics is dependent on language, the issue of shared language is even more important. The IOM recommends that an interdisciplinary group created by the Department of Health and Human Services (DHHS) develop a common language across health disciplines "on a core set of competencies that includes patient-centered care, interdisciplinary teams, evidence-based practice, quality improvement, and informatics" (2003, p. 124). Accomplishing this requires that healthcare professionals be willing to actively work together to achieve this goal. Once this is accomplished, the next major step is getting different healthcare professionals to accept a universal language. This will require compromises.

> *The data element sets and terminologies are foundational to standardization of nursing documentation and verbal communication that will lead to a reduction in errors and an increase in the quality and continuity of care. It is through standardization of nurse documentation and communication of a patient's care that the many nurses caring for a patient develop a shared understanding of that care. Moreover, the process generates the nursing data needed to develop increasingly more sophisticated decision support tools in the electronic record and to identify and disseminate best nursing practices. (ANA, 2006)*

These statements are an example of why developing and accepting a universal language is difficult but necessary. The statements are nursing focused. How to move from this approach and blend with others, such as medicine, is the challenge.

SYSTEMATIC COLLECTION OF NURSING CARE DATA: DATA ELEMENT SETS

- Nursing Minimum Data Set (NMDS): This data set describes patient problems across healthcare settings, different populations, geographic areas, and time. These clinical data also assist in identifying nursing diagnoses, nursing interventions, and nurse-sensitive patient outcomes. The NMDS is also useful in assessing resources used in the provision of nursing care. The goal is the ability to link data between healthcare organizations and providers. Data can also be used for research and healthcare policy.

- Nursing Management Minimum Data Set: This data set focuses on nursing administrative data elements in all types of settings.

INTERFACE TERMINOLOGIES

- Clinical Care Classification (CCC): The Clinical Classifications Software (CCS) for the *International Classification of Diseases, 9th Revision, Clinical Modification* (ICD-9-CM) is a diagnosis and procedure categorization scheme that can be used in many types of projects that analyze data on diagnoses and procedures. CCS is based on ICD-9-CM, a uniform and standardized coding system. The ICD-9-CM includes over 13,600 diagnosis codes and 3,700 procedure codes (ANA, 2008). CCC focuses on home care and includes diagnoses, interventions, and outcomes.

- International Classification of Nursing Practice (ICNP): This classification system is a unified nursing language system that applies to all types of nursing care. It is a compositional terminology for nursing practice that facilitates the development of, and the cross-mapping among, local terms and existing terminologies. It includes nursing diagnoses, nursing interventions, and nursing outcomes (International Council of Nurses, 2008).

- North America Nursing Diagnosis Association (NANDA), Nursing Intervention Classification (NIC), and Nursing Outcome Classification (NOC): These systems were discussed in Chapter 9. NANDA focuses on nursing diagnoses, NIC on nursing interventions, and NOC on nursing outcomes.

- Omaha System: The Omaha System is a comprehensive, standardized taxonomy designed to improve practice, documentation, and information management. It includes three components: the Problem Classification Scheme, the Intervention Scheme, and the Problem Rating Scale for Outcomes. When the three components are used together, the Omaha System offers a way to link clinical data to demographic, financial, administrative, and staffing data (Omaha System, 2005). The Omaha System is used in home health care, community health, and public health services.

- Perioperative Nursing Data Set: The Perioperative Nursing Data Set (PNDS) is a standardized nursing vocabulary that addresses the perioperative patient experience from preadmission until discharge, including nursing diagnoses, interventions, and outcomes. The PNDS was developed by a specialty organization, the members of the Association of periOperative Registered Nurses (AORN), which has been recognized by the ANA as a data set useful for perioperative nursing practice (AORN, 2008).

MULTIDISCIPLINARY TERMINOLOGIES

- ABC Codes: ABC Coding Solutions manages care, claims, and outcomes related to alternative medicine, nursing, and other integrative healthcare practices. ABC codes, paired with ABC terminology, currently describe more than 4,300 unique instances of care and services and/or supply items specific to the practice of alternative medicine, nursing, and other integrative healthcare practitioners. The codes fill the gaps left by the existing standard Health Insurance Portability and Accountability Act (HIPAA) code sets and provide for comprehensive and seamless coding (ABC Coding Solutions, 2008). This data coding system applies to nursing and other healthcare services and focuses on interventions.

- Logical Observation Identifiers Names and Codes (LOINC): This is a clinical terminology classification used for laboratory test orders and results. It is one system designated for use in U.S. federal government systems for the electronic exchange of clinical health information (National Library of Medicine, 2008a). This system can be used to collect data about assessments and outcomes for nursing and other healthcare services.

- The Current Procedural Terminology is a code used for reimbursement (Larkin, 2008).

- Systematized Nomenclature of Medicine— Clinical Terms (SNOMED CT): This is a comprehensive clinical terminology. It is one of several designated standards for use in U.S. federal government systems for the electronic exchange of clinical health information (National Library of Medicine, 2008b). This system is applicable to nursing and other healthcare services and focuses on diagnoses, interventions, and outcomes.

Informatics: Types and Methods

For informatics to be effective, three concerns must be addressed. The HCO must have effective and easily accessible IT support services. Staff must be able to pick up the telephone and get this support. Failure of the information system has major implications for patient care, so backup systems are critical. The second critical concern is staff training. This requires resources:

financial resources, trainers, and time. Staff need time to attend training, and there must be recognition that it takes time for staff to learn how to use the system. Incorporation of informatics with any of the methods described next (and others that are not included in this chapter) is a major change in care delivery. Change is stressful for staff, and it needs to be planned, representing the third concern. Too much change at one time can increase staff stress, impact the success of using more informatics in the future, decrease staff motivation to participate, and increase the risk of errors that might impact patient outcomes. It is not difficult to find nurses who will complain about a hospital's attempt to increase the use of informatics if it has been badly planned. Often, in these complaints, staff note that the system selected was not effective and that they had no part in the process. Equipment and software can be very costly, and decisions regarding these are critical. Time must be taken to evaluate equipment and software to make sure they meet the needs and demands of the organization and users such as nurses.

Automated Dispensing of Medications and Bar Coding: Pharmacies in all types of HCOs are using, or moving toward using, automatic medication dispensing systems with bar coding. These systems select the medication based on the order and prepare it in single doses for the patient. The bar code is on the packaged dose. This code can then be compared with the bar code on the patient's identification band using a handheld device. This system can decrease errors, and it supports all five rights of medication administration:

- Right drug
- Right patient
- Right amount
- Right route
- Right time

Bar coding can also be used to collect data about prescribed and administered drugs. Data can then be used for QI and for research. Bar coding systems are expensive to install and maintain, but they can make a difference in reducing errors.

Computerized Monitoring of Adverse Events: Computerized systems that monitor adverse events assist in identifying and monitoring adverse events. Developing and using a database of these events facilitates analysis of data and the development of interventions to decrease adverse events.

Electronic Medical Records: The EMR is slowly replacing the written medical record for an individual patient while he or she receives care within a specific healthcare system. A second type of electronic system is the **personal health record (PHR)**. The PHR is less common than the EMR, but there is much hope that it will become standard in the future. The PHR is a computer-based health record for which data are collected over the long term—for a lifetime. With the patient's permission, this record can be accessed easily by any provider who needs the information. To reach this point, there must be agreement on a minimum data set—that is, uniform definitions of data (i.e., standardized language) that would enable all healthcare providers to understand and use the information. There is still much to be done to make this a reality in every healthcare organization, including clinics and medical offices, but the technology is available. The EMR is a record of the patient's history and assessment, orders, laboratory results, description of medical tests and procedures, and documentation of care provided and outcomes. Care plans are included. Information can be easily input, searched, and reviewed, and reports can be printed. Data can be stored long term, which is harder to do with written records that require storage space and that may not be easy to find. In addition, written records can be less

readable over time. The hard copy record is also not always easy to access in a hospital unit. If one person is using the record, others cannot use it. With the EMR, this is not a problem as long as staff can access the computerized record system. The EMR systems do require security and backup saving systems.

Following is a summary of the advantages of EMRs (Iyer & Camp, 1999, pp. 129–130):

- Legible records
- Readily available records
- Improved nursing productivity
- Reduction in record tampering
- Support of nursing process in the system
- Reduction in redundant documentation
- Clinical prompts, reminders, and warnings
- Categorized nursing notes
- Automatically printed reports
- Documentation according to standards of care
- Improved knowledge of outcomes
- Availability of data
- Prevention of medication errors
- Facilitation of cost-defining efforts
- Printed discharge information

EMR documentation may take place at the unit work station, at a hallway computer station, or at the bedside. Bedside systems are better; they are easy to access when the nurse or other healthcare professional needs information, and point-of-care documentation is enhanced.

Professional order entry system: This system has been called the physician order entry system (POES), but this is changing to include all healthcare professionals who might write profession-specific orders, such as nursing orders. This system is included in the EMR, though it can stand alone. The healthcare provider inputs orders into the system rather than writing them. One clear advantage is legibility: Written orders are often very difficult to read because handwriting varies, and this has led to many errors. It takes time to transcribe written physician orders into a form in which the orders can be used. During this process, risk of transcription errors is increased. Typing orders into a computer can also lead to typos, but this is less of a problem. Clinical decision support systems can be included with POESs. This combination enhances the POES and can lead to improved care and a decrease in errors.

Clinical decision support systems: This type of system is leading to major changes in healthcare delivery. These systems provide immediate information that can influence clinical decisions. Some of the systems actually intervene when an error is about to be made. For example, an order for a medication is put into a patient's EMR; the computerized system indicates that the patient is allergic to that medication by immediately sending an alert, stopping the order. The nurse can get alerts that the patient is at risk for falls or decubiti. In the past, to look up information, nurses depended on textbooks or journals that the unit might have, and this was not done effectively. Easy electronic access to current information eliminates many problems related to obtaining information when needed. This, too, can improve the quality of care. EBP relies heavily on access to EBP literature, which is most easily accessible via the Internet and databases.

Use of personal digital assistants: PDAs have become popular with the general public. Many mobile telephones now have PDA capability, such as access to the Internet and storage of information. These handheld devices can hold a significant amount of information, serve as a calendar, keep contact information, and serve as an effective method for transmission of information. Nurses who use PDAs carry information with them and can look up side effects of a medication or any other type of medical information to help them as they provide care. In some cases, the nurse can access EMRs to get to patient

information through the PDA. Some textbooks can now be uploaded into PDAs, such as pharmacology and clinical laboratory resources. This is very useful information for the nurse to have available when needed, accessible in seconds at the point-of-care. Nurses who work outside a structured setting, such as in public health or in home care, find this type of system very useful for support information and for documentation needs (patient information, visit data, and so on).

Computer-based reminder systems: These systems are used to communicate with patients via e-mail to remind them of appointments and screenings and to discuss other health issues. In the future, this method will most likely take the place of telephone calls to remind patients of appointments.

Access to patient records at the point-of-care: Many hospitals are moving toward providing access to the patient records either in the patient's room or in the hallway via computers. In the future, the nurse may carry a small laptop that allows access to the EMR. This reduces time spent returning to the work station to get information. Documentation can be completed as soon as care is provided; this reduces errors and improves quality because all care providers know when care has been provided. Point-of-care access decreases the chance that something may be forgotten, documented incorrectly, or not documented at all. In addition, it saves nurses time and eliminates the need to delay doing documentation (such as in blocks in midmorning or toward end of shift)—a system that can lead to errors, incomplete data in the record if the nurse forgets information, and situations in which other providers need current patient information that has not yet been documented.

Internet prescription: There has been rapid growth in access to prescriptions via the Internet. The medications are then mailed to the patient. The consumer does have to be careful and check the legitimacy of the source to prevent errors.

Nurse call systems: Nurse call systems are a form of informatics and are very important in communication within a healthcare system. They allow for improved and efficient communication and are a great improvement on the old method of yelling out for a staff member. There are many types of nurse call systems, such as pagers, light signals, buzzers, methods that allow patients to talk directly to nurses through a direct audio system that the nurse can easily access, mobile telephones, miniature label microphones, and locater badges. The goal is to get a message to the right person as soon as possible and maintain privacy and confidentiality. This can improve care, reduce errors, and make staff more efficient, preventing the unnecessary work of trying to obtain and share information.

Voice mail: Computer-based messaging systems are found in all healthcare settings today so that staff can leave and receive voice messages. These systems can be used by staff and patients, often reducing the need for callbacks. Complicated systems can annoy consumers, and there is an impersonal quality to this form of communication, though it is part of everyday life today.

Telephone for advice and other services: Patient advice systems are used mostly by insurers and managed care. Nurses use their assessment skills and provide advice to patients who call in with questions. Typically, insurers develop standard protocols that the nurses use for common questions, but nurses must still use professional judgment when providing advice. This type of service should not become "cookbook" care in which there is no consideration of assessment and individual patient needs. Assessment is the key to successful telephone nursing in order to identify the interventions required, which may or may not be found in the guidelines. Some physician offices have telephone advice services that are manned by a physician in the practice or by a nurse. Pediatric practices are

the most common type of practice using this system. Patient advice systems via telephone require clear documentation policies and guidelines that include content related to whom is called, when, and for what reason, and the required assessment data and interventions. Telephone advice systems are typically used to answer questions, remind patients of appointments or follow-up needs, and surveillance to check in on how a patient is doing.

Hospitals are using the telephone to begin the admission process for patients with scheduled admissions. Patients are called before the admission date, asked questions related to required admission information, and told what to expect on admission. Pretesting may be scheduled prior to admission. This saves the hospital time and is more cost-effective, and pretesting can be more convenient for the patient. This method can also identify problems that may impact the needed patient care so that they can be addressed early on.

Online support groups for patients and families: These groups can focus on any problem or disease. Patients and their families can use chat rooms, e-mail, and Web sites for information sharing. Consumers gain information, education about their health and health needs, and support from others with similar problems. A healthcare provider may or may not be involved.

Internet or virtual appointment: Use of the Internet as a means of increasing accessibility to a physician or advanced practice nurse is increasing. The younger generations, as well as some senior citizens, are using the Internet to gain advice from health professionals. Family and portable family histories can be maintained in this fashion and passed on to a new primary care provider. Those patients and families who have limited resources—financial, transportation, or insurance—can more affordably receive medical advice in this format. It also keeps some employees from missing work to take a child or other family member to an appointment. Many of these sites link into cellular devices to send an alert of high importance to whomever is on call for virtual hours. This ensures that high-priority questions and advice get to the health professional quickly (Larkin, 2008). These types of services will most likely increase in the future.

The Future of Informatics and Medical Technology

The future is likely to see major expansion in the use of technology. Some of the possible technological approaches are already being used in some areas. Cutting-edge technology is sometimes hard to believe. Here are some of the possibilities.

NANOTECHNOLOGY

Nanotechnology—microscopic technology on the order of one billionth of a meter—will likely impact the diagnosis and treatment of many diseases and conditions (Gordon, Lutz, Boninger, & Cooper, 2007). Some of the pending technologies are:

- Sensing patients' internal drug levels with miniature medical diagnostic tools that circulate in their bloodstreams.
- Chemotherapy delivered directly to a tumor site, reducing systemic side effects.
- New monitoring devices for the home: a talking pill bottle that lets patients push a button to hear prescription information; bathroom counters that announce whether it is safe to mix two medications; a shower with built-in scales to calculate body mass index; measuring devices in the bathroom to track urine frequency and output and upload these data to a system or care manager; noninvasive blood glucose monitors to eliminate sticks; and sensors to compute blood sugar levels using a multiwavelength reflective dispersion photometer.

WEARABLE COMPUTING

A computer can be worn, much as eyeglasses or clothing are worn, and interactions with the user are based on the context of the situation (ANA, 2008). With heads-up displays, embedded sensors in fabrics, unobtrusive input devices, personal wireless local area networks, and a host of other context-sensing and communication tools, wearable computers can act as intelligent assistants or data collection and analysis devices. Many of these devices are available now using "smart fabrics." These wearable computer and remote monitoring systems are intertwined with the user's activity so that the technology becomes transparent. Sensors and devices can gather data during the patient's daily routine, providing healthcare providers or researchers with periodic or continuous data on the person's health while he or she is at work, at school, exercising, or sleeping, rather than the current snapshot captured during a typical hospital or clinic visit. A few applications for wearable computing include sudden infant death syndrome monitoring for infants; ambulatory cardiac and respiratory monitoring; monitoring of ventilation during exercise; activity level of poststroke patients; patterns of breathing in asthma; assessment of stress in individuals; arrhythmia detection and control of selected cardiac conditions; and daily activity monitors (Offray Specialty Narrow Fabrics, 2007).

HIPAA: Ensuring Confidentiality

The 1996 **Health Insurance Portability and Accountability Act (HIPAA)** has had a major impact on healthcare delivery systems and how they communicate. Privacy and confidentiality have long been issues in health care and were discussed in Chapter 6. Because HIPAA focuses on the issue of information and confidentiality, it applies to IT. The law also requires data security and electronic transaction standards. Why did this law become important? With the growth of information sharing, it became increasingly evident that the transactions and systems were not ensuring privacy and confidentiality, key elements that had long been part of the healthcare delivery system. Privacy is the right of a person to have personal information kept private. As discussed, this relates to professional ethics. The law requires that only *necessary* information be shared among providers, including insurers. Patients may also access their medical records. Information cannot be openly shared—for example, discussing patient information in public places, calling a patient's work or home and leaving a message that reveals information about health or health services, and so on. Carrying documents outside an HCO with patient identifier information is prohibited; this has implications for students who may take notes or have written assignments that include this information. How information is carried in PDAs or laptops is also of concern. The new technology was moving so fast that these critical issues were not addressed effectively. The law requires that staff know the key elements of HIPAA and apply them. As a result, HCOs and healthcare profession schools, such as nursing programs, are required to provide information and training about HIPAA. There are large fines if the law is broken. Consumers are informed about HIPAA when they enter the health system; they are given written information and asked to sign documents to indicate that they have been informed. Ensuring that the requirements are met must be incorporated into IT, which has become a major method for communicating health information.

Telehealth

Telehealth, or telemedicine, is the use of telecommunications equipment and communications networks for transferring healthcare information between participants at different locations. Telehealth applies telecommunication and computer technologies to the broad spectrum of public health and medicine (DHHS, 2000). This technology offers opportunities to provide care when face-to-face interaction is impossible (such as in home care, in school-based care, and in rural areas) and can be used in a variety of settings and situations as long as the equipment is available. Two-way interactive video is the most effective telehealth method. "**Telenursing** refers to the use of telecommunications technology in nursing to enhance patient care. It involves the use of electromagnetic channels (e.g. wire, radio and optical) to transmit voice, data and video communications signals. It is also defined as distance communications, using electrical or optical transmissions, between humans and/or computers" (Skiba, 1998, p. 40). Issues that arise with telehealth are cost of equipment and its use; training for staff and for consumers if they need to actively use equipment; limited or no insurance coverage for telehealth services; the need for clear policies, procedures, and protocols; privacy and confidentiality of information; and regulatory issues (e.g., a nurse who is located and licensed in one state providing telenursing for a patient in another state where he or she is not licensed). Telehealth also has implications for international health care because it provides a method for connecting expertise to patients who may need care that is not accessible in their home country.

Internet

Nurses use the Internet for information and for communication through e-mail. Patients/

consumers also use the Internet more and more. It can be an excellent source for all types of information, including health and medical information. When the Internet is used as a source of health information, it is important that nurses assess the Web sites, because they are not all of the same quality. What does a nurse need to consider when evaluating a Web site?

- The source or sponsor of the Web site; the most reliable sites are sponsored by the government, academic institutions, healthcare professional organizations, and HCOs.
- Current status of the information; when was it posted or revised?
- Accessibility of the information on the site; can you find what you need?
- References provided for content when appropriate.

Other Technology: Biomedical and Patient Care Equipment

Remote telemetry monitoring: This is technology that informs staff when a patient's condition has changed. The patient is on a monitor, and signals are sent to staff through a page system. Staff are informed of the patient's identity, heart rate, and readout of rhythm without being right next to the patient.

Robotics The use of robotics in patient care will expand (ANA, 2008). Robots have been used for many years to deliver supplies to patient care areas. Robotics enables remote surgeries and virtual reality surgical procedures. At Johns Hopkins, robots are being used as translators for patients (Greenback, 2007). Hand-assist devices help patients regain strength after a stroke ("Robotic Brace," 2007). Robots are providing a remote presence to allow physicians to virtually examine patients by manipulating remote cameras ("Telemedicine Pioneer Helps Physicians," 2007). They are being used for

microscopic, minimally invasive surgical procedures. One example is the da Vinci Surgical System, which helps surgeons perform such procedures as mitral vital repairs, hysterectomies, and prostate surgeries (da Vinci Surgery, 2008). In the future, robots may also be used in direct patient care—for instance, to help lift morbidly obese patients.

Genetics and Genomics Advances in mapping the human genome (genetics), understanding individual DNA, and examining the impact of external factors such as the environment (genomics) will have a dramatic impact on patient care (ANA, 2008). These data, especially once they are integrated into EMRs or PHRs, will lead to advances in customized patient care and medications targeted to individual responses to medications. Care and medication can be precisely customized to patients based on their unique DNA profile and how they have responded to medications and other interventions in the past; this will dramatically change how patients are managed for specific diseases and conditions, and extend into the prevention of some diseases. The inherent complexity of customized patient care will demand computerized clinical decision support. Predictive disease models based on patients' DNA profiles will emerge as clinicians better understand DNA mapping. These advances have implications for a new model of care and for the informatics nurse's participation in the development of genomic IT solutions. More than ever, patients will need to be partners in this development—patient-centered care.

High-Touch Care Versus High-Tech Care

High-touch care is what most people go into nursing for, but nursing is much more than this today. This chapter describes the increasing influence of technology on all segments of health care.

This will not decrease, but rather increase. Nurses do need to understand, and know how to use, technology that is applied to their practice areas. Nurses need to be involved in the development of this technology when possible, and they must be involved in the implementation of the technology. But there are concerns. When we talk through machines, do we lose information and the personal relationship? How can this be prevented so that we are not disconnected from our patients? How can we ensure that the information we are getting is correct and complete? Are people able to communicate fully through some of these other means? It is clear that over time, the public has become increasingly comfortable with informatics, which they are using more and more in their everyday lives. As nursing uses informatics, nurses need to keep in mind the potential for isolation and the need for effective communication, and they must not forget the need for touch and face-to-face communication.

The future will include many more new uses of technology, and change is ongoing. For example, the Iowa Medical Center has implemented an eICU (e-intensive care unit) to improve patient monitoring (Sagario, 2008). This system allows intensivists at a remote monitoring center to view patients' vital statistics, electrocardiograms, ventilators, and X-ray and lab results. The eICU includes two-way conference video capability so that patients and staff can interact when required. The system is attached to four hospitals in Iowa and their ICUs. This type of system has advantages; experts can be located in one place and then consult with multiple locations and staff. This is particularly useful in providing expert medical care for residents in rural and remote areas. There is no reason that this type of system would be limited to physician consultation; it could be used for nurses. For example, a nurse clinical specialist could view data and consult on patient care with nurses in various ICUs. The potential is there for increased access to information and expertise. The other side of this innovation is the effect on the touch side of care when the provider is not actually in the room with the patient. It is not clear how this might impact care because these types of systems are very new.

Conclusion

This chapter has explored the current and future in the world of healthcare informatics and some aspects of biotechnology. There is much more to this subject than use of e-mail, and the chapter has identified many diverse examples. The core competency to utilize informatics is critical. If graduates of the healthcare profession schools cannot understand and use informatics, the safety and quality of the care provided will be impacted. Communication, coordination, documentation, and care provision (including monitoring and decision making) are linked to informatics. However, each nurse must not get so involved in informatics and technology that the patient as a person is lost—the patient–nurse relationship is an important component of patient-centered care.

CHAPTER HIGHLIGHTS

1. The IOM describes the fifth healthcare profession core competency as: "communicate, manage knowledge, mitigate error, and support decision making using information technology" (IOM, 2003, p. 4).
2. Informatics is more than just looking at IT, but rather how that technology is used to prevent errors and improve care.
3. Informatics is used for evaluating the performance of HCOs and individual healthcare providers and has a major

impact on QI. Today, it is much easier to collect, store, and analyze large amounts of data that in the past were collected by hand.

4. Insurers rely heavily on informatics to provide insurance coverage, manage data, and analyze performance, which has a direct impact on whether care is covered for reimbursement.

5. Informatics has allowed government at all levels—local, state, national, and international—to collect data and use them for policy decision making and evaluation.

6. A clinical information system is a method of data storage that is generally used at point-of-care. It includes such things as clinical guidelines, patient information, and pharmacopedias to check for drug interactions.

7. A coding system is a mechanism for identifying treatments and procedures with specific labels in order to bill for those services.

8. Computer literacy is knowledge of basic computer technology.

9. Data mining is the ability to drill down and search through databases—for example, to determine trends in a patient or a system. Examining the data for relationships between treatment and patient outcomes is another example.

10. Decision support systems are computerized systems that assist the health professional in making clinical treatment plans.

11. Information literacy is the ability to recognize and retrieve needed data.

12. Minimum data set: The minimum categories of data with uniform definitions and categories, concerning a specific aspect or dimension of the healthcare system that meets the basic needs of multi-

ple data users. An example is the NMDS (ANA, 2008).

13. Standardized language: A collection of terms with definitions for use in informational systems databases. This enables comparisons to be made because the same term is used to denote the same condition. Standardized language is necessary for documentation in electronic health records (ANA, 2008).

14. NI is a nursing specialty that integrates nursing science, computer science, and information science to manage and communicate data, information, knowledge, and wisdom in nursing practice. It has its own sets of standards and scope of practice. There is a national certification in this specialty.

15. Informatics can directly impact care by providing data in a retrievable form for the purpose of assisting with clinical decision making. However, the data are only as reliable as the information entered in the computer.

16. Today, documentation is often in an electronic format.

17. Standardized terminology assists in promoting clearer communication across disciplines.

18. Interface terminologies include, but are not limited to, CCC, ICNP, NANDA, NIC, NOC, Omaha System, and PNDS.

19. Multidisciplinary terminologies include, but are not limited to, ABC codes, LOINC, and SNOMED CT.

20. Effective informatics is dependent on accessible IT support and adequate staff training, and change must be planned.

21. Examples of use of informatics in healthcare delivery are the automated dispensing of medications and bar coding for identification; computerized monitoring of

adverse events; use of EMRs, POESs, and clinical decision support systems; use of PDAs, and CBRS; access to patient records at the point-of-care; and Internet prescriptions, nurse call systems, voice mail, telephone for advice and other services, online support groups for patients, Internet or virtual appointments, and other examples presented in this chapter.

22. HIPAA requires that patient data be secure and private.

23. Telehealth, or telemedicine, is the use of telecommunications equipment and communications networks for transferring healthcare information between participants at different locations.

24. Robotics is the use of robots for the purposes of retrieving supplies, carrying lab specimens from one location to another, or even assisting in surgical procedures.

25. There has been expansion in the area of genomics, or the mapping of the human gene locations, as well as in looking at its environmental impact.

Linking to the Internet

- Alliance for Nursing Informatics
  http://www.allianceni.org/
- American Nursing Informatics Association
  http://www.ania.org/
- American Telemedicine Association
  http://www.atmeda.org/
- Healthcare Information and Management Systems Society
  http://www.himss.org/asp/topics_nursingInformatics.asp
- Technology Informatics Guiding Educational Reform (TIGER Initiative)
  http://www.umbc.edu/tiger/index.html

DISCUSSION QUESTIONS

1. Explain how the core competency, utilize informatics, relates to the other four IOM core competencies.
2. What is informatics, and why is it important in health care and nursing?
3. Describe the certification requirements for an informatics nurse and the role.
4. Describe four examples of healthcare informatics and implications for nursing.
5. Why is documentation important?
6. Explain how the EMR and PHR can increase quality of care and decrease errors. Provide examples.
7. Discuss issues related to confidentiality and informatics.

CRITICAL THINKING ACTIVITIES

1. Divide into small teams. Identify a healthcare organization in your local community and try to find out how it uses informatics. You can focus on the entire organization, or select a department or a unit. Are there any future plans to increase the use of informatics?
2. Interview a nurse who works in a hospital that uses an EMR. Before you conduct the interview, develop six questions that you will ask with a team of students. Each student will then interview one RN. After the interviews, combine your data and analyze the results.
3. Speak to an RN who works in staff development/education in a healthcare organization. Discuss the training that staff members receive for using informatics.
4. If you have used an EMR in clinical, what was it like for you? If you have not yet done this, interview a senior student and ask about the experience.
5. What biomedical equipment have you used or seen used? How does the use of this equipment impact care?
6. What is your opinion of the potential conflict between high-touch care and high-tech care? Discuss with your team.

CASE STUDY

A 6-year-old has come to the attention of the child welfare department as a possible victim of sexual abuse. The child lives in a very rural part of a western state. Rather than have the child travel a distance to experts, she was taken to the nearest clinic with sexual assault nurse examiners and a knowledgeable pediatrician skilled in sexual abuse examinations. At the time of the examination, pictures were taken of the child's body, including the genital area. These pictures are crucial if charges are filed. To ensure that an accurate diagnosis is made, local experts wish to have a second opinion because the physical examination was not felt to be completely clear. The experts for the second opinion were linked via the Internet and Internet video-conferencing equipment so that the two teams could talk and view de-identified (because the information was going across unsecure Internet channels) photos. Within 15 minutes, it was determined that the hymen was intact, and no penetration had occurred. Other markers indicated that there was evidence of child abuse, but none that supported sexual assault. This case used an EMR, digitized photos, and Internet consultation to arrive at a diagnosis that had both medical and legal implications.

Case Questions

1. Discuss the impact of the use of these methods in the case on the nurse–patient relationship and on patient confidentiality.

WORDS OF WISDOM

Marion J. Ball, Ed.D., Professor Emerita, Johns Hopkins University School of Nursing, Fellow, Center for Healthcare Management IBM Research

Nursing professionals are the foot soldiers of the healthcare delivery system and therefore must be well equipped to carry out the best possible care for our patients. Having a solid understanding of the use of technological enabling tools is essential to be able to give the best possible patient care. The TIGER (Technology Informatics Guiding Education Reform) initiative is working on bringing the most essential skills for the profession to the table. The nine areas TIGER is addressing are:

- Standards and interoperability
- Healthcare IT national agenda/healthcare IT policy
- Informatics competencies
- Education and faculty development

- Staff development/continuing education
- Usability/clinical application design
- Virtual demonstration center
- Leadership development

(For more information, go to http://www.tigersummit.com)

In fighting the battle of disease and suffering, nurses are the ones who can win the battle if they are well prepared. This means a good grasp of informatics is an essential ingredient.

References

ABC Coding Solutions. (2008). Retrieved March 7, 2008, from http://www.alternativelink.com/ali/abc_codes/wiify.asp

American Nurses Association. (2006). *Nursing practice information infrastructure: Glossary*. Retrieved March 5, 2008, from http://www.nursingworld.org/npii/glossary.htm

American Nurses Association. (2007). *Informatics nurse certification exam*. Retrieved March 5, 2008, from http://www.nursecredentialing.org/NurseSpecialties/Informatics.aspx

American Nurses Association. (2008). *Nursing informatics: Scope and standards of practice*. Washington, DC: Author.

Appleton, C. (1998). Nursing research: Moving into the clinical setting. *Nursing Management, 29*(6), 43–45.

Association of periOperative Registered Nurses. (2008). Retrieved March 7, 2008, from http://www.aorn.org/PracticeResources/PNDSAndStandardized Perioperative Record/

Bodenheimer, T. (2008). Coordinating care—A perilous journey through the healthcare system. *New England Journal of Medicine, 358*, 1065–1071.

da Vinci Surgery. (2008). *Surgery enabled by da Vinci®*. Retrieved March 23, 2008, from http://davincisurgery.com/surgery/index.aspx

Englebardt, S., & Nelson, R. (2002) *Healthcare informatics: An interdisciplinary approach*. St. Louis, MO: Mosby-Year Book.

Finkelman, A., & Kenner, C. (2007). *Teaching IOM*. Silver Spring, MD: American Nurses Association Publishing.

Gordon, A., Lutz, G., Boninger, M., & Cooper, R. (2007). Introduction to nanotechnology: Potential applications in physical medicine and rehabilitation. *American Journal of Physical Medicine and Rehabilitation, 86*, 225–241.

Greenback, L. (2007, January 9). Robot aids Johns Hopkins patients. *The Baltimore Examiner*. Retrieved January 9, 2007, from http://www.examiner.com/a-498079~Robot_aids_Johns_Hopkins_patients.html

Hillstead, R., Bigelow, J., Bower, A., Girosi, F., Meili, R., Scoville, R., et al. (2005). Can electronic medical record systems transform healthcare? Potential health benefits, savings, and costs. *Health Affairs, 24*(5), 1103–1117.

Institute of Medicine. (2003). *Health professions education*. Washington, DC: National Academies Press.

International Council of Nurses. (2008). *International Classification for Nursing Practice (ICNP®)*. Retrieved March 2, 2008, from http://www.icn.ch/icnp_def.htm

Iyer, P., & Camp, N. (1999). *Nursing documentation*. St. Louis, MO: Mosby.

The Joint Commission. (2002). *From practice to paper: Documentation for hospitals*. Chicago: Author.

Larkin, H. (2008). Your future chief of staff? *H&HN: Hospitals & Healthcare Networks, 82*(3), 30–34.

National Library of Medicine. (2008a). Retrieved March 12, 2008, from http://www.nlm.nih.gov/research/umls/loinc_main.html

National Library of Medicine. (2008b). Retrieved March 12, 2008, from http://www.nlm.nih.gov/research/umls/Snomed/snomed_main.html

Nelson, R. & Joos, I. (1989, fall). On language in nursing; from data to wisdom. *PLN Vision*, p. 6.

Offray Specialty Narrow Fabrics. (2007). *Smart textiles*. Retrieved October 10, 2007, from http://www.osnf.com/p_smart.html

Omaha System. (2005). *The Omaha System: Solving the clinical data-information puzzle*. Retrieved March 12, 2008, from http://www.omahasystem.org/

Richards, J. (2001). Nursing in a digital age. *Nursing Economics, 19*(1), 6–10, 34.

Robotic brace aids stroke recovery. (2007). Retrieved March 22, 2007, from Science Daily Web site: http://www.sciencedaily.com/releases/2007/03/070321105223.htm

Sagario, D. (2008, February 27). Iowa medical center implements eICU to improve patient monitoring. *Des Moines Register*.

Skiba, D. J. (1998). Health-oriented telecommunications. In M. J. Ball, K. J. Hannah, S. K. Newbold, & J. V. Douglas (Eds.), *Nursing informatics: Where caring and technology meet* (pp. 40–53). New York: Springer.

Telemedicine pioneer helps physicians on the move stay close to patients. (2007). Retrieved October 10, 2007, from Cisco Systems Web site: http://www.cisco.com/en/US/solutions/collateral/ns339/ns636/ns418/ns554/net_customer_profile0900aecd804073a3.pdf

U.S. Department of Health and Human Services. (2000). *Healthy People 2010* (2nd ed.). Washington, DC: U.S. Government Printing Office.

The Practice of Nursing Today and in the Future

Section IV concludes this textbook. It addresses two issues in nursing. The first is the nursing shortage. What are the factors that influence the critical nursing shortage, which is predicted to increase? How does the nursing shortage impact patient care? The first chapter in this section, Chapter 14, discusses these important questions and strategies that are used to cope with the shortage. Chapter 15, the last chapter, focuses on the future of nursing and discusses the transformation of nursing practice. What are our strengths as a profession, and what does the future hold for nursing and nurses?

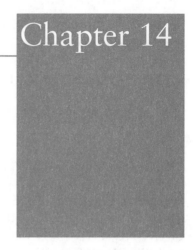

Chapter 14

Critical Healthcare Issue: Why Don't We Have Enough Nurses?

CHAPTER OBJECTIVES

At the conclusion of this chapter, the learner will be able to:

- Describe the nursing workforce profile.
- Discuss the generational issues that have an impact on the nursing workforce.
- Discuss the nursing shortage.
- Explain the impact that the nursing shortage has on health care.
- Summarize the recruitment process and issues.
- Identify key strategies to address retention.
- Describe the elements of a healthy work environment.

- Discuss strategies to address the nursing shortage.
- Critique the growth of global migration of nurses.
- Describe examples of methods for improving career development.
- Determine what criteria you would use to find the best fit for your first position as a registered nurse (RN).

CHAPTER OUTLINE

KEY TERMS

- ❑ Biosketch
- ❑ Burnout
- ❑ Career ladder
- ❑ Coaching
- ❑ Curriculum vitae
- ❑ Distribution of staff
- ❑ Flexible staffing
- ❑ Full-time equivalent (FTE)
- ❑ Mandatory overtime
- ❑ Mentoring
- ❑ Networking
- ❑ Nurse residency
- ❑ Nursing care hours
- ❑ Patient classification system (PCS)
- ❑ Portfolio
- ❑ Reality shock
- ❑ Recruitment
- ❑ Résumé
- ❑ Self-scheduling
- ❑ Staffing mix
- ❑ Student externship

Introduction

This chapter focuses on the most critical issue confronting nursing today, in both healthcare delivery and the educational system: the nursing shortage. The content discusses the history that led up to the shortage and the current shortage's impact on care. Within the context of the shortage, recruitment and retention factors are described. Staffing is related to the shortage. If there are not enough registered nurses (RNs), staffing is problematic. Strategies are outlined to resolve the shortage. Global migration of nurses is one solution to the shortage, but it can have negative consequences. This chapter also discusses how new graduates can best transition to professional practice to ensure that each nurse who graduates finds a place to work that allows him or her to stay in nursing and feel positive about the profession. Figure 14–1 identifies the many factors that impact staffing and the nursing shortage today (all are discussed in this chapter).

Workforce Profile: Current and Entering Nurses

It is important to understand the nursing workforce profile to appreciate the nursing shortage and future concerns about the shortage. Nursing is ranked as the number one growth occupation of all occupations through 2012 (U.S. Department of Labor, 2004). In May 2006, 2,417,150 RNs were employed in the United States. Their mean wages were $28.71 hourly and $59,730 annually, and their median hourly wages were

Figure 14–1 Factors affecting nurse shortage and staffing.

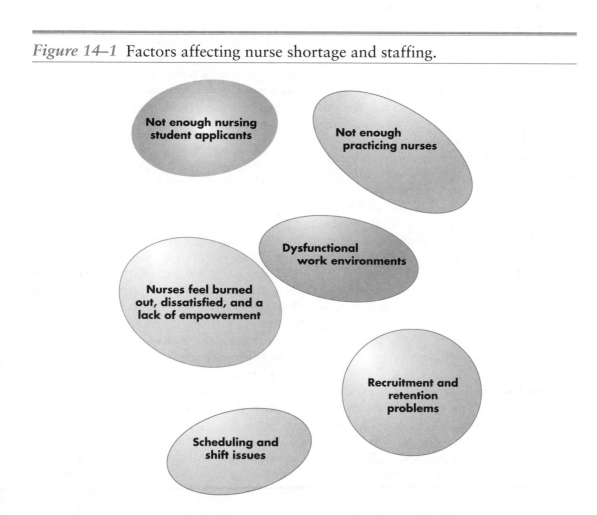

$27.54 (U.S. Department of Labor, 2007). States and regions of the country vary in the number of employed nurses and in nursing salaries. Some nurses are inactive, not employed in nursing, or not employed at all. Some of these nurses plan to return to nursing—for example, after raising a family or after younger children start school—and some do not. Some states are trying to attract these nurses back into nursing by offering transition programs to update their competencies. Some boards of nursing require completion of this type of program if a nurse has not been practicing for a specified number of years. Typically, the program includes didactic and supervised clinical instruction for several months.

Diversity

As discussed in Chapter 1, more men are needed in nursing. Data from a 2006 survey (National League for Nursing [NLN], 2008) indicate that there has been recent steady growth in the number of men graduating from nursing programs, with men representing 12.1% of nursing graduates. This is still a small percentage of men in nursing. This same survey also indicated a marked increase in graduates who are members of racial or ethnic minority groups (Asians, African Americans, Hispanics, and American Indians). The survey included data on types of degrees awarded for 2006: 59% were awarded a 2-year associate's degree; 38% were awarded a baccalaureate degree; and 8% completed a diploma program.

Despite these encouraging signs, applications to RN programs fell a notable 8.7 percent in 2005-06, down from a peak in applications a year earlier. The drop is suspected to be the result of widespread awareness of the difficulty of gaining entry to nursing school, fueled by the continuing crippling shortage of nurse educators.

By all indications, unmet demand for placement persists, with 88,000 qualified applications— one in three of all applications submitted— denied. Baccalaureate degree programs turned away 20 percent of its applications, while associate degree programs turned away 32.7 percent. (NLN, 2008, p. 1)

Generally, the workforce picture is the same, with some slight improvement in the percentage of men and members of certain racial and ethnic groups. This workforce profile is not changing rapidly.

Age

Another issue in the workforce profile is the age range of RNs. The age distribution of RNs in 2004 supports the serious future problem of retiring nurses (Division for Nursing National Sample Survey of RNs, as cited in New York Center of Health Workforce Studies [NYCHWS], 2006):

- 9% under the age of 30
- 20% 30–39 years of age
- 34% 40–49 years of age
- 28% 50–59 years of age
- 9% 60 and older

This distribution is disturbing. It indicates that 37% of nurses are quite close to retirement, and some of the RNs in the 40–49 age range are near 50 and approaching retirement as well. Retirement will have an impact on the nursing shortage, but there is another issue with this workforce profile: With a greater percentage of RNs (71%) older than 39, it is critical to consider the impact of age on the working nurse. Nursing is not an easy job; it is a physically and emotionally demanding profession. Nurses feel the impact of the care they provide, and, as is discussed later in this chapter, the work is not getting easier. Will this have an impact on how long nurses stay in nursing? Does this have an impact on errors? Does this have an impact on staff injuries? Most likely, the age of nurses does have an impact on all these issues. Exhibit 14–1 illustrates the key findings from the U.S. Health Workforce Profile (NYCHWS, 2006).

Educational Levels

Educational levels for nurses, including the issue of the entry-level degree, were discussed in Chapter 4. As was discussed, RNs can take the RN licensure exam after completion of a baccalaureate degree (BSN), an associate's degree (AD), or a diploma program. More research is being done to consider whether the degree influences patient outcomes, as is discussed later in this chapter. A recent study concluded that "the type of academic preparation nurses receive appears to be linked with work environment perceptions across the continuum of professional nursing practice. In general, BSN graduates have more positive perceptions of the work environ-

ment as compared with their AD colleagues" (Sexton, Hunt, Cox, Teasley, & Carroll, 2008, p. 105). Many AD nurses are returning to school to attend RN-BSN programs, but there are still many more who do not earn a bachelor's degree.

Generational Issues

Another important characteristic of the workforce that has an impact on how the work is done, the commitment to work, and teamwork within healthcare organizations (HCOs) is the different generations that are represented in nursing. Nursing as a profession is diverse in terms of generations, which has advantages and disadvantages. The diversity of four generations provides the profession with multiple viewpoints and approaches to solving problems. This can be positive if it does not lead to conflict. Conflict does occur when there is limited understanding of another's generation, especially how members of each generation communicate and work.

EXHIBIT 14–1 KEY FINDINGS FROM THE U.S. HEALTH WORKFORCE PROFILE, OCTOBER 2006

Nursing—Registered Nurses (RNs), Licensed Practical Nurses (LPNs), and Nurse Practitioners (NPs)

- California had more than 200,000 actively practicing RNs, the most of any state, but had the fewest RNs per capita in the nation.
- The New England census division had the most RNs per capita and 72% more than the Pacific census division, which had the fewest.
- The East South Central census division had the most LPNs per capita, more than twice as many as the Pacific census division, which had the fewest.
- More than 21% of LPNs were Black/African-American, compared to about 5% of RNs.
- Hispanics/Latinos were substantially underrepresented in nursing, comprising 6.1% of RNs and 3.2% of LPNs, even though they were nearly 13% of the general population.
- The number of RN and LPN degrees awarded increased by 18% and 22%, respectively, while the number of post-RN degrees declined by 6%.
- The New England census division had the most NPs per capita, more than three times as many as the East North Central census division, which had the fewest.

Source: The United States Health Workforce Profile, by the New York Center of Health Workforce Studies, October 2006. Report prepared for Health Resources and Services Administration (HRSA), Rensselaer, NY: Author and HRSA.

"Managing diversity here is defined as creating and maintaining an environment in which each person is respected because of his or her differences" (Davis, 2001, p. 161). We need greater dialogue and collaboration among the generations. What are the four generations present today in the nursing workforce and nursing education programs?

- *The traditional, silent, or mature generation, born between 1930 and 1940:* For the most part, this generation is no longer in practice because of their age, but it is important to recognize their impact on nursing. These nurses who were discussed in Chapter 1—those who moved nursing to a professional level in the United States and elsewhere—were committed to nursing and the HCO for which they worked. They believed in the hierarchy as an important part of the organization.
- *Baby Boomers, born between 1943 and 1960:* This generation is currently in practice, but it is also the generation approaching retirement (from practice and from nursing education). Baby boomers constitute the largest number of nurses active in the healthcare system today, so they have a major impact on healthcare delivery and the nursing profession. How is this generation described? Most nurses of this generation are women. When they entered nursing, they typically had two career choices other than being a housewife and mother—nursing or teaching. Members of this generation work independently, accept authority, cause few problems, feel that loyalty is an important work value, and are less able to cope with new technology, though many have been leaders in introducing technology to nursing. Baby Boomers are described as workaholics. This can have a

major impact on conflict with later generations, who are more interested in a balance between work and personal life (Bertholf & Kinnaird, 2001). Baby Boomer nurses prefer consensus leadership, are competitive, and are more focused on material gain (Gerke, 2001). Currently, representatives from this generation hold the major leadership positions in nursing management, nursing education, and nursing organizations. Most people expect others, even those from other generations, to respond in similar ways to themselves and have similar values; conflict can arise because this is not always true.

- *Generation X, born between 1960 and 1980:* Nurses from this generation have been replacing retiring nurses from the Baby Boomer generation. This generation has grown up in a time of major change, particularly in the area of technology. They are looking for effective, intelligent leadership and mentors. What do they want from leaders? They want to be trusted and respected by nurse leaders. This generation's key characteristics are being motivational, receptive, and positive. They are good communicators and team players, they have good people skills, and they are approachable and supportive (Wieck, Prydum, & Walsh, 2002). Some issues with this generation are not helpful to the profession. Typically, they are not as interested in groups or organizations as much as the previous generation. This will have an impact on nursing organizations that constantly struggle to maintain an active membership. Generation X nurses also do not demonstrate as much loyalty to their employers; this results in job changing, which is costly for the healthcare system and has an impact on quality care. A third issue is that this generation wants a personal life. They are not workaholics. Positive interests and qualities are diversity, technology, independence, adaptability, and creativity.

> *Generation Xers are pessimistic and rightfully so given the world they grew up in. They are loyal to themselves and the people with whom they have familial-like relationships. They like to feel that they are part of something bigger. They expect and respond well to things that contribute to their own professional knowledge and competency. Xers are flexible and very comfortable with change. . . . They are technoliterate. . . . Because Generation X often views a job as a stepping stone to the next job, benefits and rewards geared to the present rather than the future are the most valuable in recruitment and retention. (Ulrich, 2001, p. 152)*

This description of Generation X explains some of the conflicts and communication issues that have an impact on intraprofessional teams when teams of nurses must work together.

- *Generation Y, born between 1980 and 2000 (Nexters or Millennials)*: This generation is the newest to enter nursing, and many are just now entering nursing education programs. This confident group values achievement, social issues, and diversity. They are very dependent on technology (computers, cell phones, and any new communication technology that comes on the market). They can multitask and are optimistic. They are different from Generation X in that they have more trust in centralized authority (Gerke, 2001). Change is normal for them, and thus they have more experience with it.

The greatest conflict has arisen between the Baby Boomers and the entering generations. Baby Boomers are tired and have limited tolerance for different values and work ethics. Generations X and Y see this and worry about themselves as they enter the profession. Will they burn out under the stress? They complain that the "older nurses" do not support them or guide them and do not even seem to want them on the units as students. If strategies to resolve this are not initiated, this conflict will continue to cause major problems in the profession and in healthcare delivery. Understanding differences and then working toward better communication is critical to improvement. For example, Baby Boomers may wonder why newer nurses are not willing to work extra and longer hours, and Generation X and Y nurses wonder why the Baby Boomers work so hard and complain that younger nurses are not committed. Understanding takes time, but first it must begin.

The bottom line when viewing the nurse workforce profile is that

> *the success of the healthcare system is dependent on qualified personnel. Access to care, quality of care, and costs of care are all affected by the availability of properly educated and trained workers. In formulating policies, plans, and programs, health policy makers should carefully consider the supply, demand, distribution, education, and use of health workers needed to deliver essential services. (NYCHWS, 2006, p. iii)*

The Nursing Shortage

The nursing shortage has been described as part of a perfect storm in health care (Bleich et al., 2003). The three storms have combined (1) an increased demand for nurses, (2) a decreased supply of nurses, and (3) unfavorable work conditions. The shortage is influenced by several factors: (1) not enough nurses in practice, (2) not enough applicants to nursing programs, (3) not enough faculty to teach in nursing programs, and (4) the approaching retirement of an alarming number of nurses. Table 14–1 and Figure 14–2 provide some data about the shortage and employment.

Staffing: Impact on Care and the Nursing Shortage

Staffing: Impact on Care

There is an increasing amount of information about, and studies focusing on, the impact of nursing staff on care outcomes; however, much more needs to be known about this critical topic. The nursing profession needs this information to support the use of effective levels of staff and to prevent HCOs from filling RN positions with non-RNs when it may not be the best approach.

Hospitals with low nurse staffing levels tend to have higher rates of poor patient outcomes, such as pneumonia, shock, cardiac arrest, and urinary tract infections (UTIs), according to research funded by the Agency for Healthcare Research and Quality (AHRQ) and others (AHRQ, 2004). Changes in hospital care, such as new medical technologies and a declining average length-of-stay, have had an impact on patient care. New medical technologies allow many patients to receive care in outpatient settings (ambulatory case surgery) who would have previously received inpatient surgical care. Even though many patients are acutely ill, patients today tend to stay in the hospital a shorter length of time, despite their condition requiring more intense nursing care. During the period 1980–2000, the average length of an inpatient

Table 14–1 REASONS FOR THE CURRENT NURSING SHORTAGE, 2004 AND 2005

Main reasons for the current nursing shortage	RNs 2004 (N = 657) Percent	MDs 2004 (N = 445) Percent	CNOs 2005 (N = 222) Percent	CEOs 2005 (N = 142) Percent
More career options for women	32	18*	35	33
Faculty shortages in nursing schools	12	—	20	23
Salary and benefits	41	21*	14	21*
Difficult occupation/high workload/ undesirable hours	28	27	26	17*
Inadequate nursing schools/programs/ seats for students	12	3*	18	17
Nursing not seen as a rewarding career	26	—	6*	9*

—Question not asked

*Statistically significantly different from registered nurses (p = 0.05)

Source: From *The Future of the Nursing Workforce in the United States: Data, Trends and Implications*, by P.I. Buerhaus, D.O. Staiger and D.I. Auerbach, 2009, Sudbury, MA: Jones and Bartlett Publishers. Data from national surveys of RNs, physicians, and hospital executives, by Health Resources and Services Administration, Federal Division of Nursing.

Figure 14–2 Number of employed RNs using the Current Population Survey (CPS) and National Sample Survey of Registered Nurses (NSSRN), 1977–2006.

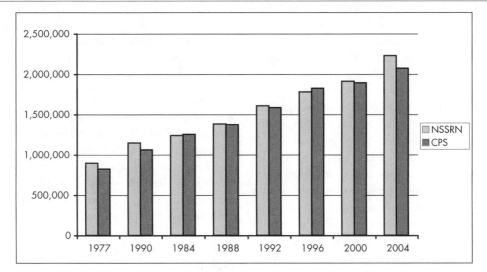

Source: From *The Future of the Nursing Workforce in the United States: Data, Trends and Implications*, by P.I. Buerhaus, D.O. Staiger and D.I. Auerbach, 2009, Sudbury, MA: Jones and Bartlett Publishers. From a current population survey, by National Sample Survey of Registered Nurses.

hospital stay decreased from 7.5 days to 4.9 days (National Center for Health Statistics, 2002). Sicker patients means an increased need for competent care that meets demand, yet the current status is that there are not enough nurses, and competency is questioned in many situations.

The Institute of Medicine (IOM) issued a report in 1996 that recognized the importance of determining the appropriate nurse–patient ratios and distribution of skills for ensuring that patients receive quality health care. The IOM's analysis of staffing and quality of care in hospitals recommended "a systematic effort . . . at the national level to collect and analyze current and relevant data and develop a research and evaluation agenda so that informed policy development, implementation and evaluation are

undertaken in a timely manner" (1996, p. 10). "Failure to rescue" (FTR) is defined as the death of a patient or a life-threatening complication for which early identification by nurses and medical staff and interventions could have influenced the risk of complication or death. The IOM report on nursing (2004) indicated that nurses are critical in decreasing failure to rescue. The number of nurses and their competency are critical factors in reducing FTR.

Nursing-sensitive outcomes, discussed in Chapter 12, are important indicators of quality of care. Some adverse patient outcomes potentially sensitive to nursing care are UTIs, pneumonia, shock, upper gastrointestinal bleeding, longer hospital stays, failure to rescue, and 30-day mortality. Most research has focused on adverse rather than positive patient outcomes because adverse outcomes are much more likely to be documented in the medical record.

The following information is from the AHRQ (2004) and highlights results from AHRQ-funded research studies about the impact of staffing on patient outcomes and quality of care. Three AHRQ-funded studies found a significant correlation between lower nurse staffing levels and higher rates of pneumonia (Cho, Ketefian, Barkauskas, & Smith, 2003; Kovner, Jones, Zhan, Gergen, & Basu, 2002; Kovner, Mezey, & Harrington, 2000). Two AHRQ-funded studies have found that when nurse staffing levels are lower, rates of 30-day mortality and the likelihood of failure to rescue are higher. Studies overall are not consistent in demonstrating that a higher nursing workload is associated with an increase in patient mortality (Aiken, Clarke, Sloane, Sochalski, & Silber, 2002; Aiken, Sloane, Lake, Sochalski, & Weber, 1999). These studies document the connection between lower levels of nurse staffing and higher rates of adverse events. Complementing those studies are a number of other studies that address the growing nurse workload and rising rates of **burnout** and job dissatisfaction. One study, jointly funded by AHRQ and the National Science Foundation, examined the relationship between nurse staffing and hospital patient acuity (the average severity of illness of the inpatient population) in Pennsylvania hospitals (Unruh, 2003). Acuity determines how much care a patient needs: The higher the acuity, the more care is required. This study found the following:

- A 21% increase in hospital patient acuity between 1991 and 1996, with no net change in the number of employed licensed nurses.
- A total decrease of 14.2% in the ratio of licensed nursing staff to acuity-adjusted

patient days of care because of the increase in patient acuity. In addition, the skill mix of the nursing staff shifted as hospitals increased the number of nurses' aides. As a result, RNs acquired more supervisory responsibilities that took them away from the bedside at a time when their patients needed more bedside nursing care.

The largest of these studies on nurse staffing—a study jointly funded by AHRQ, the Health Resources and Services Administration, the Centers for Medicare and Medicaid Services, and the National Institute of Nursing Research—examined the records of 5 million medical patients and 1.1 million surgical patients who had been treated at 799 hospitals in 1993 (Cho et al., 2003; Needleman, Buerhaus, Mattke, Stewart, & Zelevinsky, 2001). Among the study's principal findings:

- In hospitals with high RN staffing, medical patients had lower rates of five adverse patient outcomes (UTIs, pneumonia, shock, upper gastrointestinal bleeding, and longer hospital stay) than patients in hospitals with low RN staffing.
- Major surgery patients in hospitals with high RN staffing had lower rates of two patient outcomes (UTIs and failure to rescue).
- Higher rates of RN staffing were associated with a reduction in adverse outcomes of 3–12%, depending on the outcome.
- Higher staffing at all levels of nursing was associated with a reduction in adverse outcomes of 2–25%, depending on the outcome.

It is clear that nursing care has an impact on patient outcomes, though more investigation is needed to better understand the relationship and to develop improved care strategies.

Staffing: What a New Nurse Needs to Know

When a nurse takes his or her first job, it is critical that the potential new employee inquire about the staffing—who does the staffing plan; how far in advance is staffing done; what methods are used; how inadequate staffing areas are covered; and whether mandatory overtime is required. Nurses need information about staffing and what input they might have in the staffing pattern. The first step is to learn staffing terminology and about staffing methods.

AMERICAN NURSES ASSOCIATION STAFFING PRINCIPLES

The American Nurses Association (ANA) staffing principles support that adequate staffing is critical to the delivery of quality patient care (ANA, 1998). These standards are divided into three categories. The principles of the patient care unit focus on the need for appropriate staffing levels for the unit. These standards reflect both the analysis of individual patient needs and aggregate patient needs, and unit functions that are important in delivering care. The second category focuses on staff-related principles, such as the type of nurse competencies needed to provide the required care; role responsibilities are important. The third category involves institutional or organizational policies; these policies should indicate that nurses are respected, and they should state a commitment to meeting budget requirements to fill nursing positions. Competencies for all nursing staff (employees, agency, and so on) should be documented. A clear plan should describe how float staff are used and the required cross-training. Staff members need to know if they may be switched from one unit to another. There must be a clear designation of the adequate number of staff needed to meet a minimum level of qual-

ity care. The principles identify four critical elements that need to be considered when making staffing decisions (ANA, 1998, as cited in Maguire, 2002, p. 8):

1. *Patients*: Patient characteristics and number of patients for whom care is being provided.
2. *Intensity of Unit and Care*: Individual patient intensity; across the unit intensity (taking into account the heterogeneity of settings); variability of care; admissions, discharges and transfers; volume.
3. *Context*: Architecture (geographic dispersion of patients, size and layout of individual patient rooms, arrangement of entire patient care unit(s), and so forth); technology (beepers, cellular phones, computers); same unit or cluster of patients.
4. *Expertise*: Learning curve for individuals and groups of nurses; staff consistency, continuity and cohesion; cross training; control of practice; involvement in quality improvement activities; professional expectations; preparation and experience.

An example of a state's staffing principles is provided in Exhibit 14–2 (the Oklahoma Nurses Association principles).

STAFFING TERMINOLOGY

Nurse staffing not only includes RNs but may also include licensed practical nurses (LPNs)/licensed vocational nurses and unlicensed assistive personnel (UAPs), all of whom provide direct care. As discussed in earlier chapters, RNs and LPNs are licensed by the states in which they are employed. Licensure is regulated by the State Board of Nursing, as discussed in Chapter 4. RNs assess patient needs, develop patient care plans, and administer medications and treatments, and they must meet the state's nurse practice act requirements. LPNs carry out specified

EXHIBIT 14–2 OKLAHOMA NURSES ASSOCIATION POSITION STATEMENT ON STAFFING

One of the nation's greatest challenges for healthcare is nurse staffing. It is the responsibility of the employing agency to provide for adequate and competent staff to safely care for patients. Upon communication of the inability to fulfill an assignment, it becomes the responsibility of the employer to establish alternative staffing arrangements. It is the responsibility of the professional nurse to provide for the safety and well being of the patients assigned and to work collaboratively within the team to make the most of available resources. Staff concerns regarding staffing need to be communicated to management with the expectation of resolving issues.

Staffing Variability

Appropriate nurse staffing is a dynamic process affected by unpredictable changes impacting care including census, acuity and number of available skilled and experienced nursing staff.

Nurse staffing varies from practice setting to practice setting, unit to unit. Factors affecting staffing decisions include, but are not limited to:

- Patient Factors:
  - Population—age, functional status, communication skills, disease processes
  - Acuity
  - Social support
  - Psychosocial/spiritual needs and resources
  - Cultural diversity
- Organizational Factors:
  - Architecture—unit layout
  - Technology—computers, pagers, phones, monitoring, etc.
  - Support—support personnel, interdisciplinary team, manager availability
  - Number of patients
  - Medical decision support
  - Unit/department governance
- Staff Nurse Factors:
  - Experience
  - Expertise
  - Team dynamics
  - Fatigue/special needs
  - Physical/psychosocial demands of the role
  - Maturity

Macro and Micro System Planning

The staffing process is dynamic, requiring planning and vigilance in terms of short-term day-to-day fluctuations as well as accurate budgeted staffing plans.

- Staffing models and plans are developed using forecasting techniques based on historical statistics, which are only roughly predictive of staffing needs in the here and now.
- Flexibility in the staffing process is required to respond to the demands of day-to-day fluctuations in patient census and acuity in order to promote patient safety. Flexibility can be addressed through a variety of processes including:
  - Skillful adjustment of the unit staff schedule on a day-to-day basis
  - Effective use of temporary staffing services—internal or external

- Effective human resource and human capital planning to meet projected long range needs including:
  - Recruitment programs—to ensure adequate availability of staff
  - Retention programs—to maintain engagement of established staff, protect human capital investments
  - Staff education programs—to prepare staff for the changing demands of the health care environment
  - Career development programs—to address the emerging shortage of health care professionals
  - Preserving the expertise of the mature nurse workforce
  - Creating work environments that support staff with special needs
  - Staff facilitated decision making about patient care

Characteristics of effective staffing processes include:

- Staff involvement in planning on a day-to-day as well as long range basis
- Collaborative relationship among staff, front line managers and organizational leaders
- Center on the needs of the patient population served
- Address the geographic and technologic challenges of the environment
- Leverage technology to enhance communication and information management
- Flexibility to address fluctuations in census, acuity and seasonal variation
- Effective use of temporary staff
- Use unlicensed assistive staff to augment the care delivered by licensed nurses, not attempt to substitute for licensed staff
- Promote collaborative interdisciplinary support and planning

The position of the Oklahoma Nurses Association related to staffing effectiveness is:

1. There is no substitution for registered nurses.
2. Registered nurses have a positive impact on nurse sensitive patient outcomes and measures, including:
   - Failure to rescue
   - Mortality
   - Complications
     - Infection
     - DVT
     - Pneumonia
   - Pressure ulcer incidence
   - Fall rate
   - Patient Satisfaction
3. Nurse leaders are actively involved in planning operational and long range goals for effective staffing to address:
   - Impact of fatigue is associated with increased errors and nurse satisfaction
   - Maturity of the nurse, and physical demand of the role.
   - Working Hours and roles are adjusted to retain the mature workforce
4. Health care organizations facilitate collaborative relationships among staff, front line managers and organizational leaders
5. Staffing decisions are based on:
   - Needs of the patient/patient population
   - Geographic and technologic complexities are addressed in the work environment
   - Flexibility to address fluctuations related to census, acuity and seasonal variation
6. Use temporary staff and unlicensed assistive staff to augment the care delivered by licensed nurses; must be supervised by a registered nurse.

continues

Exhibit 14–2 (continued)

7. During a disaster, the mode of operation related to staffing is based on survival and strategies adopted by the federal and local authorities.

References:

American Nurses Association. (2005). Utilization Guide for the ANA Principles for Nurse Staffing. Nurse Executive Center. (2006). Towards Evidence Based Staffing: Toolkit for Optimizing Workforce Tradeoffs, Health Care Advisory Board.

Adopted 11/2006 ONA HOD

Source: Position statement on staffing, adopted by the 2006 ONA House of Delegates by Oklahoma Nurses Association, 2006, Oklahoma City, OK: Author. Reprinted with permission.

---

nursing duties under the direction of RNs. Nurses' aides typically provide nonspecialized duties and personal care activities. Some states require that UAPs complete a certification program, at which point they are referred to as certified nurse assistants. Hospitals and other HCOs have written position descriptions for RNs, LPNs, and UAPs. These descriptions should be followed. They influence staffing because the descriptions identify what staff members may do, which impacts the staff mix. Nurse staffing is measured in one of two basic ways:

- Nursing hours per patient per day
- The nurse-to-patient ratio

"Nursing hours" may refer to RNs only; to RNs and LPNs; or to RNs, LPNs, and UAPs. It is important to know which staff category is identified by the nurse staffing measurement. **Nursing care hours** refers to the number of hours of patient care provided per unit of time. However, "it is becoming increasingly clear that, when determining nursing hours of care, one size (or formula) does not fit all. In fact, staffing is most appropriate and meaningful when it is predicated on a measure of unit intensity that takes into consideration the aggregate population of patients and associated roles and responsibilities of nursing staff" (Maguire, 2002, p. 7).

The term **full-time equivalent (FTE)** is used to describe a position. An FTE is equal to 40 hours of work per week for 52 weeks, or 2,080 hours per year. One FTE can represent one staff member or several; an FTE can be divided (e.g., two staff members each working half an FTE). Many nursing units employ part-time staff.

Staffing mix describes the type of nursing staff needed to provide care. The mix should be determined by considering the type of care needed and patient status, as well as the qualification and competencies needed to provide the care. In some cases, the staff must be RNs, and in other situations, a mix of RNs, LPNs, and UAPs is needed, with the RN supervising. This issue is often a concern when the proportion of RNs is compared with other types of nursing staffing. Another factor that needs to be considered is the work level; for example, the typical time for discharges and admissions or the surgical schedule can make a difference as to when more or fewer staff members are needed (**distribution of staff**).

SCHEDULING

The shift, or typical pattern of time worked, is an important factor in scheduling. Some areas of care use multiple types of shifts, and others have only one type. Typical shifts are 8-, 10-, and 12-

hour shifts. More and more hospitals are using 12-hour shifts. Staff often prefer 12-hour shifts because of more days off (40 hours can add up quickly). However, there has been concern about 12-hour shifts and the resulting fatigue level that may lead to more errors (IOM, 2004). Other concerns are increased risk to infections for staff who are fatigued and ergonomic stressors; accidents that result from driving home tired; and responsibilities at home that further increase nurses' fatigue (Worthington, 2001). More research needs to be done to determine the impact of shifts on fatigue and errors. Split shifts are used to provide more staff at busy times of the day (such as 7:00–11:00 A.M., or later in the day). Split shifts are usually staffed by part-time staff.

The staffing schedule can contribute to many negative results. Since staff usually do not get off on time, longer shifts can compound the problems associated with 12-hour shifts. For example, when staff work 12-hour shifts instead of 8-hour shifts, staying one hour past the end of shifts can be very difficult. This is a frequent occurrence because some staff may be arriving late or not coming at all, and temporary coverage is needed until additional staff are found. This makes a 12-hour shift much longer. In some HCOs, staff are required to rotate shifts so that they may switch back and forth from the day shift to the night shift. This can be hard for many nurses, though some like to work the night shift. Exhibit 14–3 lists some tips for adjusting to the night shift.

Scheduling is not easy and causes a lot of conflict among staff. Nurses want more say in scheduling. Some organizations use computerized request systems so that staff can input their special staffing requests, and others do this in writing or orally. When staffing is posted is also of concern because staff need to make their personal plans. How far in advance is the schedule posted?

Exhibit 14–3 Tips for Working the Night Shift

- Do not exercise before you try to sleep.
- Develop a routine for your time off and sleep time, and maintain it. Set up a plan with family members so that sleep time during the day is not disrupted.
- When you get tired at work, try to do something active. If you are allowed rest time, take it.
- If you feel unusually tired and are administering medications, ask a coworker to double check dose, and so on.
- Snack foods at work are not helpful. Drink water.
- Working more than three nights in a row can cause problems with circadian rhythm.
- Eat lightly before going to sleep.
- Avoid use of sleep medications and alcohol.
- Relax a little before trying to go to sleep.
- Do not think that because you have all day open and do not have to go to work until nighttime that you have all this extra time.
- Some find it helpful to wear sunglasses on the way home from work.
- Keep a diary of your sleep pattern to see if you can find the best time for the longest daytime sleep.
- Avoid excessive use of caffeine.
- Each person's sleep is individual, so it's important to find your own pattern.

Source: Summarized information from "Surviving the Night Shift" by D. Pronitis-Ruotolo, 2001, *American Journal of Nursing, 101*(7), 63–68.

The procedures for schedule changes need to be known by all staff. The trend is for HCOs to develop staffing schedules centrally, though some may still do it unit by unit. In addition, a nonnurse scheduler is more common today (Cavouras, 2006). This model has disadvantages because it may leave out or limit important input from nurse managers. However, "one of the most important reasons that people (nurse managers) leave hospital nursing is frustration with schedules and staffing" (Cavouras, 2006, p. 36), so it is important to find a balance. Scheduling must consider patient needs, organization needs, legislative requirements, unions, shortage concerns, use of external sources for staff (e.g., agencies), and rising labor costs.

Patient classification systems (PCS) may be used to assist with staffing levels. These systems are computerized and used to identify and quantify patient needs that can then be matched with staffing level and mix. It is thought that these systems are more objective because data related to patients and their needs are input, and these data are used to determine the number and type of staff required per shift.

Some organizations or patient care units use **self-scheduling** (Hung, 2002). With this system, guidelines are developed for the schedule. Staff are then given a certain amount of time to fill in the schedule based on the guidelines. Individual staff members do need to consider the schedules that other staff members have already posted. When the designated time period is completed, the nurse manager (or a staff member who is responsible for completing the schedule) reviews it and makes any required changes or additions to ensure that staffing is adequate. This type of scheduling allows staff to feel more in control of the staffing and to work with one another to come up with the most effective arrangement. It also reduces the time that the nurse manager or another scheduler might spend

on staffing. More staff input and control over staffing usually means greater staff satisfaction and less absenteeism, which leads to greater staff empowerment.

The schedule inevitably has "holes"—positions on the schedule for which there is no staff member. What does the HCO do? One method to fill holes in the schedule is for the HCO to develop a float pool. This is a group of staff (RNs, LPNs, or UAPs) who may be moved from unit to unit based on need. This group of staff need to be competent in the relevant area of care and should be flexible and able to adjust quickly to new environments. Float pool staff are employees of the HCO who do not have a specific unit to which they are assigned. Staff who float need orientation and training related to the types of care that they will be expected to provide. Because of the nursing shortage, there is also increasing use of staff who are not employees of the organization. Agency nurses are nurses hired by a nursing agency; the agency then contracts with an HCO for specific types of staff to fill holes in the schedule. Some hospitals contract with one supplemental staffing agency, and some HCOs contract with multiple agencies to meet their staffing needs. An agency nurse is paid by the agency (typically more than usual organization staff), must be licensed, and should meet employee competency qualifications or any other criteria required by the HCO. The HCO pays the agency, and the nurse is paid by the agency. Work assignments can be for one shift, for several days, or for weeks or months. A third method for responding to incomplete schedules or lack of staff to fill all positions needed is the use of travelers. Travelers are nurses who work for an agency, but not a local agency. They are hired by the agency and then assigned to work at an HCO for a block of time (more than a few days and often several months). The nurse may come from anywhere in the United States. The agency pays the nurse's salary, benefits, moving and travel expenses, and housing. Salaries are often very high. Nurses can decline a specific assignment, and moving is required. Nurses might even be assigned a management position. Nurses who are employed by the HCO are often concerned about the pay difference; traveling nurses, as well as regular agency nurses, typically earn much more than the full-time employees, and this can cause conflict. Travelers must meet the requirements to practice in the state and the requirements of the HCO. All these nurses need orientation and should not be expected to just get to work. It is not easy to change from one HCO to another because HCOs are not all the same; the nurse has to learn quickly to work with a new team. More experienced nurses are better at making this transition, and many of these agencies hire only experienced nurses.

Mandatory overtime has become an important topic in nursing today. This is a strategy used by HCOs to fill the holes in the schedule. This strategy requires staff to work past their scheduled end time if they want to keep their job. This has serious consequences, particularly for the longer shifts (such as the 12-hour shift). It impacts fatigue, health of staff, and quality of care. Nurses need to know what their rights are in relation to overtime pay. Many states are considering legislation to stop mandatory overtime. If a nurse does not feel competent to work longer hours, he or she should say no. Nurses need to be sure that their board of nursing does not consider this action abandonment of patients (Vernarec, 2000). Working when one feels unfit can create a dangerous situation. If the nurse belongs to a union, he or she may lodge a complaint through the union.

Recruitment

Recruitment in nursing involves the recruitment of both nurses and nursing students. Some

improvement has occurred in recruitment of nurses. Much of this improvement has been stimulated by the Johnson & Johnson advertising campaign for nursing students, as discussed in Chapter 3. These multimedia campaigns highlighted the value of nursing as a profession and the need for more nurses, and they sent out a proactive message about nursing. Schools of nursing, states, and the federal government have been increasing their efforts to increase scholarship and loan funds for students. Schools of nursing have tried to expand enrollment, and many have been successful. However, there are two major roadblocks to expansion. The first is the shortage of nursing faculty, which will only increase as more faculty enter retirement. Schools are trying various strategies, such as making collaborative arrangements with hospitals and other HCOs to use their staff as clinical faculty; having nurses with BSN degrees and sufficient clinical experience assist with clinical teaching; and opening up more master's in nursing education programs. Offering these programs online and in an accelerated format can help to develop additional faculty. The second barrier is finding enough clinical sites for clinical experiences. This is a major struggle in some areas that have a lot of schools and only limited healthcare sites. The increased use of simulation labs for some of the clinical experiences decreases some of the need, but it does not solve the problem entirely.

Recruitment of staff is just as challenging. HCOs advertise in local, state, and national newspapers, on radio and television, in professional journals, and on a growing number of Internet sites that offer information about jobs. Many HCOs offer bonuses to entice new staff, though this does not guarantee that a nurse will not then seek a job elsewhere for another bonus. All specialties—not just one specialty or a few—are experiencing the shortage. Specialties that usually attract younger nurses because of the fast-paced nature of the work—such as intensive care units, emergency departments, and surgical nursing (operating room and post-anesthesia)—have had increasing difficulty attracting nurses; there simply are not enough. Nurses also listen to other nurses regarding the best places to work. Disgruntled nurses can do great damage to efforts to attract new staff. HCOs need to recognize that all aspects of recruitment can attract new nurses but also push them away. How the nurse is treated from the very beginning—on the telephone, responsiveness during the interview, whether a tour is provided, along with the opportunity to talk to staff—is very important. With so many openings, the nurse is in the "driver's seat" in the recruitment process. There are plenty of other positions to consider. The nurse's ability to relocate expands his or her opportunities. Potential new staff will also be looking at salaries and benefits, scheduling, educational benefits, orientation time, the HCO's reputation and the reputation of its nursing service, and position responsibilities. Magnet status also has become important (see Chapter 15). In last few years, new graduates have shown an increasing interest in participating in nurse residency programs, which are discussed later in this chapter.

Retention

After staff are recruited, they need to be retained. There is a great risk of job hopping with so many jobs open. New nurses and experienced nurses are leaving nursing. Nurse turnover is very costly (Jones & Gates, 2007). Turnover costs range from $22,000 to more than $64,000 per nurse (Advisory Board, 1999; Jones, 2005; O' Brien-Pallas et al., 2006; Stone et al., 2003; Waldman, Kelly, Sanjeev, & Smith, 2004). It is, however, difficult to define nurse turnover costs (and benefits). What are some of the costs and benefits of turnover (Jones & Gates, 2007)?

Nurse Turnover Costs

- Advertising and recruitment
- Vacancy costs (e.g., paying for agency nurses, overtime, closed beds, and hospital diversions when the emergency department must be closed)
- Hiring (review and processing of applicants)
- Orientation and training
- Decreased productivity (loss of staff who know routines)
- Termination (processing of termination)
- Potential patient errors; compromised quality of care
- Poor work environment and culture; dissatisfaction; distrust
- Loss of organizational knowledge (loss of staff who know the history of the organization and processes)

Nurse Turnover Benefits

- Reductions in salaries and benefits for newly hired nurses versus departing nurses
- Savings from bonuses not paid to outgoing nurses
- Replacement nurses bringing in new ideas, reality, and innovations, as well as knowledge of competitors
- Elimination of poor performers (not guaranteed, it is hoped)

Focusing on retention is more important than focusing on turnover, but there are benefits and costs related to retention as well (Jones & Gates, 2007).

Nurse Retention Benefits

- Reduction in advertisement and recruitment costs
- Fewer vacancies and reduction in vacancy costs
- Fewer new hires and reduction in hiring costs

- Fewer orientees and reduced orientation and training costs
- Maintained or increased productivity
- Fewer terminations and reduction in termination costs
- Decreased patient errors and increased quality of care
- Improved work environment and culture, and increased satisfaction, trust, and accountability
- Preserved organizational knowledge
- Easier nurse recruitment

Nurse Retention Costs

- Specific program costs (e.g., nurse residency, mentoring)
- Benefit improvements and salary increases
- Rewards and recognition events
- Ongoing education, learning and career advancement opportunities, tuition reimbursement
- Dedication of organizational leaders and staff who focus on nurse retention and building/maintaining relationships
- Bonus programs, stock options, and/or cash awards
- Mechanisms for communication and voicing concerns, such as providing anonymous suggestions, ongoing surveys, 360-degree feedback
- Promotion and career advancement opportunities
- Creative staffing and scheduling options
- Adequate nurse staffing

More research is needed to better understand turnover and retention and to "lay the foundation for estimating the economic value of nursing (e.g., that relationship between the costs of RNs relative to the quality gains derived from their employment)" (Jones & Gates, 2007, p. 1).

Strategies to Resolve the Shortage

There is no magic answer for coping with the nursing shortage, but efforts have been made to find it. California has tried to do this through its 2003 legislation that requires the state department of health to establish specific nurse-to-patient ratios in acute care hospitals. Why is this problematic? The ratio is determined by the amount of time that the RN spends on direct care activities, defined by use of patient classification systems and nursing care hours; however, neither of these has been nationally or regionally standardized. There is little to support that these ratios will be the same from one unit to the other (Upenieks et al., 2008). Upenieks et al. (2008) conducted a study to examine the implications of California's ratios. The conclusions of the study are:

- Staffing ratios may exist to guard against creating a maximum patient load per nurse, yet the mandates do not specify the ideal staffing mix. (Note that UAPs and other support staff are not factored into the ratios and, in some situations, have been reduced in number.)
- When setting statewide mandatory staffing ratios for RNs, this study suggests that it is essential to include UAP and staffing support systems (advanced nurse practitioners, intravenous therapy teams, lift teams, transporters, and orderlies) in a prescribed number because their responsibilities are an integral part of patient-centered care.
- Patient outcome evidence is insufficient for the purpose of establishing ratios as an effective way to improve patient care.

Transforming Care at the Bedside, discussed in more detail in Chapter 15, supports the perspective that "nursing productivity should be viewed as value-added care, a vision that goes beyond direct care activities and includes care measurement activities such as team collaboration, physician rounding, increased RN-to-aide communication, and patient-centeredness, all of which are crucial to both the nurse's role and the patient's well-being" (Upenieks et al., 2008, p. 294). This also is more in line with the IOM five core competencies.

Retaining staff requires planned efforts. Examples of strategies that are used today include the following (IOM, 2004; Jones & Gates, 2007):

- Improve nursing leadership
- Increase staff input into decision making
- Increase salaries and benefits (provide some choices in benefits; for example, younger nurses may be interested in child care)
- Transform the workplace environment so that the nurse is respected as a professional and as a member of the interdisciplinary team
- Redesign work spaces so that they are more ergonomic and easier to work in
- Offer **flexible staffing** schedules
- Offer innovative employment opportunities, such as job sharing and split shifts
- Develop student externship programs and nurse residency programs
- Expand educational opportunities
- Recognize achievement (degrees, certification)
- Use career ladders
- Improve quality and safety (including staff safety issues)

Workforce Commission

Over the last decade, many agencies, including state workforce centers, have examined the issue of the nursing shortage. The American Academy of Nursing held a technology conference to exam-

ine work redesign and the use of technology to transform nursing care. As this initiative evolved, a commission on the workforce was formed. Drs. Margaret McClure, Linda Burns-Bolton, and Pam Cipriano led the charge. This leadership represented practice and academe. Quickly it was recognized that this shortage must address the pipeline issue—the faculty shortage, which of course focuses on educational preparation of the workforce. Drs. Margaret McClure and Brenda Cleary headed this subcommittee. The committee's composition represented regulators from the National Council of Boards of Nursing, accreditation groups such as the NLN and the American Association of Colleges of Nursing (AACN), and officials from higher education and practice. The thrust of this work is to identify barriers to increasing enrollments and redesigning education at all levels. It is recognized that to make sweeping changes, it is necessary to have regulatory bodies in the conversations to shape the new nursing educational models of the future. The need to produce more nurses does not necessarily mean a compromise of quality, but it does mean consideration of polarities (Scott & Cleary, 2007).

Legislation Impacting the Nursing Shortage

The Nurse Reinvestment Act of 2002 is a landmark legislation that addresses the critical issue of the nursing shortage. This legislation does the following (AACN, 2005):

- Establishes nurse scholarships in exchange for commitment to serve in a public or private nonprofit health facility determined to have a critical shortage of nurses
- Establishes nurse retention and patient safety enhancement grants
- Establishes comprehensive geriatric training grants for nurses

- Establishes a faculty loan cancellation program to allow for full-time study and rapid completion of advanced degree studies; recipients are obligated to spend a certain amount of time in a faculty position at a school of nursing
- Establishes a **career ladder** grant program to assist more nurses in the workforce to obtain more education and to establish partnerships between healthcare providers and schools of nursing for advanced training
- Establishes public service announcements to advertise and promote the nursing profession and educate the public about the rewards of a nursing career

This legislation offers a multipronged approach to the shortage by establishing initiatives to increase quality of care; increase faculty; increase the education level of nurses; retain nurses in practice; increase quality of care to a growing population, the elderly; and increase the number of applicants to nursing programs. States are also passing legislation that addresses nurse staffing issues, such as mandatory overtime and ratios. California has led the way with the state ratio levels.

Global Migration of Nurses

As the nursing shortage has increased, the hospitals in the United States have relied more on hiring nurses from other countries to fill vacant positions. This is a strategy that has been used during other shortages. Some of these nurses come to the United States for a short period, such as 1–2 years, and send money home, and others want to stay. Nurses who come to the United States to practice must pass the National Council Licensure Examination (NCLEX) and obtain an RN license even if they are licensed in their home country. They must be able to speak English, though this varies and can be a major problem. The NCLEX is given in English. Foreign-educated nurses can help solve some of the shortage problems, but their employment can lead to other problems. Successful acculturation is critical for success; acculturated nurses tend to stay longer, and their care is of higher quality (Emerson, 2001).

> *The global migration of nurses is a multifactorial phenomenon. Mejia, Pizurki, and Royston (1979) described the personal, social, political, and economic conditions that drive this phenomenon as "push and pull" factors. Push factors are those conditions that are present in donor countries that drive nurses to find employment abroad while pull factors are those conditions that exist in receiving countries that entice nurses to leave their homeland. (Emerson, 2001, p. 2)*

In many countries, nurses earn very low pay and are not treated as professionals. Nurses may be compelled to work in another country for better pay to support their families, whom they leave at home. This alone is difficult for the nurses, leading to loneliness and a feeling of being disconnected from their homes and families. They enter a healthcare system in the United States that is very different from what they are used to, and there is much to adjust to in addition to culture and language. HCOs are realizing that they need to provide nurses with support services to better retain them. Some hospitals have "buddies," or RNs who volunteer to help the new RN with adjustment—not just at work, but in daily living situations and with the many questions that arise. Mentors on the job are also very important. These RNs need effective orientation programs that consider their special language and culture, and differences in how care is provided. There are ethical concerns with global migration. A critical concern is that the nurses who are migrating are often causing a shortage of nurses in their home countries. There are also concerns about how nurses are treated in some countries regarding their position, respect, and pay. Global migration is complex and not a quick fix for a worldwide growing healthcare problem—the need for more healthcare providers in all categories. Exhibit 14–4 is a letter from the president of the NLN about globalization and nursing.

Creating a Healthy Work Environment: Retaining Nurses

Working in a healthcare environment can be a very positive experience, particularly if the environment is one in which staff are respected; communication is open; staff feel empowered and part of the decision-making process; staff safety and health are considered important; and staff feel that they are making a contribution. This,

---

EXHIBIT 14–4 A LETTER FROM THE CHIEF EXECUTIVE OFFICER NATIONAL LEAGUE FOR NURSING

June 18, 2007

Dear Member:

My jet lag is almost over and I am just now thinking back to the International Council of Nurses Conference, which took place at the end of May in Yokahama, Japan. I have been to ICN conferences many times, representing the ANA and the Royal College of Nursing. But this was my first time as a representative of the NLN, our association, which is focused intently on nursing education. This was a new perspective for me, and these are some of my thoughts.

First, it is important to understand that the world is watching the United States. Representatives from 80 countries were together in Japan, and it was apparent to me that we in the US are respected for establishing the primary standards in education that are used throughout the world. Despite an underpinning of caution due to the often negative stereotypes about arrogant Americans, this respect remains strong. In many ways, it stands as a tribute to our forebears at the NLN and a reminder that as we work to reform nursing education, the consequences of our efforts will reach far beyond our borders.

And then there was the experience of being one delegate from the United States among so many countries and so many cultures. I began my career with a rather parochial point of view. I grew up in a small town in Kentucky, and I remember thinking that it was foolish to focus on problems in other parts of the world while we have so many problems at home in our own backyard. But my world expanded with education, mentors, and career opportunities, and now I believe strongly in the value of a global perspective.

A world without nursing would be a world without caring. When we meet with nurses from other parts of the world we share understanding, and that is empowering. We come to realize that we are more alike than different, and we gain insight into our own value as nurses. Living our own lives, it is easy to become discouraged. But the whole is greater than the sum of its parts. When we look around and interact with others, we take on new energy. I say we, even though these are personal responses, because I am so certain that all nurses can benefit from a global perspective, and it is important to share that vision with our students.

Nurses are in a unique position to make a difference on the global stage. We are clinicians and we provide care. Eighty percent of all care provided in the world is delivered by nurses. Nurses are researchers—we know how to use statistics and evidence to make our case for funding and support at home and overseas—and we are consultants, managers, and leaders. And colleagues, most precious to us at the NLN is that we are educators: educators who lead, manage, research, consult, and practice. When we educate our students, we as nurse educators have the ability to make a profound difference in the world. We are change agents developing an army of caring and "carers."

The next ICN conference will be in Durbin, South Africa, in 2009. I hope you will make plans to be there. Perhaps you will submit an abstract and present your work. You can be sure that others from around the world will be interested in what you have to say.

Before I close, I want to call your attention to an important ICN endeavor. The ICN is urging the United Nations to establish a women's agency that is robustly funded, operational, and with on-the-ground presence in every country. The healthy development of all citizens and communities is inextricably tied to the education and empowerment of women and the strengthening of their health. In any culture, when we touch the lives of women, we touch the lives of families. I will keep you apprised as more information becomes available.

And I also will tell you in future messages about the work of the Joint NLN/NLNAC Task Force on Creating a Global Nursing Education Community. There is so much that the NLN and the NLNAC can accomplish by working together. It is exciting to be a nurse on the global stage at this time in our history. I feel empowered to make a difference. I know you will too!

> With all my best wishes,
> Beverly Malone, PhD, RN, FAAN
> Chief Executive Officer

Source: Vol. IX, Issue No. 12, June 18, 2007. A Biweekly Publication of the National League for Nursing. NLN Member Update Index.

however, is not always the case. Staff experience stress, burnout, and conflict in the workplace. What are some signs that students and staff should watch for in themselves, in others, and in organizations?

Personal Signs

- Irritability
- Lack of sleep or too much sleep
- Complaining about many aspects of work
- Unwillingness to help others
- Desire to just get the job done and leave
- Less enjoyment during personal time
- Dreading going to work
- High frustration with management
- Angry outbursts
- Gaining or losing weight
- Lack of energy

This type of attitude and behavior impacts others too—coworkers and family. Burnout is contagious because of this impact. Morale can decrease as staff try to cope with their stress and burnout. This affects productivity and the quality of care.

Organizational Signs

- Inadequate or confused communication
- Top-down decision making, leaving staff out
- Poorly planned change that is unsuccessful
- Increase in staff complaints
- Staff–management conflict
- Distrust of staff and staff distrust of management

The American Association of Critical-Care Nurses standards for healthy work environments (2005) address the need for improved work environments:

Each day, thousands of medical errors harm the patients and families served by the American healthcare system. Work environments that tolerate ineffective interpersonal relationships and do not support education to acquire necessary skills perpetuate unacceptable conditions. So do health professionals who experience moral distress over this state of affairs, yet remain silent and overwhelmed with resignation. Consider again these all-too-familiar situations.

- A nurse chooses not to call a physician known to be verbally abusive. The nurse uses her judgment to clarify a prescribed medication and administers a fatal dose of the wrong drug.
- Additional patients are added to a nurse's assignment during a busy weekend because on-call staff are not available, and back-up plans do not exist to cover variations in patient census. Patients are placed at risk for errors and injury, and nurses are frustrated and angry.
- Isolated decision making in one department leads to tension, frustration, and a higher risk of errors by all involved. Whether affecting patient care or unit operations, decisions made without including all parties place everyone involved at risk.
- Nurses are placed in leadership positions without adequate preparation and support for their role.
- The resulting environment creates dissatisfaction and high turnover for nurse leaders and staff as well.
- Contentious relationships between nurses and administrators are heightened when managers are required to stretch their responsibilities without adequate preparation and coaching for success (American Association of Critical-Care Nurses, 2003).
- Only 65% of hospital managers are held accountable for employee satisfaction (University Health System Consortium, 2003). The standards of the American Association of Critical-Care Nurses (2005) focus on:

- **Skilled Communication**
  Nurses must be as proficient in communication skills as they are in clinical skills. *Skilled communication protects and advances collaborative relationships.*
- **True Collaboration**
  Nurses must be relentless in pursuing and fostering true collaboration. *True collaboration is an ongoing process built on mutual trust and respect.*
- **Effective Decision Making**
  Nurses must be valued and committed partners in making policy, directing and evaluating clinical care and leading organizational operations. *Advocating for patients requires involvement in decisions that affect patient care.*
- **Appropriate Staffing**
  Staffing must ensure the effective match between patient needs and nurse competencies. *Remaining focused on matching nurses' competencies to patients' needs points the way to innovative staffing solutions.*
- **Meaningful Recognition**
  Nurses must be recognized and must recognize others for the value each brings to the work of the organization. *Meaningful recognition acknowledges the value of a person's contribution to the work of the organization.*
- **Authentic Leadership**
  Nurse leaders must fully embrace the imperative of a healthy work environment, authentically live it, and engage others in its achievement. *Nurse leaders create a vision for a healthy work environment and model it in all their actions.*

An important part of any nurse's work experience is working with others—relationships—and this affects the healthy work environment. There is even more emphasis on this today, with the IOM core competency that focuses on interdisciplinary teams. Relationships with coworkers can be the deciding factor in how comfortable a nurse feels in the work environment (Trossman, 2005). These relationships take time to develop. With the hectic work environment today and shorter breaks and lunch, staff members have less time to build those relationships. Such relationships can be critical when nurses work together; working together requires communication, trust, mutual respect, and confidence that one will be supported and assisted when needed. "Positive relationships also foster loyalty to each other and to the institutions and the community [an organization] serves" (Trossman, 2005, p. 8). Staff spend a lot of time at work, and it is less stressful when one looks forward to working with the team rather than dreading work or expecting conflict. Healthy work environments are necessary to improve patient safety, staff safety, quality of care, and staff recruitment and retention, and they have an impact on the financial status of the HCO.

Career Development—First Step: First Nursing Position

Career development is a responsibility of every nurse. This process really begins before graduation from a nursing program and licensure.

From Student to Practice: Reality Shock

Reality shock has been identified in nursing as the shocklike reaction when initial education is in conflict with work-world values (Kramer, 1974). Another definition is "the incongruency of values and behaviors between the school subculture and the work subculture that leads to role deprivation or reality shock" (Schmalenberg & Kramer, 1979, p. 2). Benner (1984) identified five stages of competence: novice, advanced beginner, competent, proficient, and expert. The first three stages are affected by reality shock. Through the nursing education process, the novice nurse learns the rules for performance but has limited real-life clinical experience to apply the rules and to expand clinical reasoning and judgment. Getting the first job as a RN is a very important step in each nurse's career development. Students should take some time to begin a career plan even before graduation. The plan will change over time, but having a plan provides a guide for decisions.

Tools and Strategies to Make the Transition Easier

Where to begin? Each student should begin by developing his or her résumé, composing a biosketch, and maintaining a professional **portfolio**. A **résumé** is a one- or two-page document that describes the person's career. It includes the person's name, contact information, credentials, education, goals and objectives, and employment and relevant experience (a resumé should be kept current and not be lengthy). The **biosketch** is a paragraph that provides a short summary of the person's work history and accomplishments. It should include the person's name, credentials, and education. It is a narrative rather than a list. Later, a **curriculum vitae** can be developed. This is a more detailed accounting of information found in the résumé and includes publications, presentations, continuing education, honors and awards, community activities, and grants. The portfolio provides evidence of a person's competency. It is not always required for job applications, but sometimes it is, and in some positions, nurses are asked to maintain a portfolio for performance review. A portfolio is a collection of information that demonstrates a person's experiences and accomplishments, such as committee work, professional organization activities, presentations, development of patient education material, awards, letters of recognition, projects and grants, and so on. The portfolio should include annual goals and objectives, and review of outcomes, which should be updated annually. A professional development plan, which is based on the information in a person's résumé and portfolio, lays out the direction the person wants to take with his or her career over the next year, the next 2 years, and the next 5 years. It should include a target time frame and strategies and activities to reach the goals. Self-assessment is a critical activity for any nurse, and this assessment helps the nurse to further develop the career plan.

INTERVIEWING FOR A NEW POSITION

Interviewing for a new position as a nurse should be taken seriously. The first step is setting up the interview. As the potential employee, you should find out the time of the appointment, the location, and the length of the interview. Will there be more than one interview on the same day? Will additional interviews take place later depending on whether the person is considered for the position? Will the interview be with one person or with a group? Do your homework; find out as much as possible about the organization and people who will be at the interview, and think about the types of questions that might be asked and how to respond. Wear business dress, look neat, and be prepared. Bring a copy of your résumé and any other required documents. Make sure you know how to get to the interview, and arrive early to allow yourself time to focus on the interview. Delays can happen when you least expect it, so planning to arrive early helps to prevent lateness. During the interview, focus on the questions. Look the interviewer in the eye, take a moment to respond, and ask for clarification if you are unsure about the question. Share information about competencies and experiences—successes and challenges, and how you handled them. Ask the interviewer about the organization and the position. When the interview is completed, thank the interviewer. Follow up to thank him or her (letter, e-mail). Ask about the process—what comes next, when will the decision be made, and so on? Exhibit 14–5 provides examples questions to ask at an interview.

DETERMINATION OF THE BEST FIT: YOU AND A NEW POSITION

How does one choose a position and an organization for employment? It is not easy to know that the fit is a good one. First, know the type of nursing that interests you and why. Second,

---

EXHIBIT 14–5 QUESTIONS TO ASK DURING AN INTERVIEW FOR A HOSPITAL RN POSITION

Question
1.   Do you have an opening on one of your _____ units in this hospital?
2.   Would you hire a new BSN-prepared nurse to work in that unit? If no, why not?
3.   What skills or knowledge (beyond basic preparation) would I need?
4.   How can I obtain these skills or knowledge?
5.   What are the opportunities for advancement in the unit?
6.   What is the culture of the unit?
7.   What is the leadership style of the manager of the unit?
8.   What is the turnover rate of RNs in the unit?
9.   What is the relationship of RNs and physicians on the unit?
10.   Is a team concept practiced on the unit? If so, who are the members of the team?

Source: From *Handbook of Nursing Leadership: Creative Skills for a Culture of Safety*, by J. Milstead and E. Furlong, 2006, Sudbury, MA: Jones and Bartlett Publishers.

based on what you know about the HCOs in the location where you want to work, focus on the organizations that most interest you. Today, the Internet offers a resource for job hunting. Most HCOs, particularly hospitals, have Web sites. Explore them to learn about the organization. Talk to people who may know about the organization. Students often have clinical experiences in several HCOs, and they can use this opportunity to assess the organization. Do staff seem happy working there? What is the quality of care? What are some of the negative aspects of the organization? Salary and benefits are always an important factor. Potential employees should also consider driving distance, parking, schedules, and general work conditions. Asking about promotions and use of career ladders can yield helpful information, along with how much support is given to staff for education (i.e., orientation, staff development, continuing education, and academic degrees). Regarding education, a new employee would want to know if tuition reimbursement is available, and for whom and at what level. Is it difficult to get release time to attend classes, or is there flexible staffing to allow for this? Nurses should also ask about staff turnover, use of supplemental staffing (agency, travelers), mandatory overtime, and change in nurse leaders. Organizations that experience high turnover in staff and nurse managers are organizations that are experiencing problems. Overreliance on supplemental staff indicates that the organization is having problems retaining nurses and developing strategies to cope with the nursing shortage. Is the organization used for clinical experiences for nursing students? This usually means that the organization is interested in education, but it also means that staff need to be willing to work with students. How is medical staff coverage handled? Are there house staff? It is important to know who covers for medical issues because this has an impact on expectations of nursing staff and collaboration with others.

The HCO's top leadership, such as the chief executive officer (CEO), is an important person. The CEO signs off on the budget; if he or she does not recognize the importance of nursing to the organization and to outcomes, this can have a negative impact on how nurses are treated, and it can affect such budget issues as the number of nursing positions, salaries and benefits, and funds for education. The Forces of Magnetism, discussed in Chapter 15, have been used by nurses as criteria for evaluating an organization as an employer (hospital Magnet status).

MENTORING, COACHING, AND NETWORKING

Several methods are used in HCOs to support new staff, and **mentoring** is one of them. The mentor is more experienced and usually is selected by the staff nurse, but he or she may be assigned. The mentor acts as a role model and serves as a resource. **Coaching** is another method used for support, encouragement, and career development (e.g., how to go for a promotion or change of career ladder level, or to go back to school for a higher degree). **Networking** is a less structured method. All nurses need to learn how to network, or make connections with nurses and others who can help them. Professional organizations are good places to network and meet nurses who might provide guidance, support, and/or information. Nurses should keep contact information of potential connections even when they may not have a specific reason to make the contact; one never knows when the information may become important. Networking can also be done in non–healthcare settings that include people who may be helpful to know.

STUDENT EXTERNSHIP AND NURSE RESIDENCY PROGRAMS

Student externships are special summer programs that typically take place between the junior and senior years. In these programs, students are hired by a hospital as student externs. There is a planned program that should include some educational activities and opportunities to develop competencies. The externs work at a level above UAPs, and they are mentored by RNs. Externs are paid for their work. The student extern has the opportunity to learn more about the professional role of the RN.

Nurse residency programs are not as common as student externship programs, but they are increasing. It is clear that nursing has a major problem with retention of new graduates, particularly in the first 2 years; the current national turnover rate ranges from 35% to 60% (Cantrell & Browne, 2006). This turnover rate is associated with reality shock, as described by Kramer (1985). The increasing shortage challenges new graduates with a highly stressful, complex healthcare system, often inadequate staffing ratios, little time to adjust to full-time work, and high-acuity patients. New graduates often receive little support from experienced staff, who are already stressed with their own workloads, and the high number of older nurses who will retire in the next few years (Goode & Williams, 2004) will exacerbate the shortage problem. The Joint Commission noted that "inadequate orientation and training is a factor in 58% of serious medication errors. Staffing levels impacted 24% of 1,609 sentinel events over the past 5 years" (The Joint Commission, 2002). A report of Chicago hospitals indicated that half of the hospitals reduced orientation time to 30 days, in contrast to 3-month orientations of 5 years ago (The Joint Commission, 2002). The dissatisfaction of hospital nurses has persisted. In a recent study (Healthcare Advisory Board [HAB], 2001), 41% of working nurses reported being dissatisfied with their jobs; 43% scored high on a range of burnout measures; and 22% were planning to leave their job in the next year. Of the latter group, 33% were under the age of 30 (HAB, 2001). Others

have also commented on the serious retention problem. Aiken (2002) indicated in some of her research that 1 in 3 nurses under the age of 30 were planning on leaving their current job within 1 year (Goode & Williams, 2004; HAB, 2001). In its study, the HAB (2001) indicated that 42% of new hires by hospitals are new graduates and that they are not competent in a number of areas, such as surveillance, and recognizing safe clinical judgment and deviations from the normal (Aiken et al., 2002; Goode & Williams, 2004).

Residency programs offer the opportunity for new graduates to acquire professional values and attitudes, to develop a professional identity, and to increase competency, self-confidence, and clinical reasoning and judgment. Residency programs have demonstrated an impact on turnover rates, in some cases decreasing turnover from 36% to 14% (Beecroft, Kunzman, & Krozek, 2001). Herdrich defined a nurse residency program as "a joint partnership between academia and practice that is a learner-focused, postgraduate experience designed to support the development of competency in nursing practice" (Herdrich & Lindsay, 2006, p. 55). Residencies do not eliminate the need for orientation to the HCO, but rather should build on orientation and provide new RNs with a *graduated* transition to full practice. The Joint Commission (2002) stated,

> *Structured post-graduate training programs for nurses could provide the opportunity for skill-building in real clinical settings, just as residencies do for young physicians. Such experience would smooth the transition from nursing schools and help to build the confidence and competence of the trainees before they fully enter nursing practice. The content, length and structure of these residency programs could vary as a function of levels of undergraduate preparation as*

well as the roles eventually to be assumed by the trainees. Establishment of standardized nursing residency programs would require collaboration between schools of nursing and hospitals, the creation of an appropriate accrediting or certifying body, and identification of stable funding sources.

Residency programs range from several months to 12 months, and the longer programs appear to be more effective. Developing competency is part of a nurse residency program. Competency is the "the application of knowledge and the interpersonal, decision-making, and psychomotor skills expected for the nurse's practice role, within the context of public health, welfare, and safety" (National Council of State Boards of Nursing, 1996). Many nurse residency programs use simulation to provide greater opportunities for the nurse residents to develop their competencies and work on interdisciplinary teamwork. Nurse residents are assigned a mentor or a preceptor who works with them for the duration of the program. The program offers additional educational activities for the residents, which might be didactic classes, online courses, seminars, journal clubs, support groups, simulation labs, and the opportunity to work on evidence-based practice projects. Release time is provided to allow the residents to participate in the required educational activities. Patient workload is gradually increased during the program with guidance from the mentor or preceptor. Nurse residents are paid full-time employees. Some HCOs require that nurse residents work for the organization for a specified period after the residency is completed. Throughout the program, residents are given feedback and guidance in planning for performance improvement. Students can search the Internet and find many hospitals that offer nurse residency programs to new graduates.

Career Ladder

Many HCOs today have developed career ladder programs for their nurses. The details about these career ladders vary from organization to organization. Typically, there are levels entitled Clinician I, II, III, and so on. The first level is entry level. The levels describe the role and responsibilities, as well as the educational requirements. This type of system provides a method for promotion and an increase in salary that does not require moving to a management position, which in the past was the most common path for advancement. The career ladder structure recognizes that clinical work is important and deserves recognition. Nurses have to demonstrate that they meet the criteria for the level that they are requesting. This is the point at which a nurse might use a portfolio, and in some organizations, portfolios are required. HCOs need clear criteria and procedures for applying for a change in level within the career ladder system. Mentoring to teach staff what needs to be done to complete a successful career ladder application is also useful. Encouraging staff to participate in the career ladder offers positive outcomes for the organization, such as having motivated staff who work on improving their competencies and increasing their education level; increased efforts to improve care; an attractive recruitment strategy; and increased retention. Performance improvement should be an active part of any nursing position. Through an active, positive performance improvement program, staff can use self-assessment and assessment from supervisors to further develop their career plans.

Going Back to School, Certification, and Continuing Education

Returning to school for another degree may not be a nurse's first thought after licensure, but when a nurse develops his or her career plan, additional education should be considered. The decision should be based on goals and a timeline. One must consider the best time for additional education. Competency is a serious issue. Does the new nurse need more time to achieve competency and to further develop as a professional nurse before entering a graduate program or a specialty? This requires serious thought. Additional education assumes that the nurse is competent at his or her current level and practices effectively as a professional nurse. For many new graduates, this takes time.

Certification is another way to expand competencies and education; however, certification does require that one have a specified amount of experience before taking the examination. This means that the nurse needs to plan when he or she might apply and obtain the required experience. Specialties and certification were discussed in Chapter 4.

Continuing education (CE) is a professional responsibility. Employers may provide educational experiences that also allow nurses to earn continuing education units (CEUs), or they may cover expenses for staff to attend CE programs outside the HCO. Many professional organizations offer CE programs, and some offer Web-based programs (many CE programs are offered via the Internet). Some states require that RNs earn a certain number of CEUs prior to relicensure. Certified nurses must meet CE requirements to continue their certification. CE is more effective if the content relates to the work that the nurse does and is in alignment with his or her professional goals. Nurses should keep a file of CE activities and update their records accordingly.

Conclusion

The nursing shortage is not going to disappear, and it will get worse. All HCOs deal with this problem daily as they try to cope with daily staffing needs and develop long-term strategies to solve the problem. To meet the five IOM core competencies, it is important for HCOs to have a sufficient number of staff to complete the required work effectively. A successful work environment includes staff in planning, respects staff, provides methods for recognition of staff education and experience, and considers positive methods to address recruitment and retention.

CHAPTER HIGHLIGHTS

1. Nursing is ranked the number one growth occupation of all occupations through 2012 (U.S. Department of Labor, 2004).

2. In May 2006, 2,417,150 RNs were employed in the United States, with mean wages of $28.71 hourly and $59,730 annually, and median hourly wages of $27.54 (U.S. Department of Labor, 2007).

3. There was steady growth in the number of men graduating from nursing programs, representing 12.1 of the nursing graduates (NLN, 2008).

4. According to the NLN (2008), there has been a marked increase in graduates who are members of racial or ethnic minority groups (Asians, African Americans, Hispanics, and American Indians).

5. The NLN (2008) survey included data on types of degrees awarded for 2006: 59% earned a 2-year associate's degree; 38% earned a baccalaureate degree; and 8% graduated from a diploma program.

6. About 37% of nurses are near retirement, and some of the RNs in the age range of 40–49 are nearing 50, putting this group close to retirement (New York Center of Health Workforce Studies, 2006).

7. Generational differences can lead to conflict in the workplace and must be

considered as workforce issues are explored.

8. The perfect storm for the nursing shortage has three dimensions: (1) an increased demand for nurses, (2) a decreased supply of nurses, and (3) unfavorable work conditions. The shortage is influenced by several factors: (1) not enough nurses in practice, (2) not enough applicants to nursing programs and not enough faculty to teach in nursing programs, and (3) the approaching retirement of an alarming number of nurses.

9. Acuity levels have increased as lengths-of-stay have decreased. Staffing ratios (patients per nurse) are high.

10. Lower levels of staffing have been linked to poor patient outcomes.

11. *Nursing hours* may refer to RNs only; to RNs and LPNs; or to RNs, LPNs, and UAPs.

12. An FTE is equal to 40 hours of work per week for 52 weeks, or 2,080 hours per year.

13. *Staffing mix* describes the type of nursing staff needed to provide care.

14. PCS may be used to assist with staffing levels. These systems are computerized and used to identify and quantify patient needs and then match them with staffing level and mix.

15. Mandatory overtime has become an important topic in nursing today. This is a strategy used by HCOs to fill the holes in the schedule; it requires staff to work past their scheduled end time if they want to keep their job.

16. Nurse turnover, especially with less than 1 year on the job, is problematic and costly.

17. Workforce legislation offers a multipronged approach to the shortage by establishing initiatives to increase quality of care; increase faculty; increase the education level of nurses; retain nurses in practice; increase the quality of care to a growing population, the elderly; and increase number of applicants to nursing programs.

18. As the nursing shortage has increased, the hospitals in the United States have relied more on hiring nurses from other countries to fill vacant positions. Ethical migration must be considered.

19. Working in a healthcare environment can be a very positive experience, particularly if the environment is one in which staff are respected, communication is open, staff feel empowered and part of the decision-making process, staff safety and health are considered important, and staff feel that they are making a contribution.

20. Healthy work environments are necessary to improve patient safety, staff safety, quality of care, and staff recruitment and retention, and they have an impact on the financial status of the HCO.

21. Reality shock in nursing is a very real phenomenon. Through the nursing education process, the novice nurse learns the rules for performance but has limited real-life clinical experience to apply these rules and to expand clinical reasoning and judgment.

22. Transition to practice can be assisted with use of student externships and nurse residency programs.

23. When selecting a job, be sure to examine the type of nursing offered and how involved the nurses are in the governance structure. Determine how well these factors fit with what you are looking for in a position.

24. Mentoring, coaching, and professional networking can provide support for new nurses.

25. Career ladders offer a mechanism for advancement within an organization.
26. Continuing education and support for further education are other factors that influence the workplace environment.

Linking to the Internet

- American Nurses Association
  http://www.nursingworld.org
- American Association of Colleges of Nursing
  http://www.aacn.nche.edu
- American Association of Critical-Care Nurses
  http://www.aacn.org/
- National League for Nursing
  http://www.nln.org
- American Organization of Nurse Executives
  http://www.aone.org
- Health Resources and Services Administration
  http://www.hrsa.gov
- International Centre on Nurse Migration
  http://www.intlnursemigration.org/
- National Student Nurses Association
  http://www.nsna.org
- NurseZone.com
  http://www.nursezone.com/default.aspx?aspxerrorpath=/ads/forwork.asp?articleid=9298

DISCUSSION QUESTIONS

1. Why is there a nursing shortage?
2. What impact has the current nursing shortage had on healthcare delivery and nursing?
3. Describe two initiatives or methods for addressing the nursing shortage.
4. What are the advantages and disadvantages of global migration of nurses?
5. What is burnout? What is reality shock? Do you think they can be related, and if so, in what way?
6. Discuss strategies that might be used to develop a healthy work environment.

CRITICAL THINKING ACTIVITIES

1. How is the nursing shortage related to the five IOM core competencies?
2. In a small group, discuss the content on generational issues. What do you think about this information? How does it relate to you? How might you use this information in your practice? Summarize the key points from the group discussion.
3. Write a career plan that includes current activities, activities during the 1st year after graduation, after 3 years, and after 5 years.
4. Write a résumé for yourself and then a biosketch. Critique another classmate's résumé and biosketch, and have a discussion with the classmate who reviews your résumé and biosketch.
5. Discuss with your team observations you have made in your clinical experiences that are related to the impact of the nursing shortage.

CASE STUDY

A nursing graduate of a baccalaureate program interviewed for her first nursing position. She was told that she would have 60 days of orientation and then would be rotated to nights (12-hour shifts). She asked if there was a residency program and was told no. She asked about nurse–patient ratio, and she was told only that it varied greatly on the adult medical-surgical units. She then asked if she could talk with some newer staff nurses. This meeting was arranged. She found that the new nurses (9 months or less) were happy. They only had 60 days of orientation but were assigned a mentor who was there to help in the transition to practice. Although staffing did vary, generally the administration was very responsive to nurses' concerns, and patient outcomes were very good. What appeared on first look to be a very bad work environment for a new nurse actually was very positive. This case demonstrates the need to ask very good questions about orientation, staffing patterns, and patient outcomes, and then to follow up with actual discussions with nurses.

1. Based on this case, develop a list of questions that you would ask when applying for your first RN position.
2. How would you handle a situation in which you felt that you did not get a full answer to a question?

WORDS OF WISDOM

Geraldine Ellison, PhD, RN, Associate Professor and Director, Institute for Community and Interprofessional Alliances, University of Oklahoma College of Nursing

We've had nursing shortages before, we weathered them . . . and so we will again! The sentiments expressed in this statement reflect early reactions of many nurses—educators as well as practitioners—on the current shortage. However, these same nurse leaders quickly realized that this shortage was *not* like other shortages and so using the *same* strategies would not result in a sufficient nursing workforce (neither by numbers nor educational preparation) to meet the need. For Oklahoma nurse educators, this realization meant that we could no longer live and play within our silos of practical nursing,

AD nursing, and BSN/higher degree nursing education. For both practice and education, it meant we needed to partner together in new ways to maximize and extend the resources that we had.

Accordingly, in July of 2006, nurse educators from across all levels of nursing education in Oklahoma met for the first time in a series of nursing education summits to develop a statewide strategy for nursing education. The Institute for Oklahoma Nursing Education (IONE) grew out of these summits. For the first time in Oklahoma, an organization exists that can speak with one voice for nursing education. Its leadership comprises educators from all levels. Our strategic agenda is to create a seamless pathway in nursing education by removing or resolving barriers, expanding capacity and nursing options, sharing resources in creative ways that create win-win solutions, and creating new partnerships, collaborations, and coalitions among those involved in health care. During the same time period, the Oklahoma Hospital Association as well as other major players in health care worked with the legislature to create a Health Care Workforce Resource Center that would focus on increasing the workforce for nursing and allied health. This important center is another strong partner for nursing education and IONE as we all focus on building capacity in nursing programs and increasing career options for those interested in nursing.

We've had nursing shortages before, we weathered them . . . and so we will again! This time we are stronger because we are working together, and this time our successes will further unite and empower our profession and result in better, safer patient care.

References

Advisory Board Company. (1999). A misplaced focus: Reexamining the recruiting/retention trade-off. *Nursing Watch, 11*, 114.

Agency for Healthcare Research and Quality. (2004, March). Hospital nurse staffing and quality of care. *Research in Action* (No. 14).

Aiken, L., Clarke, S., Sloane, D., Sochalski, J., & Silber, J. (2002). Hospital nurse staffing and patient mortality, nurse burnout, and job dissatisfaction. *Journal of the American Medical Association, 288*, 1987–1993.

Aiken, L., Sloane, D., Lake, E., Sochalski, J., & Weber, A. (1999). Organization and outcomes of inpatient AIDS care. *Medical Care, 37*, 760–772.

American Association of Colleges of Nursing. (2005). *Nurse Reinvestment Act at a glance.* Retrieved March 24, 2008, from http://www.aacn.nche.edu/media/nraataglance.htm

American Association of Critical-Care Nurses. (2003). *Strategic market research study.* Aliso Viejo, CA: Author.

American Association of Critical-Care Nurses. (2005). *AACN standards for establishing and sustaining healthy work environments.* Aliso Viejo, CA: Author.

American Nurses Association. (1998). *Principles for nurse staffing.* Chevy Chase, MD: Author.

Beecroft, P., Kunzman, L., & Krozek, C. (2001). RN internship: Outcomes of a one-year pilot program. *Journal of Nursing Administration, 31*, 575–582.

Benner, P. (1984). *From novice to expert: Excellence and power in clinical nursing practice.* Menlo Park, CA: Addison-Wesley.

Bertholf, L., & Kinnaird, L. (2001). Baby boomers and Generation X: Strategies to bridge the gap. *Seminars for Nurse Managers, 9*, 169–172.

Bleich, M., Hewlett, P., Santos, S., Rice, R., Cox, K., & Richmeier, S. (2003). Analysis of the nursing workforce crisis: A call to action. *American Journal of Nursing, 103*(4), 6–74.

Cantrell, M., & Browne, A. (2006). The impact of a nurse externship program on the transition process from graduate to RN. *Journal for Nurses in Staff Development, 22*(1), 11–14.

Cavouras, C. (2006). Scheduling and staffing: Innovations from the field. *Nurse Leader, 4*(4), 34–36.

Cho, S., Ketefian, S., Barkauskas, V., & Smith, D. (2003). The effects of nurse staffing on adverse outcomes, morbidity, mortality, and medical costs. *Nursing Research,* 52(2), 71–79.

Davis, S. (2001). Diversity and Generation X. *Seminars for Nurse Managers,* 9, 161–163.

Emerson, R. (2001). Facilitating acculturation of foreign-educated nurses. *Online Journal of Nursing,* 6(1). Retrieved October 30, 2008, from http://www .nursingworld.org/MainMenuCategories/ ANAMarketplace/ANAPeriodicals/OJIN/Tableof Contents/vol132008/No1Jan08/ArticlePreviousTopic/ ForeignEducatedNurses.aspx

Gerke, M. (2001). Understanding and leading the quad matrix: Four generations in the workplace: The traditional generation, boomers, gen-X, nexters. *Seminars for Nurse Managers,* 9, 173–181.

Goode, C., & Williams, C. (2004). Post-baccalaureate nurse residency program. *Journal of Nursing Administration,* 34(2), 71–77.

Healthcare Advisory Board. (2001). *Hardwiring right retention.* Washington, DC: Author.

Herdrich, B., & Lindsay, A. (2006). Nurse residency program redesigning the transition to practice. *J ournal for Nurses in Staff Development,* 22(2), 55–62.

Hung, R. (2002). A note on nurse self-scheduling. *Nursing Economic$,* 20(1), 37–39.

Institute of Medicine. (1996). *Nursing staff in hospitals and nursing homes: Is it adequate?* Washington, DC: National Academies Press.

Institute of Medicine. (2004). *Keeping patients safe: Transforming the work environment of nurses.* Washington, DC: National Academies Press.

The Joint Commission. (2002). *Healthcare at the crossroads: Strategies for addressing the evolving nursing crisis.* Oakbrook Terrace, IL: Author.

Jones, C. (2005). The costs of nursing turnover, Part 2: Application of the nursing turnover cost calculation methodology. *Journal of Nursing Administration,* 35(1), 41–49.

Jones, C., & Gates, M. (2007). The costs and benefits of nurse turnover: A business case for nurse retention. *Online Journal of Issues in Nursing,* 12(3). Retrieved October 30, 2008, from http://www.nursingworld.org/ MainMenuCategories/ANAMarketplace/ANAPeriodic als/OJIN/TableofContents/Volume122007/No3Sept07 /NurseRetention.aspx

Kovner, C., Jones, C., Zhan, C., Gergen, P., & Basu, J. (2002). Nurse staffing and post-surgical adverse outcomes: Analysis of administrative data from a sample of U.S. hospitals, 1990–1996. *Health Services Research,* 37, 611–629.

Kovner, C., Mezey, M., & Harrington, C. (2000). Research priorities for staffing, case mix, and quality of care in U.S. nursing homes. *Journal of Nursing Scholarship, 32*(1), 77–80.

Kramer, M. (1974). *Reality shock: Why nurses leave nursing.* Saint Louis, MO: Mosby.

Kramer, M. (1985). Why does reality shock continue? In J. McCloskey & H. Grace (Eds.), *Current issues in nursing* (pp. 891–903). Boston: Blackwell Scientific.

Maguire, P. (2002). Safe staffing and mandatory overtime: Issues of concerns in today's workplace. *Ohio Nurse Review,* 77(10), 4, 7–11.

Mejia, A., Pizurki, H., & Royston, E. (1979). *Physician and nurse migration: Analysis and policy implications.* Geneva, Switzerland: World Health Organization.

National Center for Health Statistics. (2002). *Chartbook on trends in the health of Americans.* (2002). Retrieved October 30, 2008, from http://www.cdc.gov/nchs/data/hus/hus02cht_ac.pdf

National Council of State Boards of Nursing. (1996). Retrieved January, 2007, from https://www.ncsbn.org

National League for Nursing. (2008, March 3). *Number of nursing school graduates—including ethnic and racial minorities—on the rise but applications to RN programs dip, reflecting impact of tight admissions* (News Release). Retrieved March 4, 2008, from http://www.nln.org/ newsreleases/data_release_03032008.htm

Needleman, J., Buerhaus, P., Mattke, S., Stewart, M., & Zelevinsky, K. (2001). *Nurse-staffing levels and patient outcomes in hospitals: Final report for Health Resources and Services Administration* (Contract No. 230-99-0021). Boston: Harvard School of Public Health.

New York Center of Health Workforce Studies. (2006, October). *The United States Health Workforce Profile.* Report prepared for Health Resources and Services Administration. Rensselaer, NY: Author and Health Resources and Services Administration.

O'Brien-Pallas, L., Griffin, P., Shamian, J., Buchan, J., Duffield, C., Hughes, F., et al. (2006). The impact of nurse turnover on patient, nurse and system outcomes: A pilot study and focus for multicenter international study. *Policy, Politics, and Nursing Practice,* 7, 169–179.

Schmalenberg, C., & Kramer, M. (1979). *Coping with reality shock.* Wakefield, MA: Nursing Resources.

Scott, E. S., & Cleary, B. L. (2007). Professional polarities in nursing. *Nursing Outlook, 55,* 250–256.

Sexton, K., Hunt, C., Cox, K., Teasley, S., & Carroll, C. (2008). Differentiating the workplace needs of nurses by academic preparation and years in nursing. *Journal of Professional Nursing, 24,* 105–108.

Stone, P., Duffield, C., Griffin, P., Hinton-Walker, P., Laschinger, H., & O'Brien-Pallas, L. (2003, November 3). *An international examination of the cost of turnover and its impact on patient safety and outcomes.* Proceedings of the 37th biennial convention, Sigma Theta Tau International, Toronto, Ontario, Canada.

Trossman, S. (2005). Who you work with matters. *American Nurse, 37*(4), 1, 8.

Ulrich, B. (2001). Successfully managing multigenerational workforces. *Seminars for Nurse Managers, 9*, 147–153.

U.S. Department of Labor, Bureau of Labor Statistics. (2004). *Registered nurses: Occupational outlook handbook, 2004–2005 edition.* Washington, DC: Author.

U.S. Department of Labor, Bureau of Labor Statistics. (2007). *Occupational employment and wages, 2006.* Washington, DC: Author.

University Health System Consortium. (2003). *Successful practices for workplace of choice employers.* Oak Brook, IL: Author.

Unruh L. (2003). Licensed nurse staffing and adverse outcomes in hospitals. *Medical Care, 41*, 142–152.

Upenieks, V., Valda, V., Akhavan, J., Kotlerman, J., Esser, J., & Ngo, M. (2008). Value-added care: A new way of assessing nursing staffing ratios and workload variability. *Nursing Economics, 26*(5), 294–300.

Vernarec, E. (2000). Just say "no" to mandatory overtime. *RN, 63*(12), 69–74.

Waldman, J., Kelly, F., Sanjeev, A., & Smith, H. (2004). The shocking cost of turnover in healthcare. *Health Care Management Review, 29*(1), 27.

Wieck, K., Prydum, M., & Walsh, T. (2002). What the emerging workforce wants in its leaders. *Journal of Nursing Scholarship, 34*(3), 283–288.

Worthington, K. (2001). The health risks of mandatory overtime. *American Journal of Nursing, 101*(5), 96.

Transformation of Nursing Practice: Roles and Issues

CHAPTER OUTLINE

KEY TERMS

❑ Differentiated practice
❑ Forces of Magnetism

❑ Magnet hospital
❑ Practice model

Introduction

Chapter 15 is the concluding chapter in this textbook, but in another sense, it is the beginning of your professional journey. The discussion that began in Chapter 1 and continued throughout this textbook will not end with this textbook or in a course that introduces the critical elements of the nursing profession. Why is this last chapter the beginning? The content highlights the future: What will happen to nursing? Students who are using this textbook are the future of nursing. This content explores some of the newer issues, trends, and initiatives in nursing, but more change certainly is predicted for the future.

Nursing's Agenda for the Future

This chapter is organized around a report published in 2002 by the American Nurses Association (ANA), with participation from 19 nursing organizations, including the National Student Nurses Association. The vision statement in the document, **Nursing's Agenda for the Future**, describes the profession:

Nursing is the pivotal healthcare professional, highly valued for its specialized knowledge, skill and caring in improving the status of the public and ensuring safe, effective, quality care. The profession mirrors the diverse population it serves and provides leadership to create positive changes in health policy and delivery systems. Individuals choose nursing as a career and remain in the profession because of the opportunities for personal and professional growth, supportive work environments and compensation commensurate with roles and responsibilities. (ANA, 2002, p. 3)

The content in this textbook is found in this vision statement:

- Nursing as a profession
- Importance of competency
- Art (caring) and science of nursing
- Nursing specialties and multiple roles and responsibilities
- Knowledge base (education, evidence-based practice)
- Public image of nursing and nurses
- Population and individual healthcare needs and services

- The five healthcare professions core competencies
- Need for safe, effective, quality care
- Diversity (staff and patients)
- Multiple delivery systems and need for leadership
- Financially stable healthcare delivery system (effective and efficient)
- Career development
- Healthy work environments
- Health policy
- Increasing use of informatics

The content is built around the 10 domains, or areas of concern, that demand action as identified in *Nursing's Agenda for the Future*. The domains reflect the Institute of Medicine (IOM) healthcare reports that are critical for today's healthcare delivery system. The following domains are discussed, highlighting current key initiatives and the future:

1. Leadership and planning
2. Delivery systems
3. Legislation/regulation/policy
4. Professional/nursing culture
5. Recruitment/retention
6. Economic value
7. Work environment
8. Public relations/communication
9. Education
10. Diversity

Each of the domains relates to the IOM core competencies. Before you read about each domain and the new initiatives in nursing related to each domain in the following sections, first review the description of the domain found in the appendix.

Domain: *Leadership and Planning*

There is no doubt that leadership is important to the nursing profession. This textbook has highlighted leadership throughout the discussion.

Leaders in nursing are found everywhere—in practice, in administration, in education, and in policymaking areas such as the government. Leaders do not have to be in formal leadership positions. Every nurse needs to strive to develop leadership competencies and characteristics. The IOM report on nursing recommends transformation leadership as the most effective style (IOM, 2004). Transformational leaders are confident, self-directing, honest, loyal, and committed, and they have the ability to develop and implement a vision. This leader takes on change as an opportunity and does not see it as a barrier. This leader includes staff in decisions, wants to hear new ideas, and embraces the opportunity for improvement. Planning is important in leadership, but this leadership is much more than planning, as noted by the characteristics of a transformational leader. All nurses can strive to develop these characteristics.

Domain: *Delivery Systems*

This domain emphasizes that nurses influence how the healthcare delivery system works and how it changes. More nurses need to be involved in the system to actively champion nurses and nursing care and advocate for the patient. How does the system work? Some of this was discussed in Chapter 8. How nursing is delivered is also important. This issue is impacted by staff qualifications and competencies, staffing, policies and procedures, organization and structure, types of patients and needs, and leadership and management approach. What are some of the key rapidly changing areas and possible future concerns?

A PROFESSION OF MULTIPLE SETTINGS AND POSITIONS

The practice of nursing takes place in multiple settings, thus offering multiple job possibilities over a career span. Many nurses change their settings and specialties based on interest and jobs that they want to pursue. Some of the settings are:

- Hospital-based or acute care nursing: This is the area that most students think of first when considering jobs in nursing. It is what is most illustrated in the media (films, television, and so on). Within this setting are multiple specialty opportunities.
- Ambulatory care: This is a growing area for nurses, because all are community-based settings. There are many types of ambulatory care settings, such as clinics, private practice offices, freestanding ambulatory surgical centers, and diagnostic centers.
- Community health: This area, which is growing rapidly, is an important clinical site for nursing students, and within this setting are multiple opportunities. Examples are community health departments, clinics, school health facilities, tuberculosis control centers, immunization clinics, home health, and more.
- Home care: This setting is very broad in that there are numerous home health agencies across the country. Some are owned and managed by government agencies, such as city health departments. Some agencies are owned and managed by other healthcare organizations (HCOs), such as a hospital. Some home health agencies are part of national chains and are for-profit or not-for-profit HCOs. Nurses in home care practice in the patient's home.
- Hospice and palliative care: This type of setting may be partnered with home care, or it may be a separate setting. Hospice care can be associated with an agency that provides care to patients in their homes, and another possible setting is an inpatient unit that is either part of a hospital system or a freestanding facility. Hospice care has a spe-

cial mission: to include patients, families, and significant others in the dying process and to make the patient as comfortable as possible and meet his or her wishes.
- School nursing: This setting was mentioned as an example of community health nursing. The focus is on the provision of healthcare services within schools. The role of the school nurse is changing a lot. Some schools have very active clinics that provide a broad range of healthcare services to students.
- Occupational health: This is a unique setting for nursing practice. Nurses provide healthcare services in occupational or work settings. Occupational health nurses provide emergency care; provide direct care including assessment, screenings, and preventive care; provide health and safety education; and initiate referrals for additional care. Some schools of nursing offer graduate degrees in this area.
- Telehealth/telemedicine: This area was discussed in Chapter 13. Nurses work in telehealth by monitoring patients, providing patient and family education, and directing care changes. Home health also uses this method in some areas.
- Parish nursing: Parish nursing takes place in a faith-based setting, such as a church or synagogue. The nurse is often a member of the organization. Services might include screenings and prevention, health education, and referral services. The members of the faith-based organization are the population whom the nurse serves.
- Office-based nursing: Nurses work in physician practices. Some may be advanced practice nurses (APNs), but the majority are not. These nurses provide assessment and direct services, assist the physician, monitor and follow up with patients, and teach patients and families.

- Extended care and long-term care: Many nurses work in this area, though it too is experiencing a shortage. Nurses provide assessment, direct care, and support to patients, and support and education to families.
- Management positions: This is a functional position. Nurse managers are found in all HCOs. Their key responsibilities are staffing, recruitment and retention of staff, planning, budgeting, supervising, quality improvement (QI), staff education, and ensuring overall functioning of their assigned unit, division, or department.
- Nursing education (academic and staff education): This is a functional position. Academic faculty teach in a nursing program, such as a licensed practical/vocational nursing program, an Associate's Degree in Nursing (ADN) program, a Baccalaureate Degree in Nursing (BSN) program, or a graduate nursing program. Staff development and staff education focus on orientation and ongoing staff education within HCOs.
- Nursing research: Nurses are involved in nursing research and research conducted by other healthcare providers. Research was discussed in Chapter 11. Nurses have many research roles, including serving as the primary investigator leading a research study, analyzing data, and collecting data. "'Evidence-based practice [which is more than application of research results, as discussed in Chapter 11] is more than a buzz term' says Porter-O'Grady. 'It's about getting a handle on what we do that is valuable—what difference it makes. Can we do it again, and can we do it even better the next time?'" (Saver, 2006, p. 19).
- Informatics: As discussed in Chapter 13, nurses are active in the area of informatics as a specialty and as a part of their other responsibilities. A nurse might serve on the informatics committee or participate in planning for an electronic medical record.
- Nurse entrepreneurship: Nurses may serve as consultants or own a healthcare-related business. This is an area that most nursing students do not think about before learning more about the profession of nursing.
- Legal nurse consultant: This is a nurse who usually has had additional coursework related to legal issues and health care, and he or she may even be certified in this area. The nurse works with attorneys and provides advice about health issues, reviews medical records and other documents, and assists with planning responses to cases. Nurses may be expert witnesses to testify about a case. This nurse should be an expert in the area addressed in the legal case— for example, a psychiatric-mental health nurse acting as the expert witness in a case involving a patient who was injured in a mental health unit.

New roles for nurses will be developed. For example, nurses will assume more active roles in positions concerned with quality and safety, in pharmaceutical companies, in working as nurse practitioners (NPs) in clinics located in retail stores, in running research and development departments of equipment or biomedical companies, and in counseling (Saver, 2006).

What does the future hold for new settings where nursing is practiced? What new roles might nurses take on? This is unknown, but nursing history has demonstrated that the possibility of new roles is highly likely. Porter-O'Grady believes that mobility and portability will become very important in technotherapeutic interventions (Saver, 2006). Technology will extend into patients' lives, and the settings in which care is received will be less connected to hospitals. Others suggest that as patients want more control as consumers, there will be more self-diagnostic tests (Saver, 2006).

PROFESSIONAL PRACTICE MODELS

Professional practice models are discussed in the profession today, and some HCOs are developing, or have developed, their own professional practice model. **Differentiated practice,** shared governance, and collaboration are important elements of a successful professional practice model (shared governance was discussed in Chapter 8, and collaboration in Chapter 9). Differentiated practice is part of developing a professional practice model. As discussed in other chapters, the subject of the level of entry into nursing practice continues to be an issue in the nursing profession. In 1965, a decision was made to establish the BSN as the level of entry. This has not occurred. Data described in Chapter 14 indicate that ADN programs are growing faster than BSN programs; there are more ADN graduates; and more ADN graduates than BSN graduates are practicing today. All the graduates from all types of nursing programs take the same licensure exam, and this complicates the issue. RN licensure is the same

for all the graduates regardless of the type of degree earned. Boston (1990) defined differentiated nursing practice as "a philosophy that focuses on the structuring of roles and functions of nurses according to education, experience, and competence" (p. 1). This does not mean that a graduate from one program is necessarily better than another, because many individual factors would determine this, but that graduates from each program should enter practice with different competencies. This issue will not be resolved anytime soon. However, differentiated practice needs to be more evident in nursing. How do employers recognize an RN's degree? Most do not. It is rarely noted on name tags. Salaries are most likely not based on the education level of the nurse, though they should be. Much needs to be done by the profession to address this area of concern. Figures 15–1, 15–2, 15–3, 15–4, and 15–5 illustrate models that have been used in the past (some are still used today). The functional model is used less today. Total care would be used in areas such as critical care. Primary care was very popular in the 1980s but is less so now because it requires a greater number of RNs; however, some HCOs still use the primary care model today.

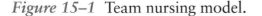

Figure 15–1 Team nursing model.

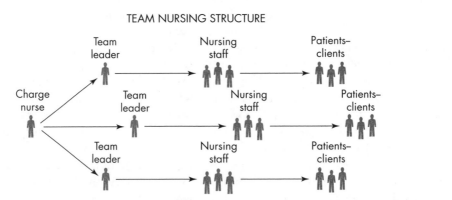

TEAM NURSING STRUCTURE

Source: From *Clinical Delegation Skills: A Handbook for Professional Practice*, by R. Hansten and M. Jackson, 2009, Sudbury, MA: Jones and Bartlett Publishers.

Figure 15–2 Functional nursing model.

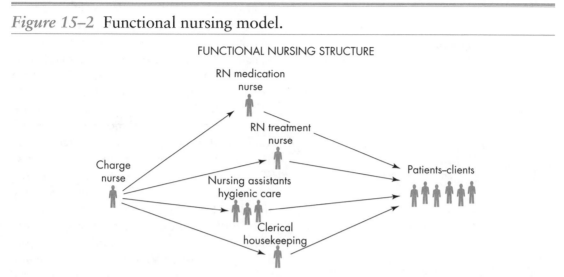

FUNCTIONAL NURSING STRUCTURE

RN medication nurse

RN treatment nurse

Charge nurse

Nursing assistants hygienic care

Patients–clients

Clerical housekeeping

Source: From *Clinical Delegation Skills: A Handbook for Professional Practice*, by R. Hansten and M. Jackson, 2009, Sudbury, MA: Jones and Bartlett Publishers.

Figure 15–3 Total patient care model.

TOTAL CARE NURSING STRUCTURE

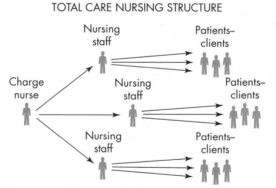

Nursing staff

Patients–clients

Charge nurse

Nursing staff

Patients–clients

Nursing staff

Patients–clients

Source: From *Clinical Delegation Skills: A Handbook for Professional Practice*, by R. Hansten and M. Jackson, 2009, Sudbury, MA: Jones and Bartlett Publishers.

One of the **Forces of Magnetism** for **Magnet hospitals** is the implementation of a professional **practice model**.

There are models of care that give nurses the responsibility and authority for the provision of direct patient care. Nurses are accountable for their own practice as well as the coordination of care. The models of care (i.e., primary nursing, case management, family-centered, district, and holistic) provide for the continuity of care across the continuum. The models take into consideration patients' unique needs and provide skilled nurses and adequate resources to accomplish desired outcomes. (American Nurses Credentialing Center, 2008)

Figure 15–4 Primary care model.

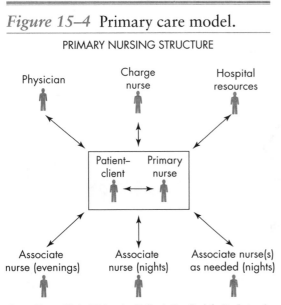

PRIMARY NURSING STRUCTURE

Source: From *Clinical Delegation Skills: A Handbook for Professional Practice*, by R. Hansten and M. Jackson, 2009, Sudbury, MA: Jones and Bartlett Publishers.

Why does an HCO need a professional practice model for nursing? The description of the magnet force provides some reasons for the need.

"Conceptual models provide an infrastructure that decreases variation among nurses, the interventions they will choose, and, ultimately, patient outcomes. Conceptual frameworks also differentiate forward thinking organization from those where nursing has less of a voice" (Kerfoot et al., 2006, p. 20). These organizations tend to have a professional rather than technical view of nursing. A model offers "a consistent way of framing the care they deliver to patients and their families" (Kerfoot et al., 2006, p. 21). The American Association of Critical-Care Nurses Synergy Model for Patient Care is one example (Kerfoot et al., 2006). This model's core premise is closely related to the IOM five core competencies, particularly with patient-centered care. The premise is that the needs of patients and families drive the characteristics and competencies of the nurse (Kerfoot et al., 2006). The model identifies eight important competencies: clinical judgment, clinical inquiry (evidence-based practice, QI, and innovative solutions), caring practices, response to diversity, advocacy and moral agency (ethics), and facilitation of learning, collaboration, and

Figure 15–5 Case management model.

CASE MANAGEMENT MODEL

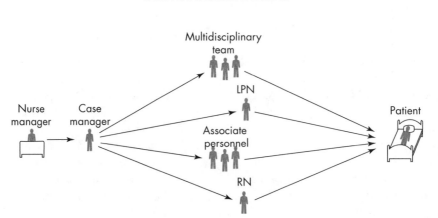

Source: From *Clinical Delegation Skills: A Handbook for Professional Practice*, by R. Hansten and M. Jackson, 2009, Sudbury, MA: Jones and Bartlett Publishers.

systems thinking. This model can be applied to all types of units, not just critical care, and many hospitals are doing this. This model identifies standards that are a part of the model. Within this model, patient characteristics are resiliency, vulnerability, stability, complexity, resource availability, participation in care, participation in decision making, and predictability. This is a good fit with the IOM core competencies.

There are other examples of new innovative models (Kimball, Cherner, Joynt, & O'Neil, 2007, pp. 393–394):

- Designing a model that provides the feel of a 12-bed hospital within a large hospital led to a model for a Primary Care Team led by a Patient Care Facilitator that monitors the nursing team. The team covers 12–16 beds. Key elements in this model are: (1) Every patient deserves an experienced RN. (2) Every novice nurse deserves mentoring. (3) Every patient should have the opportunity to participate in care. (4) Every team member is committed to the needs of the patients. (5) Each team member functions within his/her defined professional scope of practice. (6) Work intensity decreases with improved work distribution processes and team support. (7) The model of nursing care is an important element in patient safety and patient, staff, and physician satisfaction. (Baptist Hospital of Miami, Miami, Florida)
- The Collaborative Patient Care Management Model was developed by High Point Regional Health System (High Point, North Carolina). This is a multidisciplinary, population-based case management model. In this model, high-volume, high-risk, and high-cost patients in disease-specific or population-based groups are targeted to reduce length-of-stay and costs and improve patient outcomes.

- The Transitional Care Model focuses on comprehensive hospital planning, care coordination, and home follow-up of high-risk elders. (University of Pennsylvania Medical Center) APNs play a major role in this model of care, working with the elders and guiding their transition to home, plus the APN may implement the plan of care in the elder's home.

Innovative new professional practice models have common elements (Kimball et al., 2007). These elements are an elevated RN role; sharpened focus on the patient; smoothing patient transitions and handoff to decrease errors and make the patient more comfortable; leveraging technology to enable care model design, such as electronic medical records, robots, bar coding, cell phone communication, and more; and being driven by results or outcomes. The IOM core competencies also provide an effective start for a professional practice model.

TRANSFORMING CARE AT THE BEDSIDE

Transforming Care at the Bedside (TCAB) is a result of the IOM reports. This initiative began in 2003 through the Institute for Healthcare Improvement (IHI) in conjunction with the Robert Wood Johnson Foundation (Martin et al., 2007). The IHI is an effective initiative that provides multiple strategies for improving health care. "The goal is to make fundamental improvements in the healthcare delivery system that will result in safe and reliable care, vitality and teamwork, patient-centered care, and value-added care processes" (p. 445). In 2008, the TCAB initiative was implemented in 10 hospitals. Starting locally (a unit for example) and then spreading throughout the hospital is the approach taken in some of the pilots. TCAB looks not only at innovative change but also at the outcomes from the change. Did care improve? Was care monitoring used—indicators such as injury from falls, adverse events, readmission, voluntary turnover of RNs, patient satisfaction, and percentage of nurses' time in direct patient care? Examples of some of the innovative ideas being tested are (IHI, 2008):

- Use of rapid response teams to "rescue" patients before a crisis occurs
- Specific communication models that support consistent and clear communication among caregivers
- Professional support programs such as preceptorships and educational opportunities
- Liberalized diet plans and meal schedules for patients
- Redesigned workspace that enhances efficiency and reduces waste.

There is no doubt that TCAB will lead to effective innovative changes that can be used in many hospitals. The TCAB Web site listed in the Linking to the Internet section of this chapter provides information on current TCAB projects.

Domain: Legislation/Regulation/ Policy

The domain of legislation, regulation, and policy emphasizes the need for nurses to work collaboratively with other stakeholders in shaping health policy through legislation and regulation. Nurses are involved, and will continue to be involved, at the local, state, national, and international levels. The critical health policy issue coming onto the scene again is universal health coverage. This was an issue in the 2008 presidential campaign, and initiatives will be proposed to address the great need for healthcare coverage. The increasing cost of health care, the increasing number of uninsured and underinsured individuals, and the growing aging population (along with concerns about the ability of

Medicare funds to cover all) are critical healthcare issues. Any proposed initiative will impact nurses and nursing care and should include active nursing participation in the development of this important policy.

The nursing profession is committed to involvement in healthcare policy, even policy that may not be directly focused on nursing. The current federal key legislative issues in 2008 reflected common themes of interest to nurses, such as the following:

- Nurse staffing (proposed Registered Nurse Safe Staffing Act, H.R. 4138 and S.73, to hold hospitals accountable for the development of valid, reliable unit-by-unit staffing plans)
- Safe patient handling and movement (patient and staff safety; reduced work-related health injuries to nurses, other healthcare providers, and patients)
- Funding for workforce development (need to increase funding through the Health Resources and Services Administration under Title VIII of the Public Health Services Act)
- Mandatory overtime (a key concern in all states; has a negative impact on safe, quality care)

There is no doubt that safe, quality care will be major issues in legislation in the next few years. Nurses will need to be involved in these initiatives because they will directly impact nursing. Healthcare legislation at the state level is also important to nurses. Many states are trying to pass legislation related to mandatory overtime and staff–patient ratios. Some states have already passed this type of legislation.

There is a nurses' caucus in Congress made up of nurses who serve in Congress. This is an important resource for nursing. More nurses are needed to run for office at the local, state, and national levels. Nurses who have an interest in politics and health policy have to plan for this activity, particularly if they want to run for office eventually. This requires a career plan with a time frame.

Regulation is also an important issue today as change occurs within the healthcare system and with nursing. One example is the initiative to change regulation related to advanced practice registered nurses (APRNs) so that they can practice independently of physicians. This has not yet occurred.

> *The future model of APRN regulation calls for all APRNs to be regulated by boards of nursing, as independent providers, with all of the privileges and responsibilities of such. The future model requires that all APRNs demonstrate, via psychometrically sound methods, their competence as an APRN, in the role and within a population for whom they provide care, whether that be neonatal, pediatric, adult-geriatric, family, women, or mental health. APRNs will be educated to meet requirements for prescriptive authority and for reimbursement, whether or not they opt to pursue those areas. Educational programs will be required to have preapproval of each APRN program track before admitting students. All APRNs will comply with some formal mechanism for demonstrating ongoing competence in their area of practice. (Patton, 2008, p. 16)*

This represents a major change, and it will not be easy to accomplish.

Domain: Professional/Nursing Culture

The domain of professional/nursing culture focuses on the need to develop and maintain a professional culture that supports professional responsibility and accountability—collaborating, mentoring, promoting diversity, and standards and ethics.

NURSING SPECIALTIES

Nursing specialties are part of the profession and expand professionalism. There are numerous specialties in nursing, such as maternal-child (obstetrics), neonatal, pediatrics, emergency, critical care, ambulatory care, community health, home health, hospice, surgical/perioperative, psychiatric/mental health/behavioral health, management, legal nurse consulting, nursing consulting, and many more. Why did specialties develop? The most important reason is the need for focused experience and education in one area of nursing. Nursing is complex, and much knowledge is required. Nurses also become interested in a type of patient or care setting and want to learn more about it, gain more experience, and work in that area. All specialty nursing is based on core general nursing knowledge and competencies. The same specialty might practice in multiple settings—for example, a certified nurse midwife might work in a hospital in labor and delivery, in a private practice with obstetricians, in a clinic, in a freestanding delivery center, or in patients' homes, or he or she may have his or her own private practice. There are two ways to view a specialty. One is based on a nurse who works in a specialty area and thus claims that as his or her specialty (e.g., the nurse works in a behavioral health unit and is considered a psychiatric nurse). A second view, combined with the first, is that the nurse has additional education and possibly certification in a specialty. The psychiatric nurse may have a master's degree in psychiatric-mental health nursing and may or may not be certified in this specialty. The key to truly functioning as a specialty nurse is making a commitment to gaining additional education in the specialty. This also includes continuing education. As discussed earlier in this textbook, there are many titles in nursing, but they do not necessarily indicate a nurse's specialty. These titles are advanced practice nurse/nurse practitioner (APN/NP), clinical nurse specialist (CNS), clinical nurse leader (CNL), certified nurse midwife (CNM), and certified registered nurse anesthetist (CRNA). The CNM and CRNA have built-in recognition of this nurse's specialty (midwifery and anesthesia). An APN/NP may have multiple specialties, such as family APN, pediatric NP, adult health NP, and so on. A CNL is less of a clinical specialty in that it does not focus on a specific clinical group, but instead is a functional role used in any type of specialty area. For example, a CNL may serve in a medical unit, a pediatric unit, or a women's health unit. This is also true for a CNS, but the CNS master's degree does focus on a specific clinical area. Specialty education at the graduate level and certification support professionalism in nursing and help to ensure that nursing remains a profession.

Nurse leaders must continually support staff and the need for professionalism within the work setting. They do this by recognizing education and degrees through differentiated practice, encouraging ongoing staff education (continuing education and academic), ensuring that standards are maintained, working to increase staff participation in decision making, and helping staff who want to move into a management position to accomplish this (e.g., by directing staff to administration-focused education to prepare for the role). Nurse leaders also need to encourage staff to participate in professional organizations, publish in professional journals, attend professional conferences, submit abstracts for presentations, and recognize these accomplishments throughout the organization.

Magnet Nursing Services Recognition Program

Today,

the public is inundated with media coverage of changes in healthcare that could adversely affect their access to and the quality of healthcare services. Public trust in hospitals is eroding and interest in the quality of care is increasing. . . . More than 80% of the public polled in a recent survey wanted to know how to evaluate the quality of hospital care. (Aiken, Havens, & Sloane, 2000, p. 27) (Hensley, 1998; National Coalition on Healthcare, 1997)

It is important that nurses take active roles in determining the quality of care and the nurse's role in the process. Nurses run the risk of blame for some of the problems that are found in acute care today. "Politics in healthcare may not end at the bedside, but it certainly begins there. It would be a tragedy if patients and family members blamed nurses for system failures. But the more nurses detach from their patients, the easier it becomes for the rest of us (consumers) to lose sympathy" (Kaplan, 2000, p. 25). The Magnet program is one way to address this issue. What is the Magnet Nursing Services Recognition Program? What is its impact, and why is it important to new graduates? In 1981, a study was conducted that explored the issue of attracting and retaining nurses (McClure, Poulin, Sovie, & Wandelt, 1983). This was before the beginning of the major shortage that exists now; however, it has played a significant role in addressing the current shortage because it identified some methods for improving recruitment and retention of nurses. The focus of the study was to identify factors or variables that led some acute care hospitals to be more successful in recruitment and retention than other hospitals. As a result of this study, the Magnet Nursing Services Recognition Program was developed in the 1980s. The program recognizes hospitals that provide quality nursing care or excellence in nursing care.

What distinguishes a hospital that is awarded Magnet status in nursing? Management is different; it focuses more on participative management, in which staff have input into decisions, and managers listen to staff and typically use a decentralized structure. The difference is seen in the role of the nurse executive and throughout all levels of nursing management, as well as in the overall organization leadership's support of nursing. Effective leadership is present. Staff feel that nursing leaders in the organization understand their needs and provide resources and support for the work that staff do daily. Nurse managers and their roles are also critical to the success of these hospitals. Typically, these hospitals have more BSN nurses because this is a Magnet requirement, and nurses are very active in committees, projects, and so on. Clearly, staffing is of critical concern, and these hospitals use innovative methods to respond to recruitment and retention issues and to provide appropriate levels of staffing per shift. Education is valued in staff; there are opportunities for quality staff development, and staff who want to pursue additional academic degrees are encouraged to do so. Promotion can occur through the management track, the most common method, but it also should occur through the clinical track. Magnet hospitals offer both opportunities. They demonstrate higher levels of quality of care, autonomy, primary nursing, mentoring, professional recognition, and respect, and enable staff to practice nursing as it should be practiced (McClure et al., 1983).

Research in this area did not stop with the original 1981 study. Multiple studies have been conducted that support the positive impact of Magnet recognition. These hospitals have better outcomes—lower burnout rates, higher levels of job satisfaction, and higher quality of care—than non-Magnet hospitals (Laschinger, Shamian, & Thomson, 2001). Another study, *Staff Nurses Identify Essentials of Magnetism* (Kramer & Schmalenberg, 2002), reexamined 14

Magnet hospitals and identified eight variables that are important in providing quality care. Future research will undoubtedly explore these variables further (pp. 53–55):

1. Working with other nurses who are clinically competent
2. Good nurse–physician relationships
3. Nurse autonomy and accountability
4. Supportive nurse manager-supervisor
5. Control over nursing practice and practice environment
6. Support for education
7. Adequacy of nurse staffing
8. Concern for patient is paramount.

There are now significant research results that indicate that Magnet hospitals tend to provide quality care that leads to positive outcomes for patients and better work environments for nurses (Aiken, 2002).

As a result of this work and the Magnet Recognition Program, there are identified Forces of Magnetism. These variables are used to evaluate a hospital and determine if it can be designated a Magnet hospital. The variables can also be used by nurses who are considering new positions. The Forces of Magnetism can be used as a tool for learning more about the hospital and assessing whether it would be a positive workplace. If the hospital already has Magnet status, the forces should be present, but if not, the nurse applicant can still use the forces as his or her own checklist. Exhibit 15–1 describes these forces, or organizational elements of excellence in nursing care.

The Magnet Nursing Services Recognition Program for Excellence was established in 1993 and is administered by the American Nurses Credentialing Center (ANCC), the Commission on the Magnet Recognition Program. Recognition is given to acute care hospitals and long-term care facilities. Any size hospital that meets the standards may apply for Magnet status. It is

Exhibit 15-1 Forces of Magnetism

Transformational Leadership
Today's health care environment is experiencing unprecedented, intense reformation. Unlike yesterday's leadership requirement for stabilization and growth, today's leaders are required to transform their organization's values, beliefs, and behaviors. It is relatively easy to lead people where they want to go; the transformational leader must lead people to where they need to be in order to meet the demands of the future. This requires vision, influence, clinical knowledge, and a strong expertise relating to professional nursing practice. It also acknowledges that transformation may create turbulence and involve atypical approaches to solutions.

The organization's senior leadership team creates the vision for the future, and the systems and environment necessary to achieve that vision. They must enlighten the organization as to why change is necessary, and communicate each department's part in achieving that change. They must listen, challenge, influence, and affirm as the organization makes its way into the future. Gradually, this transformational way of thinking should take root in the organization and become even stronger as other leaders adapt to this way of thinking.

The intent of this Model Component is no longer just to solve problems, fix broken systems, and empower staff, but to actually transform the organizations to meet the future. Magnet-recognized organizations today strive for stabilization; however, healthcare reformation calls for a type of controlled destabilization that births new ideas and innovations.
Forces of Magnetism Represented
Quality of Nursing Leadership (Force #1)
Management Style (Force #3)

Structural Empowerment
Solid structures and processes developed by influential leadership provide an innovative environment where strong professional practice flourishes and where the mission, vision, and values come to life to achieve the outcomes believed to be important for the organization. Further strengthening practice are the strong relationships and partnerships developed among all types of community organizations to improve patient outcomes and the health of the communities they serve. This is accomplished through the organization's strategic plan, structure, systems, policies, and programs. Staff need to be developed, directed, and empowered to find the best way to accomplish the organizational goals and achieve desired outcomes. This may be accomplished through a variety of structures and programs; one size does not fit all.
Forces of Magnetism Represented
Organizational Structure (Force #2)
Personnel Policies and Programs (Force #4)
Community and the Healthcare Organization (Force #10)
Image of Nursing (Force #12)
Professional Development (Force #14)

Exemplary Professional Practice
The true essence of a Magnet organization stems from exemplary professional practice within nursing. This entails a comprehensive understanding of the role of nursing; the application of that role with patients, families, communities, and the interdisciplinary team; and the application of new knowledge and evidence. The goal of this Component is more than the establishment of strong professional practice; it is what that professional practice can achieve.
Forces of Magnetism Represented
Professional Models of Care (Force #5)
Consultation and Resources (Force #8)
Autonomy (Force #9)
Nurses as Teachers (Force #11)
Interdisciplinary Relationships (Force #13)

New Knowledge, Innovation, & Improvements
Strong leadership, empowered professionals, and exemplary practice are essential building blocks for Magnet-recognized organizations, but they are not the final goals. Magnet organizations have an ethical and professional responsibility to con-

tribute to patient care, the organization, and the profession in terms of new knowledge, innovations, and improvements. Our current systems and practices need to be redesigned and redefined if we are to be successful in the future. This Component includes new models of care, application of existing evidence, new evidence, and visible contributions to the science of nursing.

Forces of Magnetism Represented
Quality Improvement (Force #7)

Empirical Quality Results
Today's Magnet recognition process primarily focuses on structure and processes, with an assumption that good outcomes will follow. Currently, outcomes are not specified, and are minimally weighted. There are no quantitative outcome requirements for ANCC Magnet Recognition®. Recently lacking were benchmark data that would allow comparisons with best practices. This area is where the greatest changes need to occur. Data of this caliber will spur needed changes.

In the future, having a strong structure and processes are the first steps. In other words, the question for the future is not "What do you do?" or "How do you do it?" but rather, "What difference have you made?" Magnet-recognized organizations are in a unique position to become pioneers of the future and to demonstrate solutions to numerous problems inherent in our healthcare systems today. They may do this in a variety of ways through innovative structure and various processes, and they ought to be recognized, not penalized, for their inventiveness.

Outcomes need to be categorized in terms of clinical outcomes related to nursing; workforce outcomes; patient and consumer outcomes; and organizational outcomes. When possible, outcomes data that the organization already collects should be utilized. Quantitative benchmarks should be established. These outcomes will represent the "report card" of a Magnet-recognized organization, and a simple way of demonstrating excellence.

Forces of Magnetism Represented
Quality of Care (Force #6)

MODEL COMPONENTS	FORCES OF MAGNETISM
Transformational Leadership	>> Quality of Nursing Leadership *Force #1* >> Management Style *Force #3*
Structural Empowerment	>> Organizational Structure *Force #2* >> Personnel Policies and Programs *Force #4* >> Community and the Healthcare Organization *Force #10* >> Image of Nursing *Force #12* >> Professional Development *Force #14*
Exemplary Professional Practice	>> Professional Models of Care *Force #5* >> Consultations and Resources *Force #8* >> Autonomy *Force #9* >> Nurses as Teachers *Force #11* >> Interdisciplinary Relationships *Force #13*
New Knowledge, Innovations, and Improvements	>> Quality Improvement *Force #7*
Empirical Quality Outcomes	>> Quality of Care *Force #6*

Source: From *Announcing a New Model for ANCC's Magnet Recognition Program©*, by American Nurses Credentialing Center (ANCC), 2008. Retrieved on October 10, 2008, from http://www.nursecredentialing.org/Magnet/NewMagnetModel.aspx Reprinted with permission.

not an easy process to get Magnet status. The ANCC has defined

> accreditation *as a voluntary process used to validate that an organization and an approval body meets established continuing education standards.* Certification *focuses on the individual and is a process used to validate that an individual registered nurse possesses the requisite knowledge, skills, and abilities to practice in a defined practice specialty.* Recognition *is a third credentialing process operationalized in ANCC to evaluate an organization's adherence to excellence-focused standards. (Urden & Monarch, 2002, pp. 102–103)*

The Magnet Program is a recognition program. The first step for an organization that wants to apply for Magnet status recognition is for the organization to complete a self-assessment using materials provided by the program. The organization will then have a better idea about where it stands and what needs to be improved before completing the application to achieve recognition. This is not a recognition that just focuses on management; staff nurses must be involved in all steps in the process. After extensive sharing of information, an on-site survey is completed by the Magnet Recognition Program. After recognition is obtained—and not all organizations receive Magnet status—the organization must maintain standards; participate in the ANA's quality indicator study coordinated by the National Center for Nursing Quality; and provide certain annual monitoring reports that focus on the following ("New Law," 2002, p. 17):

- Notify the Magnet Recognition Program office if any of the following occurs:
  ○ a significant increase in staff turnover
  ○ a significant increase in the nurse vacancy rate
  ○ a significant decrease in nurse decision-making positions/activities
  ○ a significant negative change in the organization's nurse–patient ratio
  ○ a significant negative change in the licensed/unlicensed ratio of the nursing staff
  ○ a significant increase in the organization's nurse absentee rate
  ○ a significant amount of mandatory overtime worked by nurses reporting to the Department of Nursing
- Nursing-Sensitive Quality Indicator data that fall significantly below the threshold established by the Magnet organization
- Nursing-Sensitive Quality Indicator data that fall significantly below the national average as determined by the National Database of Nursing Quality Indicators

Recognition is not permanent, and the HCO must apply for renewal. A Web site is maintained with current information about the program (http://www.nursecredentialing.org/magnet/).

Exhibit 15–2 provides an example of how the Magnet Recognition Program is relevant to other critical concerns, such as greater use of informatics (one of the five core competencies). In this exhibit, the Technology Informatics Guiding Educational Reform Initiative in informatics asks for examples that demonstrate the forces of magnetism.

Domain: Recruitment/Retention

The domain of recruitment and retention focuses on hiring staff and keeping them (recruitment and retention were discussed in Chapter 14). These are critical issues in nursing, particularly in light of the nursing shortage. Innovative approaches to getting more nurses and keeping them will be required. There is high competition for nurses, meaning that it is the nurse who has

EXHIBIT 15–2 AN EXAMPLE: CONNECTING INFORMATICS WITH FORCES OF MAGNETISM

The Technology Informatics Guiding Educational Reform (TIGER) Initiative is collecting examples of how information technology can be used to demonstrate and support the forces of magnetism. We want to provide numerous examples to help organizations along their magnet journey. We are collecting this information to publish a "help guide" and plan to share at a pre-conference workshop at the Annual Magnet Conference this fall.

We are specifically looking for examples of how information technology enables communication, education, and the delivery of patient care and can demonstrate the forces of magnetism. Our goal is to relate these examples to the 14 forces of magnetism and to show how these examples benefit nursing. A few ideas of examples that could be used are listed below to help jog your memory, but this is certainly not an exhaustive list:

- Interdisciplinary documentation
- Evidence-based documentation
- Nursing involvement using information systems to obtain Quality Improvement measures, core measures, and other quality data
- Using information management to obtain nurse-sensitive indicators
- Nursing Informaticists or Director of Nursing Informatics positions that are an integral component of the senior nursing leadership team and report directly to the Chief Nursing Executive
- Nursing Informaticists that serve as an internal consultant to the magnet coordinators
- Active staff nurse involvement in committees that participate in system design, validation and acceptance
- Innovative education enabled by technology (e.g., e-learning)
- Technologies that improve nursing communication and nurse-to-patient communication and nurse-to-provider communication (e.g., automated nurse scheduling, voice-activated communication with patients, capacity management, message boards, etc.)
- Technologies that improve the work environment (message boards, etc.)
- Technologies that empower consumers to communicate with their families and make better healthcare decisions
- Electronic health records, computerized provider order entry, and integrated personal health records
- Technologies that improve patient safety, reduce errors, etc. (handoffs, transitions of care)
- Medication administration and other bar-coding systems
- New models of care, application of existing evidence, new evidence, and visible contributions to the science of nursing supported by technology
- Outcomes achieved as a result of the technology implemented

We will align the examples collected to the 14 Forces of Magnetism and provide this document back as part of the TIGER Initiative recommendations. We will accept any form of examples—e.g., brief description, presentation, abstract, or will be happy to interview you over the telephone to discuss your experiences. Please email your suggestions and contact information to leadership@tigersummit.com. We are working to complete our written recommendations by the end of the summer, so are collecting examples through June 13, 2008. We look forward to hearing from you and will happily share our recommendations with you. If you have any questions, please do not hesitate to reply to leadership@tigersummit.com!

Thank you in advance for your participation and your willingness to share your experiences in leveraging technology to support the Magnet journey.

Source: Technology Informatics Guiding Educational Reform, https://www.tigersummit.com/ Reprinted with permission.

the most power in a situation in which nurses are in high demand, and there are not enough of them. Openings are present across the health-care delivery continuum, from acute care to community care. Some areas of nursing prefer experienced nurses over new nurses, such as community health; however, even this is changing as the shortage grows.

The aging workforce needs to stimulate the profession and the healthcare industry to be innovative in helping staff work as long as they are able and desire to. There must be greater communication and understanding among the multiple generations represented in nursing. We need to look to technology to help find ways to make work easier and safer for nurses (Saver, 2006).

It is unclear what the future holds in this domain. HCOs are focused on recruitment and retention because of the growing nurse shortage, but there will also be shortages of other healthcare professionals such as pharmacists, physicians,

and others. Some of these healthcare professions are already experiencing shortages. HCOs have tried offering bonuses (which do not seem to retain nurses long term), innovative staffing schedules, nurse residencies (one of the newer approaches), and other methods. Competition for nurses is high. Chapter 14 discussed the issue of the nursing shortage in detail. "Patton sees opportunities in the nursing shortage. 'As difficult as it will be for us, it will help us as a profession to redefine the role of every member of the healthcare team. We'll see better utilization of nursing skills, and we could also see better access to the nurse'" (Saver, 2006, p. 20). Other healthcare professions are also experiencing shortages, an increase in aging practitioners, and an increase in the number of nurses retiring; this has an impact on all healthcare professionals and the delivery system. Exhibits 15–3 and 15–4 describe some policies that might be initiated to improve staffing and cope with the shortage.

Exhibit 15–3 Transition Policy and Strategies

Strategies	Transition Policy
	Goal: Anticipate and prepare the nurse labor market for impending shortages, thereby reducing their duration and impact and lowering the economic and noneconomic costs to patients, nurses, and hospitals.
Demand Strategies	• Speed up development and adoption of technology and use nonprofessional nursing personnel more effectively • Remove barriers to efficiency and redesign the work content and organization of nursing care • Strengthen management decision making • Avoid regulating nurse staffing
Supply Strategies	• Accommodate an older RN workforce • Accelerate improvements in working conditions • Expand the capacity of nursing education programs • Continue to inform the public about opportunities in nursing
Wage Strategies	• Assist hospitals and other healthcare employers in financing needed RN wage increases • Avoid imposing controls on RN wages

Source: From *The Future of the Nursing Workforce in the United States: Data, Trends and Implications*, by P.I. Buerhaus, D.O. Staiger and D.I. Auerbach, 2009, Sudbury, MA: Jones and Bartlett Publishers.

EXHIBIT 15–4 LONG-RUN POLICY AND STRATEGIES

Strategies	Long-Run Policy
	Goals: Expand employment of RNs in the long run by eliminating barriers that lead to an inadequate supply of RNs and by appropriately valuing the contributions of RNs.
Supply Strategies	• Remove barriers to hiring foreign-educated RNs • Remove stigmas and barriers facing men and Hispanics
Demand Strategies	• Reinforce development of pay-for-performance systems • Increase the number of nurse-sensitive outcomes included in pay-for-performance systems

Source: From *The Future of the Nursing Workforce in the United States: Data, Trends and Implications*, by P.I. Buerhaus, D.O. Staiger and D.I. Auerbach, 2009, Sudbury, MA: Jones and Bartlett Publishers.

Domain: *Economic Value*

This domain is an important one. Salaries and benefits have long been a concern of nurses. Salaries and benefits vary across the country. Some nurses have unionized to get better salaries and benefits and to have more say in the decision-making process in the work setting.

Another area related to this domain is the economic value of nurses. The nursing profession has yet to develop effective methods for determining their value in the reimbursement process. It will be important to solve this problem. How does nursing describe the value of nursing services? How does nursing identify costs of nursing services? Some efforts have been made to accomplish this, but there is much more to do.

APNs have really brought the issue of payment for nursing services to the forefront. Some examples of issues that have arisen relate to reimbursement. The Federal Employee Compensation Act (FECA) has become very important to APRNs. FECA provides healthcare services to federal employees who are injured on the job. This is one of the last major healthcare programs to deny patients access to APRNs. APRNs are covered medical providers in Medicare, Medicaid, Tri-Care, and private insurance plans, and they serve as medical providers in the Veterans Administration, the Department of Defense, and the Indian Health Service. Most federal employees have access to APRNs through their federal employee health benefit plan. Legislation was introduced in December 2007 that would allow APRNs to be reimbursed for care provided to employees with job-related injuries (H.R. 4651). This is one example of how economic value is important to nurses. The American Medical Association is asking Congress to amend these bills to restrict the scope of practice of APRNs, which prohibits them from originating and prescribing medical services. The ANA lobbied against the amendment (McKeon, 2008).

Because greater emphasis has been placed on quality and safety in health care, there may be increasing emphasis on pay for performance—third-party payers and government paying for quality care (Saver, 2006). This is already seen in the change by the Centers for Medicare and Medicaid: refusing to pay for certain complications, as was discussed in Chapter 12. This will have an impact on nursing care and on budgetary decisions related to nursing.

Domain: *Work Environment*

This domain focuses on the need for a healthy, functional work environment as discussed in Chapter 14. Key issues are staff safety; communication; collaborative, positive work relationships; work design (space/facility); work processes; infrastructures that support staff participation in decision making; and an emphasis on positive work environments that support, and seek to develop, staff.

Interdisciplinary teams are critical in today's workplace. The IOM identifies the ability to use interdisciplinary teams effectively as one of the core healthcare professions competencies. Newhouse and Mills (2002) identified key points related to nurse–physician relationships that are important in the development of effective interdisciplinary teams (pp. 64–69):

- All teams are not created equal, but careful development of working relationships and clear goals can make all the difference.
- Successful groups are composed of competent team members with the necessary skills, abilities, and personalities to achieve the desired objectives.
- Teams composed of many professional disciplines are able to expand the number and quality of actions to improve healthcare systems.
- Interdisciplinary teams work collaboratively to set and achieve goals directed toward innovative and effective care and efficient organizational systems.
- The nurse team member represents the voice of nursing as a discipline responsible for the holistic care of patients.
- Positive relationships with physicians benefit the patient and enhance the work environment for nurses.
- Nurses must develop the skills to work collaboratively as a professional member of the interdisciplinary team.

Domain: Public Relations/Communication

This domain focuses on the need to be vigilant about the image of nursing. Chapter 3 discussed the image of a nurse. Nurses are mentioned in many media forms, such as newspapers, magazines, film, television, radio, and the Internet. The profession needs to ensure that the image is positive and accurate. Every nurse is involved in public relations about nursing every day, at work and in his or her personal life. A professional always represents the profession regardless of whether he or she is at work.

Domain: Education

There is no doubt that education is very important to nursing. Earlier chapters have discussed nursing education. Changes are occurring in nursing education—from curricula with greater emphasis on the IOM core competencies, to new education programs such as the CNL and Doctor of Nursing Practice.

Distance education has been growing in nursing education for some time, and this trend will most likely continue with the growth of new technology. For example, e-books are just now coming into use; this technology has started slowly but offers many possibilities, such as dynamic graphics, interactivity, search capability, the ability to take notes and sort content, portability, and much more. Classrooms may not be so critical for many nursing courses in the future. Patient simulators are very important today, and their use is also increasing. Faculty are learning how to make the most effective use of this technology to increase interactive learning and improve competencies. Students can make mistakes and learn from them without fearing actual harm to a patient.

Greater changes may occur because of the National Nursing Education Carnegie Report spearheaded by Patricia Benner, PhD, a senior scholar with the Carnegie Foundation. This report is part of a larger study across several disciplines—medicine, nursing, clergy, engineering, and law. It is the first report since the Goldmark Report or the Flexner Report to examine professional education in such depth. According to Benner, students are educated in academic silos, when practice and emphasis on patient safety indicate the need to cross these "walls." To address these barriers, Benner suggests that three intense apprenticeships are needed. These apprenticeships are not the old form of using students as free labor, but in-depth immersion for the purpose of acquiring knowledge and skills and changing attitudes. Although three apprenticeships are described, they may be intertwined. The first is cognitive and theoretical, which focuses on teaching "nurse think." The second is skills based and teaches clinical reasoning and judgment, more in depth than critical thinking. The third apprenticeship is focused on social roles, or moral and ethical behavior. This study identifies characteristics of teaching excellence. They are (Benner, 2008):

- Have a clear vision of what kind of nurse they would like to graduate
- Place their students in a collaborative nursing role
- Ask students to answer questions about what is at stake for the patient, what the patient is experiencing, and what the next step is for the patient
- Highlight what is salient about a case or a situation and what is an appropriate response
- Seamlessly integrate the three apprenticeships to teach how to be a nurse in terms of ethical comportment, knowledge of the humanities, sciences, and social sciences, and practice skills
- Engage in dialogue with students to explore the student's thinking

This is achieved through signature pedagogies:

- *Coaching*, where instructors draw out what the student knows in a bonded clinical situation

- *Simulation*, where students use cases (manikins) to represent patients, or equipment common to particular clinical situation that allows them to practice certain skills over and over
- *Role-modeling*
- *Post-conferences*
- *Pre-clinical preparation*
- *Post-clinical conferences*
- *Articulating experiential learning*

Domain: Diversity

This domain relates directly to the IOM core competency on diversity that was discussed in Chapter 9. Disparity in health care is a growing problem. There is much more information on this topic today (for example, through the National Healthcare Disparities Report). This information can be used by nurses to improve care and reduce disparities. More of this type of information will become available. Nurses need to know how to access these data, which are available through the Internet. HCOs are also providing more staff diversity training, but much more needs to be learned about the most effective methods to improve care and reduce disparities. Health literacy is a continual problem—how to communicate healthcare information so that all patients understand it regardless of their language, education and reading levels, age, and so on. Use of interpreters is now required, but it is not easy for most HCOs to provide this service. New, innovative methods are required to meet the growing need as many communities experience a growth in diverse populations, many of whom may not speak English well.

There needs to be more representation from diverse groups in the nursing profession. As was noted in Chapter 9, there has been slight improvement, but much more is required. Nursing education programs are making efforts to attract more minority students. HCOs want to expand their staff diversity.

Moving the Profession Forward: You Are the Future of Nursing

Moving forward implies change. Many people do not like change or do not feel comfortable with it. Porter-O'Grady stated, "'Our work isn't changing. Change is our work.' He tells nurses, 'If you looked at change like that, it wouldn't be an enemy'" (Saver, 2006, p. 24.) "Patton advises, 'See opportunities instead of challenges'" (Saver, 2006, p. 24). Nurses entering the profession have before them a healthcare delivery system in need of repair, as has been noted by the IOM and reaffirmed in IOM reports. This can be seen as an impossible task or as an opportunity for nurses to step in and assume new roles, and expand old ones if need be. This all requires that nurses be educated, competent, able to communicate and collaborate with others, use political skills, and advocate for the consumer and the nursing profession. Nurses need to base their decisions on EBP, whether they are in clinical practice, nursing administration, or nursing education. Nurses need to understand the possibilities that come with technology, participate in determining how technology can be used, and then use it effectively. Change should be based on data. Data will come from QI, another area in which nurses need to step up and participate so that they are the healthcare professionals who drive nursing and how nursing care is provided. Last but not least, nurses of the future need to recognize that money drives most decisions. Understanding how money flows and how to communicate the value of nurses and nursing care is an important nursing role. Linda Burns-Bolton, RN, PhD, FAAN, vice president and chief nursing officer at Cedars-Sinai Medical Center, believes that in 5 years, "Nurses will get the evidence they need when

they need it, get information for patients when they need it, deliver safe care, communicate with team members, engage with family members, and leave work feeling satisfied" (Saver, 2006, p. 25). Her view of the future in 5 years really covers all the key elements found in this textbook.

Conclusion

This chapter concludes this textbook. The content throughout the book is an introduction to nursing as a profession, to the healthcare system, and, most important, to patients and their families. Nursing is a dynamic profession with multiple possibilities. A nurse can participate in many different nursing jobs throughout a career. Some positions require additional education, and some do not. As was described in this chapter, there are many different settings in which nurses practice. The future holds more change that will lead to new possibilities. You will have the responsibility as a nurse to participate actively in the profession and as an advocate for your patients.

CHAPTER HIGHLIGHTS

1. "Nursing is *the* pivotal healthcare professional, highly valued for its specialized knowledge, skill and caring in improving the status of the public and ensuring safe, effective, quality care" (ANA, 2002, p. 3).

2. 10 domains of nursing include current key initiatives and a desired future statement related to: leadership and planning, economic value, delivery systems/nursing models, work environment, legislation/regulation/policy, public relations/communication, professional/nursing culture, diversity, education, and recruitment/retention.

3. The IOM report on nursing recommends that transformation leadership is the most

effective style (IOM, 2004). Transformational leaders are confident, self-directed, honest, loyal, and committed, and they have the ability to develop and implement a vision.

4. The delivery systems domain emphasizes that nurses influence how the healthcare delivery system works and how it changes.

5. Nursing practice occurs in multiple settings.

6. Differentiated practice, shared governance, and collaboration are important elements of a successful professional practice model.

7. The goal of TCAB is to make fundamental improvements in the healthcare delivery system that will result in safe and reliable care, vitality and teamwork, patient-centered care, and value-added care processes (Martin et al., 2007).

8. The domain of legislation, regulation, and policy emphasizes the need of nurses to work collaboratively with other stakeholders in shaping health policy through legislation and regulation.

9. The domain of professional/nursing culture focuses on the need to develop and maintain a professional culture that supports professional responsibility and accountability—collaborating, mentoring, promoting diversity, and standards and ethics.

10. The Magnet Recognition Program recognizes hospitals that provide quality nursing care or excellence in nursing care.

11. The domain of recruitment and retention focuses on hiring staff and keeping them.

12. The domain of economic values focuses on salaries and benefits, as well as the value of nurses themselves.

13. The domain of work environment focuses on the need for a healthy, functional work environment.

14. The domain of public relations focuses on the need to be vigilant about the image of nursing.

15. Disparity in health care is a growing problem.

Linking to the Internet

- American Association of Critical-Care Nurses: Synergy Model for Patient Care
  http://web.aacn.org/WD/Certifications/content/SynModel.pcms?pid=309&
- American Nurses Association: Current Federal Legislation
  http://nursingworld.org/MainMenu Categories/ANAPoliticalPower/Federal/Issues.aspx
- Citizens Healthcare Working Group: *The Health Report to the American People*
  http://govinfo.library.unt.edu/chc/healthreport/healthreport.pdf
- Center for American Nurses
  http://centerforamericannurses.org
- Congressional Nursing Caucus
  http://rnaction.org/campaign/nurse_caucus
- Institute for Health Improvement
  http://www.ihi.org
- Magnet Recognition Program
  http://www.nursecredentialing.org/magnet/
- Massachusetts General Hospital: Clinical Recognition Program
  http://www.massgeneral.org/pcs/ccpd/Clinical_Recognition_Program/abt_Clinical_Recognition.asp
- Nurse LinkUp (online social networking for RNs)
  http://www.nurselinkup.com/
- Transforming Care at the Bedside (TCAB)
  http://www.ihi.org/IHI/Programs/StrategicInitiatives/TransformingCareAtTheBedside.htm

DISCUSSION QUESTIONS

1. What is *Nursing's Agenda for the Future*?
2. What are the 10 domains in *Nursing's Agenda for the Future*?
3. What is the Magnet Recognition Program?
4. What is a nursing model? Describe one type of model.

CRITICAL THINKING ACTIVITIES

1. How does *Nursing's Agenda for the Future* relate to the IOM five core competencies?
2. What do you think the future holds for nursing? Divide into teams and develop a vision of the future of nursing. Share your team's vision with the other teams.
3. After completing Critical Thinking Activity 2, have each team take another team's vision and decide what education issues, regulatory issues, and practice issues are involved.
4. Divide into teams, with each team assigned one of the domains from *Nursing's Agenda for the Future*. Develop a defense to support your domain as the most important. Each team should then present its defense in a creative way. Students can vote on the best defense.
5. Visit YouTube on the Internet. Search for "nursing" or "nurses." What do you find? View one of the selections and critique the image portrayed. Discuss in a team with classmates.
6. Visit the Center for American Nurses Web site (http://centerforamericannurses.org). Select and review one of the news items. What is your opinion of the item you reviewed? Does it relate to one of the five core competencies? If so, how? How does it relate to the *Nursing's Agenda for the Future*? Explore other parts of the Web site.
7. Explore the American Association of Critical-Care Nurses Synergy Model for Patient Care Web site (http://web.aacn.org/WD/Certifications/content/SynModel.pcms?pid=309&). What do you think about this model of patient care?
8. Consider how the five core competencies might be used as a framework for a professional practice model. Describe your model in narrative form and graphically.

CASE STUDY

The CNL is an example of a new role that has been created as a result of the IOM reports. The CNL functions as a care coordinator either at the unit level or in a practice. For example, Ms. Apple heads up a busy practice in a cancer institute. As a CNL, she acts as a mentor to novice nurses while coordinating care and helping patients navigate the healthcare maze. In one patient's case, she identified the need for transportation to and from radiation appointments. She also recognized financial counseling needs because the patient was no longer able to work, and her husband was on disability. Treatment plans needed to be explained, and teaching the patient about medications was necessary. A referral had been made to a radiation interventionist. The family needed much teaching and explanation about all aspects of care. The CNL pulled the interdisciplinary team together to ensure clear communication and the creation of an interdisciplinary plan of care. In some institutions, these positions are called nurse navigators, and in others, CNLs, depending on the organization's structure and needs. The CNL, having expertise in interprofessional communication, financial management, and human relations, serves the patient and family well to protect and ensure patient-focused care and promote safety.

Case Questions

1. Search the Internet to find HCOs that have CNL positions. What can you learn about this new position?
2. Find nursing programs on the Internet that offer the CNL master's. Compare and contrast them.
3. How does this new position apply or not apply to the domains in *Nursing's Agenda for the Future?* To the IOM Core Competencies?

WORDS OF WISDOM

Gloria Matthews, MSN, RN, BC, CNL, Diabetes Clinical Nurse Leader, University of Oklahoma Medical Center, Oklahoma City, Oklahoma

I have been assigned to work in conjunction with our new Glycemic Control Task Force as its co-chair. This task force is an interdisciplinary team whose purpose is to coordinate inpatient delivery systems to improve care and safety to hospitalized patients with diabetes or hyperglycemia. The goals of this team are to achieve optimal blood glucose control in hospitalized patients, to develop real-time systems to efficiently identify, track, and treat patients who experience glycemic events, and to optimize care processes to reduce complexities and variation and improve clinical workflow. This includes extensive education and training to promote cultural changes that will translate into improved quality of care and the development of evidenced-based clinical policies and protocols to improve efficiency and consistency of care. The ultimate goal of the Glycemic Task Force is to develop a comprehensive diabetes management team that daily identifies, monitors, and manages our diabetic and hyperglycemic patients and expedites the appropriate clinical interventions for those experiencing poor control.

Leslie Cooper, MSN, RN, FNP-BC, Education Coordinator, Take Care Health, Cincinnati, Ohio

I am a nurse. I have been an RN for over 30 years and a Family Nurse Practitioner for 12 of those years. Nursing has taken me places I never dreamed I would go. But I was 18 years into my career before I took the time to figure out what nursing meant to my life. I was doing a clinical rotation in a large pediatric practice for my FNP certification. One fairly slow afternoon, the founding partner in the practice and I were having a conversation about a patient we had just seen and he said to me, "You are so sharp. Have you ever thought about going to medical school?" He stopped me in my tracks. As I tried to formulate a response, I realized that he believed he was paying me a high compliment. I remember taking a deep breath, smiling, looking him in the eye and saying, "I am a nurse and I can't imagine doing anything else."

Carole Kenner, DNS, RNC-NIC, FAAN, President, Council of International Neonatal Nurses, Inc. (COINN)

We live in a global society where nursing and nursing issues are similar no matter where you live and practice. An example of building a global community to improve maternal child outcomes is the Council of International Neo-

natal Nurses, Inc. (COINN). This organization has been in existence for about 3 years. It represents over 50 countries and has influenced health policy through work with the World Health Organization and the International Council of Nurses. It has helped three organizations start. These neonatal nursing organizations have formed in South Africa, Canada, and India. Worldwide, nurses and other professionals are working together to make a difference for mothers and babies.

References

Aiken, L. (2002). Superior outcomes for Magnet hospitals: The evidence base. In M. McClure & A. Hinshaw (Eds.), *Magnet hospitals revisited* (pp. 61–81). Washington, DC: American Nurses Publishing.

Aiken, L., Havens, D., & Sloane, D. (2000). The magnet nursing services recognition program: A comparison of successful applicants with reputational magnet hospitals. *American Journal of Nursing, 100*(3), 26–35.

American Nurses Association. (2002). *Nursing's agenda for the future.* Silver Spring, MD: Author.

American Nurses Credentialing Center. (2008). *Forces of magnetism.* Retrieved April 4, 2008, from http://www.nursecredentialing.org/magnet/forces.html

Benner, P. (2008). *Study of nursing education.* Retrieved May 10, 2008, from the Carnegie Foundation for the Advancement of Teaching Web site: http://www .carnegiefoundation.org/programs/index.asp?key=1829

Boston, C. (1990). Differentiated practice: An introduction. In C. Boston (Ed.), *Current issues and perspectives on differentiated practice* (pp. 1–3). Chicago: American Association of Nurse Executives.

Hensley, S. (1998). VHA readies campaign. Proposed plan would play up local hospital's strengths. *Modern Healthcare, 28*(4), 2–3.

Institute for Healthcare Improvement. (2008). *Transforming care at the bedside.* Retrieved April 4, 2008, from http://www.ihi.org/IHI/Programs/StrategicInitiatives/ TransformingCareAtTheBedside.htm

Institute of Medicine. (2004). *Keeping patients safe: Transforming the work environment of nurses.* Washington, DC: National Academies Press.

Kaplan, M. (2000). Hospital caregivers are in a bad mood. *American Journal of Nursing, 100*(3), 25.

Kerfoot, K., Lavandero, R., Cox, M., Triola, N., Pacini, C., & Hanson, M. (2006, August). Conceptual models and the nursing organization. Implementing the AACN synergy model for patient care. *Nurse Leader,* 20–26.

Kimball, B., Cherner, D., Joynt, J., & O'Neil, E. (2007). The quest for new innovative care delivery models. *Journal of Nursing Administration, 37,* 392–398.

Kramer, M., & Schmalenberg, C. (2002). Staff nurses identify essentials of magnetism. In M. McClure & A. Hinshaw (Eds.), *Magnet hospitals revisited* (pp. 25–59). Washington, DC: American Nurses Publishing.

Laschinger, H., Shamian, J., & Thomson, D. (2001). Impact of magnet hospital characteristics on nurses' perceptions of trust, burnout, quality of care, and work satisfaction. *Nursing Economics, 19,* 209–219.

McClure, M., Poulin, M., Sovie, M., & Wandelt, M. (1983). *Magnet hospitals: Attraction and retention of professional nurses* (American Academy of Nursing Task Force on Nursing Practice in Hospitals). Kansas City, MO: American Nurses Association.

McKeon, E. (2008). Headlines from the hill. ANA works to remove legal barriers to APRN practice. *American Nurse Today, 3*(3), 18.

Martin, S., Greenhouse, P., Merryman, T., Shovel, J., Liberi, C., & Konzier, J. (2007). Transforming care at the bedside. *Journal of Nursing Administration, 37,* 444–451.

National Coalition on Healthcare. (1997). How Americans perceive the healthcare system: A report on a national survey. *Journal on Healthcare Finance, 23*(4), 12–20.

Newhouse, R., & Mills, M. (2002). *Nursing leadership in the organized delivery system for the acute care setting.* Washington, DC: American Nurses Publishing.

New law, JCAHO report recognizes success of Magnet concept. (2002). *The American Nurse, 34*(5), 16–17.

Patton, R. (2008). From your president. It was called *medicine*: Now it's called *nursing. American Nurse Today, 3*(3), 16.

Saver, C. (2006, October). Nursing—today and beyond. Leaders discuss current trends and predict future developments. *American Nurse Today,* 18–25.

Urden, L., & Monarch, K. (2002). The ANCC Magnet Recognition Program: Converting research findings into action. In M. McClure & A. Hinshaw (Eds.), *Magnet hospitals revisited* (pp. 103–116). Washington, DC: American Nurses Publishing.

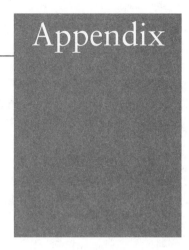

Appendix

Nursing's Agenda for the Future: Description of the 10 Domains

I. Leadership and Planning

Leadership and planning are critical to the successful development and implementation of a strategic plan to achieve nursing's desired future state. Both are required to coordinate and monitor progress on the agenda, engage external stakeholders and secure additional resources.

Desired Future Statement (Vision)

The nursing profession exhibits leadership through unified and systematic planning focused on the desired future state of the profession. This leadership behavior is driven by data/evidence and is implemented in a collaborative manner.

Four strategies were identified to achieve the vision and one of these was identified as the primary or driving strategy. They are:

- **Collaboration and accountability guide nursing in the development and implementation of its own plan:** *Nursing's Agenda for the Future.* **(Primary Strategy)**
- Unified commitment within nursing leads to success and a sense of shared accountability in accomplishing *Nursing's Agenda for the Future.*
- Decision-making and positive change are driven by reliable data.
- Well-prepared nurse leaders assume positions of power and influence on key decision-making bodies throughout the profession and health care.

II. Economic Value

How society values nursing must change to make major strides in recruiting and retaining nurses. Educating the public about nursing's pivotal role in health care will be basic to involving nurses in health care policy formulation and in key business decisions that affect nursing's future.

Desired Future Statement (Vision)

Nurses are recognized as providers of quality, cost-effective health care, compensated for their value and supported through public policy.

Five strategies were identified to achieve the vision and one of these was identified as the primary or driving strategy. They are:

- **Leadership is provided to leverage economic influence. (Primary Strategy)**
- A united profession achieves its key economic goals.
- The economic value of nursing is better understood through the use of quantified nursing data.
- Innovative compensation strategies are widely implemented.
- New and existing economic resources are applied to support nursing education.

III. Delivery Systems/Nursing Models

Nurses will aim to influence how health care is delivered through work with nurse educators, policy-makers and business leaders, armed with sound research on practice models.

Desired Future Statement (Vision)

Nurses unite to create integrated models of health care delivery through education, research, practice and public policy partnerships that improve the health of the nation.

Five strategies were identified to achieve the vision and one of these was identified as the primary or driving strategy. They are:

- **Design integrated practice models. "Integrated" practice models are: interdisciplinary, nurse led (or co-led), applied across the areas of nursing education, practice, research and policy, and blended across practice settings. (Primary Strategy)**
- Nursing practice management is redefined and reshaped for positive change.
- Strategic partnerships are created both within the profession and among influential outside groups.
- Nurse leaders contribute to shaping both public and health policy.
- Efforts are successful to advance the value and image of nursing.

IV. Work Environment

In this area so basic to nursing's future, members of the profession will work to improve nurses' work environments so that quality patient care is optimized and professional nursing staff is retained.

Desired Future Statement (Vision)

Nurses provide quality care in dynamic and satisfying environments that utilize their specialized skills and knowledge. These environments promote health and safety, appropriate staffing, shared decision-making, collaboration, mentoring and professional growth.

Six strategies were identified to achieve the vision and one of these was identified as the primary or driving strategy. They are:

- **Nurses have an effective voice in decision-making. (Primary Strategy)**
- Professional development is fostered for nurses in all roles.
- Sound methods are identified and utilized to assure appropriate staffing.
- Collaborative work relationships are actively enhanced and promoted.
- Support is demonstrated for quality of work life and safety at work.
- Practices are defined and implemented that produce quality patient care.

V. Legislation/Regulation/Policy

New collaborations will increase nursing's role in shaping public policy.

Desired Future Statement (Vision)

As leaders in the health and public policy process, nurses are unified in implementation of standards of nursing education and practice. Nurses develop evidence-based health policy (e.g., legislation, regulation) in collaboration with consumers to ensure access to health care services and safe, competent nursing care.

Five strategies were identified to achieve the vision and one of these was identified as the primary or driving strategy. They are:

- **Nurses are policy-makers at the local, state, national, and international levels. (Primary Strategy)**
- Nursing collaborates with all stakeholders for the development of public policy.
- Reliable data support all health policy formulation.
- Universal access is ensured through the delivery of outcome-driven quality health care services.
- Health policy is congruent with standards for nursing education and practice.

VI. Public Relations/Communication

Nursing's pivotal role in health care will be demonstrated on a regular basis to various publics outside of the profession.

Desired Future Statement (Vision)

Nursing is recognized as an influential, highly rewarded profession valued for its unique knowledge and expertise. It is widely known that nurses make a difference in people's lives. Four strategies were identified to achieve the vision and one of these was identified as the primary or driving strategy. They are:

- **Effectively communicate nurses' impact on the quality of care and health outcomes. (Primary Strategy)**
- Advance a valued, respected image of nursing.
- Convey nursing's influence in health care delivery and public policy-making.
- Portray nursing as a top career choice.

VII. Nursing/Professional Culture

Asserting nursing's high standards of professional practice, education, leadership and collaboration will enhance professionalism, image and career satisfaction.

Desired Future Statement (Vision)

All nurses believe they are, and all nurses are viewed to be, critical strategic health care assets valued by the public, policy-makers, employers and health care colleagues as equal partners in healthcare. Nurses embrace their professional responsibility and accountability, including: collaborating, mentoring, promoting diversity and adhering to standards and ethical codes of professional practice.

Five strategies were identified to achieve the vision and one of these was identified as the primary or driving strategy. They are:

- **Professionalism is supported by infrastructures for education and leadership development. (Primary Strategy)**
- Nurses promote a healthy environment of respect and caring for one another.
- Nurses believe, articulate and demonstrate the value of nursing.
- Collaboration is a professional imperative.
- Nurses achieve substantial external influence and recognition for their value to society.

VIII. Diversity

The profession aims for diversity that reflects the patient population, in order to better meet population needs.

Desired Future Statement (Vision)

Nursing increasingly reflects the population it serves. Our profession derives strength form its ethnic, cultural, social, economic, and gender diversity, thereby enhancing its capacity to respond to the health care needs of a diverse nation Nursing is a model for other professions in demonstrating the value of diversity.

Five strategies were identified to achieve the vision and one of these was identified as the primary or driving strategy. They are:

- **Increase health system leadership that reflects and values diversity. (Primary Strategy)**
- Create diversity and cultural competence through educational programs and standards in the workplace.
- Increase diversity of faculty, students, and curricula in all academic and continuing education.
- Focus recruitment and retention programs to greatly increase diversity.
- Target legislation and funding for diversity initiatives.

IX. Education

Stakeholders in this area will focus on reexamining and reshaping nursing education to improve nursing practice, enhance nursing's image and better meet patient care needs.

Desired Future Statement (Vision)

Nursing education is valued by the public because it prepares nurses for discrete scopes of practice and roles through programs that are accessible, affordable and flexible. Adequate numbers of nurses are attracted to faculty roles early in their careers. These highly qualified faculty engage in innovative teaching, clinical practice and research that lead to learning and work environments that are conducive to the creativity of faculty and students and promote education that is evidence-based and result in safe, quality care. Partnerships exist with other stakeholders to enhance clinical experience, meet the needs of special populations and promote professional involvement.

Five strategies were identified to achieve the vision and one of these was identified as the primary or driving strategy. They are:

- **Establish congruence between the educational enterprise and societal needs. (Primary Strategy)**
- Enrich the high caliber of nursing faculty.
- Attain clarity in education about nursing roles and scopes of practice.
- Work for universal excellence in nursing education.
- Promote the value of nursing education to the profession and the public.

X. Recruitment/Retention

Building on work in other domains, professional opportunities will be enhanced to attract and sustain excellent nurses for long, rewarding careers.

Desired Future Statement (Vision)

Nursing is comprised of a diverse body of individuals committed to promoting and sustaining the profession through addressing diversity, image, education, funding, practice models and environments, and professional development.

Five strategies were identified to achieve the vision and one of these was identified as the primary or driving strategy. They are:

- **Professional/career development opportunities are evident across the career span. (Primary Strategy)**
- Funding is secured for creative educational initiatives that support nurses across the career span.
- Nursing is seen as a highly desirable and appealing career choice.
- Nurses develop professional practice models and work environments that ensure career satisfaction.
- Comprehensive recruitment and retention strategies demonstrate nursing's strong public image and appeal to a diverse population.

Source: Nursing's Agenda for the Future: A Call to the Nation by American Nurses Association, 2002, Washington, DC: Author. Reprinted with permission.

Glossary

accountability   An obligation or willingness to accept responsibility.

accreditation   The process by which organizations are evaluated on their quality, based on established minimum standards.

acute care   Treatment of a severe medical condition that is of short duration or at a crisis level.

advance directive   A legal document that allows a person to describe his or her medical care preferences.

advanced practice nurse   A registered nurse with advanced education in adult health, pediatrics, family health, women's health, neonatal health, community health, or other specialties.

adverse event   An injury resulting from a medical intervention (in other words, an injury that is not due to the patient's underlying condition).

advertising   Methods used by employers and schools of nursing for recruitment and by professional organizations that want to make nursing more visible.

advocacy   Speaking for something important (one of the major roles of a nurse).

advocate   A nurse who speaks for the patient but does not take away the patient's independence.

annual limit   A defined maximum amount that an employee/policy holder/patient would have to pay, and after that level is reached, he or she no longer has to contribute to the payment for care.

applied research   Research designed to find a solution to a practical problem.

apprenticeship model   A nursing program developed in England that provided on-the-job training and a formal education component.

articulation   A formal agreement between two or more institutions that allows specific programs at one institution to be credited toward direct entry or advanced standing at another.

assault   The threat or use of force on another that causes that person to have a reasonable apprehension about imminent harmful or offensive contact.

assertiveness   Confronting problems in a constructive manner and not remaining silent.

Associate's Degree in Nursing   A 2-year program that includes some liberal arts and sciences curriculum but focuses more on technical nursing.

authentic leadership   Understanding your purpose, practicing solid values, leading with your heart, establishing connected relationships, and demonstrating self-discipline.

autonomy   The quality or state of being self-governing; the freedom to act on what you know.

Baccalaureate Degree in Nursing   A 4-year nursing program in a higher education institution.

basic research   Research designed to broaden the base of knowledge rather than solve an immediate problem.

battery   The actual intentional striking of someone, with intent to harm, or in a "rude and insolent manner" even if the injury is slight.

benchmarking   Measurement of progress toward a goal, taken at intervals prior to the program's completion or the anticipated attainment of the final goal.

bias A predisposition to a point of view.

bioethics Decisions and behaviors related to life and death issues.

biosketch A paragraph that provides a short summary of a person's work history and accomplishments.

blame-free environment A protected environment that encourages the systematic surfacing and reporting of serious adverse events.

breach of duty The proximate (foreseeable) cause or the cause that is legally sufficient to result in liability for harm to the patient; a breach of due care.

burnout A deterioration of attitude in which a person becomes tired, defensive, frustrated, cynical, bored, and generally pessimistic about the job; exhaustion of physical or emotional strength.

care coordination Establishment and support of a continuous healing relationship, enabled by an integrated clinical environment and characterized by a proactive delivery of evidence-based care and follow-up.

career ladder A system that provides a method for promotion and an increase in salary but does not require moving to a management position; this system provides recognition of professional achievement.

care map An innovative approach to planning and organizing nursing care.

caring Feeling and exhibiting concern and empathy for others.

case management A system of management that facilitates effective care delivery and outcomes for patients.

certification A process by which a nongovernmental agency validates, based on predetermined standards, an individual nurse's qualification and knowledge for practice in a defined functional or clinical area of nursing.

change agent Someone who engages deliberately in, or whose behavior results in, social, cultural, or behavioral change.

civil law One of two prominent legal systems; the law of private rights.

clinical The observation and treatment of patients in a variety of settings for the purpose of education and development of clinical competencies; also called practicum.

clinical data repository An "information warehouse" that stores data longitudinally and in multiple forms, such as text, voice, and images.

clinical decision support systems Computersized systems that provide immediate information that can influence clinical decisions.

clinical information system (CIS) A method of data storage generally used at the point-of-care.

clinical judgment The process by which nurses come to understand the problems, issues, and concerns of patients, to attend to salient information, and to respond to client (patient) problems in concerned and involved ways; includes both conscious decision making and intuitive response.

clinical laboratory A place that provides an opportunity for experimentation, observation, and practice in a field of study, often using simulation.

clinical nurse leader A care provider and a manager at the point-of-care to individuals and cohorts; designs, implements, and evaluates patient care by coordinating, delegating, and supervising the care provided by the healthcare team, including licensed nurses, technicians, and other health professionals.

clinical pathways Describe how care is best provided for a specific patient population with specific problem(s).

clinical reasoning The nurse's ability to assess patient problems or needs and analyze data to accurately identify and frame problems within the context of the individual patient's environment.

coaching A method used for support, encouragement, and career development, such as providing guidance about a promotion, a change of career ladder process, or returning to school for a higher degree.

Code of Ethics A list of provisions that makes explicit the primary goals, values, and obligations of the nursing profession; published by the American Nurses Association.

coding system   A set of agreed-upon symbols (frequently numeric or alphanumeric) that is used to change information into another form so that it can be better accessed and used.

collaboration   Cooperative effort among healthcare providers, staff, and multiple organizations who work together to accomplish a common mission.

colleagueship   A collaborative, professional relationship in which there is mutual trust and an understanding that each partner contributes to the relationship.

communication   The exchange of thoughts, messages, or information.

compact licensure   The mutual recognition model of nurse licensure allows a nurse to have one license (in his or her state of residency) and to practice in other states (both physical and electronic), subject to each state's practice law and regulation.

competency   The application of knowledge and the interpersonal, decision-making, and psychomotor skills expected for the nurse's practice role.

computer literacy   Knowledge of basic computer technology.

confidentiality   The responsibility to keep patient information private, except as required to communicate in the care process and with team members.

conflict   A state of opposition between persons, ideas, or interests.

conflict resolution   A process of resolving a dispute or disagreement.

consumer/customer   The ultimate user of a product or service.

continuing education   Systematic professional learning designed to augment knowledge, skills, and attitudes.

continuum of care   Care services available to assist an individual throughout the course of his or her disease.

coordination   Proactive methods to optimize health outcomes.

copayment   The fixed amount that a patient may be required to pay per service (M.D. visit, lab test, prescription, and so on).

coping   The process of managing taxing circumstances.

corporatization   Business; the business of health care.

counselor   A person who gives guidance in a specific area of expertise or knowledge.

credentialing   A process used to ensure that practitioners are qualified to perform and to monitor continued licensure.

criminal law   Those statutes that deal with crimes against the public and members of the public, with penalties and all the procedures connected with charging, trying, sentencing, and imprisoning defendants convicted of crimes.

critical thinking   Purposeful, informed, outcome-focused (results-oriented) thinking that requires careful identification of key problems, issues, and risks.

culture   The knowledge and values shared by a society.

curriculum   An integrated course of academic studies that describes the program's philosophy, level, and terminal competencies for students, or what they are expected to be able to accomplish by the end of the program.

curriculum vitae (CV)   Detailed accounting of information found in the resume but more extensive; includes publications, presentations given, continuing education completed, honors and awards, community activities, and grants.

data   Discrete entities that are described objectively without interpretation.

data analysis software   Computer software that can analyze data.

data mining   Locating and identifying unknown patterns and relationships within data.

databank   A large store of information, which may include several databases.

database   A collection of interrelated data, often with controlled redundancy, organized according to a scheme to serve one or more applications.

deductible   The part of the bill that the patient must pay before the insurer begins to pay for services.

delegatee   The person to whom someone delegates a task.

delegation   To transfer to another the responsibility to complete a task that is within the scope of that person's position.

delegator   The person who assigns responsibility or authority.

differentiated practice   A philosophy that focuses on the structuring of roles and functions of nurses according to education, experience, and competence.

Diploma in Nursing   A nursing program developed in the United States that provides on-the-job training as well as a formal education component.

disease prevention   Anticipation and/or avoidance of health problems.

disparity   An inequality or a difference in some respect.

distance education   A set of teaching and/or learning strategies to meet the learning needs of students separate from the traditional classroom and sometimes from traditional roles of faculty; for example, an online course.

distribution of staff   Allocation of staff based on patient care needs and staff competencies.

diversity   All the ways in which people differ, including innate characteristics (such as age, race, gender, ethnicity, mental and physical abilities, and sexual orientation) and acquired characteristics (such as education, income, religion, work experience, language skills, and geographic location).

Doctor of Nursing Practice   A practice-focused nursing doctoral degree program.

Do-Not-Resuscitate (DNR)   A form of advance directive that may be part of an extensive advance directive. This order means that there should be no resuscitation if the patient's condition indicates need for resuscitation.

effective care   The provision of services based on scientific knowledge (evidence-based practice) to all who could benefit, and refraining from providing services to those not likely to benefit (avoiding underuse and overuse).

efficient care   Care that avoids waste, including waste of equipment, supplies, ideas, and energy.

electronic medical record (EMR)   A medical record in a digital format.

e-mail list   A list of e-mail addresses that can be used to send one e-mail to all addresses at one time.

empowerment   To have power or authority.

encryption   Changing written information, especially patient information, into a code that protects the privacy of these data for security purposes.

entrepreneur   An innovator who recognizes opportunities to introduce a new process or an improved organization.

entry level   The first level at which a student enters professional education; positions suitable for people who do not have previous experience or qualifications in a particular area of work.

equitable care   The provision of care that does not vary in quality because of personal characteristics such as gender, ethnicity, geographic location, and socioeconomic status.

error   The failure of a planned action to be completed as intended, or the use of the wrong plan to achieve an aim; errors are directly related to outcomes.

ethical decision making   Involves ethical dilemmas that occur when a person is forced to choose between two or more alternatives, none of which is ideal.

ethical principles   A standardized code or guide to behaviors for the nursing profession.

ethnicity   A shared feeling of belonging to a group; peoplehood.

ethnocentrism The belief that one's group or culture is superior to others.

evidence-based practice (EBP) The integration of the best evidence into clinical practice, which includes research, the patient's values and preferences, the patient's history and exam data, and clinical expertise.

executive branch The branch of the U.S. government in charge of enforcing and executing the laws.

experimental design A type of research design in which the conditions of a program or experience (treatment) are controlled by the researcher and in which experimental subjects are randomly assigned to treatment conditions. This design must meet three criteria: manipulation, control, and randomization.

extended care The provision of inpatient skilled nursing care and related services to patients who require medical, nursing, or rehabilitative services.

failure to rescue The inability to recognize a patient's negative change in status in a timely manner in order to prevent patient complications and to prevent major disability or death.

flexible staffing A staffing plan that can easily be adjusted to meet patient needs.

followership The act or condition of following a leader; adherence.

Forces of Magnetism The identified effective descriptors of healthcare organizations that are designated as Magnet organizations.

for-profit An organization that must provide funds to pay stockholders or owners; this affects the availability of money for other purposes that have an impact on nurses and nursing.

fraud The deliberate deception of another for personal gain.

full-time equivalent (FTE) An equivalent to 40 hours of work per week for 52 weeks, or 2,080 hours per year.

health The state of well-being; free from disease.

Health Insurance Portability and Accountability Act of 1996 (HIPAA) An act that amended the Internal Revenue Code of 1986 to improve portability and continuity of healthcare information.

health literacy The ability to understand and use health information.

health promotion Effort to stop the development of disease; includes treatment to prevent a disease from progressing further and causing complications.

Healthy People 2010 A federal initiative to improve the health of all citizens in the United States by establishing goals and leading indicators for communities to strive for; results are monitored and then used to adjust the initiative (goals and indicators).

home care The provision of healthcare services in the home.

hospice A philosophy of care for managing symptoms and supporting quality of life as long as possible for the terminally ill.

hypothesis A formal statement in a research study describing the expected relationship or relationships between two or more variables in a specified population (the sample).

illness A sickness or disease of the mind or body.

image A representation of oneself or one's profession.

influence The power or capacity to cause an effect in indirect or intangible ways.

informatics An integration of nursing science, computer science, and information science to manage and communicate data, information, knowledge, and wisdom in nursing practice.

information Data that are interpreted, organized, or structured.

information literacy The ability to recognize when information is needed and to locate, evaluate, and effectively use that information.

informed consent Permission required by law to explain or disclose information about the medical problem and treatment or procedure so that the patient can have informed choice.

integrative review A type of EBP literature; a narrative summary of past research in which the reviewer or reviewers extract findings from original studies and use analytical reasoning to produce conclusions about the findings of a body of research.

intrapreneur One who takes direct responsibility for turning an idea into a profitable finished product through assertive risk-taking and innovation.

intuition Quick and ready insight.

The Joint Commission A major nonprofit organization that accredits more than 17,000 healthcare organizations, including hospitals, long-term care organizations, home care agencies, clinical laboratories, ambulatory care organizations, behavioral health organizations, and healthcare networks or managed care organizations.

judicial branch The branch of the U.S. government that interprets and applies laws in specific cases.

knowledge An awareness and understanding of facts.

knowledge management A method for gathering information and making it available to others.

knowledge worker A person who is effective in acquiring, analyzing, synthesizing, and applying evidence to guide practice decisions.

leadership The ability to influence group members to help achieve the goals of the group or organization.

legal issues Questions and problems concerning the protections that make laws (U.S. Congress).

legislative branch The branch of the U.S. government that hears cases that challenge or require interpretation of the legislation passed by Congress.

licensure The process by which a government authority grants permission to an individual practitioner or healthcare organization to operate or to engage in an occupation or profession.

living will A document that describes a person's wishes related to his or her end-of-life care needs.

lobbying Assembling and petitioning the government for redress of grievances.

lobbyist An individual paid to represent a special interest group, whose function is to urge support for or opposition to legislative matters.

long-term care A continuum of broad-ranged maintenance and health services delivered to the chronically ill, disabled, and the elderly.

macro consumer The major purchasers of care: the government and insurers.

Magnet hospital A hospital that demonstrates high levels of quality of care, autonomy, primary nursing care, mentoring, professional recognition, respect, and the ability to practice nursing; hospitals awarded this status meet specific standards.

malpractice An act or continuing conduct of a professional that does not meet the standard of professional competence and results in provable damages to his or her patient.

managed care A method used to reimburse or pay for healthcare services; controls the delivery services and costs.

manager A person who directs a team or group of staff.

mandatory overtime The requirement that staff work past their scheduled end time.

Master's Degree in Nursing A graduate-level nursing degree.

Medicaid The federal healthcare reimbursement program that covers health and long-term care services for children, the aged, blind persons, the disabled, and people who are eligible to receive federally assisted income maintenance payments.

medical power of attorney Also known as a durable power of attorney for health care or a healthcare agent or proxy, this person is given the right by an individual to speak for him or her if he or she cannot do so in matters related to health care.

Medicare The federal health insurance program for people aged 65 and older, persons with disabilities, and people with end-stage renal disease.

mentor A role model.

mentoring Method used in healthcare organizations to support new staff; the mentor acts as a role model and serves as a resource.

meta-analysis   A type of EBP literature; the process of using quantitative methods to appraise and summarize the results of multiple studies.

metasynthesis   A technique for drawing inferences from similar or related studies; bringing together and examining data sets.

micro consumer   The patients, families, and significant others who play a role in patient care and in the decision-making process.

minimum data set   The minimum categories of data with uniform definitions and categories; an example would be the Nursing Minimum Data Set.

misuse   An event that leads to avoidable complications that prevent a patient from receiving the full potential benefit of a service.

National Database of Nursing Quality Indicators (NDNQI)   A system in which nursing data are collected to evaluate outcomes and nursing care.

National Institute of Nursing Research (NINR)   The institute at the National Institutes of Health that supports and conducts nursing research.

near miss   An event which occurred that could have led to an adverse event but did not.

negligence   Failure to exercise the care toward others that a reasonable or prudent person would have under the same circumstances; an unintentional tort.

networking   The cultivation of productive relationships for employment or business.

nomenclature   A system of designations (terms) elaborated according to preestablished rules; an example would be the International Classification for Nursing Practice.

nonexperimental design   A research study that uses a quasi-experimental design in which there is some manipulation of the independent variable but no randomization or control.

not-for-profit   An incorporated organization whose shareholders or trustees do not benefit financially.

nurse externship   A program that offers nursing students employment (typically during the summer) and includes educational experiences such as seminars, special speakers, and simulation experiences.

Nurse Practice Act   The act that governs nursing practice in the state in which the nurse practices.

nurse residency   A special employment program that helps new RN graduates transition to practice in a structured program that provides content and learning activities, precepted experiences, mentoring, and gradual adjustment to higher levels of responsibility.

nursing   The profession of a nurse.

nursing care hours   The number of hours of patient care provided per unit of time.

nursing informatics   The specialty that integrates nursing science, computer science, and information science to manage and communicate data, information, knowledge, and wisdom in nursing practice.

nursing process   A systematic method for thinking about, and communicating how, nurses provide patient care; this includes assessment, diagnosis, planning, intervention or implementation, and evaluation.

occupational health   Health promotion, disease and illness prevention, and treatment, as well as attention to the risks of illness and injury within the work environment.

organizational culture   The values, beliefs, traditions, and communication processes that bring a group of people together and characterize the group.

organizational ethics   Organizational concerns related to the beliefs, decision making, and behavior of the organization as an entity.

outcomes   Measurable benefits of patient care.

outcomes research   Research focused on determining the effectiveness of healthcare services and patient outcomes.

overuse   The point at which the potential for harm from the provision of a service exceeds the possible benefit.

palliative care Care focused on alleviating symptoms and meeting the special needs of the terminally ill patient and the family.

patient advocacy Being active in respecting patient rights and the patient, and in ensuring that the patient has the education to understand treatment and care needs.

patient classification system (PCS) A system used to identify and quantify patient needs that can then be matched with staffing level and mix.

patient-centered care Identification of, respect, and care for patient differences, values, preferences, and needs; relief of pain; coordination of care; clear communication with and education of the patient; shared decision making; and continuous promotion of disease prevention and wellness.

personal digital assistants (PDAs) Hardware that includes information; information can be downloaded or input into the equipment; offer interactive ability to access and reconfigure information.

personal health record (PHR) Computer-based health records that collect data over a lifetime; with permission of the patient, this record can be accessed easily by any provider who needs the information.

PICO To ask a searchable and answerable question. The "P" (patient population) is specific and describes the population in terms such as age, gender, diagnosis, ethnicity, other. The "I" (intervention) relates to prognostic factors, risk behaviors, exposure to disease, clinical intervention or treatment, etc. The "C" (comparison intervention) can pertain to another treatment, no treatment, or other. The "O" (outcome) includes factors such as risk of disease, complications or side effects, or adverse outcomes.

plaintiff The party who initiates a lawsuit (also known as an action) before a court; also known as a claimant or complainant.

politics The process of influencing the authoritative allocation of scarce resources.

policy A set course of action that affects a large number of people and is stimulated by a specific need to achieve certain outcomes.

Political Action Committee (PAC) A private group that represents a specific issue or group and works to get someone elected or defeated.

portfolio A collection of information that demonstrates a person's experiences and accomplishments, such as committee work, professional organization activities, presentations, development of patient education material, awards, letters of recognition, projects and grants, etc.

power The ability to influence decisions and have an impact on issues that matter.

powerlessness The feeling that one cannot make an impact, is not listened to, or is not sought out for his or her opinion.

practicum A course that includes clinical activities and stresses the practical application of theory in a field of study.

preceptor An experienced and competent staff member (an RN or, for nurse practitioner students, possibly a nurse practitioner or physician) who has received formal training to function as a preceptor and who serves as a role model to guide student learning, serving as a resource for the nursing student.

prejudice Making assumptions or judgments about the beliefs, behaviors, needs, and expectations of other persons who are of a different cultural background than oneself because of emotional beliefs about the population; involves negative attitudes toward the "different" group.

prescriptive authority Legal authority granted to advanced practice nurses to prescribe medication.

prevention levels Levels of health promotion for the prevention, treatment, and rehabilitation of disease or condition.

private policy Policy created by non-governmental organizations.

procedures A definite statement of step-by-step actions required for a specific result.

process Particular course of action intended to achieve a result.

professional ethics Generally accepted standards of conduct and methods in the nursing profession.

professional order entry (POE)   A data entry system that allows healthcare providers to input orders into a computer system rather than writing them.

professional practice model   A system that supports nursing control over its practice and describes the framework of the structural and contextual features of nursing practice environment.

professionalism   The conduct, aims, or qualities that characterize or mark a profession.

protocols   Treatment plans.

provider of care   A healthcare staff member who provides care to patients.

proximate cause   A cause that is legally sufficient to result in liability.

Public Health Act (1944)   The act, or law, that consolidated all existing public health legislation into one law.

public policy   Policy created at the legislative, executive, and judicial branches of federal, state, and local levels of government that affects individual and institutional behaviors under the government's respective jurisdiction.

qualitative study   A systematic, subjective, methodological research approach; analysis of data that does not rely on statistics or mathematical equations.

quality   Conforming to requirements to maintain high standards.

quality improvement (QI)   An organized approach to identify errors and hazards in care, as well as improve care overall.

quantitative study   A formal, objective, systematic research process that uses statistics for data analysis.

quasi-experimental design   A research design that is similar to an experimental design but lacks the key ingredient: random assignment.

race   A biological designation of a group.

randomized controlled trial (RCT)   Often referred to as the "gold standard" in research designs, this is the true experiment in which there is control over variables, randomization of the sample with a control group and an experimental group, and an intervention(s) (independent variable).

reality shock   The reaction of students when they discover that the clinical experience does not always match the values and ideals that they had anticipated.

recruitment   Organized efforts to attract and hire new staff.

reflective thinking   Creativity and conscious self-evaluation over a period of time.

regulation   An official rule or order, based on laws, governing processes, practice, and procedures; in nursing, legal regulation governs licensure.

rehabilitation   The restoration of, or improvement of, an individual's health and functionality.

reimbursement   Payment for healthcare services.

report card   Provides specific performance data about an organization at specific intervals, with a focus on quality and safety.

research   Investigation or experimentation aimed at the discovery and interpretation of facts about a particular subject.

research analysis   The process of using methods to analyze and summarize results or data.

research design   A specific plan for conducting a study.

research problem statement   A description of the topic or subject for a research study, which provides the context for the research study and typically generates questions that the research aims to answer.

research proposal   A written document that describes recent, relevant literature on the problem area; describes the research topic/problem; and defines the processes or steps that will be followed to answer the research question(s).

research purpose   Identifies the potential uses of research results.

research question   The interrogative statement that directs a research study.

research utilization (RU)   Applying specific research results without consideration of multiple studies such as would be done with a systematic review in EBP.

researcher   A person who systematically investigates and studies materials and sources to establish facts and reach conclusions.

resilience   The ability to cope with stress.

responsibility   Moral, legal, or mental accountability.

resume   A one- or two-page document that describes a person's career; includes name and credentials, contact information, education, goals and objectives, and employment/relevant experience; not as detailed as a curriculum vitae (CV).

retention   retaining nursing staff, minimizing nursing turnover.

risk management (RM)   Maintaining a safe and effective healthcare environment and preventing or reducing financial loss to the healthcare organization.

role   Behavior oriented to the patterned expectation of others.

role transition   Gradual development in a new role.

root cause analysis   An in-depth analysis of an error to assess the event and identify causes and possible solutions.

safety   Preventing inadvertent pain, injury, or loss.

scholarship   A fund for knowledge and learning.

scope of practice   A statement that describes the who, what, where, when, why, and how of nursing practice.

security protections   Methods used to ensure that information is not read or taken by persons not authorized to access it.

self-directed learning   A process in which individuals take the initiative, with or without the help of others, in diagnosing their learning needs, formulating learning goals, identifying human and material resources for learning, choosing and implementing appropriate learning strategies, and evaluating learning outcomes.

self-management of care   The systematic provision of education and supportive interventions to increase patients' skills and confidence in managing their own health problems, including regular assessment of progress and problems, goal-setting, and problem-solving approaches.

self-scheduling   A scheduling approach in which staff complete their own schedules based on the pre-designated guidelines, coordinating with other staff schedules as needed.

sentinel event   A negative outcome with a patient, such as an unexpected death, serious physical or psychological injury, or a potentially harmful risk.

shared governance   A management model, a professional practice model, and an accountability model in which staff have direct input into decision making for educational purposes with the goal of developing competencies.

simulation   Replication of some or nearly all essential aspects of a clinical situation as realistically as possible.

social policy statement   A statement that describes the profession of nursing and its professional framework and obligations to society; published by the American Nurses Association.

Social Security Act (1935)   The act that established the U.S. Medicare and Medicaid programs, two major reimbursement programs, and also provided funding for nursing education through amendments added to the law.

software   Computer programs and applications.

staffing mix   The type of nursing staff needed to provide care.

standard   A reference point against which other things can be evaluated.

standardized language   A collection of terms with definitions for use in informational systems databases.

standards   Statements that serve as guides to practice.

status   A position in a social structure with rights and obligations.

statutory law   The body of law derived from statutes rather than constitutions or judicial decisions.

stereotype   The process by which people use social groups (such as gender and race) to gather, process, and recall information about other people; also known as labeling.

stress   A complex experience felt internally that makes a person feel a loss or threat of a loss; bodily or mental tension.

stress management   Strategies used to cope with stress to alter bodily or mental tension; reducing the negative impact of stress, improving health, and developing health-promoting behaviors.

structure   The environment in which services are provided; inputs into the system, such as patients, staff, and environments.

surveillance   Purposeful and ongoing acquisition, interpretation, and synthesis of patient data for clinical decision making.

system   The coming together of parts, interconnections, and purpose.

systematic review   A summary of evidence typically conducted by an expert or a panel of experts on a particular topic; uses rigorous process to minimize bias for identifying, appraising, and synthesizing studies to answer a specific clinical question and draw conclusions about the data gathered; different methods may be used depending on the type of review such as integrative or meta-analysis.

team   A number of persons associated in work or activity.

teamwork   Work done by several associates, with each doing a part but all subordinating personal prominence to the efficiency of the whole.

telehealth   The use of telecommunications equipment and communications networks to transfer healthcare information between participants at different locations.

telenursing   The use of telecommunications technology in nursing to enhance patient care.

theory   A body of rules, ideas, principles, and techniques that applies to a particular subject.

therapeutic use of self   The nurse's use of his or her personality consciously and in full awareness in an attempt to establish relatedness and to structure a nursing intervention.

time management   Strategies used to manage and control time productivity.

timely care   Meeting the patient's needs; providing high-quality experiences and improved healthcare outcomes when needed.

tort   A civil wrong for which a remedy may be obtained in the form of damages.

training   Activities and instruction intended to foster skilled behavior.

types of power   Include legitimate (formal), referent (informal), informational, expert, reward, and coercive power.

underuse   Failure to provide a service that would have produced a favorable outcome for the patient.

unlicensed assistive personnel (UAP)   Healthcare workers who are not licensed to perform nursing tasks but are trained and often certified.

utilization review (UR)   Evaluating necessity, appropriateness, and efficiency of healthcare services for specific patients or in patient populations.

whistle-blowing   A situation in which a person who works for an organization committing fraud and abuse reports these actions to legal authorities and shares extensive information that would be difficult for legal authorities to obtain on their own.

wisdom   The appropriate use of knowledge to solve human problems; understanding when and how to apply knowledge.

Index